Epidemiology, Biostatistics, and Preventive Medicine

Epidemiology, Biostatistics, and Preventive Medicine

SECOND EDITION

JAMES F. JEKEL, M.D., M.P.H.

Professor of Epidemiology and Public Health, Emeritus
Yale University School of Medicine
New Haven, Connecticut
Director, Griffin-Yale Residency Program in
General Preventive Medicine and Public Health
Griffin Hospital
Derby, Connecticut

DAVID L. KATZ, M.D., M.P.H.

Associate Clinical Professor of Epidemiology and
Public Health and Medicine
Yale University School of Medicine
New Haven, Connecticut
Director, Yale-Griffin Prevention Research Center
Derby, Connecticut

JOANN G. ELMORE, M.D., M.P.H.

Associate Professor of Medicine
Associate Director, Robert Wood Johnson Clinical Scholars Program
University of Washington School of Medicine
Seattle, Washington

W.B. SAUNDERS COMPANY
A Harcourt Health Sciences Company
Philadelphia   London   New York   St. Louis   Sydney   Toronto

W.B. SAUNDERS COMPANY
A Harcourt Health Sciences Company

The Curtis Center
Independence Square West
Philadelphia, Pennsylvania 19106

Library of Congress Cataloging-in-Publication Data

Jekel, James F.
   Epidemiology, biostatistics, and preventive medicine / James F. Jekel,
David L. Katz, Joann G. Elmore.—2nd ed.

      p. ; cm.

   Merger of: Epidemiology, biostatistics, and preventive medicine and
Epidemiology, biostatistics, and preventive medicine review.
   Includes bibliographical references and index.

   ISBN 0–7216–9079–3 (alk. paper)

   1. Epidemiology. 2. Medical statistics. 3. Medicine, Preventive.   I. Katz,
David L.   II. Elmore, Joann G.   III. Katz David L. Epidemiology,
biostatistics, and preventive medicine.   IV. Title.
   [DNLM: 1. Biometry.   2. Epidemiologic Methods.   3. Preventive
Medicine.   WA 950 J25e 2001]

RA652.J45   2001

614.4—dc21

                                                              2001020616

Acquisitions Editor: William Schmitt
Project Manager: Patricia Tannian
Book Design Manager: Gail Morey Hudson
Cover Designer: Teresa Breckwoldt

EPIDEMIOLOGY, BIOSTATISTICS, AND PREVENTIVE MEDICINE, Second Edition   ISBN 0-7216-9079-3

Printed in the United States of America

Last digit is the print number: 9   8   7   6   5   4   3   2   1

PREFACE

The first edition of *Epidemiology, Biostatistics, and Preventive Medicine* was written by Dr. Jekel with the collaboration of Drs. Elmore and Katz. The first edition of the companion text, *Epidemiology, Biostatistics, and Preventive Medicine Review*, which included test questions associated with each chapter, was written by Dr. Katz. Both texts were greeted with highly favorable reactions by students and faculty in public health and medicine. In particular, the texts were praised for their ability to explain difficult concepts in clear and easy-to-understand terms. While the first editions were written explicitly for use in course work and USMLE (medical board) preparation, we were gratified that both of them came to be recommended by the American Board of Preventive Medicine as tools for preparing for its core specialty examination as well.

To enhance the value of the two texts for all of our readers, we have combined them into a single text. Thus, the second edition of *Epidemiology, Biostatistics, and Preventive Medicine* includes the following study tools: an examination at the end of each chapter; a 150 question comprehensive examination; detailed explanations about why answers to test questions are correct or incorrect; and a glossary of epidemiologic and medical terms.

Our guiding principles concerning the original 21 chapters of the book were to update all of the information, to improve or retain those aspects of the chapters that worked well in the first edition, and to include coverage of additional concepts. We substantially revised and updated the information on nutrition and genetics. We also updated the information on health counseling, disease screening, and immunizations, based on the latest recommendations of the US Preventive Services Task Force, the Department of Health and Human Services, and the Centers for Disease Control and Prevention. We added information on various topics, including the calculation and interpretation of the number needed to treat and the number needed to harm; the statistical analysis of incidence density; and the role of complementary and alternative medicine in modern health care delivery.

We are grateful for the many encouraging comments and suggestions that we received from our students and colleagues, both in the USA and elsewhere, concerning the first edition texts. We wish to thank Sharon Maddox, whose editing enhanced both the accuracy and clarity of this edition. And we continue to be thankful to our spouses and families for their support of our efforts.

James F. Jekel
David L. Katz
Joann G. Elmore

PREFACE to the First Edition

Epidemiology is the basic science of preventive medicine and public health, and biostatistics is the quantitative foundation of epidemiology. To separate these fields—as is usually done in texts for students of medicine, public health, and related disciplines—incurs the risks of providing incomplete coverage of each field and failing to integrate the subject matter.

In developing this book, the goal was to present a comprehensive view of the fields of epidemiology, biostatistics, preventive medicine, and public health by showing their interrelationships and emphasizing their relevance to clinical practice, research, and public health policy. In particular, the objectives were to combine theory and application in a manner that enables readers to interpret the scientific literature with understanding; to approach clinical practice with an emphasis on prevention; and to understand the social, organizational, financial, and governmental environments in which physicians and other health professionals must practice today.

Section I, Epidemiology, reviews the many ways in which epidemiology contributes to the medical sciences; discusses the sources of health data; incorporates numerous figures and graphs to illustrate how epidemiologic measurements are made and used; outlines the steps in epidemiologic surveillance, outbreak investigation, and assessment of causation and risks; and discusses common research designs used by epidemiologists.

Section II, Biostatistics, builds on the concepts introduced in the first section and emphasizes that an understanding of biostatistics is important not only for analyzing the results of research but also for understanding and reducing errors in clinical medicine. Biostatistical tests and equations are clearly explained and easy to follow, with special "boxes" used to illustrate the steps in calculating standard errors, t values, chi-square values, and other measurements.

Section III, Preventive Medicine and Public Health, focuses on methods of primary, secondary, and tertiary prevention; provides tables with up-to-date information on immunization schedules, available vaccines and antitoxins, screening recommendations, effects of toxic exposures, and similar topics; and discusses the nutritional, environmental, and behavioral factors that have an impact on health, as well as the socioeconomic and political climate that influences health care policy.

In addition to being a textbook for medical students and others taking courses in epidemiology, biostatistics, preventive medicine, and public health, this book is a source of information for health care professionals who wish to study these topics on their own or to review them for medical board examinations. The approach taken in this book evolved from my experiences in teaching a variety of courses to both students and professionals at Yale University School of Medicine, where the Department of Epidemiology and Public Health is an accredited school of public health and also serves as a department of epidemiology, biostatistics, and preventive medicine for the medical school. As a result, I have had the privilege of teaching many of these topics to public health students for 28 years, biostatistics to medical students for 13 years, public health to medical students for 8 years, and biostatistics and related topics to specialist physicians in the Robert Wood Johnson Clinical Scholars Program for 19 years, and directing the Yale Residency Program in General Preventive Medicine and Public Health for 17 years. These varied groups of outstanding individuals, from different backgrounds and levels of training and experience, have given me the best education a teacher could obtain. Any strengths this book may have are due in significant measure to the challenges put forth by these students, who have numbered in the thousands during my three decades of university work.

I owe a tremendous debt to my collaborators, Dr. Joann Elmore and Dr. David Katz, both of whom are general internists with public health degrees and an orientation toward prevention. At first among my best students ever, they soon became trusted colleagues in teaching medical students and in research. They have achieved outstanding reputations at Yale University and are in considerable demand as teachers of medical and public health students and as research consultants. Dr. Elmore and Dr. Katz not only offered valuable suggestions regarding the book's general outlines but also provided extensive critiques of each chapter. Whenever we had differences, we resolved them in conference. For some chapters, the process of reviewing and revising was repeated several times. The final product was, therefore, a true collaboration. Any deficiencies, however, must be laid at my door alone.

Special thanks are also due to Dr. David Lane, a family practitioner and clinical epidemiologist, and to Michael Fischer, a medical student, for their insightful reviews of the epidemiology and biostatistics sections of the book. Dr. William Beckett, who has been a valued colleague for years in teaching public health to medical students, reviewed and made helpful suggestions about the information dealing with occupational health and exposure to toxins. Sharon Maddox, the book's developmental editor, made major contributions to the organization, clarity, and accuracy of the text. William Schmitt of W.B. Saunders has been a patient and supportive editor from the time he first suggested this effort.

My intellectual debts to others are countless, and unfortunately, they cannot all be acknowledged here. The late Dr. Alexander Langmuir was the inspiration for me (as for hundreds of others) to enter epidemiology and public health as a career. Dr. Steven Helgerson, another student of Dr. Langmuir, was an inspiring colleague in efforts to improve the teaching of epidemiology, particularly the investigation of acute disease outbreaks. The late Dr. Edward M. Cohart first saw that I might make an academician and persisted until I agreed to give an academic career a try. Dr. Alvan Feinstein has been a continuous inspiration by his tireless and brilliant efforts to improve clinical epidemiology and biostatistics. His 1975 request for me to assist in the Robert Wood Johnson Clinical Scholars Program at Yale University was a major stimulus to become more involved in teaching biostatistics. Dr. Lowell Levin has consistently helped me to take a wide perspective regarding the sources of health and ways to improve health. Dr. David Allen was a coinvestigator in our research into the crack cocaine problem, and he has helped me to see the mental and spiritual aspects of many health problems.

I cannot count the lessons I have learned from my parents, who at this writing are preparing to celebrate their sixty-ninth wedding anniversary, and from my wife, Jan, who has been my loving and supportive companion for 37 years. They have taught me what it means to live in an environment filled with wholeness, peace, and health, perhaps best described by the Hebrew word *shalom*.

James F. Jekel

CONTENTS

EPIDEMIOLOGY

1

Basic Epidemiologic Concepts and Principles

■ BASIC EPIDEMIOLOGIC CONCEPTS

Epidemiology has been defined in many ways. The word comes from the Greek language, in which *epi* means upon, *dēmos* denotes the population, and the combining form *-logy* means the study of. Thus, epidemiology is the study of something that afflicts (affects) a **population.** Usually, epidemiology is defined as the study of factors that determine the occurrence and distribution of disease in a population.

Epidemiology can be thought of as one of the ways in which disease is studied. In general, there are four levels at which the scientific study of disease can be approached: (1) the submolecular or molecular level (e.g., cell biology, biochemistry, and immunology);

(2) the tissue or organ level (e.g., anatomic pathology); (3) the level of individual patients (e.g., clinical medicine); and (4) the level of populations (e.g., epidemiology). Perspectives gained from these four levels are related, and research should be coordinated among the various disciplines to maximize the scientific understanding of disease.

Some people distinguish between classical epidemiology and clinical epidemiology. **Classical epidemiology,** which is population-oriented, studies the community origins of health problems, particularly those related to nutrition, the environment, human behavior, and the psychologic, social, and spiritual state of a population. Classical epidemiologists are interested in discovering risk factors that might be altered in a population to prevent or delay disease or death.

Investigators involved in **clinical epidemiology** often use research designs and statistical tools that are similar to those used by classical epidemiologists. However, clinical epidemiologists study patients in health care settings in order to improve the diagnosis and treatment of various diseases and the prognosis for patients already affected by a disease. Because clinical epidemiologists usually study people who are ill and are receiving medical attention, they must take special care to adjust for the presence of other diseases (comorbidity) and for any clinical treatments (Sackett 1969; Feinstein 1985; Sackett et al. 1991; Fletcher, Fletcher, and Wagner 1996). Because the primary goal of clinical epidemiology is to improve clinical decisions, some prefer to call clinical epidemiology **clinical decision analysis** (Last 1988), but usually this latter term has a more limited meaning.

The epidemiology section of this book is generally oriented toward classical epidemiology, although clinical examples are sometimes used. Chapters 7 and 8 discuss several topics of special interest to clinical epidemiologists. The more highly statistical parts of epidemiology are found in the biostatistics section, so that the basic concepts and methods of epidemiology can be introduced without undue complexity.

Epidemiology can also be divided into **infectious disease epidemiology** and **chronic disease epidemiology.** The former is more heavily dependent on laboratory support (especially microbiology and serology), and the latter is more dependent on complex sampling and statistical methods. This distinction is becoming less valid as molecular laboratory markers (genetic and otherwise) are being used increasingly in chronic disease epidemiology and as complex statistical analyses are being used more frequently in infectious disease epidemiology (Longini et al. 1988). Moreover, some illnesses, such as tuberculosis and acquired immunodeficiency syndrome (AIDS), may be thought of as both infectious and chronic diseases.

The name of a medical discipline indicates both a method of research into health and disease and the body of knowledge acquired by using that method of research. Thus, pathology is a field of medical research with its own goals and methods, but investigators and clinicians can also speak of the "pathology of lung cancer." Similarly, epidemiology refers to a field of research that uses particular methods, but it can also be used to denote the resulting body of knowledge about the natural history of disease—that is, about the nutritional, behavioral, environmental, and genetic sources of disease as identified through epidemiologic studies.

■ THE ETIOLOGY AND NATURAL HISTORY OF DISEASE

The progression of a disease in the absence of medical or public health intervention is often called the natural history of the disease. Public health and medical personnel take advantage of available knowledge about the stages, mechanisms, and causes of disease to determine how and when to intervene. The goal of intervention, whether preventive or therapeutic, is to alter the natural history of a disease in a favorable way.

Stages of Disease

The development and expression of a disease take place over time and can be divided into three stages: the predisease, latent, and symptomatic stages. During the **predisease stage** (before the pathologic process begins), early intervention may avoid exposure to the agent of disease (e.g., lead or a microbe), thereby preventing the disease process from starting; this is called **primary prevention.** During the **latent stage** (when the disease has begun but is still asymptomatic), the process of screening and instituting appropriate treatment may prevent the progression to symptomatic disease; this is called **secondary prevention.** During the **symptomatic stage** (when disease manifestations are evident), intervention may arrest, slow, or reverse the progression of disease; this is called **tertiary prevention.** These concepts are discussed in more detail in Chapter 14 and subsequent chapters of the book.

Mechanisms and Causes of Disease

When discussing the etiology of disease, epidemiologists make a distinction between the **biologic mechanisms** of disease and the **social and environmental causes of disease.** In a study of osteomalacia, for example, investigators might explore the mechanisms of this bone disease, as well as its causes and consequences in a specific social context, such as among women who observe the custom of purdah. In keeping with this custom, which is generally observed among Muslims and some Hindus in countries such as India, women who have reached puberty avoid public observation by spending most of their time indoors and by wearing clothing that covers virtually all of the body when they go outdoors. By blocking the action of the sun's radiation on the skin, these practices prevent the irradiation of ergosterol, which is one of the D vitamins necessary for growth. If, as often happens, the diet of these women is also deficient in vitamin D during the rapid growth period of puberty, they may develop osteomalacia as a result of insufficient calcium absorption. Osteomalacia can affect future pregnancies by causing the pelvis to become distorted (more pear-shaped), thereby making the pelvic opening too small for the fetus to pass through during delivery. If such problems should arise, a female surgeon or obstetrician must be available, because it would be unthinkable under purdah for a male physician to attend the birth. In this example, the social and nutritional *causes* set in motion the biochemical and other biologic *mechanisms* of osteomalacia that may lead to maternal and infant mortality.

Likewise, excessive fat intake, smoking, and lack of exercise are social factors that contribute to biologic mechanisms of atherogenesis, such as elevated blood levels of low-density lipoprotein cholesterol (LDL) and very low density lipoprotein cholesterol (VLDL), as well as reduced blood levels of high-density lipoprotein cholesterol (HDL).

Epidemiologists attempt to go as far back as possible to discover the societal causes of disease, which offer clues to methods of prevention. Hypotheses introduced by epidemiologists frequently guide laboratory scientists as they seek biologic mechanisms of disease, which may in turn suggest methods of treatment.

Host, Agent, and Environment

The causes of a disease are often considered in terms of a triad of factors: the host, the agent, and the environment. For many diseases, it is useful to add a fourth factor, the vector (Fig. 1–1). In measles, the host is a human being who is susceptible to measles infection, the agent is a highly infectious virus that can produce serious disease in human beings, and the environment enables susceptible people to be exposed to infectious persons. In malaria, the host, agent, and environment are all important, but the vector, the *Anopheles* mosquito, is also critical.

Host factors are responsible for the degree to which the individual is able to adapt to the stressors produced by the agent. Host resistance is influenced by a person's genotype, nutritional status, immune system, and social behavior. General resistance in people without immunodeficiency depends partly on good nutrition. This is evident in the fact that measles is seldom fatal in well-nourished children, even in the absence of measles immunization and modern medical care. In contrast, up to 25% of children with ma-

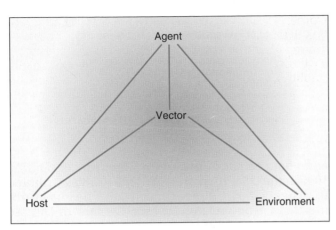

FIGURE 1–1   Factors involved in the natural history of disease.

rasmus (starvation) or kwashiorkor (protein-calorie malnutrition, usually related to weaning) die from complications of measles. The fact that social behavior has an effect on disease spread is also seen in the case of dysentery caused by the organism *Shigella.* This type of dysentery is seldom spread by person-to-person contact where proper hygiene is maintained, but it can spread rapidly via this method in homes for mentally retarded individuals. Behavior such as smoking can also be considered a host factor.

Agents of disease or illness can be divided into several categories. **Biologic agents** include allergens, infectious organisms (e.g., bacteria and viruses), and sometimes even vaccines, antibiotics, and foods (e.g., a high-fat diet). **Chemical agents** include chemical toxins (e.g., lead) and dusts, which can cause either acute or chronic illness. **Physical agents** include kinetic energy (e.g., in cases involving bullet wounds, blunt trauma, and vehicular injuries), radiation, heat, cold, and noise. Epidemiologists are now studying the extent to which **social and psychologic stressors** can be considered agents in the production of health problems.

The **environment** influences the probability and circumstances of contact between the host and the agent. For example, poor restaurant sanitation increases the probability of patrons being exposed to *Salmonella* infections. Poor roads and bad weather conditions increase the number of automobile collisions and airplane crashes. But the environment also includes social, political, and economic factors: crowded homes and schools make exposure to measles and other infectious diseases more likely, and the political structure and economic health of a society partly determine the nutritional status of the members of that society.

Vectors of disease commonly include insects (e.g., mosquitoes associated with the spread of malaria), arthropods (e.g., ticks associated with Lyme disease), and animals (e.g., raccoons associated with rabies in the eastern USA). The concept of the vector, however, can be applied more widely to include groups of human beings (e.g., vendors of heroin and cocaine) and even objects (e.g., contaminated needles associated

with hepatitis and AIDS). A vector may be considered part of the environment, or it may be treated separately, as shown in Fig. 1–1. To be an effective transmitter of disease, the vector must have a specific relationship to the agent, the environment, and the host.

In the case of human malaria, mentioned briefly above, the vector is a mosquito of the genus *Anopheles;* the agent is a parasitic organism of the genus *Plasmodium;* the host is a human being; and the environment enables the mosquito to breed and to come into contact with the host. Specifically, the parasitic organism must go through part of its life cycle in the mosquito; the climate must be relatively warm and have standing water in which the mosquito can breed; the mosquito must be willing to bite human beings and must be able to spread the disease; the host must be bitten by an infected mosquito (in the case of malaria, usually the biting occurs in houses at night); and the host must be susceptible to the disease.

In the case of Lyme disease, human beings are an accidental host. The agent is the spirochete *Borrelia burgdorferi,* which is normally found in the deer mouse. The spirochete is spread by the vector, an *Ixodes* tick, from mouse to mouse in the spring and early summer and is spread to deer by the mature ticks. The environment is usually a wooded area that permits these animals to coexist with human beings, who are bitten by infected ticks.

Risk Factors: The "BEINGS" Model

Risk factors and preventable causes of disease, particularly life-threatening diseases such as cancer, have been the subject of much epidemiologic research. In 1964, an expert committee of the World Health Organization (WHO) estimated that "the majority" of cancer cases were potentially preventable and were due to "extrinsic factors." In the same year, the US Surgeon General released a report that indicated that the risk of death from lung cancer among smokers was almost 11 times that among nonsmokers (US Surgeon General 1964).

In their 1981 book entitled *The Causes of Cancer,* two leading epidemiologists, Richard Doll and Richard Peto, praised the 1964 WHO report and made the following argument (p. 1197):

In the years since that report was published, advances in knowledge have consolidated these opinions and few if any competent research workers now question its main conclusion. Individuals, indeed, have gone further and have substituted figures of 80% or even 90% as the proportion of potentially preventable cancers in place of the 1964 committee's cautious estimate of "the majority."

Unfortunately, the phrase "extrinsic factors" (or the phrase "environmental factors," which is often substituted for it) has been misinterpreted by many people to mean only "man-made chemicals," which was certainly not the intent of the WHO committee. The committee included, in addition to man-made or natural carcinogens, viral infections, nutritional deficiencies or excesses, reproductive activities, and a variety of other factors determined wholly or partly by personal behavior.

Given the many different cell types of cancer and the fact that there are many causal factors to be considered, how do epidemiologists estimate the percentage of deaths caused by cancer?

According to one method, the first step is to look at each type of cancer and determine (from epidemiologic studies) the percentage of cases having an identifiable and preventable cause. These percentages are then added up in a weighted manner to determine the total percentage having identifiable causes.

A second method requires the use of annual age- and sex-specific cancer incidence rates from countries that have the lowest rates of a given cell type of cancer and that also have good medical care to ensure a reasonable level of accuracy in detecting the presence of disease. For a particular cell type of cancer, a low rate in such a country presumably is due to a low prevalence of the risk factors for that type of cancer. After epidemiologists have gathered the necessary data concerning other countries, they could calculate the number of cases of each type of cancer that would be expected to occur annually in each age and gender group in the USA if the lowest globally observed rates had been true for the US population. Next, they would add up the expected numbers for the various cancer types and groups in the USA. Finally, they would compare this total number of expected cases with the total number of cases actually diagnosed in the US population. Using this method, epidemiologists have found that the USA has about five times as many total cancer cases as would be expected. Presumably, the excess cancer cases in the USA are due to a high prevalence of risk factors for cancer, such as smoking.

The acronym "BEINGS" serves as a helpful device for remembering the major categories of risk factors for disease. Some of these factors, which are listed in Table 1–1 and discussed below, are easier to change or eliminate than others. Currently, genetic factors are among the most difficult to change, although this field is rapidly developing and becoming more important to both epidemiology and prevention. Immunologic factors are often the least difficult to change because of effective immunization programs.

"B"—Biologic Factors and Behavioral Factors

The risk for particular diseases may be influenced by gender, age, weight, bone density, and numerous other biologic factors. In addition, human behavior is a central factor in health and disease. The most obvious example of a behavioral risk factor is smoking, which contributes to a variety of health problems, including myocardial infarction; lung, esophageal, and nasopharyngeal cancer; and chronic obstructive pulmonary disease. According to the US Surgeon General (1964), cigarettes are responsible for about 50% of the cases of myocardial infarction among smokers

TABLE 1–1   "BEINGS": An Acronym for Remembering the Categories of Preventable Causes of Disease

Biologic factors and **B**ehavioral factors
Environmental factors
Immunologic factors
Nutritional factors
Genetic factors
Services, **S**ocial factors, and **S**piritual factors

and about 90% of the cases of lung cancer. During 1995 in the USA, there were 482,185 deaths attributed to ischemic heart disease and 156,073 deaths attributed to lung and related cancers (Centers for Disease Control and Prevention 1996a). Based on the percentages noted above, this means that cigarettes were responsible for more deaths from heart disease (241,093 deaths) than they were for deaths from lung cancer (140,466 deaths) during 1995.

Multiple behavioral factors are associated with the spread of some diseases. In the case of AIDS, for instance, the spread of type 1 human immunodeficiency virus (HIV-1) can result from male homosexual activity and from intravenous drug abuse, which are the two predominant routes of transmission in the USA. It can also result from heterosexual activity, which is the predominant route of spread in Africa and many other countries and is becoming more important in the USA.

Although epidemiologic studies were the first to suggest how to prevent both cigarette-related diseases and HIV-1 infection, satisfactory clinical treatments for these diseases are still lacking.

Among the many other examples of behavior that can lead to disease, injury, or premature death (i.e., death before the age of 65 years) are excessive intake of alcohol, abuse of illegal drugs, driving while intoxicated, and homicide and suicide attempts. In each of these cases, as in cigarette smoking and HIV-1 infection, changes in behavior could prevent the untoward outcomes.

Many of the efforts in health promotion depend heavily on the modification of human behavior, which is discussed in detail in Chapter 15.

"E"—Environmental Factors

To everyone's surprise, early epidemiologic studies suggested that the outbreak of sometimes-fatal pneumonia among members of the American Legion who were attending a 1976 conference in Philadelphia was caused by an infectious agent distributed through the air-conditioning and ventilation systems of the primary hotels hosting the conference. Only later, after *Legionella pneumophila* was identified, was the discovery made that this small bacterium actually thrives in air-conditioning cooling towers and in warm water systems. It also has been shown that respiratory therapy equipment that is merely rinsed with water can become a reservoir for *Legionella*, causing hospital-acquired legionnaires' disease.

Early epidemiologic research concerning an illness that was first reported in 1975 in Old Lyme, Connecticut, suggested that the arthritis, rash, and other symptoms of the illness were caused by infection with an organism transmitted by a tick. This was enough information to enable preventive methods to be started. By 1977, it was clear that the disease, called Lyme disease, was spread by *Ixodes* ticks, and this opened the way for more specific prevention and research. Not until 1982, however, was the causative agent, *Borrelia burgdorferi,* discovered and shown to be spread by the *Ixodes* tick.

As a "first responder" in the investigation of new health problems such as legionnaires' disease and Lyme disease, epidemiologists are involved in describing the patterns of disease in the population, developing hypotheses about causal factors, and introducing methods to prevent further cases of disease.

"I"—Immunologic Factors

Smallpox is the first infectious disease known to have been eradicated from the globe (although samples of the causative virus remain stored in laboratories in the USA and in the former Soviet Union). Smallpox eradication was possible because vaccination against the disease conferred individual immunity and also produced herd immunity. Discussed in greater detail later in this chapter, **herd immunity** results when a vaccine not only prevents the vaccinated person from contracting the disease but also prevents him or her from spreading the disease. A reduction in the number of people able to spread disease results in reduced disease transmission.

Most people now think of AIDS when they hear of a deficiency of the immune system, but **immunodeficiency** also may be caused by genetic abnormalities or by other factors. For example, transient immune deficiency has been noted following some infections and after the administration of certain vaccines. An important example concerns measles and live measles vaccine, both of which produce a temporary immune deficiency that is potentially serious, especially in malnourished children.

"N"—Nutritional Factors

In the 1950s, it was shown that Japanese-Americans living in Hawaii had a much higher rate of myocardial infarction than did persons of the same age and sex in Japan, and Japanese-Americans in California had a still higher rate of this disease than did similar persons in Japan (Gordon 1957; Keys 1966, 1970; Reed 1990). The investigators believed that a difference in diet was the single most important factor producing these differences in disease, and their beliefs generally have been supported by subsequent research.

Before his death, Denis Burkitt, the physician after whom Burkitt's lymphoma was named, spent many years doing epidemiologic research on the critical role that dietary fiber plays in good health. During a lecture at Yale University in 1989, he made some stunning statements that included the following: (1) "By world standards, the entire United States is constipated." (2) "Don't diagnose appendicitis in Africa unless the patient speaks English." (3) "African medical students go through 5 years of training without seeing coronary heart disease or appendicitis." (4) "Populations with large stools have small hospitals. Those with small stools have large hospitals."

Based on his cross-cultural studies, Burkitt observed that many of the diseases commonly seen in the USA were rarely encountered in indigenous populations of tropical Africa (Table 1–2). This observation was true even of areas with good medical care, such as Kampala, Uganda, at the time Burkitt was there—a fact suggesting that these diseases were not being missed because of lack of diagnosis. Nor were these differences primarily genetic in origin, because African-Americans in the USA suffer from these diseases at roughly the same rate as other groups in the USA. If the diseases listed in Table 1–2 suddenly disappeared, most US hospitals and many US physicians would be at risk of bankruptcy, unless these diseases were quickly replaced by others. The cross-cultural differences suggest that the current heavy burden of these diseases in the USA is *not* inevitable. Indeed, Burkitt proposed mechanisms by which a high intake of dietary fiber could prevent these diseases or markedly reduce their incidence (Kellock 1985).

The Framingham Heart Study showed that an elevated blood cholesterol level was associated with an elevated risk for myocardial infarction (for a description of the study's inception, see Dawber, Meadors, and Moore 1951). This study and others led to laboratory research into the behavior of blood lipids, and now, decades later, much of the pathogenesis of atherosclerosis and coronary artery disease has been worked out. Only recently have effective medical interventions to prevent myocardial infarction been developed, yet the death rates from this health problem have been falling for two decades, partly because of societal improvements in diet and exercise and the reduction of cigarette smoking, all of which had been suggested by epidemiologic studies in the past.

"G"—Genetic Factors

It is well established that the genetic inheritance of individuals interacts with diet and environment in complex ways to promote or protect against a variety of illnesses, including heart disease and cancer. Genetic epidemiology is a growing field of research. Population genetics and genetic epidemiology are concerned with, among other things, the distribution of normal and abnormal genes in the population and

TABLE 1–2 Diseases That Are Rare in the Indigenous Populations of Tropical Africa

Appendicitis	Diverticulitis
Breast cancer	Gallstones
Colon cancer	Hemorrhoids
Coronary heart disease	Hiatal hernia
Diabetes mellitus	Varicose veins

Source of data: Burkitt, D. Lecture at Yale University School of Medicine, New Haven, Conn., April 28, 1989.

whether or not these are in equilibrium. According to experts, population gene frequencies appear to be stable (Scriver 1988). Genetic epidemiology is also concerned with gene mutation rates, which do not appear to be changing. Considerable research involves studying the possible interaction of various genotypes with environmental, nutritional, and behavioral factors and investigating the extent to which environmental adaptations can reduce the burden of diseases with a heavy genetic component.

Genetic disease now accounts for a higher proportion of disease than in the past, not because the incidence of genetic disease is rising but because the incidence of noninherited disease is falling. This point is illustrated in the following discussion by Scriver (1988):

> Heritability refers to . . . the contribution of genes relative to all determinants of disease. Rickets, a genetic disease, recently showed an abrupt fall in incidence and an increase in heritability in Quebec. The fall in incidence followed universal supplementation of dairy milk with calciferol. The rise in heritability reflected the disappearance of a major environmental cause of rickets (vitamin D deficiency) and the persistence of Mendelian disorders of calcium and phosphate homeostasis without a change in their incidence.

Scriver lists other genetic problems for which the environmental, nutritional, and behavioral components have been reduced, with little or no fall in the genetic disease in the same area. For example, as a result of the control of paralytic poliomyelitis through immunization, juvenile musculoskeletal disorders show an increased **heritability**—that is, an increased proportion of cases having genetic causes.

Genetic screening is important for identifying a few problems in newborns (such as phenylketonuria and congenital hypothyroidism) for which therapy can be extremely beneficial if instituted early enough in life. Screening is also important for identifying other genetic disorders for which genetic counseling can be beneficial. Nevertheless, the greatest future health improvements in the genetic area may evolve from a better understanding of how identification of individual genotypes can lead to special protection for people who are particularly susceptible to environmental problems at home and at work or for those who cannot tolerate certain foods, medicines, or behaviors. Major screening efforts for "susceptibility genes" will undoubtedly increase in the future, but there are ethical concerns about potential problems, such as medical insurance carriers hesitating to insure individuals with known genetic risks. For more on the prevention of genetic disease, see Section III, particularly Chapter 19.

"S"—Services, Social Factors, and Spiritual Factors

Medical care services may be quite beneficial to health, but they can also be dangerous. One of the important tasks of epidemiologists is to determine the value of medical care in different settings. Approximately 5% of hospitalized patients acquire a hospital infection (Inlander, Levin, and Weiner 1988), and 3.7% of hospitalized patients suffer "adverse events" (medical errors) other than infection (Leape et al. 1991). Other medical care–related causes of illness include unnecessary and inappropriate diagnostic or surgical procedures.

The effects of **social and spiritual factors** on disease and health have been less intensively studied than have the effects of other causal factors. However, evidence is accumulating that personal beliefs concerning the meaning and purpose of life, access to forgiveness, and the support received from members of a social network are powerful influences on health. Studies have shown that both experimental animals and human beings are better able to resist noxious stressors when they are in the presence of other members of the same species. Social support may be achieved through the family, friendship networks, and membership in various groups, such as clubs and churches. Larson, Sawyers, and McCullough (1998) have reviewed the literature concerning the association of religious faith with generally better health.

Many investigators have explored factors related to health and disease in Mormons and Seventh-Day Adventists. Both of these religious groups have been shown to have lower than average age-adjusted death rates from many common types of disease and specifically from heart disease, cancer, and respiratory disorders (Berkman and Breslow 1983). Part of their protection undoubtedly arises from the behaviors proscribed or prescribed by the groups. For example, Mormons prohibit the use of coffee, tea, alcohol, and tobacco. Seventh-Day Adventists likewise tend to avoid alcohol and tobacco, and in addition they strongly encourage (but do not require) their members to eat a vegetarian diet. However, as Berkman and Breslow (1983:62) indicated, it is not clear that these behaviors are solely responsible for the health differences: "It is difficult . . . to separate the effects of health practices from other aspects of life-style common among those belonging to such religions, for example, differing social stresses and network systems."

In an earlier study, Berkman and Syme (1979) showed that for all age groups, the greater one's participation in churches and other groups and the stronger one's social networks, the lower the mortality that was observed.

The work of the psychiatrist Frankl (1963) also documented the importance of a person's having a meaning and purpose in life, which can be useful in the treatment of distressed persons and in promoting a reduction of emotional problems. Such factors are increasingly being studied as important in understanding the web of causation of diseases.

■ ECOLOGIC ISSUES IN EPIDEMIOLOGY

Some epidemiologists see their field as "human ecology," "medical ecology," or "geographic medicine"

(Kilbourne and Smillie 1969). This is because an important characteristic of epidemiology is its ecologic perspective. People are seen not only as individual organisms, but also as members of communities, in a social context. The world is understood as a complex ecosystem in which disease patterns vary greatly from one country to another. In fact, the types and rates of diseases in a country are a kind of "fingerprint" that indicates the per capita income (a proxy for the standard of living), the life-style, the predominant occupations, and the climate, among other things. Owing to the tremendous growth in world population (reaching 6 billion in 1999) and the rapid technologic developments in the 20th century, human beings have had a profound impact on the global environment, often with deleterious effects. The existence of great biodiversity, which helps to provide the planet with greater adaptive capacity, has become increasingly threatened. Every action that affects the ecosystem (even an action whose goal is to increase the health and well-being of humans) produces a reaction in the system, and the result is not always positive. Several examples are given below.

The Solution and Unintended Creation of Problems

One of the most important insights of ecologic thinking is that as people change one element in a system, they inevitably change other parts. Thus, an epidemiologist will constantly be alert for possible negative side effects that a medical or health intervention might produce. For example, in the USA, the reduction of mortality in infancy and childhood has increased the prevalence of chronic degenerative diseases, because now the majority of people live to retirement age. Medically, nobody would want to go back a hundred years or more. Nevertheless, the control of infectious diseases has produced another set of problems. Table 1–3 shows some of the new health and societal problems introduced by the solution of earlier health problems.

Vaccination and Patterns of Immunity

Understanding **herd immunity** is essential to thinking about the ecologic problems in immunization today. If herd immunity is present, not only will an immunized individual be protected, but he or she will be unable to transmit the disease to others, and this will cause the prevalence of the organism in the population to decline.

Herd immunity is illustrated in Fig. 1–2, where it is assumed that each infected person comes into sufficient contact with two other persons to expose both of them to the disease if they are susceptible. Under this assumption, if there is no herd immunity against the disease and everyone is susceptible, the number of cases will double every "disease generation" (see Fig. 1–2A). If there is 50% herd immunity against the disease, the number of cases will be small and will remain approximately constant (see Fig. 1–2B). If there is greater than 50% herd immunity, as would be true in a well-immunized population, the infection should eventually die out. Obviously, the degree of immunity necessary to eliminate a virus from a population varies depending on the type of virus, the time of year, and the density and social patterns of the population.

It may seem that immunization is simple: immunize essentially everybody in childhood, and there will be no problems from the targeted diseases. Although there is some truth to this way of thinking, in reality the control of diseases by immunization is more complex. In this section, the examples of diphtheria, smallpox, poliomyelitis, and syphilis are used to illustrate some of the current issues concerning vaccination programs and population immunity.

Diphtheria. Vaccine-produced immunity in individuals tends to decrease over time. This phenomenon has a different impact today, when infectious diseases such as diphtheria are less common, than it did in the past. When diphtheria was a more common disease, people who had been vaccinated against it were exposed more frequently to the causative agent, and this exposure could result in a mild reinfection. The reinfection would produce a "natural booster effect" and maintain a high level of immunity. As diphtheria became less common because of immunization programs, fewer people were exposed and there were fewer subclinical "booster" infections. Today, the less recently immunized people tend to be more susceptible to infection.

This is demonstrated by events in the newly independent states (NIS) of the former Soviet Union, where despite the wide availability of diphtheria vaccine, many adults who had not recently been in the

---

TABLE 1–3   **Examples of Negative Ecologic Side Effects from the Solution of Earlier Health Problems**

Initial Health Problem	Solution	Negative Ecologic Side Effects
Childhood infections	Vaccination.	Decrease in the level of immunity during adulthood, owing to a lack of repeated exposures to infection.
High infant mortality rate	Improved sanitation.	Increase in the population growth rate; appearance of epidemic paralytic poliomyelitis; and appearance of epidemic hepatitis A infection.
Sleeping sickness in cattle	Control of the tsetse fly (the disease vector).	Increase in the area of land subject to overgrazing and drought, owing to an increase in the cattle population.
Malnutrition and the need for larger areas of tillable land	Erection of large river dams (e.g., on the Aswan and Senegal Rivers).	Increase in the rates of some infectious diseases, owing to water system changes that favor the vectors of disease.

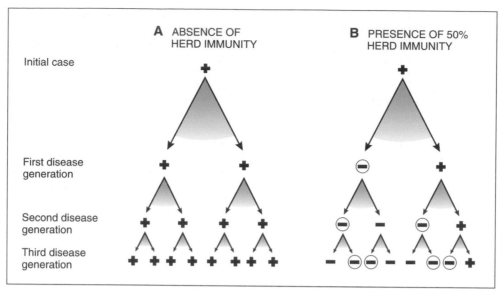

A ABSENCE OF HERD IMMUNITY

B PRESENCE OF 50% HERD IMMUNITY

Initial case

First disease generation

Second disease generation

Third disease generation

FIGURE 1–2   **The effect of herd immunity on the spread of infection.** The diagrams illustrate how an infectious disease, such as measles, could spread in a susceptible population if each infected person were exposed to two other persons. In the absence of herd immunity (diagram A), the number of cases doubles each disease generation. In the presence of 50% herd immunity (diagram B), the number of cases remains constant. The plus sign represents an infected person; the minus sign represents an uninfected person; and the circled minus sign represents an immune person who will not pass the infection to others.

military were found to be susceptible to the diphtheria organism (Rappuoli, Perugini, and Falsen 1988). Beginning in 1990, a major epidemic of diphtheria appeared in the NIS. By 1992, about 72% of the reported cases were found to be among people over 14 years of age. This was not due to lack of initial immunization, because more than 90% of the adults in the NIS had been fully immunized against diphtheria when they were children. The disease in older people apparently was due to a decline in the adult immunity levels. By 1995, the epidemic produced more than 125,000 cases of diphtheria and caused 4000 deaths (Centers for Disease Control and Prevention 1996b).

Smallpox. As mentioned earlier in this chapter, the goal of worldwide eradication of smallpox has been met by immunizing people against the disease. There were some potential risks in the attempt to eradicate the disease, however. The dominant form of smallpox in the 1970s was variola minor (alastrim). This was a relatively mild form of smallpox which, although often disfiguring, had a low mortality rate. Yet alastrim provided individual and herd immunity against the much more disfiguring and often fatal variola major form of the disease (classical smallpox). If the immunization program were to eradicate variola minor but not variola major, in time some populations might become susceptible to the more severe form of the disease. To eliminate alastrim and instead get variola major would have been a poor exchange. Fortunately, the smallpox vaccine was effective against both forms of smallpox, and the immunization program was successful in eradicating both variola minor and variola major.

Poliomyelitis. The need for herd immunity was also demonstrated by poliomyelitis. The Salk (injected) polio vaccine, which became available in 1955, provided protection to the immunized individual but did not produce herd immunity. Although it stimulated the production of blood antibodies against poliovirus, it did not produce cell-mediated immunity in the intestine, where the polioviruses multiplied. Because of this, it did little to interrupt viral replication in the intestine. Declining rates of paralytic poliomyelitis lulled many people into lack of concern, and immunization rates for newborn children dropped. Unfortunately, this led to recurrent cases and periodic small epidemics of poliomyelitis in the late 1950s and early 1960s.

The live, attenuated Sabin oral polio vaccine (OPV) was approved in the early 1960s. The OPV produced cell-mediated immunity, thus preventing the poliovirus from replicating in the intestine, and therefore it provided herd immunity. After the widespread use of OPV in the USA, the prevalence of all three types of the wild poliovirus declined rapidly, as monitored in waste sewage. As the wild polioviruses became scarce in the environment, even children who were not given polio vaccine usually were protected, because they were not exposed to the virus (herd immunity). Poliovirus now appears to have been eradicated from the western hemisphere, where the last known case of paralytic poliomyelitis caused by a wild poliovirus was confirmed in Peru in August 1991 (see Centers for Disease Control and Prevention 1994b).

It might appear from this information that the OPV is always superior, but that is not true. When the health department for the Gaza Strip used only the

OPV in its polio immunization efforts, many cases of paralytic poliomyelitis occurred among Arab children. Because of inadequate sanitation, the children often had other intestinal infections when they were given the OPV, and these infections interfered with the OPV infection in the gut. Because the oral vaccine often did not "take," many children were still unprotected (Lasch 1979). The health department subsequently switched to an immunization program in which children were first injected with Salk vaccine to produce adequate blood immunity. Later, they were given OPV as a booster vaccine to achieve herd immunity.

Now that the OPV has succeeded in eradicating wild poliovirus from the western hemisphere, the only indigenous cases of paralytic poliomyelitis occurring in the USA since 1979 have been due to this oral (live, attenuated) vaccine itself, which produces about one case per 2.4 million vaccine doses. In 1997, to reduce this number of cases, the Advisory Committee on Immunization Practices (ACIP) of the Centers for Disease Control and Prevention recommended that infants be given the injected (killed) vaccine before the OPV. This approach was accepted, and the vaccination levels were maintained. Then in 1999, the ACIP recommended that the use of OPV be discontinued and that infants be given only the killed vaccine, starting in January of 2000 (see Centers for Disease Control and Prevention 1999a, 1999b). Some oral vaccine will still be held in reserve for outbreaks or other special purposes.

Syphilis. Syphilis has several stages. In the primary and secondary stages, the lesions are highly contagious, but they subside spontaneously. Next is a latent period, after which a tertiary stage may occur. The immunity that develops from an untreated infection is not absolute. It does not protect the individual from progressive damage to his or her own body. It does, however, provide herd immunity by making the infected person unlikely to develop another highly infectious primary chancre (the initial ulcer of syphilis infection, which is filled with spirochetes) if he or she is exposed to syphilis again (Jekel 1968). When penicillin came into general use, syphilis infections were killed so quickly that "chancre immunity" did not develop, and high-risk persons continued to reacquire and spread the disease.

Effects of Sanitation

In the 19th century, diarrheal diseases were the biggest killer of children, and tuberculosis was the leading cause of adult mortality. The sanitary revolution, which began in England about the middle of the century, was the most important single factor in reducing the infant mortality rate. However, the reduction of infant mortality contributed in a major way to increasing the effective birth rate and, hence, the rate of population growth. The sanitary revolution was therefore one of the causes of today's worldwide population problem. The magnitude of the world population, which reached 6 billion people late in 1999, has a profound and often unappreciated impact on global health through its impact on environmental pollution, fish supply, available land for cultivation, forest devastation, and as still yet poorly understood influences on climate (Ehrlich and Ehrlich 1990).

In discussing this phenomenon, care must be taken to avoid oversimplifying the relationships among the factors involved. On the one hand, the reduction of the infant mortality rate temporarily helps to produce a big difference between the birth and death rates of a society and results in rapid population growth (the so-called **demographic gap**). On the other hand, the control of infant mortality also appears to be necessary for cultures to accept population control. In a time when the infant mortality rate is high, a family needs to have a large number of children to ensure that one or two will survive to adulthood. This is not true in a time when the infant mortality rate is low. Therefore, although it may seem to be contradictory, the reduction of the infant mortality appears to be both a cause of the population problem and a necessity for population control.

In addition to affecting population growth, the sanitary revolution during the 19th century affected disease patterns in unexpected ways. The improvement in sanitation also was a fundamental cause of the appearance of epidemic paralytic poliomyelitis late in the 19th century. Before polio vaccine was introduced, epidemics of paralytic poliomyelitis tended to appear as a nation's infant mortality rate dropped, usually to about 70 or 80 deaths per 1000 live births. The relationship of paralytic poliomyelitis to improvement in sanitation seems counterintuitive, but it illustrates the importance of an ecologic perspective and offers an example of the iceberg phenomenon discussed later in this chapter. The three polioviruses are enteric viruses transmitted by the fecal oral route. People who have developed antibodies to all three types of poliovirus are immune to their potentially paralytic effects and thus show no symptoms or signs of clinical disease if they are exposed. Newborn infants have passive antibodies from their mothers, and these maternal antibodies normally prevent polioviruses from invading the central nervous system early in an infant's first year of life. Thus, exposure of a young infant to polioviruses rarely results in paralytic disease but instead leads to a subclinical (largely asymptomatic) infection, which causes the infant to produce his or her own active antibodies and cell-mediated immunity.

Although improved sanitation reduced the proportion of people who were infected with polioviruses, it also delayed, on the average, the time when an infant or child was exposed to the polioviruses. More children were exposed after they were no longer protected by maternal immunity, with the result that a higher percentage of them suffered from the paralytic form of the disease. *Epidemic* paralytic poliomyelitis, therefore, can be seen as an unwanted side effect of the sanitary revolution. Because members of the upper socioeconomic groups had the best sanitation, they were hit first and hardest, at least until polio vaccine became available.

A similar phenomenon occurred with hepatitis A, another virus spread by the fecal-oral route. In young children, hepatitis A is normally mild or asymptomatic. In adults, hepatitis A infection usually causes symptoms; rarely, it even causes death. Improved sanitation caused a delay in exposure to the hepatitis A virus, so that epidemic hepatitis A can also be seen as a side effect of improved sanitation.

Vector Control and Land Use Patterns

Sub-Saharan Africa is one of the more disturbing examples of how negative side effects can come from an attempt to do good. A successful effort was made to control the tsetse fly, which is the vector of African sleeping sickness in cattle and sometimes in people. Control of the vector enabled herders to keep larger numbers of cattle, and this in turn led to overgrazing. The overgrazed areas have been subjected to frequent droughts, and some have become dust bowls (Ormerod 1976).

River Dam Construction and Patterns of Disease

For a time, it was fashionable for Western nations to build large river dams for developing countries to enable them to increase the amount of available farmland by irrigation. During this period, the warnings of epidemiologists about potential negative side effects went unheeded, and as the epidemiologists predicted, the number of cases of schistosomiasis increased in the areas supplied by the Aswan High Dam after it was erected in Egypt. An increase in the number of cases of mosquito-borne diseases (malaria, Rift Valley fever, and dengue fever) also occurred after the main dam and several tributary dams of the Senegal River Project were built in western Africa, and cases of schistosomiasis also developed. Before the dams were erected in Senegal, during the dry season the sea would move far inland and mix with the fresh water, making the water too salty to support the larvae of the blood flukes responsible for schistosomiasis or the mosquitoes that transmit malaria, Rift Valley fever, and dengue fever (Patton 1992).

Synergism of Factors Predisposing to Disease

There may be a synergism between diseases or between factors predisposing to disease, so that each makes the other worse or more easily acquired.

Sexually transmitted diseases, especially those which produce open sores, predispose to the spread of type 1 human immunodeficiency virus (HIV-1). This is thought to be a major factor in countries where HIV-1 is usually spread through heterosexual activity. AIDS, in turn, predisposes to the reactivation of previously latent infections, such as tuberculosis, and this is partly responsible for the current resurgence of tuberculosis.

The relationship between malnutrition and infection is also complex. Not only does malnutrition make infections worse, but infections make malnutrition worse. A malnourished child has more difficulty making antibodies and repairing tissue damage, and this makes him or her less resistant to infectious diseases and their complications. This is seen, for example, in the case of measles. In isolated societies without medical care or measles vaccine, fewer than 1% of well-nourished children may die from measles, whereas as many as 25% of malnourished children may die from measles infection or its complications.

There are several reasons why infection can make malnutrition worse. First, infection puts greater demands on the body, so the relative deficiency of nutrients becomes greater. Second, infection tends to reduce the appetite, and this in turn reduces the intake. Third, in the presence of infection, the diet is frequently changed to emphasize bland foods, which often are deficient in proteins and vitamins. And, finally, in cases of gastrointestinal infection, the food is rushed through the irritated bowel at a faster pace (causing diarrhea), and this allows fewer nutrients to be absorbed.

A final example of synergism concerns how ecologic and genetic factors can interact to produce new strains of influenza virus. Some people wonder why many of the new, epidemic strains of influenza virus have had names from China (Hong Kong flu, Beijing flu, etc.). In rural China, pigs are in close contact with both ducks and people. Both the duck and human strains of influenza infect pigs, and in the pigs the genetic material of the two influenza strains may mix, producing a new variant of influenza. The new strains produced in the pigs can then infect human beings (Shope 1992). If the genetic changes in the influenza virus are major, this is called an **antigenic shift,** and the new virus may produce a worldwide outbreak (pandemic) of influenza. If the genetic changes in the influenza virus are minor, the phenomenon is called an **antigenic drift,** but this can still produce major regional outbreaks of influenza.

■ CONTRIBUTIONS OF EPIDEMIOLOGISTS TO THE MEDICAL SCIENCES

Investigating Epidemics and New Diseases

Using the surveillance and investigative methods discussed in detail in Chapter 3, epidemiologists have often provided the initial hypotheses for others to test in the laboratory. Since 1975, epidemiologic methods have suggested the probable type of agent and modes of transmission for the diseases listed in Table 1–4, usually within months of their recognition as new or emergent diseases. Knowledge of the modes of transmission in turn led epidemiologists to suggest ways to prevent each of these diseases before the causative agents were determined or extensive laboratory results were available. Laboratory work to identify the causal agents, clarify the pathogenesis, and develop vaccines or treatments for most of these

TABLE 1–4 Some Recent Diseases Whose Natural History and Methods of Prevention Were the Subjects of Early Hypotheses by Epidemiologists

Disease	Date of Appearance	Epidemiologic Hypotheses	
		Agent and Route of Spread	Methods of Prevention
Lyme disease	1975	Infectious agent, spread by ticks.	Avoid ticks.
Legionnaires' disease	1976	Small infectious agent, spread via air-conditioning systems.	Treat the water in air-conditioning systems.
Toxic shock syndrome	1980	Staphylococcal toxin, associated with the use of tampons, especially the Rely brand of tampons.	Avoid using long-lasting tampons.
Acquired immunodeficiency syndrome (AIDS)	1981	Viral agent, spread via sexual activity, especially male homosexual activity, and via sharing of needles and exchange of blood and blood products during intravenous drug use and transfusions.	Use condoms; avoid sharing needles; and institute programs to exchange needles and screen blood.
Eosinophilia-myalgia syndrome	1989	Toxic contaminant, associated with the use of dietary supplements of L-tryptophan.	Change methods of product manufacturing.
Hantavirus pulmonary syndrome	1993	Hantavirus, spread via contact with the contaminated droppings of deer mice.	Avoid contact with excreta of deer mice.
New-variant Creutzfeldt-Jakob disease	1996	Prions, spread via ingestion of beef infected with bovine spongiform encephalopathy.	Avoid eating infected beef; avoid feeding animal remains to cattle.

diseases still continues many years after this basic epidemiologic work was done.

Concern about the many recently discovered and resurgent diseases, although not new, is at a peak because of a variety of newly emerging disease problems (see Jekel 1972; Institute of Medicine 1992; Gibbons 1993; Centers for Disease Control and Prevention 1994a). The rapid growth in population, increased travel and contact with new areas such as jungles, declining effectiveness of antibiotics and insecticides, and many other factors encourage the development of new diseases or the resurgence of older ones.

Studying the Biologic Spectrum of Disease

The first identified cases of a new disease are often fatal or severe, which leads observers to conclude that the disease is always severe. However, as more becomes known about the disease, less severe (and even asymptomatic) cases are usually discovered. In infectious disease, asymptomatic infection may be uncovered either by finding elevated antibody titers to the organism in clinically well people or by culturing the organism from them.

This variation in severity of a disease process is referred to as the **biologic spectrum of disease,** or the **iceberg phenomenon** (Morris 1967). The latter term is appropriate because most of an iceberg remains unseen, below the surface, as do most asymptomatic and mild cases of disease. An outbreak of diphtheria will illustrate the point. In 1962 and 1963, when one of the authors (JFJ) worked with the Centers for Disease Control, he and a colleague were assigned to investigate an epidemic of diphtheria in a county in

Alabama. In addition to causing 2 deaths, the diphtheria caused symptoms of clinical illness in 12 children who recovered with or without sequelae. It also caused known asymptomatic infection in 32 children, some of whom had even been immunized against diphtheria. The 32 cases of asymptomatic infection were discovered by an extensive campaign of culturing the throats of the school-age children in the outbreak area as well as the home contacts of any infected child. In this "iceberg" (Fig. 1–3), 14 infections were visible, but the 32 asymptomatic carriers would have remained invisible without the extensive use of culturing and epidemiologic surveillance (Jekel, Zatlin, and Gay 1970).

The iceberg phenomenon is extremely important to epidemiology, because studying only symptomatic individuals may produce a misleading picture of the disease pattern and severity (Evans 1987).

Surveillance of Community Health Interventions

Field trials are an important phase of evaluating a new vaccine before it is given to the community at large, but field trials are only one phase of the evaluation of immunization programs. After the introduction of a vaccine, ongoing surveillance of the disease and vaccine side effects is essential to ensure the continued safety and effectiveness of the vaccine.

The importance of continued surveillance can be illustrated in the case of immunization against poliomyelitis. In 1954, large-scale field trials of the Salk inactivated polio vaccine were done, and these confirmed the value and safety of the vaccine (Francis et al. 1955). In 1955, the polio surveillance program of the Centers for Disease Control discovered an out-

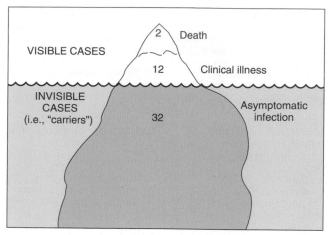

FIGURE 1–3 The iceberg phenomenon, as illustrated by a diphtheria epidemic in Alabama. In epidemics, the number of people with severe forms of the disease (the tip of the iceberg) may be much smaller than the number of people with mild or asymptomatic clinical disease. (Source of data: Jekel, J. F., G. S. Zatlin, and O. F. Gay. *Corynebacterium diphtheriae* survives in a partly immunized group. Public Health Reports 85:310, 1970.)

break of vaccine-associated poliomyelitis, which was linked to vaccine from Cutter Laboratories (Langmuir 1963). Ultimately, 79 vaccinated individuals and 105 of their family members were found to have developed poliomyelitis. Apparently, a slight change from the recommended procedure for producing the vaccine had allowed clumping of the poliovirus to occur, and this enabled some of the virus particles in the center of the clumps to avoid being killed by formaldehyde during vaccine production. Because of this faulty processing, some people were vaccinated with a vaccine containing live virus. It was only because of the vaccine surveillance program that the problem was detected quickly and the dangerous vaccine removed from use.

Likewise, ongoing surveillance programs were responsible for detecting outbreaks of measles that occurred in 1971, 1977, and 1990, after impressive initial progress against the disease. Epidemiologists were able to show that much of the unexpected disease occurred in college students and other people who had received only one dose of measles vaccine, which had been administered in the period before the 12th month of life, during which time the persistence of maternal antibody may have reduced the antigenicity of the vaccine (Marks, Halpin, and Orenstein 1978). Such findings have led to the current recommendations to give measles vaccine initially at 15 months of age, to give a booster dose of measles vaccine before primary school entry, and to ensure that students entering college have had at least two doses of measles vaccine (see Centers for Disease Control and Prevention 1999b).

Setting Disease Control Priorities

Disease control priorities should be based not only on the currently existing size of the problem but also on the potential of a disease to spread to others, its likelihood of causing death and disability, and its cost to individuals, families, and society. Unfortunately, legislatures often fund disease control efforts inappropriately, by considering only the number of cases reported, as was illustrated by the federal government's support for syphilis control in the USA (Jekel 1968).

In the mid-1980s, the potential threat that AIDS posed to society was recognized as being far greater than was suggested by the absolute numbers and costs involved at that time. Because of this, a much larger portion of national resources was allocated to the study and control of AIDS than to efforts focused on other diseases affecting similar numbers of patients. Special concerns with AIDS included the rapid increase in the number of cases reported during such a brief period, the high case fatality ratio, the huge medical care and social costs, the transmissibility of the disease, and the fact that known methods of prevention were not being well applied.

Improving the Diagnosis, Treatment, and Prognosis of Clinical Disease

The application of epidemiologic methods to clinical questions has improved research concerning the diagnosis, therapy, and prognosis of disease (Feinstein 1985). This application is the domain of clinical epidemiology.

Epidemiologic methods are used to improve disease **diagnosis** through the selection of the best diagnostic tests, the determination of the best cutoff points for diagnostic tests, and the development of strategies to use in screening for disease (Sackett et al. 1991). These issues are discussed in Chapters 7 and 8 and in the preventive medicine section of this book.

Epidemiologic methods are frequently used to determine the most effective **treatment** in a given situation. For example, Bracken et al. (1990) used a randomized controlled clinical trial in many centers around the USA to test the hypothesis that methylprednisolone reduced spinal cord damage and improved residual motor function following acute spinal cord injury. The hypothesis was confirmed.

Epidemiologic methods also help improve **prognosis.** For example, Horwitz, Cicchetti, and Horwitz (1984) used a case-control study to compare two different coronary prognostic indices, analyze their weaknesses, and suggest ways in which prognostication could be enhanced. Individual patients want to know their prognoses, and such knowledge also helps investigators stratify patients into groups with similar disease severity in clinical trials and other research to evaluate treatments.

Improving Health Services Research

The principles as well as the methods of epidemiology are used in health services research (Spitzer, Feinstein, and Sackett 1975; Holland and Karhausen

1979; Knox 1979; Levine and Lilienfeld 1987). In health planning, epidemiologic measures are employed to determine the level of community health needs, both present and future. Demographic projection techniques enable good estimations to be made of the size of different age groups in the future, and the analysis of patterns of disease frequency and services use can estimate the level of services that will be required in the future (see, for example, Connecticut Hospital Association 1978). Both in health program evaluation and in the broader field of cost-effectiveness analysis and cost-benefit analysis, epidemiologic methods are used to determine the effects of medical care. It is usually more difficult to determine the effect of a program or a policy than to determine its cost.

Providing Expert Testimony in Courts of Law

Increasingly, epidemiologists are being called upon to testify regarding the state of knowledge about product hazards and the probable risks and effects of various environmental exposures. Among the many kinds of lawsuits that may rely on epidemiologic data are those involving claims of damage from general environmental exposures (e.g., the possible association of magnetic fields and brain cancer); occupational illness claims (e.g., occupational lung damage from workplace asbestos); medical liability (e.g., adverse effects of vaccines); and product liability (e.g., the association of lung cancer with tobacco use and the association of toxic shock syndrome with tampon use). Frequently, the answers to the questions posed are unknown or can only be estimated. Greenland (1999) has described some of reasons that a high level of epidemiologic expertise is needed for such testimony.

■ SUMMARY

Epidemiology is a branch of medical science that relates what is happening in the lives of individuals and society to the occurrence and distribution of diseases, injuries, and other health problems. As such, it is concerned with all of the biologic, social, behavioral, spiritual, and psychologic factors that may increase the frequency of disease or offer opportunities for prevention. Epidemiologic methods are often the first scientific methods applied to a new health problem in order to define its pattern in the population and to develop hypotheses about its causes and methods of transmission.

Epidemiologists generally describe the causes of a disease in terms of the host, agent, and environment, sometimes adding the vector as a fourth factor for consideration. In exploring the means to prevent a given disease, they look for possible behavioral, genetic, and immunologic causes, which are usually associated with the host. They also look for biologic and nutritional causes, which are usually considered under the agent. And they consider the environment in which the disease occurs. The acronym "BEINGS" is useful in remembering these categories of preventable causes of disease (see Table 1–1).

Epidemiology is concerned with human ecology and, in particular, the impact that health interventions have on disease patterns and on the environment. Knowing that the solution of one problem tends to create new problems, epidemiologists are particularly concerned to look for undesirable side effects of medical and public health interventions.

The contributions of epidemiologists to the medical sciences include the following: (1) investigating epidemics and new diseases; (2) studying the biologic spectrum of disease; (3) instituting surveillance of community health interventions; (4) setting disease control priorities; (5) improving the diagnosis, treatment, and prognosis of clinical disease; (6) improving health services research; and (7) providing expert testimony in courts of law.

■ QUESTIONS

Directions (Items 1–10). Each of the numbered items or incomplete statements in this section is followed by answers or by completions of the statement. Select the ONE lettered answer or completion that is BEST in each case. Correct answers and explanations are given at the end of the chapter.

1. Epidemiology is broadly defined as the study of factors that influence the health of populations. The application of epidemiologic findings in populations to decisions in the care of individual patients is
   - (A) generally inappropriate
   - (B) known as clinical epidemiology
   - (C) limited to chronic disease epidemiology
   - (D) limited to infectious disease epidemiology
   - (E) subject to the ecologic fallacy

2. The "BEINGS" model is a useful paradigm for
   - (A) allocating public health resources
   - (B) assessing the impact of herd immunity
   - (C) determining the role of social policy on public health
   - (D) establishing the importance of social contacts
   - (E) evaluating etiologic factors in disease

3. The "BEINGS" model provides a list of factors in disease causality. Which of the following factors are explicitly included in the list?
   - (A) Behavioral, ecologic, idiopathic, nutritional, genetic, and social factors
   - (B) Behavioral, environmental, iatrogenic, nutritional, genetic, and selective factors
   - (C) Behavioral, environmental, immunologic, nutritional, genetic, and social factors
   - (D) Biologic, environmental, immunologic, nutritional, genetic, and synergistic factors
   - (E) Biologic, environmental, innate, nutritional, genetic, and synergistic factors

4. For an infectious disease to occur, there must be interaction between
   (A) behavioral factors and genetic factors
   (B) the agent and the vector
   (C) the host and the agent
   (D) the vector and the environment
   (E) the vector and the host

5. Widely publicized fatalities associated with an "emerging" disease (e.g., hantavirus pulmonary syndrome) may be an example of
   (A) active surveillance
   (B) case finding
   (C) iatrogenesis
   (D) the first responder effect
   (E) the iceberg phenomenon

6. Which of the following activities is beyond the scope of activities undertaken by epidemiologists?
   (A) Analyzing cost-effectiveness
   (B) Establishing modes of disease transmission
   (C) Preventing disease
   (D) Providing data for genetic counseling
   (E) Rationing health care resources

7. Herd immunity refers to
   (A) genetic resistance to species-specific disease
   (B) immunity naturally acquired in a population
   (C) the high levels of antibody present in a population following an epidemic
   (D) the prevention of disease transmission to susceptible individuals through acquired immunity in others
   (E) the vaccination of domestic animals to prevent disease transmission to humans

8. Attempts to eradicate a disease through widespread immunization programs are associated with potential adverse effects. Which of the following effects is correlated with the efficacy of the vaccine?
   (A) The emergence of resistant strains
   (B) The loss of the natural booster effect
   (C) The occurrence of allergic reactions
   (D) The occurrence of infection in younger age groups
   (E) The occurrence of neurologic complications

9. Which of the following phenomena resulted from attempts to solve a public health problem?
   (A) Antigenic drift in the influenza virus
   (B) Desertification in sub-Saharan Africa
   (C) Reactivation of latent tuberculosis in individuals with human immunodeficiency virus (HIV) infection
   (D) Spread of *Legionella pneumophila* through air-conditioning systems

   (E) Transmission of hepatitis C via blood transfusions

10. Evaluation of which of the following potentially preventable causes of disease is most likely to raise ethical concerns?
    (A) Dietary intake
    (B) Genetic susceptibility
    (C) Immunization status
    (D) Smoking history
    (E) Social support networks

■ ANSWERS AND EXPLANATIONS

1. **The answer is B: known as clinical epidemiology.** Clinical practice is devoted to the care of individual patients. However, outcomes in individual patients in response to clinical interventions cannot be known until after the interventions have been tried. Therefore, the basis for choosing therapy (or, for that matter, for choosing diagnostic tests) is prior experience in similar patients, rather than knowledge of what will work best for the individual. The use of clinically applied statistics, probability, and population-based data to inform medical decisions is known as clinical epidemiology, the newest of the epidemiology branches. Clinical epidemiology pertains to all clinical care. Its findings and applications are therefore not limited to infectious diseases or chronic diseases. Far from being inappropriate, the application of epidemiologic principles to patient care is fundamental to evidence-based practice and is supportive of robust clinical decisions. It is not subject to the ecologic fallacy; this fallacy is the belief that two variables associated in a population are necessarily associated within individuals in that population.

2. **The answer is E: evaluating etiologic factors in disease.** "BEINGS" is an acronym that stands for the factors that may play a role in disease development: B = biologic and behavioral factors; E = environmental factors; I = immunologic factors; N = nutritional factors; G = genetic factors; and S = services, social factors, and spiritual factors. Often, several of these factors interact to produce illness.

3. **The answer is C: behavioral, environmental, immunologic, nutritional, genetic, and social factors.** The "BEINGS" model explicitly includes the factors listed in the answer to question 2 (see above). Although iatrogenic factors (i.e., causes of illness produced by the physician or health care system) are implicitly included in the "BEINGS" model under the rubric "environment," iatrogenesis is not an explicitly distinguished category of disease etiology. The "BEINGS" model summarizes features of the host, agent, and envi-

ronment that may interact to produce disease. By identifying individual components that contribute to disease causation, the model is useful in suggesting opportunities for disease prevention.

4. **The answer is C: the host and the agent.** The minimum requirement for disease transmission to occur is the interaction of the agent and the host in an environment that enables them to come together. A vector of transmission may or may not be involved. Behavioral factors are intrinsic to the host, and genetic factors may be included under both host and agent.

5. **The answer is E: the iceberg phenomenon.** When a new disease (e.g., hantavirus pulmonary syndrome) emerges, the first cases that are reported tend to be the most severe cases. Continued investigation reveals that these cases are merely the "tip of the iceberg." Many more cases that are generally less severe are initially hidden from view, just as the bulk of an iceberg lies below the water and is not initially seen. Active surveillance is generally initiated only after the threat of a transmissible disease has been exposed, and case finding is an effort to detect occult disease in a clinical setting as part of a medical evaluation.

6. **The answer is E: rationing health care resources.** While the responsibilities of epidemiologists may include recommending cost-effective allocation of health care resources, the rationing of these resources is a political task and falls outside the purview of epidemiologists. Establishing modes of disease transmission and identifying means of preventing disease spread are integral aspects of epidemiology. Genetic epidemiologists participate in genetic counseling.

7. **The answer is D: the prevention of disease transmission to susceptible individuals through acquired immunity in others.** Herd immunity not only prevents the immunized individuals in a population from contracting a disease, but it also prevents them from spreading the disease to nonimmunized individuals in the population. In other words, herd immunity prevents disease transmission to susceptible individuals as a result of acquired immunity in others. The characteristics of a particular infection and a particular population determine the level of prevailing immunity required to limit the spread of a disease. For example, the presence of a highly infectious illness (e.g., measles) in a population with multiple exposures (e.g., college students) requires that nearly everyone be immunized to prevent transmission.

8. **The answer is B: the loss of the natural booster effect.** When an infectious disease is common, a large number of people become infected and develop immunity to the causative agent. When their immunity begins to wane and they come into contact with infected individuals, they are reexposed to the causative agent. This environmental reexposure "boosts" their immune system so that their protective immunity is maintained. The phenomenon is called the natural booster effect. One of the potential adverse effects associated with a widespread immunization program is the loss of the natural booster effect. This loss is correlated with the efficacy of the vaccine. If a vaccine is highly efficacious, it will markedly reduce the chances of exposure to the causative agent in the environment. If exposure does occur after the vaccine's effect in an individual has declined with time, the vaccinated individual will be at risk for infection. This is why booster vaccines are given at specified intervals. Other potential adverse effects associated with widespread immunization, such as allergic reactions and neurologic complications, are rare and idiosyncratic and are unlikely to be correlated with the efficacy of the vaccine. Widespread vaccination tends to delay exposure to the wild type pathogen and therefore tends to shift the disease to older age groups, rather than younger ones. Like antibiotics, vaccines are ineffective in some individuals. Unlike antibiotics, which act by killing or arresting the growth of pathogens, vaccines act by sensitizing the immune system to pathogens and do not promote the emergence of resistant strains.

9. **The answer is B: desertification in sub-Saharan Africa.** In Africa, the tsetse fly transmitted often-fatal illness to domestic cattle. Tsetse fly control was therefore thought to represent a significant advance. However, the uncontrolled growth of domestic cattle herds led to the overgrazing of arable land and the subsequent desertification in sub-Saharan Africa. This desertification contributes to mass malnutrition and starvation. As this example shows, the solutions to public health problems often harbor unanticipated consequences. Antigenic drift and shift in influenza virus strains do not result from any particular effort to control influenza but instead seem to derive from viral properties and environmental conditions, especially in China, where viruses from humans and ducks may mingle in pigs. The spread of *Legionella pneumophila* through air-conditioning systems did not result from an attempt to solve a public health problem, although it was facilitated by environmental modification. The transmission of hepatitis C virus via blood transfusions was due to an inability to detect the virus, not to any public health effort. The blood supply in the USA

is now reliably screened for hepatitis C. The reactivation of latent tuberculosis in individuals who become infected with the human immunodeficiency virus (HIV) is an example of synergism.

10. The answer is B: genetic susceptibility. Social support networks, immunization status, dietary intake, and smoking status are all factors that can be modified to prevent disease. The currently available technology permits the identification of genetic susceptibility to some diseases (e.g., colon cancer). However, since the ability to modify genetic risk is not nearly as great as the ability to recognize it, ethical concerns have been raised. Little good may come from informing people about a risk that they cannot readily modify, while harm, such as anxiety or increased difficulty and expense involved in obtaining medical insurance, might result.

References Cited

Berkman, L. F., and L. Breslow. Health and Ways of Living: The Alameda County Study. New York, Oxford University Press, 1983.

Berkman, L. F., and L. S. Syme. Social networks, host resistance, and mortality: a nine-year follow-up of Alameda County residents. American Journal of Epidemiology 109:186–204, 1979.

Bracken, M. B., et al. A randomized controlled trial of methylprednisolone or naloxone in the treatment of acute spinal cord injury. New England Journal of Medicine 322:1405–1411, 1990.

Burkitt, D. Lecture at Yale University School of Medicine, New Haven, Conn., April 28, 1989.

Centers for Disease Control and Prevention. Addressing Emerging Infectious Disease Threats. Atlanta, Centers for Disease Control and Prevention, 1994a.

Centers for Disease Control and Prevention. Births and Deaths: United States, 1995. Monthly Vital Statistics Report 45(supplement 2), 1996a.

Centers for Disease Control and Prevention. Progress toward global eradication of poliomyelitis, 1988–1993. Morbidity and Mortality Weekly Report 43:499–503, 1994b.

Centers for Disease Control and Prevention. Recommendations of the Advisory Committee on Immunization Practices: revised recommendations for routine poliomyelitis vaccination. Morbidity and Mortality Weekly Report 48:590, 1999a.

Centers for Disease Control and Prevention. Recommended childhood immunization schedule, United States. Morbidity and Mortality Weekly Report 48:12–16, 1999b.

Centers for Disease Control and Prevention. Update: diphtheria epidemic in the newly independent states of the former Soviet Union, January 1995–March 1996. Morbidity and Mortality Weekly Report 45:693–697, 1996b.

Connecticut Hospital Association. Impact of an aging population on utilization and bed needs of Connecticut hospitals. Connecticut Medicine 42:775–781, 1978.

Dawber, T. R., G. F. Meadors, and F. E. Moore, Jr. Epidemiologic approaches to heart disease: the Framingham Study. American Journal of Public Health 41:279–286, 1951.

Doll, R., and R. Peto. The Causes of Cancer. Oxford, Oxford University Press, 1981.

Ehrlich, P. R., and A. H. Ehrlich. The Population Explosion. New York, Simon and Schuster, 1990.

Evans, A. S. Subclinical epidemiology. American Journal of Epidemiology 125:545–555, 1987.

Feinstein, A. R. Clinical Epidemiology: The Architecture of Clinical Research. Philadelphia, W. B. Saunders Company, 1985.

Fletcher, R. H., S. W. Fletcher, and E. H. Wagner. Clinical Epidemiology: The Essentials, 3rd ed. Baltimore, Williams and Wilkins Company, 1996.

Francis, T., Jr., et al. An evaluation of the 1954 poliomyelitis vaccine trials. American Journal of Public Health, April supplement, 1955.

Frankl, V. E. Man's Search for Meaning: An Introduction to Logotherapy. New York, Washington Square Press, 1963.

Gibbons, A. Where are "new" diseases born? Science 261:680–681, 1993.

Gordon, T. Mortality experience among the Japanese in the United States, Hawaii, and Japan. Public Health Reports 72:543–553, 1957.

Greenland, S. Relation of probability of causation to relative risk and doubling dose: a methodologic error that has become a social problem. American Journal of Public Health 89:1166–1169, 1999.

Holland, W. W., and L. Karhausen, eds. Health Care and Epidemiology. Boston, G. K. Hall and Company, 1979.

Horwitz, R. I., D. V. Cicchetti, and S. M. Horwitz. A comparison of the Norris and Killip coronary prognostic indices. Journal of Chronic Disease 37:369–375, 1984.

Inlander, C., L. S. Levin, and E. Weiner. Medicine on Trial. New York, Prentice-Hall, 1988.

Institute of Medicine. Emerging Infections. Washington, D. C., National Academy Press, 1992.

Jekel, J. F. Communicable disease control and public policy in the 1970s: hot war, cold war, or peaceful coexistence? American Journal of Public Health 62:1578–1585, 1972.

Jekel, J. F. Role of acquired immunity to Treponema pallidum in the control of syphilis. Public Health Reports 83:627–632, 1968.

Jekel, J. F., G. S. Zatlin, and O. F. Gay. Corynebacterium diphtheriae survives in a partly immunized group. Public Health Reports 85:310, 1970.

Kellock, B. The Fiber Man: The Life Story of Dr. Denis Burkitt. Belleville, Mich., Lion Publishing Corporation, 1985.

Keys, A. The peripatetic nutritionist. Nutrition Today 13(4):19–24, 1966.

Keys, A. Summary: coronary heart disease in seven countries. Circulation 42(supplement 1):186–198, 1970.

Kilbourne, E. D., and W. G. Smillie. Human Ecology and Public Health, 4th ed. London, Macmillan Company, 1969.

Knox, E. G., ed. Epidemiology in Health Care Planning. Oxford, Oxford University Press, 1979.

Langmuir, A. D. The surveillance of communicable diseases of national importance. New England Journal of Medicine 268:182–192, 1963.

Larson, D. B., J. P. Sawyers, and M. E. McCullough, eds. Scientific Research on Spirituality and Health: A Consensus Report. Rockville, Md., National Institute for Healthcare Research, 1998.

Lasch, E. [Former health officer in the Gaza Strip.] Personal communication, 1979.

Last, J. M. What is "clinical epidemiology"? Journal of Public Health Policy 9:159–163, 1988.

Leape, L. L., et al. Adverse events and negligence in hospitalized patients. Iatrogenics 1:17–21, 1991.

Levine, S., and A. Lilienfeld, eds. Epidemiology and Health Policy. New York, Tavistock Publications, 1987.

Longini, I. M., Jr., et al. Statistical inference for infectious diseases. American Journal of Epidemiology 128:845–859, 1988.

Marks, J. S., T. J. Halpin, and W. A. Orenstein. Measles vaccine efficacy in children previously vaccinated at 12 months of age. Pediatrics 62:955–960, 1978.

Morris, J. N. The Uses of Epidemiology. Edinburgh, E. and S. Livingstone Ltd., 1967.

Ormerod, W. E. Ecological effect of control of African trypanosomiasis. Science 191:815–821, 1976.

Patton, C. L. [Professor of Epidemiology, Yale University School of Medicine, New Haven, Conn.] Personal communication, 1992.

Rappuoli, R., M. Perugini, and E. Falsen. Molecular epidemiology of the 1984–1986 outbreak of diphtheria in Sweden. New England Journal of Medicine 318:12–14, 1988.

Reed, D. The paradox of high risk of stroke in populations with low risk of coronary heart disease. American Journal of Epidemiology 131:579–588, 1990.

Sackett, D. L. Clinical epidemiology. American Journal of Epidemiology 89:125–128, 1969.

Sackett, D. L., et al. Clinical Epidemiology: A Basic Science for Clinical Medicine, 2nd ed. Boston, Little, Brown, and Company, 1991.

Scriver, C. R. Human genes: determinants of sick populations and sick patients. Canadian Journal of Public Health 79:222–224, 1988.

Shope, R. [Professor of Epidemiology, Yale University School of Medicine, New Haven, Conn.] Personal communication, 1992.

Spitzer, W. O., A. R. Feinstein, and D. L. Sackett. What is a health care trial? Journal of the American Medical Association 233:161–163, 1975.

US Surgeon General. Smoking and Health. Public Health Service publication No. 1103. Washington, D. C., US Government Printing Office, 1964.

Selected Readings

Feinstein, A. R. Clinical Epidemiology: The Architecture of Clinical Research. Philadelphia, W. B. Saunders Company, 1985. [Complex, research-oriented clinical epidemiology.]

Fletcher, R. H., S. W. Fletcher, and E. H. Wagner. Clinical Epidemiology: The Essentials, 3rd ed. Baltimore, Williams and Wilkins Company, 1996. [Simple, clinically oriented epidemiology.]

Gerstman, B. B. Epidemiology Kept Simple. New York, Wiley-Liss, 1998. [Good, but not as simple as the title suggests.]

Gordis, L. Epidemiology. Philadelphia, W. B. Saunders Company, 1996. [An excellent text.]

Hennekens, C. H., and J. E. Buring. Epidemiology in Medicine. Boston, Little, Brown, and Company, 1987. [Classical epidemiology.]

Institute of Medicine. Emerging Infections. Washington, D. C., National Academy Press, 1992. [Medical ecology.]

Kelsey, J. L., et al. Methods in Observational Epidemiology, 2nd ed. New York, Oxford University Press, 1996. [Classical epidemiology.]

Levine, S., and A. Lilienfeld, eds. Epidemiology and Health Policy. New York, Tavistock Publications, 1987. [Epidemiology and health services.]

Sackett, D. L., et al. Clinical Epidemiology: A Basic Science for Clinical Medicine, 2nd ed. Boston, Little, Brown, and Company, 1991. [Moderately complex, clinically oriented epidemiology.]

US Surgeon General. The Health Consequences of Smoking: Cardiovascular Disease. Public Health Service publication No. 84-50204. Washington, D. C., US Government Printing Office, 1984.

2 Epidemiologic Data Sources and Measurements

■ SOURCES OF HEALTH DATA

Epidemiologists rely on a variety of sources for obtaining data to analyze health-related rates and risks. Data for the rates used in epidemiologic studies can be discussed in terms of **denominator data,** which define the population at risk, and **numerator data,** which define the events or conditions of concern. Census statistics are often used in the denominator, and statistics gathered from a wide range of health and disease surveys and registries are used in the numerator.

International Census and Health Data

Most nations conduct **censuses** periodically (e.g., every 10 years) to obtain data on the number and characteristics of members of the population. They also use continuous registration (reporting) systems to collect data about the number and characteristics of births and deaths in the population. These systems, which are called **vital statistics registration systems,** use recent census data for the denominators of birth and death rates. Not all countries have effective disease reporting systems, and the accuracy of the census and vital statistics data varies from country to country. The collection of these data is a national responsibility, but most countries also report their data to the United Nations, which then publishes large compendia of national statistics, such as the *Demographic Yearbook* and *World Health Statistics Annual.* Today, the fastest way to obtain the statistics is to consult the World Wide Web. Access to recent statistics of various countries is crucial for making comparisons, for example, of infant mortality rates.

US Census and Health Data

In the USA, most of the birth and death data, as well as many other types of health-related statistics, come from public data systems. The collection of data frequently involves local, state, and national agencies. For example, data on births, deaths, causes of death, fetal deaths, marriages, and divorces are initially collected locally by the registrar of vital statistics for the municipality or county involved. Birth certificates are completed by a physician or other birth attendant, and death certificates are completed by a physician, medical examiner, or coroner. The local jurisdiction then sends the original birth and death certificates to the state government, which is responsible for maintaining the permanent records. The state governments (often the state health departments) prepare summaries of these data. The states then send copies of the birth and death certificates to the **National Center for Health Statistics (NCHS),** a federal agency that prepares national summaries.

US Census

In the USA, the census is undertaken by the federal government. A complete population census, effective the first day of April, is done every year ending in 0. Findings from the census taken in the year 2000 will begin to be published 1 or 2 years later. Population projections are used to estimate the size of the population between censuses and beyond the most recent census.

US Health Data Bases

In clinical epidemiology, health-related data usually come from examination of the patient, from clinical records, or from special questionnaires containing indexes that the investigator creates to answer specific research questions. In monitoring the health of large populations, however, as much use as possible is made of existing data bases, because this reduces the costs. The following are some of the most important ongoing US health data bases.

US Vital Statistics System. The federal government collates data on births, deaths, causes of death, fetal deaths, marriages, and divorces in the USA and its territories. These data are initially obtained by local and state representatives, as discussed above. Because analyses are, at best, only as good as the data on which they are based, great care is used to make the vital statistics system as accurate as possible. Nevertheless, there are many potential sources of error in these data, including unreported births and deaths, inaccurate death certificate diagnoses, and erroneous demographic and clinical data on the birth and death certificates. This is illustrated in the following discussion of the process followed to record the causes of death on death certificates in the USA.

When the numbers of deaths in the USA are categorized by cause of death and reported in government publications, the cause of death given is the **underlying cause of death,** not necessarily the **immediate cause of death.** If a person dies without medical attention or if foul play is suspected, a medical examiner or coroner decides the cause of death for that person. Otherwise, the attending physician is responsible for completing the information on the cause of death.

The cause-of-death portion of the death certificate is shown in Fig. 2–1. If a person dies of pneumonia following a cerebral hemorrhage, the physician probably would put "pneumonia" on line (a) and "cerebral hemorrhage" on line (b). The cerebral hemorrhage would then be considered the underlying cause of death. If, however, the physician decided that the person's coexistent hypertension caused the cerebral hemorrhage, then "hypertension" would be put on line (c), and that would now become the underlying cause of death. On the other hand, the physician might decide that the hypertension was too mild to cause the stroke and enter "hypertension" under "Other Significant Conditions," in which case the cerebral hemorrhage would be the underlying cause of death.

The complications of deciding and recording the underlying cause of death do not end here. There are also complex rules used by the people who make the final determination about which numbered codes will be used for each death and about how to proceed with the coding if what they see does not fit certain expectations. In hospitals, death certificates are often completed at night by sleepy interns who are not the patients' primary physicians. Now there is a provision for a second signature, allowing funeral directors to contact the attending physician for any changes in the cause of death.

The death certificate data concerning the underlying cause of death are sufficiently accurate for purposes of setting many national priorities, but there is

FIGURE 2–1   Facsimile of the cause-of-death portion of death certificates used in the USA. The form also requests information regarding autopsy, referral to a medical examiner or coroner, homicide investigation, and so forth.

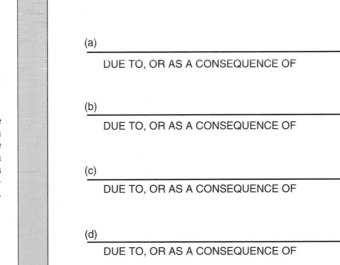

DEATH CERTIFICATE

PART I

IMMEDIATE CAUSE [Enter only one cause per line for (a), (b), (c), and (d).]

(a) _____   Interval between onset and death

DUE TO, OR AS A CONSEQUENCE OF

(b) _____   Interval between onset and death

DUE TO, OR AS A CONSEQUENCE OF

(c) _____   Interval between onset and death

DUE TO, OR AS A CONSEQUENCE OF

(d) _____   Interval between onset and death

DUE TO, OR AS A CONSEQUENCE OF

PART II

OTHER SIGNIFICANT CONDITIONS Conditions contributing to death but

not related to cause given in part I(a) _____

_____

serious doubt about whether they are good enough for most epidemiologic research. Studies in the USA have suggested that 80–85% of diagnoses either were probably correct or at least were reasonable, while serious questions remained about the other 15–20% of diagnoses on death certificates (Moriyama 1966, 1989).

National Notifiable Disease Surveillance System. Physicians, hospitals, clinics, and laboratories in the USA are required to report all cases of many types of infectious diseases to local and state health departments, who in turn report them to the Centers for Disease Control and Prevention (CDC), the federal agency in Atlanta, Georgia. Epidemiologic investigation of possible disease outbreaks is done, as needed, by representatives of the local, state, or federal public health agencies. Reporting requirements also apply to some noninfectious diseases, such as lead poisoning in children. Although there is considerable agreement among states regarding the diseases to be reported, some variation exists from state to state. Table 2–1 shows the infectious diseases that the CDC monitors and that must be reported in most states.

Only a fraction of the disease cases are actually reported, but this fraction tends to vary with the seriousness of the disease. Most of the extremely serious diseases, such as paralytic poliomyelitis, tend to be recognized and reported, but even here epidemiologists must be wary of the numbers reported. For example, one study indicated that only about 58% of the cases of acquired immunodeficiency syndrome (AIDS) in South Carolina were reported (Conway et al. 1989). Part of the problem may be underdiagnosis, and part may be hesitancy to report something that could bring social isolation if discovered by others. Underreporting also applies to other serious infectious diseases, including tuberculosis.

Underreporting is even more frequent for the common and less serious diseases, such as chickenpox. This does not mean that the statistics on chickenpox have no value. As long as the proportion of cases reported remains constant, the pattern revealed by the reporting is useful, because it may reflect actual trends in the occurrence and distribution of the disease.

Studies of the National Center for Health Statistics (NCHS). The NCHS carries out many important studies in the USA on topics such as the current levels of illness and disability, the practice of preventive health services, the population's use of preventive measures and medical care, and the ways in which sampling methods and instrument design for health surveys can be improved. In addition, the NCHS carries out surveys on a variety of topics. In the past, these have included hospital discharges, ambulatory medical care, and long-term care services (Jekel 1984). Newer surveys include information about family growth and use of preventive health measures. Among the surveys that are done on an ongoing basis are the following: (1) the **National Health Interview Survey (NHIS)** to determine yearly changes in acute and chronic illness and disability in the USA; (2) the **National Health and**

TABLE 2–1 Infectious Diseases That Are Reportable to the Centers for Disease Control and Prevention (CDC)*

Acquired immunodeficiency syndrome (AIDS)	Legionellosis
Anthrax	Lyme disease
Botulism	Malaria
Brucellosis	Measles (rubeola)
Chancroid	Meningococcal disease
Chlamydia trachomatis infection, genital	Mumps
Cholera	Pertussis
Coccidioidomycosis	Plague
Congenital rubella syndrome	Poliomyelitis, paralytic
Congenital syphilis	Psittacosis
Cryptosporidiosis	Rabies, animal
Diphtheria	Rabies, human
Encephalitis, California	Rocky Mountain spotted fever
Encephalitis, eastern equine	Rubella
Encephalitis, St. Louis	Salmonellosis
Encephalitis, western equine	Shigellosis
Escherichia coli O157:H7 infection	Streptococcal disease, invasive, group A
Gonorrhea	Streptococcal toxic shock syndrome
Haemophilus influenzae disease, invasive	*Streptococcus pneumoniae* infection, drug-resistant
Hansen's disease (leprosy)	Syphilis
Hantavirus pulmonary syndrome	Tetanus
Hemolytic-uremic syndrome, postdiarrheal	Toxic shock syndrome
Hepatitis A	Trichinosis
Hepatitis B	Tuberculosis
Hepatitis C/non-A, non-B	Typhoid fever
Human immunodeficiency virus infection, pediatric (i.e., in persons <13 years old)	Yellow fever

Source: Centers for Disease Control and Prevention. Summary of notifiable diseases, United States, 1997. Morbidity and Mortality Weekly Report 46(54):iv, 1997.
*Although varicella (chickenpox) is not included in this list, the Council of State and Territorial Epidemiologists recommends that cases of varicella also be reported to the CDC.

Nutrition Examination Surveys (NHANES), in which a large probability sample of the US population participates in health interviews and physical examinations; and (3) the **National Health Care Survey** to monitor the use of medical care in the USA. A detailed list of current surveys is provided at the back of NCHS reports. Tapes or compact discs containing data from most NCHS surveys can be purchased from the NCHS for a reasonable fee.

Behavioral Risk Factor Surveillance System (BRFSS). In this system, ongoing surveys of behavioral risk factors in the US population are carried out by state health departments in cooperation with the CDC. When the BRFSS was begun in 1981 by the CDC, only a few states participated. By 1990, however, 45 states and the District of Columbia, which together account for 90% of the US population, were participating. In the behavioral surveys, a random sample of the population is interviewed by telephone and questioned about a variety of behaviors that have an effect on health and well-being, including exercise, smoking, obesity, alcohol consumption, drinking and driving, and use of automobile seat belts and child restraints.

Disease Registries. In some states and regions of the USA, government agencies or authorities have established special registries to record information concerning specific diseases, such as cancer, tuberculosis, and birth defects. For example, the oldest population-based cancer registry in the USA is the **Connecticut Tumor Registry,** which is maintained by the Connecticut State Department of Health and Addiction Services. The name of every Connecticut resident in whom cancer has been diagnosed since 1935 has been reported to the registry, and data have been collected from patient records, including extensive clinical, pathologic, and risk factor data. The state has established an extensive surveillance program to ensure complete reporting of cancers.

The National Cancer Institute sponsors the surveillance, epidemiology, and end results (SEER) program and supports a network of cancer registries, including the Connecticut Tumor Registry and eight other regional, population-based cancer registries in the USA (Young et al. 1981). Investigators involved in the SEER program have studied trends in the incidence and treatment of cancer and have analyzed treatment results over time.

Cancer registries are valuable aids for determining the effectiveness of cancer screening programs, because the rate of subsequent cancer deaths can be determined both in those who are screened and in those who are not screened. The registries are also valuable for determining whether new practices are linked with cancer. For example, Jekel, Freeman, and Meigs (1978) used the Connecticut Tumor Registry to study whether the introduction of alum-adsorbed allergenic extracts used in "allergy shots" was associated with the subsequent occurrence of soft tissue sarcomas or other cancers at the injection sites.

Data from Third-Party Payers. Over the years, medical care insurance carriers and other third-party payers, such as Medicare and the Veterans Administration, have collected increasing amounts of clinical data for payment purposes. These data are sometimes used by clinical epidemiologists and health care researchers who are concerned with the patterns and cost-effectiveness of medical care.

■ EPIDEMIOLOGIC MEASUREMENTS

Clinical phenomena must be measured accurately in order to develop and test hypotheses. Because epidemiologists study phenomena in populations, they need measures that summarize what has happened in populations. The fundamental epidemiologic measure is the frequency with which an event of interest (e.g., disease, injury, or death) occurs in the population to be studied.

Frequency

The frequency of a disease, injury, or death can be measured in different ways, and it can be related to different denominators, depending on the purpose of the research and the availability of data. The concepts of incidence and prevalence are of fundamental importance to all of epidemiology.

Incidence (Incident Cases)

Incidence is the frequency (number) of new occurrences of disease, injury, or death—that is, the number of transitions from well to ill, from uninjured to injured, or from alive to dead—in the study population *during the time period being examined.* The term *incidence* is sometimes incorrectly used to mean incidence rate, so that to avoid confusion, it is sometimes better to use the term *incident cases* rather than incidence. Fig. 2–2 shows the annual number of incident cases of AIDS by year of report for the USA, beginning in 1981.

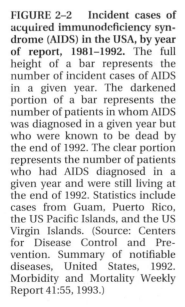

FIGURE 2–2 **Incident cases of acquired immunodeficiency syndrome (AIDS) in the USA, by year of report, 1981–1992.** The full height of a bar represents the number of incident cases of AIDS in a given year. The darkened portion of a bar represents the number of patients in whom AIDS was diagnosed in a given year but who were known to be dead by the end of 1992. The clear portion represents the number of patients who had AIDS diagnosed in a given year and were still living at the end of 1992. Statistics include cases from Guam, Puerto Rico, the US Pacific Islands, and the US Virgin Islands. (Source: Centers for Disease Control and Prevention. Summary of notifiable diseases, United States, 1992. Morbidity and Mortality Weekly Report 41:55, 1993.)

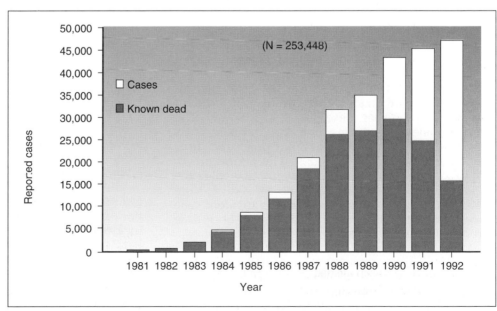

Prevalence (Prevalent Cases)

Prevalence (sometimes called point prevalence) is the number of persons in a defined population who have a specified disease or condition *at a point in time,* usually the time a survey is done. The term *prevalence* is sometimes incorrectly used to mean prevalence rate, so to avoid confusion, the somewhat awkward term *prevalent cases* usually is preferable to the term *prevalence.*

Difference Between Point Prevalence and Period Prevalence

In this text, when the term *prevalence* is used, **point prevalence** is meant (i.e., prevalence at a point in time). Some articles in the literature will discuss **period prevalence,** which refers to the number of persons who had the disease at any time during the specified time interval. Period prevalence is the sum of the point prevalence at the beginning of the interval plus the incidence during the interval. Because period prevalence is a mixed measure, composed of both point prevalence and incidence, it is not recommended for scientific work.

Illustration of Morbidity Concepts

The concepts of incidence (incident cases), point prevalence (prevalent cases), and period prevalence are illustrated in Fig. 2–3, based on a method devised by Dorn (1957). The figure provides data concerning eight persons who have a given disease in a defined population in which there is no emigration or immigration. Each person is assigned a case number (case no. 1 through case no. 8). A line begins when a person becomes ill and ends when that person either recovers or dies. The symbol t_1 is the beginning and t_2 is the end of the study period (i.e., a calendar year).

In case no. 1, the patient was ill when the year began and was still alive and ill when it ended. In case nos. 2, 6, and 8, the patients were ill when the year began but recovered or died during the year. In case nos. 3 and 5, the patients became ill during the year and were still alive and ill when the year ended. And in case nos. 4 and 7, the patients became ill during the year, and both of them either recovered or died during the year.

On the basis of this illustration, the following calculations can be made: There were four incident cases during the year (case nos. 3, 4, 5, and 7). The point prevalence at t_1 was four (the prevalent cases were nos. 1, 2, 6, and 8). The point prevalence at t_2 was three (case nos. 1, 3, and 5). The period prevalence is equal to the point prevalence at t_1 plus the incidence between t_1 and t_2, or here 4 + 4 = 8. Note that whereas a case could only be an incident case once, a case could be a prevalent case at both time intervals (as with case no. 1 in this figure).

The Relationship Between Incidence and Prevalence

Fig. 2–2 provides some data from the CDC concerning the incidence and prevalence of AIDS in the USA

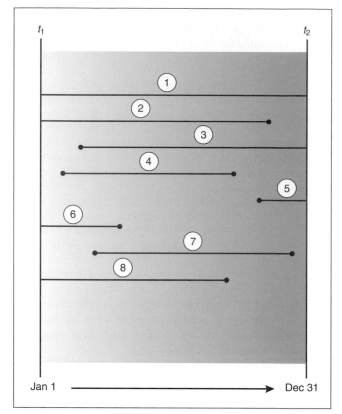

FIGURE 2–3 Illustration of several concepts in morbidity. Lines indicate when eight persons became ill (start of a line) and when they recovered or died (end of a line) between the beginning of a year (t_1) and the end of the same year (t_2). Each person is assigned a case number, which is circled in this figure.

during the first 12 years it was known (i.e., 1981–1992). In this figure, the full height of each year's bar shows the total number of new AIDS cases reported to the CDC for the year. The darkened part of each bar shows the number of patients in whom AIDS was diagnosed in that year but who were known to be dead by December 31, 1992. Therefore, the clear space in each bar represents the number of patients in whom AIDS was diagnosed in that year and who were, presumably, still alive on December 31, 1992; these are the prevalent cases as of that date. Of the patients whose AIDS had been diagnosed between 1990 and 1992 and who had suffered from the disease for a relatively short time, a fairly high proportion were still alive at the cutoff date, partly because of the recency of their infection and partly because of improved treatment. However, almost all of those in whom AIDS was diagnosed in the first 6 years of the epidemic had died.

The total number of cases of an epidemic disease reported by a given time is the **cumulative incidence.** For example, according to the CDC, the cumulative incidence of AIDS cases in the USA through December 31, 1991, was 206,392, and the number known to have died was 133,232 (see Centers for Disease Control and Prevention 1992). Therefore, at the close of 1991, there were 73,160 prevalent cases of AIDS (206,392 minus 133,232). When these patients with

AIDS died in subsequent years, they would be removed from the prevalent cases category.

On January 1, 1993, the CDC made a major change in the criteria for defining AIDS. A backlog of patients whose disease manifestations met the new criteria were included in the counts for the first time in 1993, and this resulted in a sudden, huge spike in the number of reported AIDS cases (Fig. 2–4). Because of this change in criteria and reporting, the more recent AIDS data are not as satisfactory as the older data for illustrating the relationship between incidence and prevalence. Nevertheless, the more recent AIDS data provide a vivid illustration of how important a consistent definition of a disease is to epidemiologists.

Prevalence is the result of many factors: the periodic (annual) number of new cases, the immigration and emigration of persons with the disease, and the **duration of the disease,** which is defined as the time from the onset of the disease until death or healing occurs.

The following is an approximate general formula for prevalence that seldom can be used for detailed scientific estimation but that is conceptually important for understanding and predicting the **burden of disease** on a society:

$$\text{Prevalence} = \text{Incidence} \times \text{(Average) Duration}$$

This simplified formula works well only if the incidence of the disease and its duration in individual persons are stable for an extended time. The implication of the formula, however, is that the prevalence of a disease, such as AIDS, could increase as a result of either (1) an increase in the yearly numbers of new cases or (2) an increase in the length of time that symptomatic patients survive before dying (or recovering, if that becomes possible). Note that AIDS is a clinical syndrome, and the discussion here is about the prevalence of AIDS rather than the prevalence of type 1 human immunodeficiency virus (HIV-1) infec-

tion. The incidence of AIDS in the USA has started to decline, but the duration of life of persons with AIDS is increasing with the use of antiviral agents and other new methods of treatment and prophylaxis. New treatments have increased the length of survival proportionately more than the decline in incidence, so there continues to be an increase in the prevalent cases of AIDS in the USA. In fact, it appears from Fig. 2–2 that this has already occurred. The rapid increase in AIDS prevalence has led to an increase in the **burden of care** of patients, both in terms of demand on the medical care system and in terms of the dollar cost to society.

Risk

Definition of Risk

Epidemiologically, risk is defined as the proportion of persons who are unaffected at the beginning of a study period but who undergo the risk event during the study period. The **risk event** may be death, disease, or injury, and the persons at risk for the event are called a **cohort,** which is a clearly defined group of persons studied over time. If an investigator follows all of the persons in a cohort over a several-year period, the denominator for the risk of an event will not change (unless persons are lost to follow-up). For example, in a cohort, the denominator for a 5-year risk of death or disease is the same as for the 1-year risk, because in both situations the denominator is the number of persons entered at the beginning of the study.

Care is needed when applying actual risk estimates (which are derived from populations) to an individual patient. If death, disease, or injury occurs to an individual patient, for that person the risk is 100%. The best way to approach patients' questions regarding, say, the risk related to surgery is probably not to give them a number (e.g., "Your chances of survival

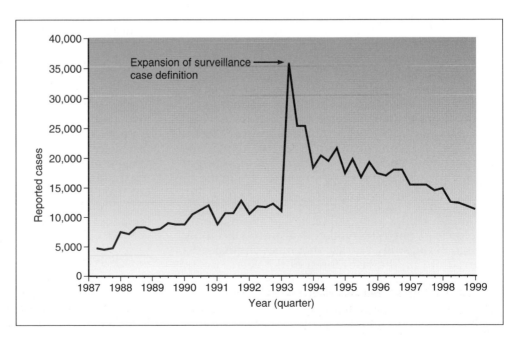

FIGURE 2–4 Incident cases of acquired immunodeficiency syndrome (AIDS) in the USA, by quarter of report, 1987–1998. Statistics include cases from Guam, Puerto Rico, the US Pacific Islands, and US Virgin Islands. Note that on January 1, 1993, the Centers for Disease Control and Prevention changed the criteria for defining AIDS. The expansion of the surveillance case definition resulted in a huge spike in the number of reported cases. (Source: Centers for Disease Control and Prevention. Summary of notifiable diseases, United States, 1998. Morbidity and Mortality Weekly Report 47(53):20, 1999.)

are 99%"). They will worry about whether they will be the 1% or the 99%. Rather, it is better to put the risk of surgery in the context of the many other risks they may take frequently, such as those related to long automobile trips. The real issue is whether they are willing to take any risk in order to achieve the potential benefit of surgery. In other cases as well, it is generally better to interpret the risks of a negative outcome in terms other than numbers.

Limitations of the Concept of Risk

Often it is difficult to be sure of the correct denominator for a measure of risk. Who is truly at risk? This may be especially difficult to know for infectious diseases, unless the number of people in the population who lack protective antibodies is known. Ideally, in a risk or rate, only the **susceptible population**—i.e., those without antibody protection—would be counted in the denominator, but antibody levels are usually unknown. Therefore, as a compromise, the denominator will usually consist of either the total population of an area or those in an age group who probably lack antibodies.

The risk of death from an infectious disease, although appearing simple, is actually quite complex. This is because it is the product of many different proportions, as can be seen in Fig. 2–5. There are numerous **subsets of the population** to consider. Those who **die** of an infectious disease are a subset of those who are **ill,** who in turn are a subset of those who are **infected,** who are a subset of those who are **exposed** to the infection, who are a subset of those who are **susceptible,** who are a subset of the **total population.**

The proportion of the clinically ill persons who die is called the **case fatality ratio.** The higher the case fatality ratio, the more **virulent** the infection is. The proportion of infected persons who are clinically ill is often called the **pathogenicity** of the organism. The proportion of exposed persons who become infected is sometimes called the **infectiousness** of the organism, but this is also influenced by the conditions of exposure. A full understanding of the epidemiology of an infectious disease would require knowledge of all the ratios shown in Fig. 2–5.

The concept of risk has other limitations. For example, assume that three different populations of the same size have the same overall risk of death (say, 10%) in the same year (e.g., from January 1 to December 31, 2000). Yet the deaths in the three populations may occur in very different patterns. Suppose that population A suffered a bad influenza epidemic in January (the beginning of the study year) and that most of those who died during the year died in the first month of the year. Suppose that the influenza epidemic did not hit population B until December (the end of the study year) so that most of the deaths occurred during the last month of the year. Finally, suppose that population C was not hit with the epidemic and that its deaths occurred (as usual) somewhat evenly throughout the year. The 1-year risk (10%) would be the same in all three populations, but

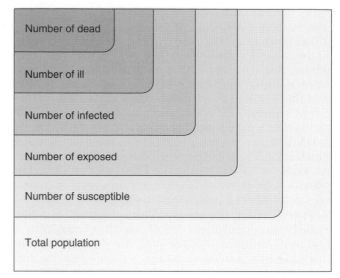

FIGURE 2–5 **Illustration of why the death rate from an infectious disease is the product of many proportions.** The formula may be thought of as follows:

$$\frac{\text{Number of dead}}{\text{Total population}} = \frac{\text{Number of dead}}{\text{Number of ill}} \times \frac{\text{Number of ill}}{\text{Number of infected}} \times \frac{\text{Number of infected}}{\text{Number of exposed}} \times \frac{\text{Number of exposed}}{\text{Number of susceptible}} \times \frac{\text{Number of susceptible}}{\text{Total population}}$$

If each of the five fractions to the right of the equal sign were 0.5, the persons who were dead would represent 50% of those who were ill; 25% of those who were infected; 12.5% of those who were exposed; 6.25% of those who were susceptible; and 3.125% of the total population.

the **force of mortality** would not be the same. The force of mortality would be strongest in population A, weakest in population B, and intermediate in population C. Because the measure of risk cannot distinguish between these three patterns, a more precise measure—namely, the rate—is usually used instead. After a brief description of rates, the discussion will return to this example.

Rates

Definition of Rate

A rate is the frequency (number) of events that occur in a defined time period, divided by the average population at risk. Because the midperiod population usually can be considered a good estimate of the average number of people at risk for the outcome during the time period, the midperiod population is often used as the denominator of a rate. The formal structure of a rate is described in the following equation:

$$\text{Rate} = \frac{\text{Numerator}}{\text{Denominator}} \times \text{Constant multiplier}$$

Risks and rates usually have values less than 1, and decimals are awkward to think about and discuss. It is particularly awkward to talk about fractions of a death (e.g., "one one-thousandth of a death per year"). Therefore, rates are usually multiplied by a **constant multiplier,** either 100 (to make a percentage) or else 1000, 10,000, or 100,000, in order to make the numerator larger than 1 and therefore easier to discuss (e.g., "one death per thousand people per year"). When a constant multiplier is used, both the numerator and the denominator are multiplied by the same number, so the value of the ratio is not changed.

An example in which a constant multiplier is customarily used is in the calculation of the crude death rate. In 1995, this rate in the USA was about 0.0088 per year, but it is easier to multiply this by 1000 and express it as 8.8 deaths per 1000 individuals in the population per year. The general form for calculating the rate in this case is as follows:

$$
\text{Crude death rate} = \frac{\substack{\text{Number of deaths} \\ \text{(defined place and time period)}}}{\substack{\text{Midperiod population} \\ \text{(same place and time period)}}} \times 1000
$$

Rates can be thought of somewhat in the same way as velocity. It is possible to talk about **average rates** or average velocity for a period of time. The average velocity is obtained by dividing the miles traveled (e.g., 55) by the time required (e.g., 1 hour), in which case the car averaged 55 miles per hour. This does not mean that the car was traveling at exactly 55 miles per hour for every instant during that hour. In a similar manner, the average rate of an event (e.g., death) is equal to the total number of events for a defined time (e.g., 1 year) divided by the population exposed to that event (e.g., 12 deaths per 1000 persons per year).

A rate, like a velocity, also can be thought of as describing reality at an instant in time, when it is sometimes called an **instantaneous death rate** or **hazard rate.** However, because death is a discrete event rather than a continuous function, instantaneous rates cannot be measured at an instant of time; they can only be estimated. The rates discussed in this book will be average rates unless otherwise mentioned.

The Relationship Between Risk and Rate

In an example presented in an earlier section (see Limitations of the Concept of Risk), populations A, B, and C each had a 10% overall risk of death in the same year, but their patterns of death differed greatly. Fig. 2–6 shows the three different patterns and illustrates how in this example the concept of rate is superior to the concept of risk in demonstrating the differences in the **force of mortality.**

Because most of the deaths in population A occurred before July 1, the midyear population of the cohort would be the smallest of the three, and the resulting death rate would be the highest (because the denominator is the smallest and the numerator is the same size for all three populations). In contrast, because most of the deaths in population B occurred at the end of the year, the midyear population of the cohort would be the largest of the three and the death rate would be the lowest. The number of deaths before July 1, and therefore the death rate for population C, would be intermediate between those of A and B. Thus, although the 1-year risk did not demonstrate differences in the force of mortality, rates were able to do so by reflecting more accurately the mortality experience of the three populations. This quantitative result agrees with the graph and with intuition, because assuming that the quality of life was reason-

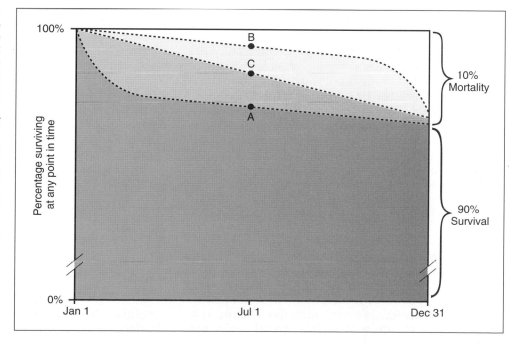

FIGURE 2–6   Illustration of circumstances under which the concept of rate is superior to the concept of risk. Assume that populations A, B, and C are three different populations of the same size; that 10% of each population died in a given year; and that most of the deaths in population A occurred early in the year, most of the deaths in population B occurred late in the year, and the deaths in population C were fairly evenly distributed throughout the year. In all three populations, the risk of death would be the same— that is, 10%—even though the patterns of death differed greatly. However, the rate of death, which is calculated using the midyear population as the denominator, would be the highest in population A, the lowest in population B, and intermediate in population C, reflecting the relative magnitude of the force of mortality in the three populations.

ably good, most people would prefer to be in population B. More days of life are lived by those in population B during the year, owing to the lower force of mortality.

A rate is often used to estimate risk. A rate is a good approximation of risk if (1) the event in the numerator occurs only once per individual during the study interval; (2) the proportion of the population affected by the event is small, e.g., less than 5%; and (3) the time interval is relatively short. If the time interval is long or the percentage who die is large, the rate will be noticeably larger than the risk. If the event in the numerator occurs more than once during the study period—as can occur, for example, with ear infections or with asthmatic attacks—a related statistic called **incidence density** (see below) should be used instead of a rate.

Note that although the denominator for the 5-year risk is the same as for the 1-year risk in a cohort study, that would not be true for a rate. The denominator for a rate is constantly changing. It will decrease as some people die and others emigrate from the population. The denominator will increase as some immigrate and others are born into the population. In most real populations, all four of these changes are occurring at the same time. The rate reflects these changes by using the midperiod population as an estimate of the average population at risk.

The Quantitative Relationship Between Risk and Rate

As noted above, a rate is a good approximation of the risk if the time interval in a study is short. If the time interval is long, the rate will be higher than the risk, because the denominator is reduced by the number of risk events (e.g., deaths) that occur up to the midperiod. When the rate and risk are small, the differences between the rate and the corresponding risk are also small. These principles can be demonstrated by examining the relationship between the **mortality rate** and the **mortality risk** in population C in Fig. 2–6. Population C had an even mortality risk throughout the year and a total yearly mortality risk of 10%. By the middle of the year, death had occurred in 5%. Therefore, the mortality rate would be $0.10/(1-0.05) = 0.10/0.95 = 0.1053 = 105.3$ per 1000 persons per year. In this example, the denominator is 0.95 because 95% of population C was still living at midyear to form the denominator. The yearly rate is somewhat higher than the yearly risk, because the **average population** at risk is smaller than the **initial population** at risk.

What would be the **cumulative mortality risk** for population C at the end of 2 years, assuming a **constant yearly mortality rate** of 0.1053? It could not be calculated by simply multiplying 2 years times 10%, because the number still living and subject to the force of mortality by the beginning of the second year would be smaller (i.e., it would be 90% of the original population). Likewise, the cumulative risk of death over 10 years could not be calculated by simply multiplying 10 years times 10%; this would mean that

100% of population C would be dead, and intuition suggests that at least some of the population would live more than 10 years. In fact, if the mortality rate remains constant, the cumulative risks at 2 years, 5 years, 10 years, and 15 years would be 19%, 41%, 65%, and 79%, respectively. As described in Box 2–1, there is a straightforward way to determine the cumulative risk for any number of years, and the calculations can easily be done on most hand-held calculators.

Criteria for the Valid Use of the Term *Rate*

To be valid, a rate must meet certain criteria with respect to the correspondence between numerator and denominator. First, all the events counted in the numerator must have happened to persons in the denominator. Second, all of the persons counted in the denominator must have been at risk for the events in the numerator.

Before comparisons of rates can be made, the following must be true: The numerators for all groups being compared must be defined or diagnosed in the same way; the constant multipliers being used must be the same; and the time intervals must be the same. These criteria may seem obvious, but it is easy to overlook real problems related to comparisons over time and comparisons between populations.

Numerators may not be easy to compare if the quality of medical diagnosis differs over time. For example, in the late 1800s there was no diagnostic category called myocardial infarction, but many persons were dying of acute indigestion. By 1930, the situation was reversed: almost nobody died of acute indigestion, but many died of myocardial infarction. It might be tempting to say that the acute indigestion of the late 1800s was really myocardial infarction, but there is no certainty that this is true.

Another example of problems in studying causes of disease over time relates to changes in the classification systems commonly used. In 1948, there was a major revision in the *International Classification of Diseases* (ICD), the international coding manual for classifying diagnoses. This revision of the ICD was followed by sudden, major changes in the reported numbers and rates of many diseases.

Not only is it difficult to track changes in causes of death over time, but it is difficult to make fair comparisons of cause-specific rates of disease between populations, especially between countries. Different nations have different degrees of access to medical care and different levels in the quality of medical care available to most of those who are dying, as well as different styles of diagnosis. It is not easy to determine how much of any apparent difference in reported causes of death is real and how much of the difference is due to variation in diagnostic styles and quality of care around the time of death.

Definitions of Specific Types of Rates

Earlier in the chapter, the concepts of incidence (incident cases) and prevalence (prevalent cases) were

---

BOX 2–1   Calculation of the Cumulative Mortality Risk in a Population with a Constant Yearly Mortality Rate

Part 1   Beginning data (see Fig. 2–6)

Population C in Fig. 2–6 had an even mortality risk throughout the year and a total yearly **mortality risk** of 10%. By the middle of the year, death had occurred in 5%. Therefore, the **mortality rate** would be $0.10/(1 - 0.05) = 0.10/0.95 = 0.1053 = 105.3$ per 1000 persons per year. If this rate of 0.1053 remained constant, what would be the cumulative mortality risk at the end of 2 years, 5 years, 10 years, and 15 years?

Part 2   Formula

$R(t) = 1 - e^{-\mu t}$,

where R = risk; t = number of years of interest; e = the base for natural logarithms; and μ = the mortality rate

---

Part 3   Calculation of the cumulative 2-year risk

$R(2) = 1 - e^{-(0.1053)(2)}$

$\quad = 1 - e^{-0.2106}$

    Exponentiate the second term (i.e., take the anti–natural logarithm, or anti-ln, of the second term)

$\quad = 1 - 0.8101$

$\quad = 0.1899$

$\quad = $ **19% risk** of death in 2 years

Part 4   Calculation of cumulative risks on a hand-held calculator

To calculate cumulative risks on a hand-held calculator, the calculator must have a key for natural logarithms (i.e., a key for logarithms to the base $e = 2.7183$). The logarithm key will be labeled "ln" (not "log," which is a key for logarithms to the base 10).

Begin by entering the number of years (t), which in the above example is 2. Multiply the number by the mortality rate (μ), which is 0.1053. The product will be 0.2106. Hit the "+/–" button to change the sign to negative. Then hit the "INV" (inverse) button and the "ln" (natural log) button. The result at this point will be 0.810098. Hit the "M in" (memory) button to put this result in memory. Clear the register. Then enter 1 minus "MR" (memory recall) and hit the "=" button. The result should be 0.189902. Rounded off, this is the same 2-year risk shown above (19%).

Calculations for 5-year, 10-year, and 15-year risks can be made in the same way, yielding the following results:

Number of Years	Cumulative Risk of Death
1	0.100 (10%)
2	0.190 (19%)
5	0.409 (41%)
10	0.651 (65%)
15	0.794 (79%)

As these results demonstrate, the cumulative risk cannot be calculated or accurately estimated by merely multiplying the number of the years by the 1-year risk. If it could, then at 10 years, the risk would be 100%, rather than 65%. It is worth emphasizing, however, that the results shown here are based on a constant mortality rate. Because in reality the mortality rate increases with time (particularly for an older population), the longer-term calculations are not as useful as the shorter-term calculations. The techniques described here are most useful for calculating a population's cumulative risks for intervals of up to 5 years.

---

discussed. Now that the concept of a rate has also been reviewed, it is appropriate to define different types of rates.

Incidence Rate. The incidence rate is calculated as the number of incident cases over a defined study period, divided by the population at risk at the midpoint of that study period. An incidence rate is usually expressed per 1000, per 10,000, or per 100,000

population. Fig. 2–7 shows the incidence rate of AIDS per 100,000 adult population in the USA, by age and gender groups, in 1992.

Prevalence Rate. The so-called prevalence rate is actually a proportion and not a rate. However, the term is in common use and will be used here to indicate the proportion (usually the percentage) of persons with a defined disease or condition at the time they

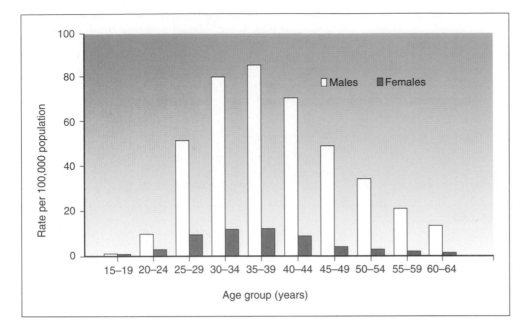

FIGURE 2–7 Incidence rate of acquired immunodeficiency syndrome (AIDS) per 100,000 adult population in the USA, by age and gender groups, 1992. Denominators for computing rates are based on 1992 population estimates from the US Bureau of Census. (Source: Centers for Disease Control and Prevention. Summary of notifiable diseases, United States, 1992. Morbidity and Mortality Weekly Report 41: 55, 1993.)

are studied. For example, the 1990 Behavioral Risk Factor Survey reported that the prevalence rate of overweight status in adults—that is, the proportion of adults who were overweight by self-report over the telephone—ranged from 16.3% in Colorado to 27.4% in the District of Columbia, with the median state estimate being 22.7% (see Centers for Disease Control 1991).

Prevalence rates can be applied to risk factors as well as to diseases or other conditions. For example, in the USA in 1997, the prevalence rate of current smoking among high school students varied from 16.4% in Utah to 47.0% in Kentucky and Michigan (see Centers for Disease Control and Prevention 1998).

Incidence Density. Incidence density refers to the frequency (density) of new events per **person-time** (such as per person-months or person-years). For example, suppose that three patients were followed after tonsillectomy and adenoidectomy for recurrent ear infections. If one patient were followed for 13 months, one for 20 months, and one for 17 months and if 5 ear infections occurred in these three patients during this time, the incidence density would be 5 infections per 50 person-months of follow-up, or 10 infections per 100 person-months.

Incidence density is especially useful when the event of interest (such as colds, otitis media, or myocardial infarction) can occur in a person more than once during the period of study. For example, in a study of the impact of breast feeding versus formula feeding on the rate of infections in normal newborns in Copenhagen, Denmark, Rubin et al. (1990) recorded monthly data on the occurrence of infectious diseases and then compared them by month for the first year. Because infections often occurred more than once per month in infants and certainly more than once over the study year, the authors used inci-

dence density to measure the frequency of the target events. For methods of statistical comparison of two incidence densities, see Chapter 11.

Special Issues Concerning the Use of Rates

Rates or risks are usually used to make one of three types of comparison.

The first type is a comparison of an observed rate (or risk) with a target rate (or risk). For example, the USA set national health goals for the year 2000, including expected rates of various types of death, such as the infant mortality rate (see US Department of Health and Human Services 1990). When the final year 2000 statistics are published, the observed infant mortality rates for the nation and for subgroups will be compared with the target objectives set by the government.

The second type is the comparison of two different populations at the same time. This is probably the most common type. One example involves comparing the rates of death or diseases in two different countries, states, or ethnic groups for the same year. Another example involves comparing the results in treatment and control groups participating in randomized clinical trials (e.g., in trials of thrombolytic therapy versus a placebo following a myocardial infarction). A major research concern is to make sure that the two populations are similar and are measured in exactly the same way, especially when comparing different countries, where diagnostic styles and quality may differ.

The third type consists of a comparison of the same population at two different time periods. This is used for studying time trends. Because there are also trends over time in the composition of a population (such as the increasing proportion of older people in the US population), adjustments must be made for such changes before concluding that there are real differences over time in the disease rates. Another concern is the change over time (usually improvement) in diagnostic capabilities.

Use of Crude Rates Versus Specific Rates

There are three broad categories of rates: crude, specific, and standardized. Rates that apply to an entire population, without reference to any characteristics of the individuals in it, are **crude rates.** When a population is divided into more homogeneous subgroups based on a particular characteristic of interest (e.g., age, sex, race, risk factors, or comorbidity) and rates are calculated within these groups, the rates are called **specific rates** (age-specific rates, sex-specific rates, etc.). Standardized rates are discussed in the next section.

Crude rates are valid rates, but they are often misleading, which may be why they were named "crude." Here is a quick challenge: Try to guess which of the following three countries—Sweden, Colombia, and the USA—has the highest and which has the lowest crude death rate. Those who guessed that Colombia has the highest and Sweden the lowest crude death rate have the sequence exactly reversed. The actual crude death rates and the corresponding life expectancy at birth are found in Table 2–2. At the end of the 1980s, Colombia had the lowest crude death rate and Sweden the highest, even though Colombia had the highest age-specific mortality rates and the shortest life expectancy, and Sweden had just the reverse.

This seeming anomaly occurs primarily because the crude death rates do not take age into account. For a population with a young age distribution, such as Colombia, the birth rate is likely to be relatively high and the crude death rate is likely to be relatively low, even though the age-specific death rates (ASDRs) for each age group may be fairly high. In contrast, for an older population, such as Sweden, a low crude birth rate and a high crude death rate would be expected. This is because age has such a profound influence upon the force of mortality that an old population, even if it is relatively healthy, will inevitably have a high overall death rate, and vice versa. The huge impact that age has on death rates can be seen in Fig. 2–8, which shows data on ASDRs in the USA in 1991. As a general principle, investigators should never make comparisons of the risk of

death or disease between populations without controlling for age. Sometimes other characteristics must be controlled for as well.

Why not avoid crude rates altogether and just use specific rates? There are many circumstances when it is not possible to use specific rates: (1) if the frequency of death or disease (i.e., the numerator) is not known for the subgroups of the population; (2) if the size of the subgroups (i.e., the denominator) is not known; or (3) if the numbers of persons at risk are too small to provide stable estimates of the specific rates. However, if the number of persons at risk is large in each of the subgroups of interest, specific rates provide the most information, and they should be sought whenever possible.

Although the biasing effect of age can be controlled in several ways, the simplest (and usually the best) method is to calculate the ASDRs, so that the rates can be compared in similar age groups. The formula is as follows:

$$\text{Age-specific death rate} = \frac{\begin{array}{c}\text{Number of deaths to people}\\\text{in a particular age group}\\\text{(defined place and time period)}\end{array}}{\begin{array}{c}\text{Midperiod population}\\\text{(same age group, place, and}\\\text{time period)}\end{array}} \times 1000$$

Crude death rates are the result of the ASDRs in each of the age groups, weighted by the relative size of each age group. The underlying formula for any summary rate is as follows:

$$\text{Summary rate} = \Sigma w_i r_i$$

where w_i represents the individual weights (proportions) of each age-specific group, and r_i represents the rates for the corresponding age group.

This formula is useful for understanding why crude rates can be misleading. In studies involving two populations, if the relative weights for the high and low age-specific death rates differ, the ASDRs will be mixed differently, and no fair comparison can be made. This general principle applies not only to demography and population epidemiology, where investigators are interested in comparing the rates of large groups, but also to clinical epidemiology, where investigators may wish to compare the risks or rates of two patient groups that have different proportions of severely ill, moderately ill, and mildly ill patients (Chan et al. 1988).

A similar problem occurs when investigators interested in measuring the quality of care try to compare death rates in various hospitals. To make fair comparisons among hospitals, investigators must make some adjustment for differences in the types and severity of illness in the people being treated. Otherwise, the hospitals that care for the sickest people would be at an unfair disadvantage in such a comparison.

TABLE 2–2   Crude Death Rate and Life Expectancy for Three Countries

Country (Year)	Crude Death Rate	Life Expectancy at Birth
Colombia (1985–1989)	7.4 per 1000	63.4 years
USA (1988)	8.8 per 1000	71.3 years
Sweden (1989)	10.8 per 1000	74.2 years

Source: United Nations. Demographic Yearbook. New York, United Nations, 1990.

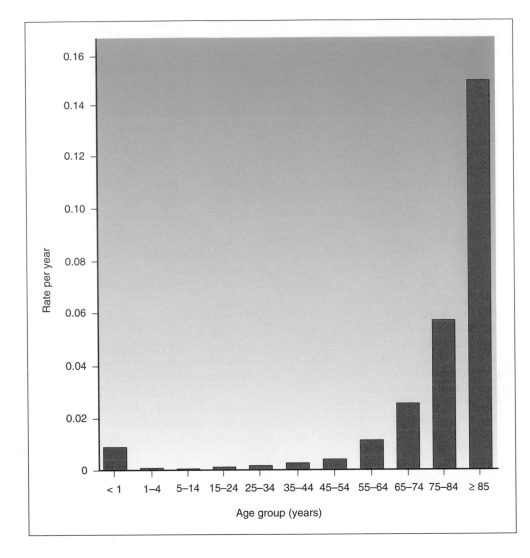

FIGURE 2–8   Age-specific death rates (ASDRs) for deaths from all causes in the USA, 1991. The figure illustrates the profound impact that age has on death rates. (Source of data: National Center for Health Statistics. Health, United States, 1993. Washington, D. C., US Government Printing Office, 1994.)

Standardization of Death Rates

Standardized rates, which are also called **adjusted rates,** are crude rates that have been modified (adjusted) to control for the effects of age or other characteristics and thereby allow for valid comparisons of rates. Standardization is usually applied to death rates but may be used to adjust any type of rate.

In the case of death rates, the comparison of many age-specific death rates (ASDRs) can become unwieldy. Therefore, to obtain a summary death rate that is free from age bias, investigators can age-standardize (age-adjust) the crude death rates by a direct or an indirect method.

Direct Standardization. Direct standardization is the most commonly used method to remove the biasing effect of the differing age structure of different populations. In the direct method of standardization, the ASDRs of the two (or more) populations to be compared are applied to a single standard population. This is done by multiplying each ASDR from a population to be compared by the number of persons in the corresponding age group in the **standard population.** Because the age structure of the standard population is the same for all of the death rates applied to

it, the distorting effect of having different age distributions in the different real populations is eliminated. Overall death rates can then be compared without age bias.

The standard population may be any real (or any realistic) population, and it is often a larger population of which the populations to be compared are a part. Thus, the death rates of two cities in a state can be compared using the state's population as the standard population. Likewise, the death rates of states may be standardized using the population of the USA.

The direct method shows the total number of deaths that *would have occurred* in the standard population *if* the ASDRs of the individual populations had occurred. The total expected number of deaths from each of the comparison populations is then divided by the standard population to give a standardized "crude" death rate, which may be compared with any other death rate standardized using the same standard population. The direct method may be applied to compare incidence rates of disease or injury as well as deaths.

Standardized rates are *fictitious.* They are only

"what if" rates, but they do allow investigators to make fairer comparisons of death rates than would be possible with crude rates. A simplified example is shown in Box 2–2, where two populations, A and B, are divided into "young," "middle-aged," and "older" people, and the ASDR for each age group in population B is twice as high as that for each age group in population A. Population A has a higher overall crude death rate (4.51%) than population B (3.08%), despite the fact that the ASDRs in B are twice those in A. After the death rates are standardized (here the standard population is simply the sum of the two individual populations), the adjusted death rate for population B correctly reflects the fact that its ASDRs are twice as high as those of population A.

Indirect Standardization. Indirect standardization is used if ASDRs are not available in the population whose crude death rate is to be adjusted. It is also used if the population to be standardized is small, which makes the ASDRs statistically unstable. The indirect method uses **standard rates** and applies them to the known age (or other stratum) groups in the population to be standardized.

Suppose, for example, that an investigator wanted to see if the death rates for male workers in a particular company were similar to or greater than the death rates for males in the US population. To start, the investigator would need the observed crude death rate and the ASDRs for US males for a similar year.

These would serve as the **standard death rates.** Next, the investigator would determine the number of workers in each of the same age categories that were used in the US male population. Then the investigator would determine the observed total deaths for 1 year for all of the male workers in the company.

The first step in calculation is to multiply the standard death rates from each age group in the standard population times the number of workers in the corresponding age groups in the company. This gives the number of deaths that would be expected in each age group of workers if they had the death rates of the standard population. The expected numbers of worker deaths for the various age groups are then added to obtain the total number of deaths that would be expected if the ASDRs in the company were the same as those in the standard population. Next, the number of *observed* total deaths among the workers is divided by the *expected* total deaths among the workers to obtain a ratio called the **standardized mortality ratio** (SMR). Finally, the SMR is multiplied by 100 to get rid of fractions, so that the expected mortality rate among the standard population equals 100. If the employees in this example had an SMR of 140, it means that their mortality was 40% greater than was expected on the basis of the ASDRs of the standard population. (For further discussion, see Chan et al. 1988.) An illustration of indirect standardization is presented in Box 2–3.

BOX 2–2 Direct Standardization of Crude Death Rates of Two Populations, Using the Averaged Weights as the Standard Population (Fictitious Data)

Part 1 Calculation of the crude death rates

Age Group	Population A				Population B			
	Population Size	Age Specific Death Rate		Expected Number of Deaths	Population Size	Age-Specific Death Rate		Expected Number of Deaths
Young	1,000	× 0.001	=	1	4,000	× 0.002	=	8
Middle-aged	5,000	× 0.010	=	50	5,000	× 0.020	=	100
Older	4,000	× 0.100	=	400	1,000	× 0.200	=	200
Total	10,000			451	10,000			308
Crude death rate	451/10,000 = 4.51%				308/10,000 = 3.08%			

Part 2 Direct standardization of the above crude death rates, with the two populations combined to form the standard weights

Age Group	Population A				Population B			
	Population Size	Age-Specific Death Rate		Expected Number of Deaths	Population Size	Age-Specific Death Rate		Expected Number of Deaths
Young	5,000	× 0.001	=	5	5,000	× 0.002	=	10
Middle-aged	10,000	× 0.010	=	100	10,000	× 0.020	=	200
Older	5,000	× 0.100	=	500	5,000	× 0.200	=	1,000
Total	20,000			605	20,000			1,210
Standardized death rate	605/20,000 = 3.03%				1,210/20,000 = 6.05%			

BOX 2–3 Indirect Standardization of the Crude Death Rate for Males in a Company, Using the Age-Specific Death Rates for Males in a Standard Population (Fictitious Data)

Part 1 Beginning data

Age Group	Males in the Standard Population				Males in the Company			
	Proportion of Standard Population	Age-Specific Death Rate		Observed Death Rate	Number of Workers	Age-Specific Death Rate		Observed Number of Deaths
Young	0.40	× 0.0001	=	0.00004	2,000	× ?	=	?
Middle-aged	0.30	× 0.0010	=	0.00030	3,000	× ?	=	?
Older	0.30	× 0.0100	=	0.00300	5,000	× ?	=	?
Total	1.00			0.00334	10,000			48
Observed death rate		0.00334, or 334/100,000				48/10,000, or 480/100,000		

Part 2 Calculation of the expected death rate, using indirect standardization of the above rates and applying the age-specific death rates from the standard population to the numbers of workers in the company

Age Group	Males in the Standard Population				Males in the Company			
	Proportion of Standard Population	Age-Specific Death Rate		Observed Death Rate	Number of Workers	Standard Death Rate		Expected Number of Deaths
Young	0.40	× 0.0001	=	0.00004	2,000	× 0.0001	=	0.2
Middle-aged	0.30	× 0.0010	=	0.00030	3,000	× 0.0010	=	3.0
Older	0.30	× 0.0100	=	0.00300	5,000	× 0.0100	=	50.0
Total	1.00			0.00334	10,000			53.2
Expected death rate						53.2/10,000, or 532/100,000		

Part 3 Calculation of the standardized mortality ratio (SMR)

$$SMR = \frac{\text{Observed death rate for males in the company}}{\text{Expected death rate for males in the company}} \times 100$$

$$= \frac{0.00480}{0.00532} \times 100$$

$$= (0.90)(100) = 90$$

= Males in the company actually had a death rate that was only 90% of the value that would be expected, based on the death rates in the standard population

Cause-Specific Rates

Whereas creating age-specific or sex-specific death rates makes the denominators of the rates homogeneous, cause-specific death rates make the numerators homogeneous according to diagnosis. Comparing cause-specific death rates over time or between countries is often risky, because there may be differences in diagnostic styles or efficiency between countries. For example, in countries with inadequate medical care, 10–20% of deaths may be signed out as "symptoms, signs, and ill-defined conditions." This also happens among people who die without adequate medical care in the USA (Becker et al. 1990).

Cause-specific death rates have the following general form:

Cause-specific death rate =

$$\frac{\begin{array}{c}\text{Number of deaths due to} \\ \text{a particular cause} \\ \text{(defined place and} \\ \text{time period)}\end{array}}{\begin{array}{c}\text{Midperiod population} \\ \text{(same place and time period)}\end{array}} \times 1000$$

Table 2–3 provides data on the leading causes of death in the USA for 1950 and 1994, as reported by the National Center for Health Statistics (NCHS) based on the underlying cause of death indicated on death certificates. These data are rarely accurate enough for epidemiologic studies of causal factors (Burnand and Feinstein 1992), but they are useful for understanding how important the different disease groups are relative to each other. They are also useful for studying trends in causes of death over time. For example, it appears that the rates for deaths caused by diseases of the heart and deaths caused by cerebrovascular disease have been dropping steadily for approximately two decades, whereas the rate for deaths caused by malignant neoplasms has remained approximately constant and the rate for deaths caused by AIDS has been rising rapidly.

Commonly Used Rates That Reflect Maternal and Infant Health

Many of the rates commonly used in public health, especially the infant mortality rate, reflect the health of mothers and infants. The definitions used for terms relating to the reproductive process are especially important to have clearly in mind.

Definitions of Terms

The official international definition of a **live birth** is the delivery of a product of conception that shows any sign of life after complete removal from the mother. A **sign of life** may consist of a breath or a cry, any spontaneous movement, a pulse or a heartbeat, or pulsation of the umbilical cord.

Fetal deaths are categorized as early, intermediate, or late fetal deaths. An **early fetal death,** which is better known as a **miscarriage,** occurs when a dead fetus

is delivered within the first 20 weeks of gestation. According to international agreements, an **intermediate fetal death** is one in which a dead fetus is delivered between 20 and 28 weeks of gestation. A fetus born dead at 28 weeks of gestation or greater is a **late fetal death,** better known as a **stillbirth.** Because it is easier just to fill out a fetal death certificate than both a birth certificate and a death certificate for an infant, if there is any doubt about the presence of signs of life, an infant barely alive at birth might be treated as a late fetal death. It is not known how often this happens, nor is it known whether any fetuses delivered by induced abortion have any sign of life after birth.

An **infant death** is the death of a live-born child before that child's first birthday.

Definitions of Specific Types of Rates

Crude Birth Rate. The crude birth rate is the number of live births divided by the midperiod population:

Crude birth rate =
$$\frac{\text{Number of live births}}{\text{(defined place and time period)}} \times 1000$$
Midperiod population (same place and time period)

Crude Death Rate and Age-Specific Death Rate. These are discussed earlier in this chapter (see Use of Crude Rates Versus Specific Rates, above).

Infant Mortality Rate. Because the health of infants is unusually sensitive to maternal health practices (especially maternal use of tobacco, alcohol, and illegal drugs), environmental and nutritional factors, and the quality of health services, the infant mortality rate (IMR) is often used as an overall index of the health status of a nation. The IMR has the added advantages of being available for most countries and of being age-specific. Moreover, both the numerator and the denominator of the IMR are obtained from the same kind of data collection system (vital statistics reporting), so that in areas where infant deaths are reported, births are also likely to be reported, and in areas where reporting is poor, this should affect both births and deaths. The formula for the IMR is as follows:

Infant mortality rate =
$$\frac{\text{Number of deaths to infants under 1 year of age (defined place and time period)}}{\text{Number of live births (same place and time period)}} \times 1000$$

Most infant deaths occur in the first month (in fact, in the first week) of life and are due to prematurity and the resulting immaturity, which often lead to respiratory failure. Some infant deaths in the first month are due to congenital anomalies.

A subtle point, which is seldom of concern in large populations, is that for any given year—for example, 2000—there is not an exact correspondence between the numerator and denominator of the IMR. This is

TABLE 2–3 **Age-Adjusted Death Rates for Selected Causes of Death in the USA, 1950 and 1994**

Cause of Death	Age-Adjusted Death Rate per 100,000 per Year	
	1950	1994
Diseases of the heart	307.2	140.4
Malignant neoplasms	125.3	131.5
Unintentional injuries	57.5	30.3
Cerebrovascular disease	88.6	26.5
Chronic obstructive pulmonary disease	4.4	21.0
Acquired immunodeficiency syndrome (AIDS)	—	15.4
Influenza and pneumonia	26.2	13.0
Diabetes	14.3	12.9
Suicide	11.0	11.2
Homicide	5.4	10.3
Chronic liver disease and cirrhosis	8.5	7.9
Other causes	192.1	87.0
All causes	840.5	507.4

Sources: (1) National Center for Health Statistics. Health, United States, 1993. Washington, D. C., US Government Printing Office, 1994. (2) National Center for Health Statistics. Advance report of final mortality statistics, 1994. Monthly Vital Statistics Report 45(3), Supplement, 1996.

because some of the infants born in 2000 will not die until 2001, and some of the infants dying in 2000 were born in 1999. Although this does not ordinarily influence the rate of a large population, it could do so in a small population. For studies of small populations, taking the average of 3 or 5 years is better. For detailed epidemiologic studies of causation, it is necessary to link each infant death with the corresponding birth.

Neonatal and Postneonatal Mortality Rates. Epidemiologists distinguish between neonatal and postneonatal mortality. Neonatal deaths are those occurring in infants under 28 days of age, whereas postneonatal deaths are those occurring in infants from the 28th day of life to the first birthday. The formulas for the rates are as follows:

Neonatal mortality rate =

$$\frac{\substack{\text{Number of deaths to infants} \\ \text{under 28 days of age} \\ \text{(defined place and time period)}}}{\substack{\text{Number of live births} \\ \text{(same place and time period)}}} \times 1000$$

Postneonatal mortality rate =

$$\frac{\substack{\text{Number of deaths to infants} \\ \text{between 28 and 365 days of age} \\ \text{(defined place and time period)}}}{\substack{\text{Number of} \\ \text{live births} \\ \text{(same place and} \\ \text{time period)}} - \substack{\text{Number of} \\ \text{neonatal deaths} \\ \text{(same place and} \\ \text{time period)}}} \times 1000$$

The formula for the neonatal mortality rate is fairly obvious, because it is so close to that for the infant mortality rate. For the postneonatal mortality rate, however, investigators must keep in mind the criteria for a valid rate, especially the criterion that all those in the denominator must be at risk for the numerator. Infants born alive are not at risk for dying in the postneonatal period if they die during the neonatal period. Therefore, the correct denominator for the postneonatal mortality rate is the number of live births *minus* the number of neonatal deaths. When the number of neonatal deaths is small, however, as is true in the USA (with fewer than 6 per 1000 live births), there is little difference between the two formulas, and the following approximate formula is perfectly adequate for almost all purposes:

$$\substack{\text{Approximate} \\ \text{postneonatal} \\ \text{mortality rate}} = \substack{\text{Infant} \\ \text{mortality} \\ \text{rate}} - \substack{\text{Neonatal} \\ \text{mortality} \\ \text{rate}}$$

As a rough general rule, the neonatal mortality rate provides a better reflection of the quality of medical services and of maternal prenatal behavior (smoking, alcohol, drugs, etc.), whereas the postneonatal mortality rate offers a better reflection of the quality of the home environment.

Perinatal Mortality Rate and Ratio. The use of the infant mortality rate has its limitations, not only because the probable causes of death change rapidly as the time from birth progresses but also because the number of infants born alive is influenced by the effectiveness of prenatal and perinatal care. It is conceivable that an improvement in care could actually increase the infant mortality rate; this would occur, for example, if the improvement keeps very sick fetuses alive long enough to be born, so that they die after being born and are counted as infant deaths rather than as stillbirths. In order to avoid this problem, the **perinatal mortality rate** was developed. This rate is defined slightly differently from country to country. In the USA, it is defined as follows:

Perinatal mortality rate =

$$\frac{\substack{\text{Number of} \\ \text{stillbirths} \\ \text{(defined place} \\ \text{and time period)}} + \substack{\text{Number of deaths} \\ \text{to infants under} \\ \text{7 days of age} \\ \text{(same place} \\ \text{and time period)}}}{\substack{\text{Number of} \\ \text{stillbirths} \\ \text{(same place} \\ \text{and time period)}} + \substack{\text{Number of} \\ \text{live births} \\ \text{(same place} \\ \text{and time period)}}} \times 1000$$

Perinatal means "around the time of birth." In the formula shown here, stillbirths are included in the numerator to capture the deaths around the time of birth. The stillbirths are included in the denominator because of the criteria for a valid rate and, more specifically, because all of those fetuses who reach the 28th week of gestation are at risk for being late fetal deaths, and their number is equal to those who die before birth (the stillbirths) plus those who are born alive (the live births).

An approximation of the perinatal mortality rate is the **perinatal mortality ratio,** in which the denominator does not include the stillbirths. In another variation, the numerator uses neonatal deaths instead of deaths under 7 days of life (hebdomadal deaths). The primary use of the perinatal mortality rate is to evaluate progress in prenatal and perinatal care of pregnant women and their infants.

Maternal Mortality Rate. Although pregnancy is generally considered a "normal" biologic process, there is no question that it puts considerable strain on the pregnant woman and places her at risk for a number of hazards that she would not usually face otherwise, such as hemorrhage, infection, and toxemia of pregnancy. Pregnancy complicates the course of other conditions, such as heart disease, diabetes, and tuberculosis. Therefore, a useful measure of the progress of a nation in providing adequate nutrition and medical care for pregnant women is the maternal mortality rate (MMR), calculated as follows:

Maternal mortality rate =

$$\frac{\substack{\text{Number of pregnancy-related deaths} \\ \text{(defined place and time period)}}}{\substack{\text{Number of live births} \\ \text{(same place and time period)}}} \times 100{,}000$$

Note that the equation is based on the number of **pregnancy-related (puerperal) deaths.** The death of a pregnant woman or of a woman who was recently delivered is not pregnancy-related in the case of an automobile injury, homicide, and so forth, but care must be taken here. For example, was a suicide pregnancy-related, or was a cancer made worse by the pregnancy?

Technically, the denominator of the equation should be the number of pregnancies rather than live births, but this number is not easy to obtain in any country, and therefore the number of live births is used instead. The constant multiplier used is usually 100,000, because in recent decades the MMR in many countries has dropped below 1 per 10,000 live births. For example, the MMR for the USA in 1994 was 8.3 per 100,000 live births, although the rates were lower for whites (6.2) than for all other races combined (16.2) (see National Center for Health Statistics 1996).

■ SUMMARY

Many of the data for epidemiologic studies are collected routinely by various levels of government and are made available to local, state, federal, and international groups. The USA and most other countries undertake a complete population census on a periodic basis. The census in the USA, for example,

---

BOX 2–4 Definitions of Basic Epidemiologic Concepts and Measurements

Incidence (incident cases): The frequency (number) of new occurrences of disease, injury, or death—that is, the number of transitions from well to ill, from uninjured to injured, or from alive to dead—in the study population during the time period being examined.

Point prevalence (prevalent cases): The number of persons in a defined population who had a specified disease or condition at a particular point in time, usually the time a survey was done.

Period prevalence: The number of persons who had a specified disease at any time during a specified time interval. Period prevalence is the sum of the point prevalence at the beginning of the interval plus the incidence during the interval. Because period prevalence combines incidence and prevalence, it must be used with extreme care.

Incidence density: The frequency (density) of new events per **person-time** (such as person-months or person-years). Incidence density is especially useful when the event of interest (such as colds, otitis media, or myocardial infarction) can occur in a person more than once during the period of study.

Cohort: A clearly defined group of persons who are studied over a period of time to determine the incidence of death, disease, or injury.

Risk: The proportion of persons who are unaffected at the beginning of a study period but who undergo the **risk event** (death, disease, or injury) during the study period.

Rate: The frequency (number) of new events that occur in a defined time period, divided by the average population at risk. Often, the midperiod population is used as the average number of persons at risk (see Incidence rate, below). Because a rate is almost always less than 1.0 (unless everybody dies or has the risk event), a **constant multiplier** is used to increase both the numerator and the denominator to make the rate easier to think about and discuss.

Incidence rate: A rate calculated as the number of incident cases (see above) over a defined study period, divided by the population at risk at the midpoint of that study period. Rates of the occurrence of births, deaths, and new diseases are all forms of an incidence rate.

Prevalence rate: The proportion (usually the percentage) of a population that has a defined disease or condition at a particular point in time. Although usually called a rate, it is actually a proportion.

Crude rates: Rates that apply to an entire population, without reference to any characteristics of the individuals in it. Crude rates are generally not useful for comparisons, because populations may differ greatly in composition, particularly with respect to age.

Specific rates: Rates that are calculated after a population has been categorized into groups with a particular characteristic. Examples include age-specific rates and sex-specific rates. Specific rates are generally needed for valid comparisons.

Standardized (adjusted) rates: Crude rates that have been modified (adjusted) to control for the effects of age or other characteristics and thereby allow for valid comparisons of rates.

Direct standardization: The preferred method of standardization if the specific rates come from large populations and the needed data are available. The direct method of standardizing death rates, for example, applies the age distribution of some population—the **standard population**—to the actual age-specific death rates of the different populations to be compared. This removes the bias that would occur if an old population was compared to a young population.

Indirect standardization: The method of standardization used either when the populations to be compared are small (so that age-specific death rates are unstable) or when age-specific death rates are not available from one or more populations but data concerning the age distribution and the crude death rate are available. Here **standard death rates** (from the standard population) are applied to the corresponding age groups in the different population or populations to be studied. The result is an "expected" (standardized crude) death rate for each population under study. These "expected" values are those which would have been expected if the standard death rates had been true for the populations under study. Then the standardized mortality ratio is calculated.

Standardized mortality ratio (SMR): The **observed crude death rate** divided by the **expected crude death rate.** The SMR is generally multiplied by 100, with the standard population having a value of 100. If the SMR is greater than 100, the **force of mortality** is higher in the study population than in the standard population. If the SMR is less than 100, the force of mortality is lower in the study population than in the standard population.

BOX 2–5   Equations for the Most Commonly Used Rates from Population Data

(1) Crude birth rate

$$= \frac{\text{Number of live births (defined place and time period)}}{\text{Midperiod population (same place and time period)}} \times 1000$$

(2) Crude death rate

$$= \frac{\text{Number of deaths (defined place and time period)}}{\text{Midperiod population (same place and time period)}} \times 1000$$

(3) Age-specific death rate

$$= \frac{\text{Number of deaths to people in a particular age group (defined place and time period)}}{\text{Midperiod population (same age group, place, and time period)}} \times 1000$$

(4) Cause-specific death rate

$$= \frac{\text{Number of deaths due to a particular cause (defined place and time period)}}{\text{Midperiod population (same place and time period)}} \times 1000$$

(5) Infant mortality rate

$$= \frac{\text{Number of deaths to infants under 1 year of age (defined place and time period)}}{\text{Number of live births (same place and time period)}} \times 1000$$

(6) Neonatal mortality rate

$$= \frac{\text{Number of deaths to infants under 28 days of age (defined place and time period)}}{\text{Number of live births (same place and time period)}} \times 1000$$

(7) Postneonatal mortality rate

$$= \frac{\text{Number of deaths to infants between 28 and 365 days of age (defined place and time period)}}{\text{Number of live births (same place and time period)} - \text{Number of neonatal deaths (same place and time period)}} \times 1000$$

(8) Approximate postneonatal mortality rate

$$= \text{Infant mortality rate} - \text{Neonatal mortality rate}$$

(9) Perinatal mortality rate*

$$= \frac{\text{Number of stillbirths (defined place and time period)} + \text{Number of deaths to infants under 7 days of age (same place and time period)}}{\text{Number of stillbirths (same place and time period)} + \text{Number of live births (same place and time period)}} \times 1000$$

(10) Maternal mortality rate

$$= \frac{\text{Number of pregnancy-related deaths (defined place and time period)}}{\text{Number of live births (same place and time period)}} \times 100,000$$

*Several similar formulas are in use around the world.

is taken every 10 years, on April 1 of every year ending in 0.

Community-wide epidemiologic measurement depends on accurate determination and reporting of (1) numerator data, especially events such as births, deaths, becoming ill (incident cases), and recovery from illness; and (2) denominator data, especially the census. Prevalence data are determined by surveys. These types of data then are used to create community rates and ratios for planning and evaluating health progress. The collection of such health data is the responsibility of individual countries. Most countries report their data to the United Nations, which then publishes large compendia such as the *Demographic Yearbook* and the *World Health Statistics Annual.* The data can also be found on the World Wide Web.

In large-scale population studies, as much use as possible is made of existing data bases. Some of the most important ongoing health data bases in the USA are the US Vital Statistics System, the National Notifiable Disease Surveillance System, the studies of the National Center for Health Statistics (NCHS), and disease registries, such as the Connecticut Tumor Registry.

In contrast to the types of data above, the data in clinical epidemiologic studies usually come from examination of patients; laboratory, x-ray, and special studies; clinical records; special questionnaires; or summaries of these data in large insurance carrier data bases.

Box 2–4 offers definitions of the basic epidemiologic concepts and measurements discussed in this chapter, while Box 2–5 lists the equations for the most commonly used population rates.

To be valid, a rate must meet certain criteria with respect to the denominator and numerator. First, all of the people counted in the denominator must have been at risk for the events counted in the numerator. Second, all of the events counted in the numerator must have happened to people included in the denominator. Moreover, before comparisons of rates can be made, the following must be true: the numerators for all groups being compared must be defined or diagnosed in the same way; the constant multipliers being used must be the same; and the time intervals being studied must be the same.

■ QUESTIONS

Directions (Items 1–4). Each of the numbered items or incomplete statements in this section is followed by answers or by completions of the statement. Select the ONE lettered answer or completion that is BEST in each case. Correct answers and explanations are given at the end of the chapter.

1. A study involves tracking a condition that can recur in individuals over time. Which of the following measures would allow the authors of the study to make full use of their collected data?
   (A)   Attributable risk
   (B)   Incidence density
   (C)   Period prevalence
   (D)   Point prevalence
   (E)   Proportional hazards

Items 2–4

During a given year, 12 cases of disease X are detected in a population of 70,000 college students. Many more students have mild symptoms of the disease, such as persistent daydreams about selling coconuts on a Caribbean beach.

2. Of the detected cases, 7 result in death. The ratio of 7/12 therefore represents
   (A)   the case fatality ratio
   (B)   the crude death rate
   (C)   the pathogenicity
   (D)   the standardized mortality ratio
   (E)   1 – prevalence

3. To report the incidence rate of disease X, it would be necessary to know
   (A)   nothing more than the data provided
   (B)   the age distribution of the population
   (C)   the case fatality ratio
   (D)   the duration of the clinical illness
   (E)   the midyear population at risk

4. To report the prevalence of disease X, it would be necessary to know
   (A)   the cure rate
   (B)   the duration of illness
   (C)   the number of cases at a given time
   (D)   the number of losses to follow-up
   (E)   the rate at which new cases developed

Directions (Items 5–15). The set of matching questions in this section consists of a list of lettered options followed by several numbered items. For each numbered item, select the ONE lettered option that is most closely associated with it. To avoid spending too much time on matching sets with large numbers of options, it is generally advisable to begin each set by reading the list of options. Then, for each item in the set, try to generate the correct answer and locate it in the option list, rather than evaluating each option individually. Each lettered option may be selected once, more than once, or not at all.

Items 5–15

(A) Age-specific death rate
(B) Case fatality ratio
(C) Cause-specific death rate
(D) Crude birth rate
(E) Direct standardization of death rate
(F) Incidence rate
(G) Indirect standardization of death rate
(H) Infant mortality rate
(I) Prevalence rate
(J) Standardized mortality ratio
(K) Standardized rate

For each of the following descriptions, select the corresponding rate or measure.

5. This is calculated after the two populations to be compared are "given" the same age distribution, which is then applied to the observed age-specific death rates of each population.

6. This is the number of new cases over a defined study period, divided by the midpoint population at risk.

7. This is used if age-specific death rates are not available in the population whose crude death rate is to be adjusted.

8. This is not a true rate; it is actually a proportion.

9. This is the observed total deaths in a population, divided by the expected deaths in that population, multiplied by 100.

10. This is useful for studying trends in the causes of death over time.

11. This is often used as an overall index of the health status of a nation.

12. This is a fictitious rate.

13. This is the proportion of individuals with a given condition who die of the condition.

14. This is the number of live births, divided by the midperiod population.

15. This provides the death rate within a defined age range.

■ **ANSWERS AND EXPLANATIONS**

1. **The answer is B: incidence density.** Incidence density is reported in terms of the frequency (density) of a condition per person-time (such as person-months or person-years). It is a composite measure of the number of individuals observed and the period of observation contributed by each. For example, 10 individuals observed for 1 year each would represent 10 person-years of observation, as would 1 individual observed for 10 years. Incidence density allows all data to be captured and reported, even when some individuals are lost to follow-up before the end of the observation period. This measure is particularly useful when an event can recur in an individual during the observation period. Period prevalence and point prevalence fail to capture recurrent events over time, because they describe events during a given period (period prevalence) or at a given point in time (point prevalence). Propor-

tional hazards is a statistical method used to characterize the effects of multiple variables on the risk of a binary outcome, such as survival. Attributable risk expresses the extent to which a single factor is responsible for a particular outcome in a population.

2. **The answer is A: the case fatality ratio.** The case fatality ratio for a particular condition is the number of deaths caused by the condition, divided by the total number of identified cases of the condition in a specified population. In this instance, the case fatality ratio is 7/12; or expressed as a percentage, it is 58.3%. The crude death rate is the number of deaths caused by the condition, divided by the midperiod population. Pathogenicity is indicated by the proportion of infected persons with clinical illness. The standardized mortality ratio is the number of observed deaths in a population subgroup, divided by the expected deaths based on a reference population. The term (1 – prevalence) is not meaningful.

3. **The answer is E: the midyear population at risk.** The incidence rate is the number of new cases in a specified population, during a specified period of time, divided by the midperiod population at risk. In the information provided, it does not say whether 70,000 represents the population at the midpoint or at the beginning of the observation period, nor does it say whether the entire population is at risk for disease X. Sometimes, incidence rates are based on the total population, even though not everyone is at risk, because there is no convenient way to distinguish the susceptible from the immune. An example would be incidence rates of hepatitis B in the USA; only the unimmunized would truly be at risk, but the rate might be reported with the total population in the denominator.

4. **The answer is C: the number of cases at a given time.** By definition, the prevalence of a condition is the number of cases in a specified population at a particular time. If this information is known, nothing else is required to report the prevalence. However, the prevalence is influenced by the duration of illness, the cure or recovery rate, and the cause-specific death rate, as well as by immigration and emigration. These are factors that influence the number of cases in the study population at any particular time.

5. **The answer is E: direct standardization of death rate.** In direct standardization, the age-specific death rates (ASDRs) are available for the populations to be compared. The age distribution of a hypothetical "standard" population (often consisting of the sum of the populations under comparison) is derived. The ASDRs from each of the populations are applied to the hypothetical age

distribution, and these summary rates may be compared because they are free of age bias. As is indicated in the text, crude death rates may be low in developing countries because the population is relatively young. Age standardization is required to demonstrate that in particular age groups, mortality rates tend to be higher in developing countries than in industrialized countries.

6. **The answer is F: incidence rate.** Incidence, or incident cases, is merely the number of new cases. To generate a rate, the number of new cases over a specified period of time is divided by the population at risk at the midpoint of the study period (recall the differences between risks and rates) and then multiplied by a constant, such as 1000 or 10,000, to facilitate expression.

7. **The answer is G: indirect standardization of death rate.** When the age-specific death rates are not known for the populations to be compared, direct standardization of rates is not feasible. Indirect standardization applies the rates from a reference population (e.g., the USA) to the study populations. The reference rates are applied to the age distribution of the study populations, and the number of deaths expected in each group is calculated by assigning the reference population mortality rates to the study population. The actual death rates in the study groups are then compared with the expected rates.

8. **The answer is I: prevalence rate.** As defined in the text, the prevalence rate is not a true rate. It is actually just the proportion, or percentage, of persons in a specified population with a defined condition at the time of study.

9. **The answer is J: standardized mortality ratio.** The standardized mortality ratio is often derived from indirect standardization methods. The observed number of deaths in a population subgroup (e.g., an age group) is divided by the expected number of deaths in that subgroup, based on the reference population. This figure is usually multiplied by 100 to generate a percentage (the percentage of the reference mortality rate experienced by the study group).

10. **The answer is C: cause-specific death rate.** For rates to be compared, the denominators (or populations) must be comparable. In order to compare events that are similar, the numerators must be derived in the same way. Cause-specific rates provide homogeneous numerator data based on diagnosis. Death rates may be similar in two populations, but the deaths may be due to different conditions, with differing implications for public health management. Cause-specific rates would be useful in attempting to define appropriate allocation of public health resources.

11. **The answer is H: infant mortality rate.** The infant mortality rate is influenced by various aspects of maternal and fetal care, including nutrition, access to prenatal medical care, maternal substance abuse, the home environment, and social support networks. The rate is often used as an overall index of the health status of a nation. If infants are able to thrive, the overall health of a nation is thought to be adequate, whereas if infants are failing and the resulting infant mortality rate is high, improvements in basic health care are generally needed.

12. **The answer is K: standardized rate.** Standardized rates are derived from a hypothetical age distribution that does not truly exist in the populations being compared. These rates permit valid comparisons but are, in fact, fictitious.

13. **The answer is B: case fatality ratio.** Although the case fatality ratio is commonly used to describe the deaths attributable to specific infectious diseases, it can also be used to describe the deaths attributable to any condition. The measure requires that both the number of affected individuals and the number of deaths attributable to the condition be known.

14. **The answer is D: crude birth rate.** The crude birth rate, by convention, is calculated as the number of live births, divided by the midperiod population. This is an unusual rate, because not everyone in the denominator can truly be said to be "at risk" for the numerator event (i.e., only women of childbearing age are at risk for bearing children).

15. **The answer is A: age-specific death rate.** Age is one of the strongest predictors of mortality. Therefore, death rates that do not reflect the experience of particular age groups are difficult to interpret. Age-specific death rates use the population within a particular age range as the denominator and use deaths within that group as the numerator.

References Cited

Becker, T. M., et al. Symptoms, signs, and ill-defined conditions: a leading cause of death among minorities. American Journal of Epidemiology 131:664–668, 1990.

Burnand, B., and A. R. Feinstein. The role of diagnostic inconsistency in changing rates of occurrence for coronary heart disease. Journal of Clinical Epidemiology 45:929–940, 1992.

Centers for Disease Control. Behavioral risk factor surveillance, 1986–1990. Morbidity and Mortality Weekly Report 40(SS-4):1–47, 1991.

Centers for Disease Control and Prevention. The second 100,000 cases of acquired immunodeficiency syndrome: United States, June 1981 to December 1991. Morbidity and Mortality Weekly Report 41:28–29, 1992.

Centers for Disease Control and Prevention. Youth risk behavioral surveillance, United States, 1997. Morbidity and Mortality Weekly Report 47(SS-3):51, 1998.

Chan, C. K., et al. The value and hazards of standardization in clinical epidemiologic research. Journal of Clinical Epidemiology 41:1125–1134, 1988.

Conway, G. A., et al. Underreporting of AIDS cases in South Carolina, 1986 and 1987. Journal of the American Medical Association 262:2859–2863, 1989.

Dorn, H. F. A classification system for morbidity concepts. Public Health Reports 72:1043–1048, 1957.

Jekel, J. F. Publications of the National Center for Health Statistics and their relevance for chronic disease. Jounal of Chronic Disease 37:681–688, 1984.

Jekel, J. F., D. H. Freeman, and J. W. Meigs. A study of trends in upper arm soft tissue sarcomas in Connecticut following the introduction of alum-adsorbed allergenic extracts. Annals of Allergy 40:28–31, 1978.

Moriyama, I. M. Inquiring into the diagnostic evidence supporting medical certification of death. *In* Lilienfield, A. M., and A. J. Gifford, eds. Chronic Diseases and Public Health. Baltimore, Johns Hopkins University Press, 1966.

Moriyama, I. M. Problems in measurement of accuracy of cause-of-death statistics. American Journal of Public Health 79: 1349–1350, 1989.

National Center for Health Statistics. Advance report of final mortality statistics, 1994. Monthly Vital Statistics Report 45(3), Supplement, 1996.

Rubin, D. H., et al. The relationship between infant feeding and infectious illness: a prospective evaluation of infants during the first year of life. Pediatrics 85: 464–471, 1990.

US Department of Health and Human Services, Public Health Service. Healthy People 2000: National Health Promotion and Disease Prevention Objectives. Washington, D. C., US Government Printing Office, 1990.

Young, J. L., Jr., et al. Surveillance, epidemiology, and end results: incidence and mortality data, 1973–1977. National Cancer Institute Monograph 57. Washington, D. C., US Government Printing Office, 1981.

Selected Readings

Centers for Disease Control and Prevention. International Health Data Reference Guide, 1993. Publication No. (PHS)94-1007. Hyattsville, Md., US Department of Health and Human Services, 1994. [International data.]

Chan, C. K., et al. The value and hazards of standardization in clinical epidemiologic research. Journal of Clinical Epidemiology 41:1125–1134, 1988. [Standardization of rates.]

Elandt-Johnson, R. C. Definition of rates: some remarks on their use and misuse. American Journal of Epidemiology 102:267–271, 1975. [Risks, rates, and ratios.]

Gable, C. B. A compendium of public health data sources. American Journal of Epidemiology 131:381–394, 1990. [General information.]

3 Epidemiologic Surveillance and Outbreak Investigation

■ THE SURVEILLANCE OF DISEASE

Responsibility for Surveillance in the USA

Surveillance is the entire process of collecting, analyzing, interpreting, and reporting data concerning the incidence of death, diseases, and injuries and the prevalence of certain conditions whose knowledge is considered important for promoting the health of the public.

In the USA, the Centers for Disease Control and Prevention (CDC) in Atlanta, Georgia, is the federal agency responsible for the surveillance of most types of acute diseases and, if deemed necessary, the investigation of outbreaks. Data for disease surveillance are passed from local and state governments to the CDC, which then evaluates the data and works with the state and local agencies regarding further investigation and control of problems discovered.

According to the US Constitution, the federal government has jurisdiction over matters concerning in-terstate commerce, including disease outbreaks with **interstate implications** (outbreaks that originated in one state and have spread to other states or have the potential to do so). Each state government has jurisdiction over disease outbreaks with **intrastate implications** (i.e., an outbreak confined within one state's borders). If a disease outbreak has interstate implications, the CDC is a first responder and takes immediate action, rather than waiting for a request for assistance from a state government.

Creating a Surveillance System

The development of a surveillance system requires clear objectives regarding the diseases or conditions to be covered (e.g., infectious diseases, side effects of vaccines, elevated lead levels, or pneumonia-related deaths in patients with influenza) and the purposes for which the surveillance is to be done (e.g., surveillance of varicella [chickenpox] to determine if the varicella vaccine program is effective, to look for possible side effects of the vaccine or vaccine program, or to determine if the nation is meeting its health objectives for the year 2010).

To enable the development of standardized reporting procedures and reporting forms, the criteria for defining a case of the reportable disease or condition must be known. As discussed later in this chapter, the case definition is usually based on clinical findings, laboratory results, and epidemiologic data concerning the time, place, and persons affected. The intensity of the planned surveillance (active versus passive) and duration of the surveillance (ongoing versus time-limited) must be known in advance. Special methods, such as the use of sentinel clinicians or institutions for regular reporting, should be considered.

The items of data to be collected and the manner in which each item will be used in the analysis must be carefully determined. The kinds of analyses needed (e.g., analyses of incidence, prevalence, case fatality ratios, years of potential life lost [YPLL], quality-adjusted life years [QALY], and costs) should be stated in advance. In addition, there should be plans for dissemination of findings.

The above objectives and methods should be developed with the aid of those who will collect, report, and use the data. A pilot test should be performed and evaluated in the field, perhaps in one or a few demonstration areas, before the full system is attempted. When the full system is operational, it too should be subjected to continual evaluations. The CDC has extensive information on surveillance at its web site (www.cdc.gov).

Purposes and Methods for the Surveillance of Disease

Surveillance, generally considered the foundation of public health disease control efforts, has various interrelated functions. A distinction must be made between passive surveillance and active surveillance. Most of the surveillance done on a routine basis is **passive surveillance,** in which those who are required to report disease, such as physicians, laboratories, and hospitals, are given the appropriate mailing forms and instructions, with the expectation that they will report all of the cases of reportable disease that come to their attention. **Active surveillance** requires periodic (usually weekly) telephone calls or personal visits to the reporting individuals and institutions to obtain the required data. Active surveillance is obviously more labor-intensive and costly, and it is seldom done on a routine basis.

The percentage of reportable disease cases that are actually reported to public health authorities varies considerably. Harkess et al. (1988) estimated that the percentage reported to state-based passive reporting systems varied from 30% to 62% of cases. These same authors, however, found that 81% of the culture-confirmed cases of shigellosis that occurred in Oklahoma over a 6-month period were reported to the passive surveillance system in that state.

Sometimes a change in medical care practice will uncover a problem that was previously invisible. This occurred, for example, when one hospital in Connecticut began reporting many cases of pharyngeal gonorrhea in young children. This apparent localized outbreak was investigated by a student-faculty rapid response team from Yale University School of Public Health, which discovered that the cases began to appear only after the hospital started examining all throat cultures in children for gonococci as well as for beta-hemolytic streptococci (Helgerson, Jekel, and Hadler 1988).

In contrast to the reporting of infectious diseases, the reporting of most other diseases, injuries, and conditions is less likely to be rapid or nationwide, and surveillance systems tend to develop on a problem-by-problem basis. Without significant support and funding from the federal government, surveillance systems are difficult to develop. Even with such support, most systems tend to begin as demonstration projects in which a few states participate. Later, the systems expand to include participation by all states. This occurred, for example, when a surveillance system for emergency events involving hazardous substances was developed by the Agency for Toxic Substances and Disease Registry of the Environmental Protection Agency (see Centers for Disease Control and Prevention 1994).

As discussed in Chapter 2, several states and regions have cancer registries, but there is no national cancer registry. Fatal diseases can be monitored to some extent by death certificates, but the diagnoses are often inaccurate and reporting is seldom rapid enough for the detection of disease outbreaks. The reporting systems for occupational and environmental diseases and injuries are discussed in Section III of this book.

Establishment of Baseline Data

Usual (baseline) rates and patterns of diseases can be known only if there is a regular reporting and surveillance system. Epidemiologists study the patterns of diseases by the time of occurrence of cases, the geo-

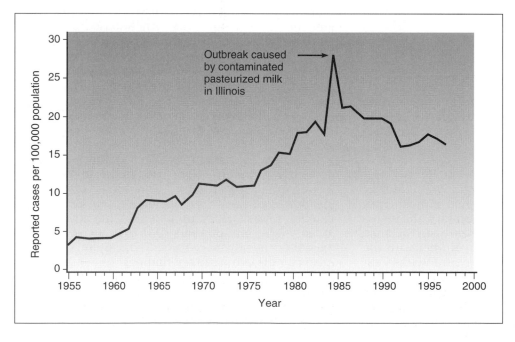

FIGURE 3–1 **Incidence rates of salmonellosis (excluding typhoid fever) in the USA, by year of report, 1955–1997.** (Sources: Centers for Disease Control and Prevention. Summary of notifiable diseases, United States, 1992. Morbidity and Mortality Weekly Report 41:41, 1992. Centers for Disease Control and Prevention. Summary of notifiable diseases, United States, 1997. Morbidity and Mortality Weekly Report 46: 18, 1998.)

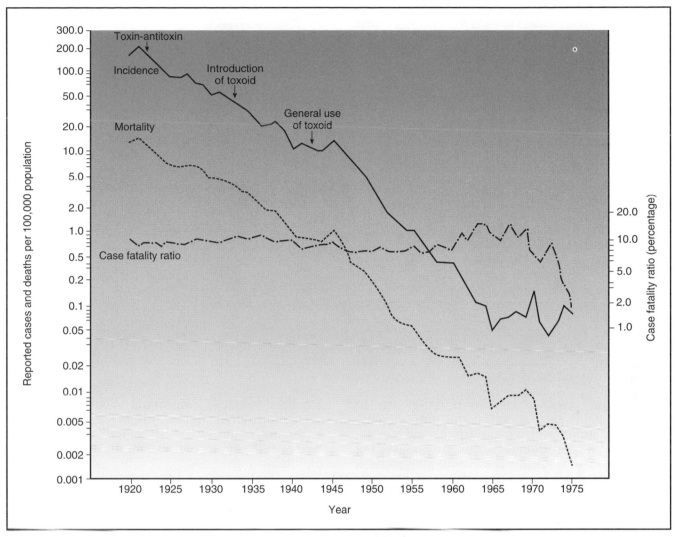

FIGURE 3–2   Incidence rates, mortality rates, and case fatality ratios for diphtheria in the USA, by year of report, 1920–1975. (Source: Centers for Disease Control. Diphtheria Surveillance Summary. Publication No. (CDC)78-8087. Atlanta, Centers for Disease Control, 1970.)

graphic location of cases, and the characteristics of the persons involved. Continued surveillance allows epidemiologists to detect deviations from the usual pattern of data, which prompts them to explore whether an epidemic (i.e., an unusual incidence of disease) is occurring or whether other factors (such as an alteration in reporting practices) are responsible for the observed changes.

Evaluation of Time Trends

Long-Term Secular Trends. The implications of long-term secular (time) trends of disease are usually different from those of outbreaks or epidemics, and they are often of greater significance. For example, the graph in Fig. 3–1, taken from a CDC surveillance report about salmonellosis, shows that a rise in the number of reported cases of salmonellosis in the USA has been seen over time. The first question to be asked is whether the trend could be explained by changes over time in disease detection, disease re-

porting, or both, which often happens when an apparent outbreak of a particular disease is reported. When a real or suspected outbreak is announced, this may increase the index of suspicion of physicians practicing in the community and may thereby lead to increased diagnosis and to increased reporting of cases that are diagnosed.

Because there have been increasing numbers of outbreaks and because the trend has continued over an extended time period, epidemiologists considered that most of the observed increase in salmonellosis from 1955 to 1985, as shown in Fig. 3–1, was real. This was especially true for New England and the East Coast, where a sharp increase in outbreaks caused by *Salmonella enteritidis* was noted beginning about 1977. A long-term increase in a disease in one region of the country, particularly when it is related to one serotype, is usually of greater public health significance than is a localized outbreak, because it suggests the existence of a more widespread problem.

Fig. 3–2 shows the decline in the reported inci-

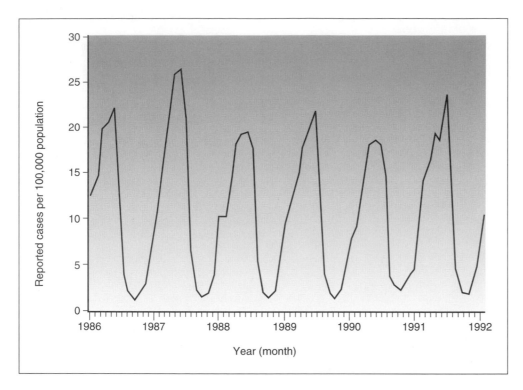

FIGURE 3–3 **Incidence rates of varicella (chickenpox) in the USA, by month of report, 1986–1992.** (Source: Centers for Disease Control and Prevention. Summary of notifiable diseases, United States, 1992. Morbidity and Mortality Weekly Report 41:53, 1992.)

dence and mortality from diphtheria in the USA. The data in this figure are presented in the form of a **semi-logarithmic graph,** with a **logarithmic scale** used for the *y*-axis and an **arithmetic scale** for the *x*-axis. Fig. 3–2 illustrates one advantage of using a logarithmic scale: the lines showing incidence and mortality demonstrate an approximately parallel decline. On a logarithmic scale, this means that the decline in rates was proportional, so that the percentage of cases that resulted in death—i.e., the **case fatality ratio—**

remained relatively constant at about 10% over the years shown in the figure. This, in turn, suggests that prevention of disease, rather than treatment of those who were ill, was responsible for the improvement in diphtheria in the USA.

Seasonal Variation. When determining the usual number of cases or rate of disease, epidemiologists must incorporate the expected seasonal variation into their calculations. Many infectious diseases show a strong seasonal variation, with periods of

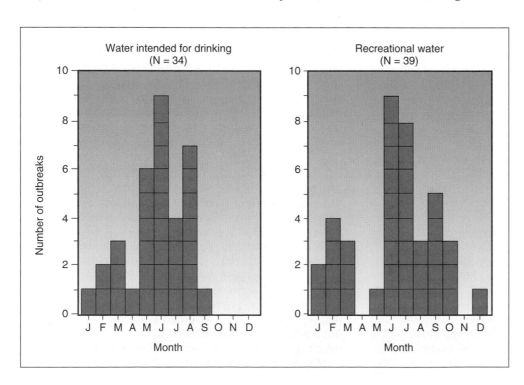

FIGURE 3–4 **Incidence of waterborne outbreaks of gastrointestinal disease in the USA, by month of report, 1991–1992.** (Source: Centers for Disease Control and Prevention. Surveillance for waterborne disease outbreaks, United States, 1991–1992. Morbidity and Mortality Weekly Report 42(SS-5):1–22, 1993.)

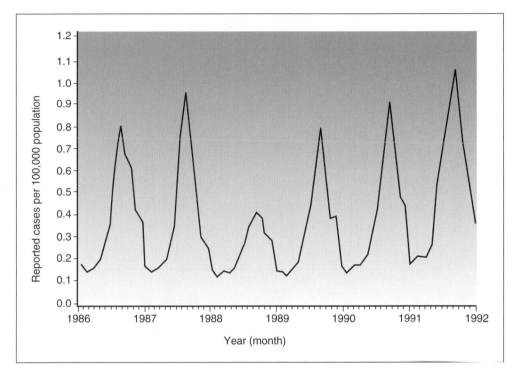

FIGURE 3–5   Incidence rates of aseptic meningitis in the USA, by month of report, 1986–1992. (Source: Centers for Disease Control and Prevention. Summary of notifiable diseases, United States, 1992. Morbidity and Mortality Weekly Report 41:20, 1992.)

highest incidence usually depending on the **route of spread.**

Infectious diseases that are spread by the **respiratory route,** such as influenza, colds, measles, and varicella (chickenpox), have a much higher incidence in the winter and early spring months in the northern hemisphere. For example, Fig. 3–3 shows the seasonal variation for varicella in the USA by month during the period 1986–1992. Notice the peaks after January and before summer of each year. This pattern is thought to occur because people spend most of their time close together in indoor environments where the air changes slowly. The drying of mucous membranes, which also occurs in the wintertime because of low humidity and indoor heating, may play a role in promoting respiratory infections. Diphtheria, on the other hand, when it was common, tended to strike especially in the early autumn, perhaps related to the return of children to school.

Diseases that are spread by **insect or arthropod vectors** (such as viral encephalitis from mosquitoes) have a strong predilection for the summer or early autumn. Lyme disease, spread by *Ixodes* ticks, is usually acquired in the late spring or summer, a pattern explained by the seasonally related life cycle of the ticks and the outdoor activity of people with less protective clothing at that time of the year.

Infectious diseases that are spread by the **fecal-oral route** are most common in the summer, partly because of the ability of the organisms to multiply more rapidly in food and water during warm weather. Fig. 3–4 shows the summer seasonal pattern of waterborne outbreaks of gastrointestinal disease. The peak frequency of outbreaks from drinking water sources occurs from May to August, whereas that for recreational water sources (such as lakes, rivers, and

swimming pools) is from June to October. The presence of flies during the summer also contributes to the spread of enteric diseases during this season.

Fig. 3–5 shows a late summer peak for aseptic meningitis, which is usually due to viral infections spread by the fecal-oral route or by insects. Fig. 3–6, which shows a pattern that is similar but has sharper and narrower peaks in late summer and early autumn, describes a known arthropod-borne viral infection caused by California-serogroup viruses of the central nervous system.

For reasons that usually are obscure, some noninfectious diseases have a higher incidence during certain seasons. For example, peptic ulcer disease has classically had a higher incidence in the spring and autumn, but the reasons for this are unknown (Harrison et al. 1958). Although peptic ulcers used to be considered a noninfectious disease, the newest hypothesis is that they are frequently caused by the bacterium *Helicobacter pylori,* which would make some peptic ulcers an infectious disease. The reasons for the seasonal pattern still are unknown, however.

Because the peaks of different patterns occur at different times, the CDC sometimes shows the incidence of diseases by what it calls an epidemiologic year. Unlike the **calendar year,** which runs from January of one year to January of the next year, the **epidemiologic year** for a given disease runs from the month of lowest incidence in one year to the same month in the next year. The advantage of using the epidemiologic year when plotting the incidence of a disease is that it puts the high-incidence months near the center of a graph and avoids having the high-incidence peak split between the two ends of the graph, as would occur with many respiratory diseases if they were graphed for a calendar year.

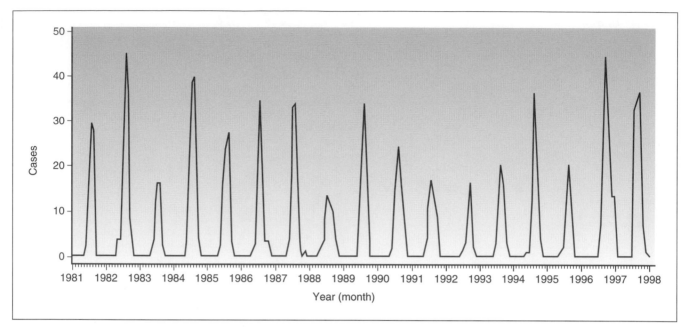

FIGURE 3–6   Incidence of central nervous system infections caused by California-serogroup viruses in the USA, by month of report, 1981–1997. (Sources: Centers for Disease Control and Prevention. Summary of notifiable diseases, United States, 1992. Morbidity and Mortality Weekly Report 41:18, 1992. Centers for Disease Control and Prevention. Summary of notifiable diseases, United States, 1997. Morbidity and Mortality Weekly Report 46:20, 1998.)

Other Types of Variation. Health problems can vary by the day of the week, as is illustrated in Fig. 3–7, which shows that recreational drownings are much more frequent on weekends than during the week.

Identification and Documentation of Outbreaks

An **epidemic,** or **disease outbreak,** is the occurrence of disease at an unusual (unexpected) frequency. Be-

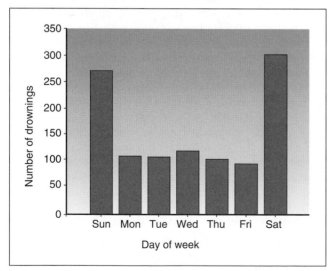

FIGURE 3–7   Number of drownings at the recreation facilities of the US Army Corps of Engineers, by day of week of report, 1986–1990. (Source: Centers for Disease Control and Prevention. Drownings at U.S. Army Corps of Engineers recreation facilities, 1986–1990. Morbidity and Mortality Weekly Report 41:331–333, 1992.)

cause the word *epidemic* tends to create fear in a population, that term is usually reserved for a problem of wider than local implications, and the term *outbreak* is usually used for a localized epidemic. Nevertheless, the two terms are often used interchangeably.

Whether the level of disease is unusual can be determined only if the usual rates of the disease are known and if reliable surveillance shows that the current rates are in considerable excess of those ordinarily expected. For example, in order to determine when and where influenza and pneumonia outbreaks occur, the CDC uses a seasonally adjusted *expected* number of influenza and pneumonia deaths in the USA—a number called the **epidemic threshold**—to compare with the reported number of cases. (Pneumonias are included because influenza-induced pneumonias often are signed out on the death certificate just as pneumonia, with no mention of influenza.)

Fig. 3–8 provides data concerning the expected proportion of deaths caused by pneumonia and influenza in 122 US cities for 1994–2000. The lower sine wave is the seasonal baseline, which is the expected proportion of pneumonia and influenza deaths per week in these cities. The upper sine wave is the epidemic threshold, as discussed above. There was essentially no influenza outbreak in the winter of 1994–1995. There was a moderate influenza outbreak in the winter of 1995–1996, and there were major outbreaks in the winters of 1996–1997, 1997–1998, and 1998–1999 and in the autumn of 1999. No other disease has a prediction model as sophisticated as this one, but the basic principles apply

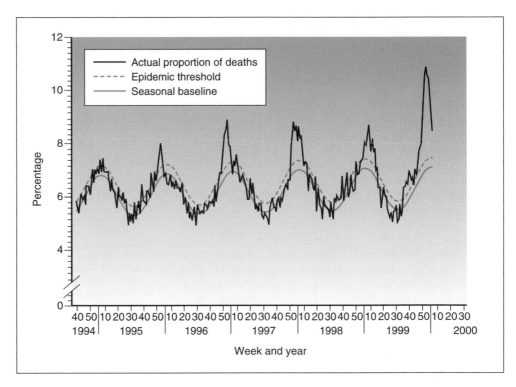

FIGURE 3–8 Epidemic threshold, seasonal baseline, and actual proportion of deaths caused by pneumonia and influenza in 122 US cities, 1994–2000. The epidemic threshold is 1.645 standard deviations above the seasonal baseline. The expected seasonal baseline is projected using a robust regression procedure in which a periodic regression model is applied to observed percentages of deaths from pneumonia and influenza since 1983. (Source: Centers for Disease Control and Prevention. Update: influenza activity—United States and worldwide, 1999–2000. Morbidity and Mortality Weekly Report 49:174, 2000.)

to determining whether or not an outbreak is occurring.

Evaluation of Disease Interventions

The introduction of major interventions, especially vaccines, is monitored by looking for changes in long-term disease patterns. Fig. 3–9 shows the impact that the two types of polio vaccine—the inactivated (Salk) vaccine and the oral (Sabin) vaccine—had on the reported incident cases of poliomyelitis. Note

that the large graph in this figure has a logarithmic scale on the y-axis. It is used here because the drop in the poliomyelitis incidence rate was so steep that on an arithmetic scale, no detail would be visible at the bottom after the early 1960s. A logarithmic scale compresses the high rates on a graph compared with lower rates, so that the detail of the latter can be seen.

Fig. 3–9 shows that after the inactivated vaccine was introduced in 1955, the rates of paralytic disease dropped quickly. Unfortunately, the public tended to think the problem had gone away, and many parents

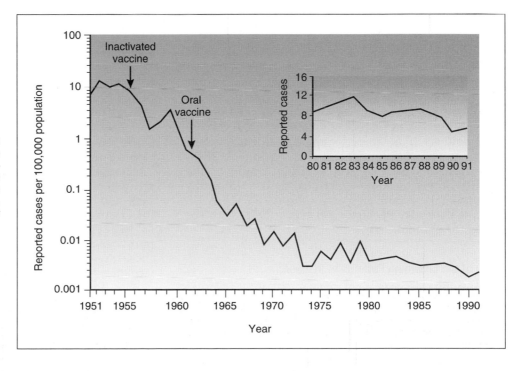

FIGURE 3–9 Incidence rates of paralytic poliomyelitis in the USA, by year of report, 1951–1991. (Source: Centers for Disease Control. Summary of notifiable diseases, United States, 1991. Morbidity and Mortality Weekly Report 40:37, 1991.)

became less concerned about immunizing newborn children. However, because the inactivated vaccine did not provide herd immunity, the unimmunized newborns were very much at risk. Fig. 3–9 shows a recurrent poliomyelitis spike in 1958 and 1959. At that time, most of the new cases of paralytic poliomyelitis were among young children who had not been immunized. The rates dropped again in 1960 and thereafter, both because the public was shaken out of its complacency to obtain vaccine and because a newer vaccine was introduced. This live, attenuated oral vaccine provided herd immunity as well as individual immunity. (For a discussion of herd immunity, see Chapter 1 and Fig. 1–2.)

The failure of a vaccine to produce immunity or the failure of people to use the vaccine can be detected by one of the following: (1) a lack of change in disease rates; (2) an increase in disease rates following an initial fall, as occurred in the example of the polio vaccine just discussed; or (3) an increase in disease rates in a recently vaccinated group, as occurred following the use of bad lots of inactivated polio vaccine manufactured by Cutter Laboratories in the 1950s (see Chapter 1).

The importance of surveillance was underscored recently through continued evaluation and close surveillance of measles rates in the USA. Investigators were able to detect the failure of the initial measles vaccines and vaccination schedules to provide long-lasting protection (see Chapter 1). Research into this problem led to a new set of recommendations for immunization against measles. According to the 1999 recommendations (see Centers for Disease Control and Prevention 1999b), two doses of measles vaccine should be administered to young children. The first dose should be given when the child is between 12 and 15 months of age (to avoid the greater failure rate if given earlier), and a second dose should be given when the child is between 4 and 6 years old, before school entry.

Setting of Disease Control Priorities

The patterns of diseases for the current time and recent past help governmental and voluntary agencies establish priorities for disease control efforts. This is not a simple counting procedure. A disease will be of more concern if its rates rise rapidly—as was the case with acquired immunodeficiency syndrome (AIDS)—than if its rates are steady or declining. Moreover, the severity of the disease is a critical feature, and this usually can be established by good surveillance. AIDS gets high priority because of its severity and its potential for epidemic spread.

Study of the Changing Patterns of Diseases

By studying the patterns of occurrence of a particular disease over time in populations and in subpopulations, epidemiologists can better understand the changing patterns of the disease.

Data derived from the surveillance of syphilis cases in New York City during the 1980s proved valu-

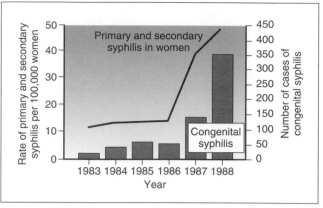

FIGURE 3–10   Incidence of congenital syphilis in infants under 1 year of age (bars) and incidence of primary and secondary syphilis in women (line) in New York City, by year of report, 1983–1988. (Source: Centers for Disease Control. Congenital syphilis, New York City, 1983–1988. Morbidity and Mortality Weekly Report 38:825–829, 1989.)

able in suggesting the source of changing patterns of acquired and congenital syphilis. As shown in Fig. 3–10, there was a substantial increase in the reported number of cases of primary and secondary syphilis among women beginning in 1987, soon after the epidemic of "crack" cocaine began in the city. The rise in congenital syphilis was strongly associated with the women's use of cocaine (trading sex for drugs) and with their lack of prenatal care (a lack that allowed their syphilis to go undetected and untreated).

A new pattern of occurrence may be more ominous than a mere increase in the incidence of disease. In the case of tuberculosis in the USA, for example, the yearly incidence fell steadily from 1953 (when reporting began) to 1985, when 22,201 cases were reported. After this, the yearly incidence began to rise again. Of special concern was the association of this rise with the increasing impact of the AIDS epidemic and the increasing resistance of *Mycobacterium tuberculosis* to antimicrobial agents. This concern led to greater efforts to detect tuberculosis in AIDS patients and to use directly observed therapy (DOT) to prevent antimicrobial resistance. Tuberculosis rates peaked in 1992, when 26,673 cases were reported, and then began falling again. In 1997, the number of cases reported was 19,855 (see Centers for Disease Control and Prevention 1993, 1999a).

Changes in the virulence of infectious organisms are also of concern to epidemiologists. For example, beta-hemolytic streptococci are causing more severe infections again after almost a century of behaving as less virulent organisms. This phenomenon is poorly understood and raises the question of whether these organisms have a regular long-term cycle of virulence.

■ THE INVESTIGATION OF EPIDEMICS
The Nature of Epidemics

The common definition of an **epidemic** is an unusual or unexpected occurrence of disease. The term comes from the Greek language and means "upon the population."

Although people usually think of an epidemic as something that involves large numbers of people, it is possible to name circumstances under which just *one* case of a disease could be considered an epidemic. For example, because smallpox has been eradicated from the world, a single case would represent a smallpox epidemic. Similarly, if a disease has been eradicated from a particular region (for example, paralytic poliomyelitis in the western hemisphere) or if a disease is approaching elimination from an area and has the potential for spread (as is the case with measles in the USA), the report of even one case in the geographic region is "unexpected" and is cause for concern. Under these circumstances, any occurrence of the disease can be considered an epidemic.

When a disease in a population is occurring regularly and at about its usual level, it is said to be **endemic.** This term, also from the Greek language, means "within the population."

Epidemiologists also distinguish between usual and unusual patterns of diseases in animals. If there is a disease outbreak in an animal population, it is said to be **epizootic** ("upon the animals"), or if a disease is deeply entrenched in a wild animal population but not changing much, it is said to be **enzootic** ("within the animals").

Investigators of acute disease outbreaks ordinarily use a measure of disease frequency called the **attack rate,** particularly when the period of exposure is short (i.e., considerably less than a year). Rather than being a true rate, the attack rate is really the proportion of exposed persons that becomes ill. It is calculated as follows:

$$\text{Attack rate} = \frac{\text{Number of new cases of a disease}}{\text{Number of persons exposed in a}} \times 100$$
$$\text{particular outbreak}$$

In this equation, 100 is used as the constant multiplier so that the rate can be expressed as a percentage. (For a discussion of other measures of disease frequency, see Chapter 2.)

Procedures for Investigating an Epidemic

If a disease epidemic occurs, it suggests that something in the equilibrium of factors for and against the occurrence of that particular disease has been disrupted, rather suddenly and probably rather recently. The goal is to discover and correct the recent changes so the balance can be restored and the epidemic controlled. The physician who is alert to possible epidemics will not only be concerned to give the correct treatment to individual patients prospectively (i.e., from the time of disease onset forward) but will also ask the following retrospective question: Why did *this* patient become sick with *this* disease at *this* time and place?

Outbreak investigation is somewhat like crime investigation in that both require a lot of "shoe leather" (for good examples of epidemic investigation, see Roueché 1991). Although there is no simple way to teach imagination and creativity in the investigation of disease outbreaks, there is an organized way of approaching and interpreting the data that assists in the solution of problems. This section outlines the series of steps to follow in investigating a disease outbreak.

Establish the Diagnosis

Establishing the diagnosis may seem obvious, but it is surprising how many people start investigating an outbreak without taking this first step. Many cases are "solved" just by making the correct diagnosis and thereby demonstrating that the disease occurrence was not unusual after all. For example, a health department in North Carolina received panic calls from numerous people who lived in a small town and were concerned about the occurrence of smallpox in their county. A physician working in the local health department was assigned to investigate the matter and quickly discovered that the reported case of smallpox was actually a typical case of chickenpox in a young child. The child's mother did not speak English well, and the neighbors heard the word "pox" and panicked. The "outbreak" was stopped by a correct diagnosis.

Establish the Epidemiologic Case Definition

The case definition is the list of specific criteria used to decide whether or not a person has the disease of concern. The epidemiologic case definition does not make a clinical diagnosis; rather, it establishes consistent criteria that enable epidemiologic investigations to proceed before definitive diagnoses are available. Establishing a case definition is especially important if the disease is unknown, as was the case in the early investigations of legionnaires' disease, AIDS, hantavirus pulmonary syndrome, and eosinophilia-myalgia syndrome, among others. For example, the CDC case definition for eosinophilia-myalgia syndrome includes (1) a total eosinophil count greater than $1000/\mu L$; (2) generalized myalgia at some point during the course of the illness of sufficient severity to limit the ability to pursue normal activities; and (3) exclusion of other neoplastic or infectious conditions that could account for the syndrome. By use of these epidemiologic and clinical criteria, the source of the outbreak was discovered (Slutsker et al. 1990).

No case definition will be perfect, because there will always be some **false positives** (i.e., individuals wrongly included in the group considered to have the disease) and **false negatives** (i.e., diseased individuals wrongly included in the unaffected group). Nevertheless, the case definition should be developed carefully and adhered to in the collection and analysis of data. Using a generally established case definition also permits epidemiologists to make more accurate comparisons among the findings from many different outbreak investigations (see Centers for Disease Control and Prevention 1997).

Determine Whether an Epidemic Exists

Even if there are proven cases, are they sufficient in number to constitute an epidemic? As emphasized above, it is difficult to answer this question unless the "usual" number of cases is known by ongoing surveillance. However, it may be assumed that a completely new disease or syndrome meets the criteria for an epidemic.

Characterize the Epidemic by Time, Place, and Person

The epidemic should be characterized using the criteria in the case definition. It is unwise to start the data collection until the case definition has been established, because the case definition determines the data needed to classify persons as affected or unaffected.

Time. The time dimension of the outbreak is best described by an **epidemic time curve.** This is a graph with time on the *x*-axis and the number of new cases on the *y*-axis. The epidemic time curve should be created so that the units of time on the *x*-axis are considerably smaller than the expected incubation period, and the *y*-axis is simply the *number* of cases that became symptomatic during the time interval. Rates are not used in creating the epidemic time curve.

The epidemic time curve provides several important clues about what is happening in an outbreak and helps the epidemiologist answer the following questions: What was the **type of exposure** (i.e., common source or propagated)? What was the **route of spread** (respiratory, fecal-oral, skin-to-skin contact, exchange of blood or body fluids, or via insect or animal vectors)? When were the affected persons exposed? What was the incubation period? In addition to **primary cases** (persons infected initially by a common source), were there **secondary cases** (which represent person-to-person transmission of disease from primary cases to other persons, often members of the same household)?

In a **common source exposure,** many people come into contact with the same source, such as contaminated water or food, usually over a short period of time. If an outbreak is due to this type of exposure, the epidemic curve usually has a sudden onset, a peak, and a rather rapid decline. If the outbreak is due to **person-to-person spread,** however, the epidemic curve usually has a prolonged, irregular pattern. The latter kind of outbreak is often referred to as a **propagated outbreak.**

Fig. 3–11 shows the epidemic time curve from an outbreak of gastrointestinal disease caused by a common source exposure to *Shigella boydii* at Fort Bliss in Texas. In this outbreak, spaghetti was contaminated by a food handler. The time scale in this figure is shown in 12-hour periods. Note the rapid increase and rapid disappearance of the outbreak.

Fig. 3–12 shows the epidemic time curve from a propagated outbreak of bacillary dysentery due to *Shigella sonnei,* which was transmitted from person to person at a school for mentally retarded people in Vermont. In this outbreak, the spread of disease was

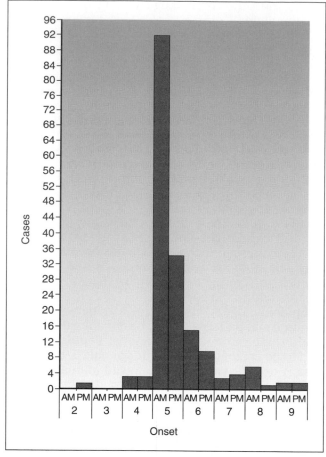

FIGURE 3–11   Epidemic time curve showing the onset of cases of gastrointestinal disease caused by *Shigella boydii* in Fort Bliss, Texas, in November 1976. Note that the onset is shown in 12-hour periods for dates in November. (Source: Centers for Disease Control. Food and Waterborne Disease Outbreaks: Annual Summary, 1976. Atlanta, Centers for Disease Control, 1977.)

through contamination of persons, clothing, bedding, and the school environment with feces. The time scale here is shown in 5-day periods. Note the ongoing, "dragged-out" appearance of the outbreak.

If conditions are right, a respiratory disease spread by the person-to-person route may produce an epidemic time curve that looks almost like that of a common source epidemic. Fig. 3–13 shows the spread of measles in an elementary school. A widespread exposure apparently occurred in the school assembly, so that the air in that assembly can almost be thought of as a common source. The initial case in this situation is called the **index case**—i.e., the case that introduced the organism into the population. However, sequential individual cases can be seen every 12 days or so during the prior 2 months. The first of these measles cases should have warned school and public health officials to immunize all of the school children immediately. If that had been done, the outbreak would probably have been avoided.

Sometimes an epidemic will have more than one peak, either because of multiple common source exposures or because of secondary cases. This is illustrated in Fig. 3–14, which shows the epidemic time

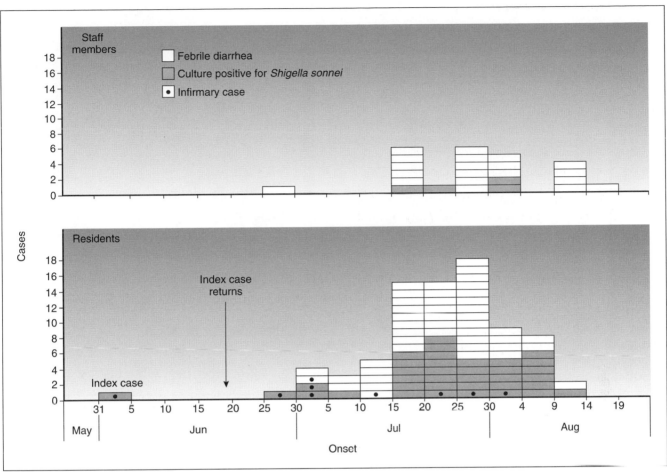

FIGURE 3–12 Epidemic time curve showing the onset of cases of bacillary dysentery caused by *Shigella sonnei* at a training school in Brandon, Vermont, from May to August 1974. Note that the onset is shown in 5-day periods for dates in May, June, July, and August. (Source: Centers for Disease Control. *Shigella* Surveillance. Report No. 37. Atlanta, Centers for Disease Control, 1976.)

curve for an outbreak of shigellosis among students who attended a camp in the eastern USA. The campers who drank contaminated water on a trip were infected with *Shigella* organisms. After they returned home, they infected others with shigellosis.

Epidemiologists occasionally encounter situations in which there are two different common source outbreaks that had the same time and place of exposure but had different incubation periods. Say, for example, that a group of people is exposed to contaminated shellfish in a restaurant. The exposure might cause an outbreak of shigellosis in 24–72 hours and also cause an outbreak of hepatitis A about 2–4 weeks later in the same population.

Not only is the epidemic time curve useful in ascertaining the type of exposure, but also it is useful in determining when the affected persons were exposed. If the causative organism is known and the exposure appears to be a common source, the epidemiologist can use knowledge about that organism's usual incubation period to determine the probable time of exposure. Two methods are commonly used. The data in Fig. 3–14, which pertain to *Shigella* infection among campers, will serve as the basis for illus-

trating each of these methods of determining the probable time of exposure.

Method 1 involves taking the shortest and longest known incubation period for the causative organism and calculating backward in time from the first and last cases. If these estimates are reasonably close together, they bracket the probable time of exposure. For example, the incubation period for *Shigella* organisms is usually from 1 to 3 days (from 24 to 72 hours), but it may be as short as 12 hours or as long as 96 hours (Benenson 1995). Fig. 3–14 shows that the first two cases of shigellosis occurred after noon on August 17. If these cases had a 12-hour incubation period, the exposure was sometime before noon on August 17 (without knowing the exact hours, it is not possible to be more specific). The longest known incubation period for *Shigella* is 96 hours, and the last camper case was August 21 after noon. Ninety-six hours before that would be August 17 after noon. The most probable exposure time, therefore, was either before noon or after noon on August 17. If the same procedure is used but applied to the *most common* incubation period (from 24 to 72 hours), the result is an estimate of after noon on August 16 (from

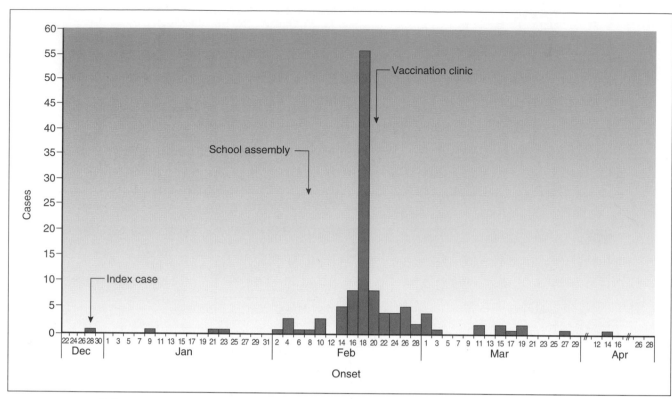

FIGURE 3–13 **Epidemic time curve showing the onset of cases of measles at an elementary school from December 1975 to April 1976.** Note that the onset is shown in 2-day periods for dates in December 1975 and in January, February, March, and April 1976. (Source: Centers for Disease Control. *Measles Surveillance, 1973–1976.* Report No. 10. Atlanta, Centers for Disease Control, 1977.)

the early cases) and an estimate of after noon on August 18 (from the last case). These two estimates still center on August 17, so it is reasonable to assume that the campers were exposed sometime during August 17.

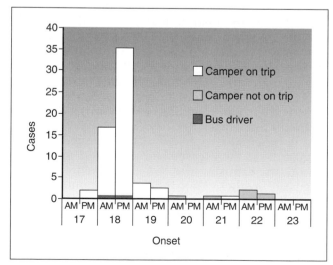

FIGURE 3–14 **Epidemic time curve showing the onset of cases of shigellosis in campers from New Jersey and New York in August 1971.** Note that the onset is shown in 12-hour periods for dates in August. (Source: Centers for Disease Control. *Shigella* Surveillance: Annual Summary, 1971. Atlanta, Centers for Disease Control, 1972.)

Method 2 is closely related to the above method but involves taking the average incubation period and measuring backward from the epidemic peak, if that was clear. In Fig. 3–14, the peak is after noon on August 18. An average of 48 hours (2 days) earlier would be after noon on August 16, slightly earlier than the previous estimates. Therefore, the most probable time of exposure was either after noon on August 16 or anytime during August 17. It is probable that the exposure occurred whenever a camper happened to drink water on August 16 or 17.

Place. The accurate characterization of an epidemic involves defining the geographic location of cases. A geographic clustering of cases may give important clues to what is going on. Usually, however, the geographic picture is not sufficient by itself but needs other data to complete the interpretation.

Sometimes a **spot map** showing where each affected person lives or works will be helpful to the solution of an epidemic puzzle. One of the best examples came from a study done in the 1850s in London by John Snow, who showed that most of the persons affected by an outbreak of cholera lived in the blocks immediately surrounding the Broad Street water pump. Based on this information, Snow had the pump removed from service.

The use of spot maps is limited in outbreak investigations nowadays, because these maps show only the numerator (the number of cases) and do not provide information on the denominator. Epidemiolo-

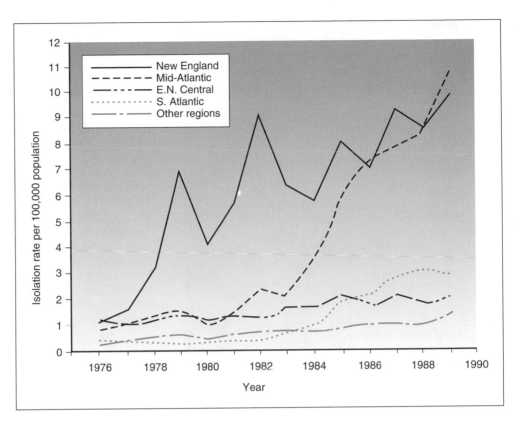

FIGURE 3–15   Isolation rate of *Salmonella enteritidis* infections per 100,000 population in various regions of the USA, by year of report, 1976–1989. (Source: Centers for Disease Control. Update: *Salmonella enteritidis* infections and shell eggs, United States, 1990. Morbidity and Mortality Weekly Report 39:909–912, 1990.)

gists usually prefer to show **incidence rates by location,** such as by hospital ward (in a hospital infection outbreak), by work area or classroom (in an occupational or school outbreak), or by block or section of a city (in a community outbreak). For example, Roueché (1991) described an outbreak of respiratory fungal infection in an Arkansas school and showed how classroom incidence rates provided a clue to the cause of the outbreak. All but one of the classrooms had 3 or fewer cases each. The exception, a room named the Liberace Room, had 14 cases. This room was located directly over the coal chute, and coal had been dumped on the ground and then shoveled into the chute over several windy days. The Liberace Room had become very dusty from the coal, which had come from a strip mine and had become contaminated with *Histoplasma capsulatum* in the soil before it was delivered to the school. The children had inhaled the dust and become ill with histoplasmosis.

When epidemiologists wish to determine the general location of a disease and how it is spreading, they may compare trends in incidence rates in different regions. For example, Fig. 3–15 shows the rates of reported *Salmonella enteritidis* infections by region in the USA for the period 1976–1989. According to this figure, there was an unusually high rate for the New England region from 1978 to 1989. Beginning in about 1984, the mid-Atlantic states also began to show an excessive rate of salmonellosis from the same serotype, suggesting that the problem was spreading down the East Coast. Fig. 3–16 uses a map to demonstrate the spread of epidemic cholera in

South and Central America from January 1991 through July 1992.

A special type of investigation problem in recent years has been reports of clusters of cancer or other types of disease in neighborhoods or other small areas. From the theory of random sampling, epidemiologists would expect clusters of disease to happen by chance alone, but that does not comfort the people involved.

Distinguishing **"chance" clusters** from **"real" clusters** is often difficult, but the types of cancer in a cluster may help epidemiologists decide fairly quickly whether or not the cluster might be an environmental problem. If the types of cancer in the cluster vary considerably and are of the more common cell types (lung, breast, colon, prostate, etc.), the cluster probably is not due to a hazardous local exposure (see Brooks-Robinson, Helgerson, and Jekel 1987; Jacquez 1993; and National Conference on Clustering of Health Events 1990). If, however, most of the cases are of only one type or are of a limited number of related types of cancer (especially leukemia or brain cancer), a more intensive investigation is indicated.

The next step is to begin at the time the "cluster" is reported and observe the situation prospectively. The hypothesis is that the unusual number of cases will not continue. Because this is a prospective hypothesis, as will be explained in Chapter 10, an appropriate statistical test can be used to decide whether the number of cases continues to be excessive. If the answer is "yes," there may be a true environmental problem in the area.

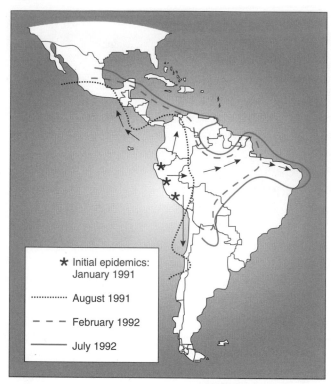

FIGURE 3–16 **Map showing the spread of epidemic cholera in Latin America from January 1991 to July 1992.** (Source: Centers for Disease Control and Prevention. Update: cholera, western hemisphere. Morbidity and Mortality Weekly Report 41:667–668, 1992.)

Person. Knowing the characteristics of persons affected by an outbreak may help clarify the problem and its cause. Among the important characteristics are age; sex; race; religion; source of water, milk, and food; immunization status; type of work or schooling; and contacts with other affected persons.

Figs. 3–17 and 3–18 illustrate the value of analyzing the personal characteristics of affected individuals for clues regarding the cause of the outbreak. Fig. 3–17 shows the age distribution of measles cases among children in the Navajo nation, while Fig. 3–18 shows the age distribution of measles cases among residents of Cuyahoga County, Ohio. The fact that measles in the Navajo nation tended to occur in very young children is consistent with the hypothesis that the outbreak in this instance was due to lack of immunization of young preschool children. In contrast, the fact that very young children in Cuyahoga County were almost exempt from measles and that school-aged children tended to be the ones infected suggests that the young children had been immunized and that the outbreak in this instance was due to failure of measles vaccine to produce long-lasting immunity. If they were not immunized early, the children of Cuyahoga County probably would have had measles earlier in life and would therefore have been immune by the time they entered school. This type of outbreak has been almost eliminated by the requirement that children receive a booster dose of measles vaccine before entering school.

Develop Hypotheses Regarding Source, Type, and Route of Spread

The **source of infection** is the person (the index case) or vehicle (e.g., food, water) that brought the infection into the affected community in the first place. For example, the source of infection in the outbreak of gastrointestinal illness at Fort Bliss (see Fig. 3–11) was an infected food handler, who contaminated spaghetti that was eaten by many persons more or less simultaneously.

The **pattern of spread** is the pattern by which infection can be spread from the source to those infected. The primary distinction is between a **common source pattern,** such as occurs when contaminated water is drunk by many people in the same time period, and a **propagated pattern,** in which the infection "propagates itself" by spreading directly from person to person over an extended period of time. There is also a **mixed pattern,** in which persons acquire a disease through a common source and then spread it to family members or others (the secondary cases) by personal contact.

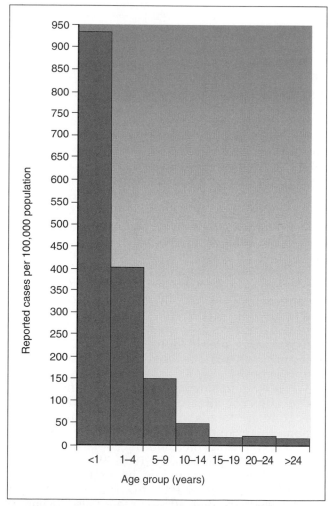

FIGURE 3–17 **Incidence rates of measles in members of the Navajo nation, by age group, 1972–1975.** (Source: Centers for Disease Control. Measles Surveillance, 1973–1976. Report No. 10. Atlanta, Centers for Disease Control, 1977.)

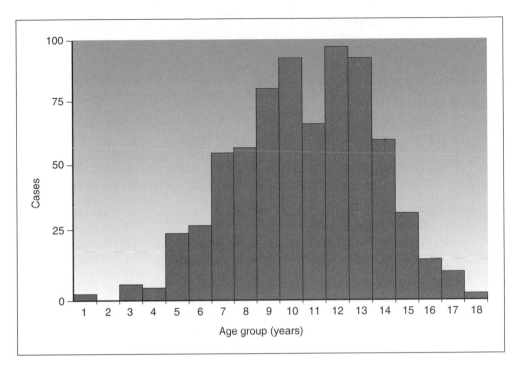

FIGURE 3–18   Incidence of measles in residents of Cuyahoga County, Ohio, by age group, from October 1973 to February 1974. (Source: Centers for Disease Control. Measles Surveillance, 1973–1976. Report No. 10. Atlanta, Centers for Disease Control, 1977.)

Affected persons in common source outbreaks may have just one short **point source exposure,** or they may have a **continuous common source exposure.** In the Fort Bliss outbreak, the infected spaghetti was the point source. In Milwaukee in 1993, an epidemic of *Cryptosporidium* infection was caused by contamination of the public water supply for the southern part of the city over a several-day period (MacKenzie et al. 1994), and this was an example of a continuous common source exposure.

Many types of infections have more than one pattern of spread. *Shigella* infection, for example, can be spread through contaminated water (a common source) or through person-to-person contact (propagation). The human immunodeficiency virus (HIV) can be spread to many intravenous drug users through the sharing of one infected needle and syringe (a common source), or it can be passed from one person to another through sexual contact.

The **mode of transmission** of epidemic disease may be respiratory, fecal-oral, vector-borne, skin-to-skin, or via exchange of serum or other body fluids. In some cases, transmission is via contact with fomites—that is, objects that can passively carry organisms from one person to another, such as unclean sheets or bedside water containers in hospitals.

Test the Hypotheses

Laboratory studies are important in testing the hypotheses and may include one or more of the following: (1) cultures from patients and, if appropriate, from possible vehicles such as food or water; (2) stool examinations for ova and parasites; (3) serum tests for antibodies to the organism suspected of causing the disease (e.g., tests of ''acute'' and ''convales-

cent'' serum samples to determine if there has been a rise in antibodies to the organism over time); and (4) tests for nonmicrobiologic agents, such as toxins or drugs.

A common, efficient way of testing hypotheses is to do **case-control studies** (see Chapter 5). For example, if there has been a food-borne outbreak of disease, the investigator assembles the persons who have the disease (the cases) and a sample of the persons who ate at the same place at the suspected time of exposure but did not have the disease (the controls). Then the investigator looks for what exposures (e.g., food items eaten) were considerably more common in the cases than in the controls. Both groups are questioned regarding the specific foods they did or did not eat prior to the outbreak. For each item of food and drink, the percentage of controls who consumed it is subtracted from the percentage of cases who consumed it. The food or drink showing the greatest difference in percentage is the most likely suspect. The case-control study can be used in an epidemic of noninfectious disease as well. Herbst, Ulfelder, and Poskanzer (1971) noted that 8 young women with adenocarcinoma of the vagina were treated at one hospital between 1966 and 1969. Because of the rarity of this type of cancer, the number of cases would qualify as an outbreak. When the investigators did a case-control study, they used 32 controls (4 matched controls for every case). They were able to demonstrate that the only significant difference between the 8 cases and 32 controls was that 7 of the 8 cancer patients had been exposed to diethylstilbestrol (DES) in utero. Their mothers had been given DES, a synthetic estrogen, during the first semester of pregnancy in an effort to prevent miscarriage or premature labor. In contrast, none of the 32 controls were the offspring of mothers given DES during pregnancy. The probability of finding this distribution by chance alone was infinitesimal. DES is no longer used for any purpose during pregnancy.

Initiate Control Measures

When an outbreak occurs, there is usually a general outcry that something be done immediately. It may be necessary to begin control measures before the source of the outbreak and other pertinent details are known for certain. If at all possible, the measures should be initiated in such a way as not to interfere with the investigation of the outbreak.

There are four common types of intervention. The first is **sanitation,** which often involves modification of the environment. Sanitation efforts may consist of removing the pathogenic agent from the sources of infection (water, food, etc.); removing the human source of infection from where he or she can spread it to others; or removing susceptible people from the environment. The second type is **prophylaxis,** which implies putting a barrier to the infection within the susceptible hosts. While a variety of immunizations are recommended for the entire population and are usually begun during infancy, other measures that offer short-term protection are also available for people who plan to travel to other countries. Examples include antimalarial drugs and hyperimmune globulin against hepatitis A. The third type of intervention consists of **diagnosis and treatment** of those who are infected (such as in outbreaks of tuberculosis, syphilis, and meningococcal meningitis) so that the infected persons cannot spread the disease to others. The fourth type of intervention involves **control of disease vectors,** such as mosquitoes (involved in malaria, dengue, or yellow fever) and *Ixodes* ticks (involved in Lyme disease).

Although an outbreak may require one or more of the above interventions, sometimes an outbreak may simply fade away if enough people have been infected that there is a lack of susceptible individuals.

One important aspect of the control effort is the written and oral communication of findings to the appropriate authorities, the appropriate health professionals, and the public. This enables local and state authorities to assist in disease control, contributes to the professional fund of knowledge about the causes and control of outbreaks, and also adds to the information regarding prevention that the public has at its disposal.

Initiate Specific Follow-Up Surveillance to Evaluate the Control Measures

No medical or public health intervention is adequate without follow-up surveillance of the disease or problem that initially caused the outbreak. The importance of a sound surveillance program is not only to detect subsequent outbreaks but also to evaluate the effect of the control measures. If possible, the surveillance following an outbreak should be active surveillance (defined at the beginning of this chapter).

A Brief Example of the Investigation of an Outbreak

In January 1991, a liberal arts college with a population of about 400 students reported 82 cases of acute gastrointestinal illness, mostly among students, over a period of 102 hours. The president of this small college in New England sought help from local and state health authorities to determine whether the college cafeteria should be closed or even whether the entire college should be closed and the students sent home, which would have been terribly disruptive to their academic year.

Initial investigation focused on making a diagnosis. Clinical data suggested that the illness was of short duration, with most students found to be essentially well in 24 hours. The data also suggested that the illness was relatively mild. Only one student was hospitalized, and the need for hospitalization in this case was uncertain. In most cases, the symptoms consisted of nausea and vomiting, with little or no diarrhea and only mild systemic symptoms such as headache and malaise. Examination revealed only a low-grade fever. Initial food and stool cultures for pathogenic bacteria yielded negative results.

Based on this information, the investigating team developed a case definition. A case was defined as any person in the college who complained of either diarrhea or vomiting between Monday, January 28, and Thursday, January 31, 1991. The large percentage of cases over this short time made it clear that the situation was unusual and that the problem could be considered a disease outbreak.

The people meeting the criteria of the case definition included resident students, commuter students, and employees. When the investigating team interviewed samples of these groups of affected people, they found that most, but not all, of the resident students had eaten only at the campus cafeteria. The epidemic time curve (Fig. 3–19) suggested that if cafeteria food were the source, one or more meals on 2 days in January could have been responsible, although a few cases had occurred before and after the peak of the outbreak. Near the beginning of the outbreak, two food handlers had worked while feeling ill with typical symptoms. Health department records, however, revealed that the school cafeteria had always received high scores for sanitation, and officials who conducted an emergency reinspection of the facilities and equipment during the outbreak found no change. They detected no problem with sanitary procedures, except for the food handlers working while not feeling well.

Most of the commuter students with symptoms had brought food from home during the time of question. Almost none of them had eaten at the college cafeteria, although a few had eaten at an independently run snack bar in the student center. Further questioning revealed that the family members of several of the affected commuter students had also

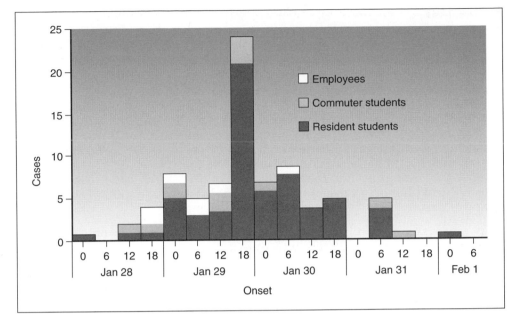

FIGURE 3-19 Epidemic time curve showing the onset of cases of gastroenteritis in a small college in New England from January 28 to February 1, 1991. Note that the onset is shown in 6-hour periods for dates in January and February.

had a similar illness during the weeks preceding the outbreak or concurrent with it. One public school in a nearby town had closed briefly because of a similar illness in the majority of the children and staff members.

Although a college-wide questionnaire was distributed and analyzed, this took several days, and the president wanted some answers as soon as possible. Within 2 days of being summoned, the investigation team was able to make the following recommendations: the college, including the cafeteria, should remain open; college-wide assemblies and indoor sports events should be canceled for 2 weeks; and no person should be allowed to work as a food handler while ill. To demonstrate their confidence in the cafeteria, the members of the investigation team ate lunch there and sat in a prominent place. The outbreak quickly faded away, and the college schedule was able to proceed more or less normally.

Why was the investigation team able to make these recommendations so quickly? While the epidemic time curve and information gathered from interviews offered numerous clues, past knowledge gained from similar outbreaks, from disease surveillance, and from research concerning the natural history of diseases all helped the investigators make their recommendations with confidence. In addition, the following observations made the diagnosis of bacterial infection unlikely: the self-limiting, mild course of disease; the lack of reported diarrhea, even though it was in the original case definition; and the fact that no bacterial pathogens could be cultured from the food and stool samples that had been collected. A staphylococcal toxin was considered initially, but the consistent story of a low-grade fever made a toxin unlikely; fever is a sign of infection but not of an external (ingested) toxin.

The clinical and epidemiologic pattern was most

consistent with an outbreak caused by a Norwalk-like viral agent, the laboratory demonstration of which is exceedingly difficult and costly. For Norwalk-like agents, the fecal-oral route of spread has been demonstrated for both food and water, but many outbreaks show a pattern also suggesting a respiratory route of spread, although that has not been confirmed. The latter was the reason for suggesting cancellation of assemblies and indoor sports events.

The outbreak investigation team was comfortable in recommending that the cafeteria remain open, because the commuters who had become ill had not eaten at the cafeteria and because a similar illness was reported in the surrounding community. These factors made it unlikely that the cafeteria was the only source of infection, although there was a possibility that the ill food handlers had spread their disease to some. The short duration and mild nature of the illness meant that there was no need to close the college, even though there probably would be a certain amount of disruption and class absenteeism for a few more days.

Continued surveillance was established at the college, and this confirmed that the outbreak was dying out. Cultures continued to yield negative results for bacterial pathogens, and the analysis of the major questionnaire survey did not change any conclusions. This outbreak illustrates, among other things, that even without a definitive diagnosis, epidemiologic evidence enabled the investigators to rule out the biggest concern, bacterial food contamination, with a high degree of probability. In contrast to viral gastroenteritis, bacterial gastroenteritis is often quite serious, requiring hospitalization. In outbreaks, negative evidence (i.e., evidence that shows what the problem is not) often can permit epidemiologists to calm a nervous population.

■ SUMMARY

Surveillance is the foundation of public health control of disease. It may be active or passive. Its functions are varied and include determining the baseline rates of disease, detecting outbreaks, and evaluating control measures. Surveillance data are used for setting disease control policy.

The investigation of disease outbreaks is one of the primary functions of public health agencies, but the practicing physician has the important roles of detecting and reporting disease and assisting in the investigation. The approach to the investigation of disease outbreaks has been developed and standardized during the last century. The procedure involves making a diagnosis, establishing a case definition, and determining whether or not there is a definite outbreak.

If an outbreak is occurring, the cases of disease are characterized by time (especially using an epidemic time curve), place (usually determining rates in people who live and work in different locations), and person (determining the personal characteristics and patterns of the persons involved in the outbreak and ascertaining how they differ from those of persons not involved). This is followed by the development and testing of hypotheses regarding the source of the infection, the pattern of spread, and the mode of transmission. These hypotheses are tested with cultures, paired sera, analysis for toxins, or case-control studies, depending on the hypotheses. Control measures are initiated as soon as practicable, and follow-up surveillance is initiated to evaluate the control measures.

■ QUESTIONS

Directions (Items 1–12). Each of the numbered items or incomplete statements in this section is followed by answers or by completions of the statement. Select the ONE lettered answer or completion that is BEST in each case. Correct answers and explanations are given at the end of the chapter.

1. An outbreak of disease should be reported to the local or state health department
   - (A) if the diagnosis is uncertain
   - (B) if the disease is infectious
   - (C) if the disease is serious
   - (D) if the outbreak involves at least 10 people
   - (E) under all circumstances

2. Arizona, Colorado, and New Mexico report cases of an unexplained respiratory tract illness with a high case fatality ratio. Which of the following is most reliably true regarding this event?
   - (A) It is an epidemic
   - (B) It is an example of active surveillance
   - (C) It is appropriately investigated by the Centers for Disease Control and Prevention (CDC)
   - (D) It is attributable to improved surveillance
   - (E) It is not an outbreak, since the condition may be endemic

3. Cases of "flesh-eating" group A streptococcal disease are reported in a defined population. Which of the following types of information would be most helpful for determining whether these cases represent a disease outbreak?
   - (A) The clinical features and methods of diagnosing the disease
   - (B) The disease vector and reservoir
   - (C) The exact location and timing of disease onset
   - (D) The incubation period and pattern of disease transmission
   - (E) The usual disease patterns and reporting practices

4. An official from the state department of public health visits outpatient clinics and emergency rooms to determine the number of cases of postexposure prophylaxis for rabies. The official's action is an example of
   - (A) active surveillance
   - (B) case finding
   - (C) outbreak investigation
   - (D) screening
   - (E) secondary prevention

5. An article highlighting the long-term consequences of inadequately treated Lyme disease is published in a medical journal. After a summary of the article appears in popular newspapers and magazines, patients with joint pains begin insisting that their physicians test them for Lyme disease. Cases in which the test results are positive are reported as cases of Lyme borreliosis. This represents
   - (A) a change in reporting that will underestimate prevalence
   - (B) a change in surveillance that will have an unknown effect
   - (C) a change in surveillance that will overestimate the likelihood of an outbreak
   - (D) active surveillance
   - (E) recall bias

Items 6–12

A Democratic president invites a dozen or so of his dearest friends, prominent Republican legislators, to a formal luncheon at the White House. The salmon mousse is even more popular than highlights from the campaign finance reform movement. Within 24 hours, 11 of the 17 diners experience abdominal pain, vomiting, and diarrhea. The president, who happens not to like salmon because it deadens the taste buds to the subtleties of beef jerky, feels fine. In fact, he goes jogging. Of the 11 symptomatic guests, 4 have fever and 7 do not; 5 have an elevated white blood cell count and 6 do not; 6 ate shrimp bisque and 5 did not; 9 ate salmon mousse and 2 did not; and 1 goes on to have surgery for acute cholecystitis resulting from an impacted calculus (stone) in the common bile duct. Of the 11 symptomatic guests, 10 recover within 3 days; the exception is the senator who underwent surgery and recovered over a longer period of time. The guests at this luncheon had shared no other meals at any time recently.

6. The phenomenon described
   - (A) is a coincidence until proved otherwise
   - (B) is a disease outbreak
   - (C) is attributable to bacterial infection
   - (D) is not an outbreak, because the usual pattern of disease is not known
   - (E) should be investigated by the Centers for Disease Control and Prevention (CDC)

7. The attack rate is
   - (A) 4/11
   - (B) 5/11
   - (C) 11/13
   - (D) 1/17
   - (E) 11/17

8. An early priority in investigating the phenomenon would be to
   - (A) close the kitchen temporarily
   - (B) define a case
   - (C) perform a case-control study
   - (D) perform stool tests
   - (E) submit food samples to the laboratory

9. The best case definition for the guests' disease would be
   - (A) abdominal pain, vomiting, and diarrhea within 24 hours of the state luncheon
   - (B) acute viral gastroenteritis
   - (C) staphylococcal food poisoning
   - (D) the onset of abdominal pain and fever following the state luncheon
   - (E) vomiting, diarrhea, and an elevated white blood cell count

10. Suspecting that the disease is the result of a common source exposure involving contaminated food, the investigators attempt to determine which food is responsible. Their initial task is to
    - (A) analyze food specimens in the laboratory
    - (B) close the White House kitchen
    - (C) examine the food preparers
    - (D) interview the symptomatic guests to find out what they ate
    - (E) perform a case-control study

11. The investigators are unable to identify a single food that was eaten by every symptomatic guest. Therefore, they should
    - (A) abandon the investigation, since the disease is not very serious
    - (B) conclude that the disease was not food-borne
    - (C) conclude the investigation but without identifying the source
    - (D) implicate the food least eaten by those without symptoms
    - (E) implicate the food most eaten by those with symptoms

12. The investigators suspect that the salmon mousse is the source of the disease. To confirm or refute their suspicion, they should
    - (A) conduct a prospective study
    - (B) identify the causative agent
    - (C) initiate active surveillance
    - (D) perform a case-control study in which the cases are the guests who ate salmon mousse and the controls are those who did not
    - (E) perform a case-control study in which the cases are the guests who became ill and the controls are those who did not

■ ANSWERS AND EXPLANATIONS

1. **The answer is E: under all circumstances.** By definition, an outbreak represents a deviation from the expected pattern of health and disease in a population. Any outbreak may therefore reveal a new health threat or point to the breakdown of some aspect of the system designed to protect health in the population. Outbreaks of both infectious and noninfectious disease may be equally dangerous and important, and a seemingly mild disease may represent a serious health threat to certain vulnerable populations. Therefore, all suspected outbreaks should be reported to local public health officials to facilitate efficient characterization and control of the threat.

2. **The answer is C: it is appropriately investigated by the Centers for Disease Control and Prevention (CDC).** The respiratory tract illness described in the question is the hantavirus pulmonary syndrome. Because fatalities were reported from more than one state, the investigation of the illness would fall within the jurisdiction of the CDC. Because the case reports were unsolicited, they would be an example of passive surveillance, rather than active surveillance. The question does not provide enough information to determine whether any of the other options are true. To know whether the reported cases constitute an epidemic or an outbreak, the illness would need to be sufficiently characterized to ascertain whether a sudden change in the pattern of disease had occurred. Even if the condition were endemic, this would not exclude the possibility of an outbreak. It is not possible to say whether the case reporting was attributable to improved surveillance, because no information about previous surveillance methods and reporting practices was supplied.

3. **The answer is E: the usual disease patterns and reporting practices.** Steps in the evaluation of an outbreak include the following: establishing a di-

agnosis; developing a case definition; determining whether an outbreak exists; characterizing the outbreak by time, place, and person; developing and testing hypotheses; initiating control measures; and initiating follow-up surveillance. To complete all of these steps, considerable information about the disease in question is required. However, an early determination about the probability of an outbreak is most dependent on knowing the usual disease patterns and knowing the reporting practices that bring the disease to attention. In this case, if group A streptococcal fasciitis does not generally occur at all in the population, then the occurrence of even one correctly reported case might represent an outbreak. Because the disease is severe, the regular occurrence of unreported cases would be unlikely, so even without active surveillance, reporting would probably be fairly reliable and complete. Therefore, although the information provided is extremely limited, this scenario would strongly suggest the occurrence of an outbreak.

4. **The answer is A: active surveillance.** Whenever a public health official visits health care delivery sites to assess the pattern of a disease or condition, the assessment constitutes active surveillance. The question does not provide enough information to determine whether an "outbreak" of rabies exposure is under consideration. Case finding refers to testing a group of patients for a disease that is not yet clinically apparent; an example is taking chest x-rays or electrocardiograms in a group of patients being admitted to the hospital without cough or chest pain. Screening is an effort to identify occult (asymptomatic) disease or risk factors in a population. While case finding takes place in a clinical setting, screening takes place in a community setting. Secondary prevention is an effort to prevent clinical consequences of a disease once the disease is identified. The administration of postexposure rabies vaccines might qualify as secondary prevention, but a public health official's review of cases in which the vaccines were given would not qualify as secondary prevention.

5. **The answer is B: a change in surveillance that will have an unknown effect.** Whenever public attention is focused on a particular health problem, there is likely to be a rise in the number of reported cases of the problem. However, when the available diagnostic tests are imperfect, as is almost always true and is certainly true for Lyme disease, some of the cases reported will be false-positive cases. The number of false-positive cases will rise as more people with vaguely characterized clinical syndromes are tested. In this example, the increased testing may be identifying previously undiagnosed cases of Lyme disease, or it may be producing false-positives. To

distinguish between the two, it would be necessary to know a great deal about the operating characteristics of the tests employed, as well as something about the patients who are insisting that they be tested. Without this additional information, it can only be concluded that surveillance has changed but that the effect of the change is as yet unknown.

6. **The answer is B: is a disease outbreak.** Although there is no formal surveillance of state luncheons, clearly the situation described represents the unexpected occurrence of disease. The usual pattern of disease in this case does not derive from surveillance. Instead, it derives from common experience: nobody expects disease to follow lunch. The Centers for Disease Control and Prevention (CDC) would not investigate so small and localized an outbreak unless for some reason it were invited to do so by local public health officials. Perhaps the Republicans would want the Federal Bureau of Investigation to look over the White House kitchen.

7. **The answer is E: 11/17.** The attack rate is the proportion of those exposed who become ill. As the investigation of this outbreak begins, the exposure is likely to be defined as participation in the luncheon. Of the 17 who dine together, 11 become ill. As the outbreak investigation proceeds, the definition of exposure could change if a particular food, such as the salmon mousse, were implicated. Then the denominator used to calculate the attack rate might change to represent only those exposed to the contaminated food. However, since that information is not yet available, 11/17 represents the best estimate of the attack rate.

8. **The answer is B: define a case.** Establishing a diagnosis or a case definition is the earliest priority in an outbreak investigation. Laboratory tests, control measures, and case-control studies are usually performed later in an investigation, after hypotheses have been generated regarding transmission and cause.

9. **The answer is A: abdominal pain, vomiting, and diarrhea within 24 hours of the state luncheon.** The case definition is required to distinguish between cases and noncases of the disease under investigation. The ideal case definition would permit the inclusion of all cases and the exclusion of all noncases, thereby providing perfect sensitivity and specificity (see Chapter 7). In this instance, the case definition includes the salient clinical features of most affected individuals from the exposed group. It might miss mild forms of the illness or might include in the group of cases someone ill for reasons other than the outbreak exposure. The other answers, however, either invoke a specific diagnosis prematurely or

include clinical features absent in most of the affected cohort.

10. **The answer is D: interview the symptomatic guests to find out what they ate.** Even before developing hypotheses about the source of infection, investigators would have to characterize this outbreak by time, place, and person. In this fairly simple example, virtually all of that information is contained in the case definition, but that is usually not so. The time and place of exposure were the lunch hour at the White House, and the cases were the symptomatic guests. With enough information to generate the hypothesis that this outbreak is due to contaminated food, the investigators can determine what food to implicate. To do so, they must find out what foods were eaten preferentially by the symptomatic guests. A simple interview would be the initial step.

11. **The answer is E: implicate the food most eaten by those with symptoms.** The methodology detailed in the text provides the basic means to conduct an outbreak investigation. There is, however, no substitute for rigorous thinking. At the stage of hypothesis generation, it is rare for the exact source of the outbreak to be completely obvious. Often, even if a particular food is suspected in an outbreak such as this one, the suspected food will have been eaten by some people who avoided becoming ill (the noncases) and will have been avoided by some of the people who did become ill (the cases). Avoidance of illness could occur if the contaminated food were not uniformly contaminated, with some portions free or relatively free of the pathogenic agent. Illness in those avoiding the contaminated food could occur if this food came into contact with other foods on a platter. An outbreak investigation is usually conducted while the outbreak is occurring and before it is clear how severe or protracted the outbreak will be. Therefore, if possible, the investigation should be conducted to its conclusion. The food least eaten by noncases would be a possible source of the outbreak only if that food were eaten by the majority of cases. (Otherwise, it might simply be a dish that no one liked.)

12. **The answer is E: perform a case-control study in which the cases are the guests who became ill and the controls are those who did not.** A case-control study is one in which the cases have the disease under investigation, the controls do not, and both groups are then assessed for prior exposures (see Chapter 5). Cases, as stipulated by the case definition, are luncheon participants who had abdominal pain, vomiting, and diarrhea within 24 hours of the state luncheon. Controls would be luncheon participants who did not become ill. Both groups would be interviewed about the consumption of particular foods, including the salmon mousse. If it turned out that most cases and few controls had eaten this dish, the hypothesis would be supported. An additional, important means of testing the hypothesis would be to analyze the suspected food in the laboratory and look for a pathogen or toxin that would explain the clinical syndrome. This step is usually done to confirm a diagnosis and facilitate control measures, rather than to establish the source of the outbreak.

References Cited

Benenson, A. S. Control of Communicable Diseases in Man, 16th ed. Washington, D. C., American Public Health Association, 1995.

Brooks-Robinson, S., S. D. Helgerson, and J. F. Jekel. An epidemiologic investigation of putative cancer clusters in two Connecticut towns. Journal of Environmental Health 50:161–164, 1987.

Centers for Disease Control and Prevention. Case definitions for infectious conditions under public health surveillance. Morbidity and Mortality Weekly Report 46(RR-10), 1997.

Centers for Disease Control and Prevention. Expanded tuberculosis surveillance and tuberculosis morbidity in the United States, 1993. Morbidity and Mortality Weekly Report 43:361–366, 1993.

Centers for Disease Control and Prevention. Progress toward the elimination of tuberculosis, United States, 1998. Morbidity and Mortality Weekly Report 48:732–736, 1999a.

Centers for Disease Control and Prevention. Recommended childhood immunization schedule, United States, 1999. Morbidity and Mortality Weekly Report 48:12–16, 1999b.

Centers for Disease Control and Prevention. Surveillance for emergency events involving hazardous substances, United States, 1990–1992. Morbidity and Mortality Weekly Report 43(SS-2): 1–6, 1994.

Harkess, J. F., et al. Is passive surveillance always insensitive? American Journal of Epidemiology 128:878–881, 1988.

Harrison, T. R., et al. Principles of Internal Medicine, 3rd ed. New York, McGraw-Hill Book Company, 1958.

Helgerson, S. D., J. F. Jekel, and J. L. Hadler. Training public health students to investigate disease outbreaks: examples of community service. Public Health Reports 103:72–76, 1988.

Herbst, A. L., H. Ulfelder, and D. C. Poskanzer. Adenocarcinoma of the vagina: association of maternal stilbestrol therapy with tumor appearance in young women. New England Journal of Medicine 284:878–881, 1971.

Jacquez, G. M., ed. Workshop on Statistics and Computing in Disease Clustering. Statistics in Medicine 12:1751–1968, 1993.

MacKenzie, W. R., et al. A massive outbreak in Milwaukee of *Cryptosporidium* infection transmitted through the public water supply. New England Journal of Medicine 331:161–167, 1994.

National Conference on Clustering of Health Events. American Journal of Epidemiology 132:S1–202, 1990.

Roueché, B. The Medical Detectives. New York, Truman Talley Books, 1991.

Slutsker, L., et al. Eosinophilia-myalgia syndrome associated with exposure to tryptophan from a single manufacturer. Journal of the American Medical Association 264:213–217, 1990.

Selected Readings

Centers for Disease Control. Guidelines for evaluating surveillance systems. Morbidity and Mortality Weekly Report 37(S-5):1–19, 1988. [Surveillance.]

Centers for Disease Control and Prevention. Case definitions for infectious conditions under public health surveillance. Morbidity and Mortality Weekly Report 46(RR-10), 1997. [Surveillance.]

Epidemiology Program Office, Centers for Disease Control and Prevention. Principles of Epidemiology: Self-Study Course 3030-G, 2nd ed. Atlanta, Centers for Disease Control and Prevention, 1992. [Outbreak investigation.]

Goodman, R. A., J. W. Buehler, and J. P. Koplan. The epidemiologic field investigation: science and judgment in public health practice. American Journal of Epidemiology 132:9–16, 1990. [Outbreak investigation.]

Gregg, M. B., and J. Parsonnet. The principles of an epidemic field investigation. *In* Holland, W. W., et al., eds. Oxford Textbook of Public Health, 2nd ed. Oxford, Oxford University Press, 1991. [Outbreak investigation.]

Kelsey, J. L., et al. Methods in Observational Epidemiology, 2nd ed. New York, Oxford University Press, 1996. [Outbreak investigation; see especially Chapter 11, entitled Epidemic Investigation.]

Langmuir, A. D. The surveillance of communicable diseases of national importance. New England Journal of Medicine 268: 182–192, 1963. [Surveillance.]

Rhot, L. H., et al. Principles of Epidemiology: A Self-Teaching Guide. New York, Academic Press, 1982. [Outbreak investigation.]

4 The Study of Causation in Epidemiologic Investigation and Research

Epidemiologists are frequently involved in studies to determine causation—that is, to find the specific cause or causes of a disease. This is a more difficult and elusive task than might be supposed, and it leaves considerable room for obfuscation, as was demonstrated in an article in *The New York Times* (September 24, 1991) that focused on cigarette smoking. In this article, Thomas Lauria, a spokesman for the Tobacco Institute (a trade association for cigarette manufacturers) was quoted as saying that he did "not deny that smoking was a risk factor, though not a cause, of a variety of diseases."

Is a risk factor, then, a cause, or is it not? To answer this question, this chapter begins with a review of basic concepts concerning causation.

◼ TYPES OF CAUSAL RELATIONSHIP

Most scientific research seeks to identify causal relationships. The three fundamental types of causation, which are discussed below in the order of decreasing strength or sufficiency as a cause, are (1) a sufficient cause, (2) a necessary cause, and (3) a risk factor (Box 4–1).

Sufficient Cause

A sufficient cause precedes a disease and has the following relationship with it: if the cause is present, the disease will always occur. Examples in which this proposition holds true are rare, apart from certain genetic abnormalities that, if homozygous, inevitably lead to a fatal disease (e.g., Tay-Sachs disease).

Smoking is not a sufficient cause of bronchogenic lung cancer, because many people who smoke do not acquire lung cancer before they die of something else. It is not known whether all smokers would get lung cancer if they lived and smoked long enough, but within the human life span, smoking cannot be considered a sufficient cause of lung cancer.

Necessary Cause

A necessary cause precedes a disease and has the following relationship with it: the cause must be present for the disease to occur. However, the necessary cause may be present without the disease occurring. For example, in the absence of the organism *Mycobacterium tuberculosis*, the disease tuberculosis cannot occur. Therefore, *M. tuberculosis* can be called a necessary cause, or prerequisite, of tuberculosis. It cannot be called a sufficient cause of tuberculosis, however, because it is possible for people to carry the organism in their bodies for decades and yet have no symptoms of the disease.

The initial exposure to *M. tuberculosis* usually leads to a primary infection with few or no symptoms. Primary tuberculosis commonly leaves a healed lesion filled with dormant mycobacteria at the initial infection site in the lungs, in the hilar lymph nodes, or in both locations. The mycobacteria remain alive for the rest of the infected person's life, as demonstrated by the results of skin testing with purified protein derivative (PPD). The mycobacteria usually remain dormant, held in check by the cell-mediated immunity that developed during the first infection. If there is a decline in cell-mediated immunity against the mycobacteria, however, the organisms may reactivate and cause a recurrence of clinical disease, although this may be decades after the original infection.

Cigarette smoking is not a necessary cause of bronchogenic lung cancer, because lung cancer can and does occur in the absence of both active and pas-

---

> **BOX 4–1   Types of Causal Relationship**
>
> **Sufficient cause:** If the factor (cause) is present, the effect (disease) will always occur.
>
> **Necessary cause:** The factor (cause) must be present for the effect (disease) to occur. However, a necessary cause may be present without the disease occurring.
>
> **Risk factor:** If the factor is present, the probability that the effect will occur is increased.
>
> **Directly causal association:** The factor exerts its effect in the absence of intermediary factors (intervening variables).
>
> **Indirectly causal association:** The factor exerts its effect via intermediary factors.
>
> **Noncausal association:** The relationship between two variables is statistically significant, but no causal relationship exists, either because the temporal relationship is incorrect (the presumed cause comes after, rather than before, the presumed effect) or because another factor is responsible for both the presumed cause and the presumed effect.

---

sive cigarette smoking. Furthermore, exposure to other agents, such as radon gas, radiation, arsenic, asbestos, chromium, nickel, coal tar, and some organic chemicals, has been shown to be associated with lung cancer, even in the absence of cigarette smoking (Doll and Peto 1981).

Risk Factor

A risk factor is a characteristic that, if present and active, clearly increases the probability of a particular disease in a group of persons who have the risk factor compared with an otherwise similar group of persons who do not. A risk factor, however, is neither a necessary cause nor a sufficient cause of the disease. Even though smoking is the most important risk factor for bronchogenic carcinoma, producing up to 20 times as high a risk of lung cancer in males who are heavy smokers as in males who are nonsmokers, smoking is neither a sufficient cause nor a necessary cause of lung cancer.

What about the quotation cited above, in which the spokesman from the Tobacco Institute did "not deny that smoking was a risk factor, though not a cause, of a variety of diseases"? If by "cause" the speaker includes only necessary and sufficient causes, he is correct. If, however, the concept of causation includes those situations in which the presence of the risk factor clearly increases the probability of the disease, he is wrong. The overwhelming proportion of scientists who have studied the question of smoking and lung cancer (98% of them, according to the article in *The New York Times*) believe that cigarette smoking is a cause of lung cancer and, in fact, is the most important cause, despite the fact that it is neither a necessary nor a sufficient cause of the disease.

Causal and Noncausal Associations

The first and most basic requirement for a causal relationship to exist is that there must be an **association** between the outcome of interest (e.g., a disease or death) and the presumed cause. This means that the outcome must occur either clearly more often or clearly less often in individuals who are exposed to the presumed cause than in those who are not exposed to it. In other words, exposure to the presumed cause must make a difference, or it is not a cause. Some difference would be expected to occur as a result of random variation; therefore, in order to be a **statistically significant association,** the difference must be large enough to be "unlikely" if the exposure really had no effect. As discussed in Chapter 10, "unlikely" is usually defined as being likely to occur no more than 1 time in 20 opportunities (i.e., 5% of the time, or 0.05) by chance alone.

If an association is causal, the causal pathway may be direct or indirect. The classification here depends on the absence or presence of **intermediary factors,** which are called **intervening variables.**

A **directly causal association** occurs when the factor under consideration exerts its effect without intermediary factors. For example, a severe blow to the head will cause brain damage and death without other external causes being required.

An **indirectly causal association** occurs when one factor influences one or more other factors that are, in turn, directly causal. For example, poverty per se may not cause disease and death, but by preventing adequate nutrition, housing, and medical care, it may lead to ill health and premature death. In this case, the nutrition, housing, and medical care would be called intervening variables. Education appears to lead to better health indirectly, presumably because it increases the amount of knowledge about health, the level of motivation to maintain health, and the extent of financial resources.

A statistical association may be strong and yet not be causal; in this case, it would be called a **noncausal association.** One of the most important principles of data analysis is that association does *not* prove causation. If a statistically significant association is found between two variables but the presumed cause occurs after the effect (rather than before it), the association is not causal. Likewise, if a statistically significant association is found between two variables but some other factor causes both the presumed cause and the effect, the association is not causal. For example, baldness may be associated with the risk of coronary artery disease, but it is probably a noncausal association, because both baldness and coronary artery disease are functions of age and gender.

■ STEPS IN THE DETERMINATION OF CAUSE AND EFFECT

Investigators must have a model of causation to guide their thinking. The scientific method for determining causation can be summarized as having three steps, which should be considered in the following order: (1) investigation of the statistical association, (2) investigation of the temporal relationship, and (3) elimination of all known alternative explanations (Bauman 1980). These steps in epidemiologic studies are similar in many ways to the steps followed in murder investigations, as discussed below.

Investigation of the Statistical Association

Investigations may test hypotheses about risk factors or protective factors. For causation to be identified, the presumed **risk factor** must be present significantly more often in persons with the particular disease of interest than in persons without the disease. Moreover, this difference must be large enough to be considered statistically significant in order to eliminate most chance differences. Conversely, the presumed **protective factor** must be present significantly less often in those with the disease than in those without it. When the presumed factor (either a risk factor or a protective factor) is not associated with a different frequency of disease, the factor cannot be considered causal. It might be argued that something else could be obscuring a real association between the factor and the disease. If that occurs, however, this principle is not violated, because proper research design and statistical analysis would demonstrate the real association.

While the first step in an epidemiologic study is to demonstrate statistical association between the presumed risk or protective factor and the disease, the equivalent first step in a murder investigation is to demonstrate a geographic and temporal association between the accused murderer and the victim—that is, to show that both were in the same place at the same time or that the murderer was in a place from which he or she could have caused the murder.

The relationship between smoking and lung cancer provides an example of how an association can lead to the understanding of causation. The earliest epidemiologic studies showed that smokers had an average overall death rate approximately 2 times that for nonsmokers, and the studies also indicated that the death rate for lung cancer among all smokers was approximately 10 times that among nonsmokers (see US Surgeon General 1964). These studies led to other research efforts, which clarified the role of cigarette smoking as a risk factor for lung cancer and for many other diseases as well.

In epidemiologic studies, the research design must allow a statistical association to be shown, if it exists. This usually means comparing the rate of disease before and after an intervention or comparing groups with and without the exposure or the treatment. Statistical analysis is needed to demonstrate that the difference associated with the intervention or exposure is greater than would be expected by chance alone, as well as to estimate how large this difference is. Research design and statistical analysis, therefore, work

closely together. (For a detailed discussion of the types of research design, see Chapter 5.)

If a statistically significant difference in risk of disease or rate of recovery is seen, the investigator must first consider the direction and extent of the difference: Did the therapy make the patients better or worse, on the average? Was the difference large enough to be etiologically or clinically important? Even if the difference observed is real and large, statistical association does not prove causation. It may initially appear that an association is causal, when in fact it is not. For example, in the era before antibiotics were developed, syphilis was treated with arsenic compounds (e.g., salvarsan), despite their toxicity. An outbreak of fever and jaundice occurred in many of the patients treated with arsenicals (see Anderson, Arnstein, and Lester 1962). At the time, it seemed obvious to those concerned that the outbreak was due to the arsenic. Many years later, however, medical experts realized that the outbreak of fever and jaundice was most likely due to an infectious agent—probably hepatitis B or C virus—spread via the use of inadequately sterilized needles during the administration of the arsenic compounds.

There are several criteria that, if met, increase the probability that a statistical association is causal (Susser 1973). Many of the criteria can be traced back to the philosopher John Stuart Mill (1856) and are often called **Mill's canons.** In general, an association is more likely to be causal if the following are true: (1) The association shows **strength**—i.e., the difference is large. (2) The association demonstrates **consistency**—i.e., the difference is always observed if the risk factor is present. (3) The association shows **specificity**—i.e., the difference does not appear if the risk factor is not present. (4) The association has **biologic plausibility**—i.e., it makes sense, based on what is known about the natural history of the disease. (5) The association exhibits a **dose-response relationship**—i.e., the risk of disease is greater with stronger exposures to the risk factor (Box 4–2).

An example of a dose-response relationship is shown in Fig. 4–1 and is based on an early study of cigarette smoking and lung cancer. In this study, Doll and Hill (1956) found the following rates of lung cancer deaths, expressed as the number of deaths per 100,000 population per year: 7 deaths in men who did not smoke; 47 deaths in men who smoked about one-half pack of cigarettes a day; 86 deaths in men

---

BOX 4–2   Statistical Association and Causality

The following factors increase the likelihood that a statistical association is causal:

(1) the **strength** of the association
(2) the **consistency** of the association
(3) the **specificity** of the association
(4) the **biologic plausibility** of the association
(5) the presence of a **dose-response relationship**

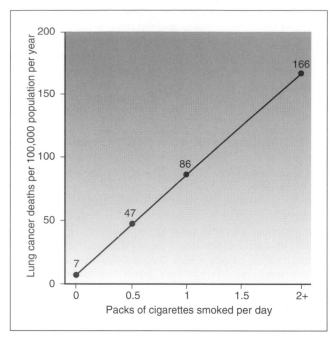

FIGURE 4–1   An example of a dose-response relationship in epidemiology. The *x*-axis is the approximate "dose" of cigarettes per day, and the *y*-axis is the rate of deaths from lung cancer. (Source of data: Doll, R., and A. B. Hill. Lung cancer and other causes of death in relation to smoking. British Medical Journal 2:1071, 1956.)

who smoked about one pack a day; and 166 deaths in men who smoked two or more packs a day.

Even if all of the above-mentioned criteria for an association hold true, the proof of a causal relationship will also depend on the demonstration of the necessary temporal relationship and the elimination of alternative explanations, which are the next two steps discussed below.

Investigation of the Temporal Relationship

Although some philosophical traditions consider time as circular, Western science assumes that time runs only one way. To demonstrate causation, the suspected causal factor must have occurred or been present before the effect (e.g., the disease) developed. This is more complex than it might seem unless **experimental control**—i.e., randomization followed by measurement of the risk factor and disease in both groups before and after the experimental intervention—is possible.

With chronic diseases, the onset of the "effect" is often unclear: When did atherosclerosis begin? When did the first bronchial cell become cancerous? Likewise, the onset of the risk factor may be unclear: When did the blood pressure begin to rise? When did the diet first become unhealthy? Because of long but varying **latent periods** between the onset of risk factors and the onset of the diseases they cause, the temporal relationships may be obscured.

Research design has an important role in determining the temporal sequence of cause and effect (see Chapter 5). If information on both the cause and the effect is obtained simultaneously, as in a survey, it is difficult to decide whether the presumed cause or the effect began first. On the one hand, basic demographic variables such as gender and race—factors that are present from birth—presumably would have begun to have an effect before diseases caused by external risk factors began. On the other hand, it is often impossible in a survey or in a single medical visit to determine which variables occurred first.

With respect to temporal relationships, parallels can again be drawn between epidemiologic investigations and murder investigations. In the case of a murder, the accused individual not only must have been with the victim at some time but also must have been with the victim immediately preceding the death (unless some remote technique was used). In murder mysteries, the innocent but accused individual often stumbles onto the scene immediately after the murder has taken place and is discovered there bending over the body. The task of the attorney is to demonstrate that the accused individual actually appeared after the murder and that someone else was there at the time of the murder.

The following discussion of prenatal care illustrates the difficulties that epidemiologists encounter when trying to determine the temporal relationship of events. Essentially every analysis of prenatal care in the literature demonstrates a direct (positive) association between the number of prenatal visits and the health of the infant, whether health is measured in terms of birth weight or survival (which are closely associated), and this relationship holds even if maternal socioeconomic status and education are controlled. This would seem to provide direct evidence of the benefit of prenatal care on the pregnancy and infant, but a major problem arises. Prenatal visits are made with increasing frequency as the pregnancy nears term, often weekly in the last 4 weeks and biweekly in the 2 months before that. A pregnancy that terminates at 36 weeks of gestation will, on the average, have had 4 fewer prenatal visits than a pregnancy that terminates at 40 weeks of gestation, regardless of the reason that the pregnancy ended early. Therefore, any cause that induces preterm delivery will also produce a reduced number of prenatal visits (Fig. 4–2). Studies that attempted to control for this problem have suggested that prenatal care does provide some benefits to the child, but the magnitude of these benefits is smaller than the crude association would suggest.

Elimination of All Known Alternative Explanations

In a murder case, the verdict of "not guilty"—i.e., "not proved beyond a reasonable doubt"—can usually be obtained for the accused person if that person's attorney can demonstrate that there are other possible scenarios for what happened and that one of them is at least as likely as the scenario that implicates his or her client. For example, evidence that another person was at the scene of the crime and had a murder motive as great as or greater than that of the accused person would usually cast sufficient doubt on the guilt of the latter to result in an acquittal.

In the case of an epidemiologic investigation concerning the causation of disease, even if the presumed causal factor is associated statistically with the disease and occurs before the disease appears, it is necessary to demonstrate that there are no other likely explanations for the association.

On the one hand, proper research design can reduce the likelihood of competing causal explanations. For example, randomization, if done correctly, ensures that neither self-selection nor investigator bias will influence the allocation of subjects into experimental and control groups. Randomization also means that the treatment and control groups should be reasonably comparable with regard to disease susceptibility and disease severity. Hard work by the investigator can reduce measurement bias (discussed in detail below) and other potential problems, such as a difference between the number of subjects lost during the follow-up of each group.

On the other hand, the criterion that all alternative explanations be eliminated can *never* be fully met for all time, because it is violated as soon as someone proposes a new explanation that fits the data and cannot be ruled out. For example, the classic theory of the origin of peptic ulcers (stress and hypersecretion) has been challenged by the theory that *Helicobacter pylori* infection is an important cause of these ulcers. The fact that scientific explanations are always tentative—even when they seem perfectly satisfactory and meet the criteria concerning statistical association, timing, and elimination of known

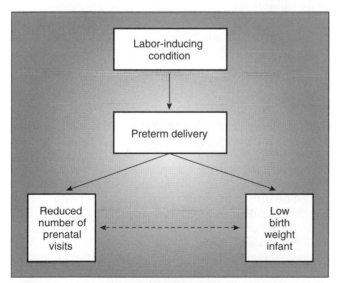

FIGURE 4–2 An illustration of causal association (arrows with solid lines) and possible noncausal association (arrow with dotted lines) in studies of infant birth weights and prenatal care.

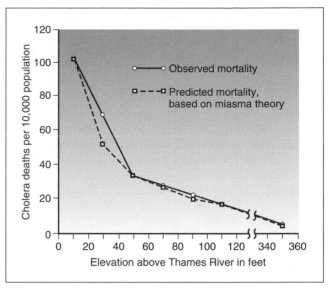

FIGURE 4–3 Predicted and observed cholera rates at various levels of elevation above the Thames River in London, England, in 1849. (Reproduced with permission from Langmuir, A. D. Epidemiology of airborne infection. Bacteriological Reviews 24: 173–181, 1961.)

alternatives—is demonstrated in the following additional examples concerning the causation of cholera, coronary heart disease, and eosinophilia-myalgia syndrome.

An Alternative Explanation for Cholera in 1849

In 1849, there was an almost exact correspondence between the predicted cholera rates and the observed cholera rates in London, England, at various levels of elevation above the Thames River, as shown in Fig. 4–3. The accuracy of the prediction of cholera rates in London was hailed as an impressive confirmation of miasma theory, on which the rates had been based (Langmuir 1961). According to this theory, cholera was due to "miasmas" (noxious vapors), which have their highest and most dangerous concentrations at low elevations. Subsequently, the germ theory of cholera became popular, and this theory is held to the present. Although nobody accepts the miasma theory today, it would be difficult to improve on the 1849 prediction of the cholera rates that were based on that theory.

Alternative Explanations for Coronary Heart Disease

Several recent studies of atherosclerosis and myocardial infarction have questioned the adequacy of the reigning paradigm of hyperlipidemia, hypertension, and smoking as the causes of coronary heart disease.

A few years ago, the primary challenge to the hyperlipidemia hypothesis was that excess levels of iron in the body caused coronary atheromas by oxidizing cholesterol (Sullivan 1981; Salonen et al. 1992). However, the fact that treatment of hyperlipidemia with the so-called statin drugs (e.g., atorvastatin, fluvastatin, lovastatin, pravastatin, and simvastatin) reduced the number of negative cardiac events has convinced most investigators that iron is not an important factor in coronary heart disease.

Newer hypotheses concern the role of chronic inflammation in the development of coronary atheromas (Danesh, Collins, and Peto 1997). Chronic inflammation can produce endothelial damage, with thrombi forming on the damaged vessel walls. It can also produce hypercoagulability and cause activation of macrophages. Once atheromatous plaques have formed, chronic infection can produce plaque instability. In experimental studies, Fabricant et al. (1978) showed that when germ-free chickens were infected with a bird herpesvirus, they developed atherosclerosis-like arterial disease. More recently, investigators have found higher rates of coronary artery disease in patients who have evidence of one of several types of infection, particularly infection with a gram-negative bacterium (such as *Chlamydia pneumoniae* or *Helicobacter pylori)* or with certain herpesviruses (especially cytomegalovirus). They have also found higher rates of coronary artery disease in patients with chronic periodontal infection and in patients who have certain blood factors that are associated with acute or chronic infection (such as C-reactive protein and serum amyloid A protein). In a randomized clinical trial of antibiotic treatment for *C. pneumoniae* infection, Gurfinkel et al. (1997) showed that treatment with roxithromycin reduced the number of negative cardiac events in patients with unstable angina or non–Q-wave myocardial infarction.

Reigning hypotheses are always open to challenge. Whether or not the chronic inflammation hypothesis is supported by further research, the cholesterol hypothesis can be expected to face challenges by other hypotheses in the 21st century.

Alternative Explanations for Eosinophilia-Myalgia Syndrome

Another example of an explanation that met the causal criteria of association and temporal sequence and yet was replaced by a better hypothesis was the association of eosinophilia-myalgia syndrome (EMS) with the use of dietary supplements of L-tryptophan, an amino acid.

Initially, investigators thought that high doses of the amino acid were responsible for EMS. Subsequently, however, this hypothesis was replaced by a new one, based on the discovery that essentially all of the EMS patients had used L-tryptophan from only one of the two primary chemical companies making the supplements, the Showa-Denka Company in Japan, which had switched to a new strain of bacteria in the company's fermentation process. This new strain, investigators discovered, produced an unknown substance or substances (called "peak E" in chromatographic studies) that were contained in the L-tryptophan pills and were probably responsible for the EMS (Slutsker et al. 1990; Belongia et al. 1990; Philen et al. 1993).

> **BOX 4–3   Common Pitfalls in Causal Research**
>
> **Bias:** A differential error that usually produces findings consistently distorted in one direction, owing to nonrandom factors.
> **Random error:** A nondifferential error that produces findings that are too high and too low in approximately equal amounts, owing to random factors.
> **Confounding:** The confusion of two supposedly causal variables, so that part or all of the purported effect of one variable is actually due to the other.
> **Synergism:** The interaction of two or more presumably causal variables, so that the total effect is clearly greater than the sum of the individual effects.
> **Effect modification (interaction):** A phenomenon in which a third variable alters the direction or strength of association between two other variables.

■ COMMON PITFALLS IN CAUSAL RESEARCH

Among the most frequently encountered pitfalls in causal research are bias, random error, confounding, synergism, and effect modification, each of which is defined in Box 4–3 and discussed below.

Bias

Bias, also known as **differential error,** is a dangerous source of error in epidemiologic research. Bias usually produces deviations or distortions that tend to go in one direction. Bias becomes a problem when it weakens a true association, produces a spurious association, or distorts the apparent direction of association between variables.

So many sources of bias in research have been identified that a list of them can be somewhat overwhelming. It is easiest to think of the chronologic sequence of a clinical trial (see Chapter 5) and categorize biases as forms of assembly bias or detection bias.

Assembly Bias

The first step in a clinical trial involves assembling the groups of subjects to be studied. If the characteristics of the intervention group and those of the control group are not comparable at the start, then differences in the results (outcomes) seen in the groups might be due to assembly bias instead of being due to the intervention itself. Assembly bias may take the form of selection bias or allocation bias.

Selection Bias. Selection bias results when subjects are self-selected into study groups. If subjects are allowed to choose which study group they will be in, those who are more educated, more adventuresome, or more health-conscious may want to try a new therapy or preventive measure. Differences subsequently found may be partly or entirely due to differences between the subjects rather than to the effect of the intervention.

Selection bias may be found in studies of treatment methods for terminal diseases. In such studies, the most severely ill patients are often the ones who are the most willing to try a new treatment, despite its known or unknown dangers. This is presumably because these patients believe that they have little to lose. Because of self-selection, a new treatment might be given to the patients who are sickest, with relatively poor results. These results could not be fairly compared with those among patients who were not as sick.

Allocation Bias. Allocation bias may occur if investigators choose a nonrandom method of assigning subjects to study groups. It may also occur if a random method is chosen but not followed by everyone involved in a clinical trial. In one study, for example, the investigators thought that patients were being randomly assigned to care on the teaching service or the nonteaching service of a university-affiliated hospital, but when early data were analyzed, it was discovered that the randomization process tended to be bypassed, particularly at night, to ensure that "interesting" patients were allocated to the teaching service (Garrell and Jekel 1979). In clinical trials, maintaining the randomization process also requires resisting the pressures of study subjects who want to be placed in the group that will receive a new form of treatment or preventive care (Lam, Hartwell, and Jekel 1994).

Associated Problems of Validity. Randomized clinical trials must allow potential study subjects to participate or not, as they choose. This introduces an element of self-selection into the participant group before randomization into study groups even takes place. Because of randomization, the results are presumed to have **internal validity** (i.e., validity for participants in the study). However, it may be unclear to whom the results can be generalized, because the self-selected study group is not really representative of any population. In other words, the study may lack **external validity.**

A good illustration of these problems occurred in the 1954 polio vaccine trials, which involved one intervention group and two control groups (Francis et al. 1955). Earlier studies of paralytic poliomyelitis had shown that the rates of this disease were greater in upper socioeconomic groups than in lower socioeconomic groups. When a polio vaccine was first developed, some parents (usually those with more education) wanted their children to have a chance to receive the vaccine, so they agreed to let their children be randomly assigned to either the intervention group (the group to be immunized) or the primary control group (control group I), who received a placebo injection. Other parents (usually those with less education) stated that they did not want their children to be "guinea pigs" and receive the vaccine; their children were followed as a secondary control group (control group II). The investigators correctly predicted that the rate of poliomyelitis would be greater in control group I, whose parents were of a higher socioeconomic level, than in control group II, whose socioeconomic status was lower. During the study period, the rate of paralytic poliomyelitis was 0.057% in control group I but only 0.035% in control group II.

Questions of generalizability (external validity) have arisen in regard to the Physicians' Health Study, a costly but well-performed field trial involving the use of aspirin to reduce cardiovascular events and the use of beta-carotene to prevent cancer (see Physicians' Health Study Steering Committee 1989). The approximately 22,000 participants in the study were US physicians who were men between 40 and 75 years of age and met the exclusion criteria (baseline criteria) of never having had heart disease, cancer, gastrointestinal disease, a bleeding tendency, or an allergy to aspirin. The early participants had agreed to take part in the study, but after a trial period, those with poor compliance were dropped. To what group of people in the population can investigators generalize the results obtained from a study of predominantly white, exclusively male, compliant, middle-aged or older physicians who were in good health at the start? The results certainly cannot be generalized to women and young men, and they probably cannot be generalized to nonwhite individuals, to members of the lower socioeconomic groups, or to persons with the excluded health problems.

Detection Bias

Once a clinical study is under way, the investigators focus on detecting and measuring causal factors (e.g., high-fat diet or smoking) and the outcomes of interest (e.g., disease or death) in the study groups. Care must be taken to ensure that the differences observed in the groups are not attributable to measurement bias or recall bias (discussed below) or other forms of detection bias.

Detection bias may simply be the result of failure to detect a case of disease, a possible causal factor, or an outcome of interest. For example, in a study of a certain type of lung disease, if the case group consists of individuals receiving care in the pulmonary service of a hospital while the control group consists of individuals in the community, early disease among the controls may not be detected because they did not receive the intensive medical evaluation that the hospitalized patients received. This might reduce the apparent effect of a true cause of the disease. There may also be detection bias if the groups of study subjects have large differences in their rates of loss to follow-up. In some clinical trials, those who are lost to follow-up may be sicker than those who remain under observation; in other clinical trials, those who are lost to follow-up may be the healthiest subjects.

Measurement Bias. Measurement bias may occur in collecting baseline data or follow-up data. Bias could result, for example, from measuring the height of patients with their shoes on, in which case all the heights would be too great, or measuring the weight of patients with their clothes on, in which case all the weights would be too large. Even this is complicated, because the heels of men's shoes may differ in height from those of women's shoes and also because there will be variation in heel size within each group. Nevertheless, all people measured with their shoes on will be overmeasured to some extent.

In the case of blood pressure values, bias can occur if some investigators or some study sites have blood pressure cuffs that measure incorrectly and cause the measurements to be higher or lower than the true values. Chemistry data from various medical laboratories are subject to bias. Some laboratories consistently report higher or lower values than other laboratories because of the use of different methods. Clinical investigators who collect laboratory data over time in the same institution or who compare laboratory data from different institutions must obtain the normal standards for each laboratory at the appropriate times and adjust their findings accordingly. For example, differences in reported blood glucose levels are meaningful only if adjusted to the same level of "normal." The differences in laboratory standards are a potential source of bias that can be corrected by the investigator.

Recall Bias. Recall bias may occur when people who have experienced an adverse event, such as a disease, cogitate more about why the event might have happened and therefore are more likely to recall previous risk factors than people who have never experienced the event. All study subjects may forget some information, but bias results when the members of one study group are more likely to remember events than are members of the other study group. Recall bias is a major problem in research into causes of congenital anomalies. For example, mothers who give birth to abnormal infants tend to think more about their pregnancy and are more likely to remember infections, medications, and injuries. This may produce a spurious (falsely positive) association between a risk factor (such as respiratory infections) and the outcome (congenital abnormality).

Random Error

Random error, also known as **nondifferential error,** produces findings that are too high and too low in approximately equal amounts, owing to random factors. Even though it is a serious problem, random error is ordinarily less serious than bias because it is less likely to distort (i.e., reverse the direction of) findings. It does, however, decrease the probability of finding a real association by reducing the statistical power of a study (Kelsey et al. 1996).

Confounding

Confounding (from the Latin meaning "to pour together") is the confusion of two supposedly causal variables, so that part or all of the purported effect of one variable is actually due to the other. For example, the percentage of gray hairs on the heads of adults is associated with the risk of myocardial infarction, but presumably that is not a causal association. Age increases both the proportion of gray hairs and the risk of myocardial infarction.

The next example is similar but concerns the risks of breast cancer. Women who had high parity (had given birth to many children) were found to have lower rates of breast cancer, and investigators assumed that childbearing was protective against subsequent breast cancer. Later, it was discovered that the best predictor was childbearing at an early age. When the woman's age at the time of her first delivery was entered into statistical analyses, the number of offspring no longer predicted the rate of breast cancer. As Fig. 4–4 shows, because childbearing at a young age was associated with high parity, there was an association between parity and breast cancer, but apparently it was not causal (Kelsey et al. 1996).

Confounding can also obscure a true causal relationship, as illustrated by a final example. In the early 1970s, one of the authors (JFJ) and a colleague were involved in a study of the predictors for educational success among teenage mothers. Analysis of the data concerning these young women revealed that both their age and their grade level were positively associated with their ultimate educational success: the older a young mother was and the higher her grade level in school, the more likely she was to stay in school and graduate. But age was strongly associated with grade level in school (the older she was, the more likely she was to be in a high grade). When the effect of age was studied *within* each grade level, age was shown to be negatively associated with educational success. That is, the older a teenage mother was for a given grade level, the less successful she was (Klerman and Jekel 1973). This was apparently due to the fact that a woman who was old for a given grade level had been kept back because of academic or social difficulties, which were negative predictors of success. Thus, one important aspect of the association of age and educational success was obscured by its confounding with grade level.

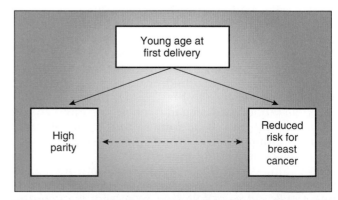

FIGURE 4–4   An illustration of causal association (arrows with solid lines) and noncausal association (arrow with dotted lines) in studies of childbearing and breast cancer.

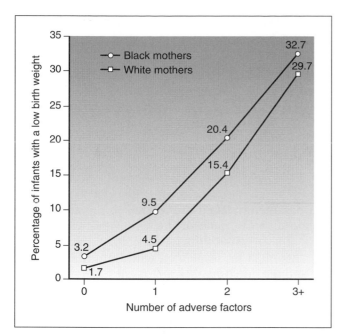

FIGURE 4–5   Relationship between the percentage of infants with a low birth weight and the number of adverse factors present during the pregnancy. Low birth weight was defined as 2500 g or less, and examples of adverse factors were teenage pregnancy and maternal smoking. (Source of data: Miller, H. C., and J. F. Jekel. Incidence of low birth weight infants born to mothers with multiple risk factors. Yale Journal of Biology and Medicine 60:397–404, 1987.)

Synergism

Synergism (from the Greek meaning "to work together") is the interaction of two or more presumably causal variables, so that the combined effect is clearly greater than the sum of the individual effects. For example, the risk of lung cancer is greater when a person has exposure to both asbestos and smoking than would be expected on the basis of summing the observed risks from each factor acting alone (Hammond, Selikoff, and Seidman 1979).

Fig. 4–5 shows the relationship between the percentage of infants with a low birth weight and the number of adverse factors present during the pregnancy. Low birth weight in this study was defined as 2500 g or less, and examples of adverse factors were teenage pregnancy and maternal smoking. For infants with white mothers, the risk was 1.7% (12/708) if no adverse factor was present; 4.5% (32/715) if one adverse factor was present; 15.4% (35/228) if two adverse factors were present; and 29.7% (19/64) if three or more adverse factors were present (Miller and Jekel 1987). Similarly, for infants with black mothers, the figure shows how adverse factors interacted synergistically to produce low birth weight infants.

Effect Modification (Interaction)

Sometimes the direction or strength of association between two variables will differ depending on the value of a third variable. This is usually called **effect modification** by epidemiologists and **interaction** by biostatisticians.

A biologic example of effect modification is seen in the ways in which Epstein-Barr virus infection is manifested in different geographic areas. While the virus usually results in infectious mononucleosis in the USA, it often produces Burkitt's lymphoma in African regions where malaria is endemic. To test whether malaria modifies the effects of Epstein-Barr virus, investigators instituted a malaria suppression program in an African region where Burkitt's lymphoma was usually found and followed the number of new cases. They reported that the incidence of Burkitt's lymphoma fell after malaria was suppressed, although other factors appeared to be involved as well (Geser, Brubaker, and Draper 1989).

A quantitative example of effect modification can be seen in the reported rates of hypertension among white men and women surveyed in the USA in 1991 (see National Center for Health Statistics 1993). In both men and women, the probability of hypertension rose with age. In the group aged 30–44 years, men were somewhat more likely than women to have hypertension. However, in older groups, the reverse was true. In the group aged 45–64 years, women were somewhat more likely than men to have hypertension, and in the group aged 65 years and older, women were much more likely than men to have hypertension. Gender did not reverse the trend of rising rates of hypertension with increasing age, but the rate of increase did depend on the gender. Gender modified the effect of age on blood pressure. Statistically, there was an interaction between age and gender as predictors of blood pressure.

■ IMPORTANT REMINDERS ABOUT RISK FACTORS AND DISEASE

While it is essential to avoid the specific types of pitfalls described above, it is also necessary to keep two important concepts in mind.

First, one causal factor may increase the risk for several different diseases. For example, cigarette smoking is a risk factor for cancer of the lungs, larynx, mouth, and esophagus, as well as for chronic bronchitis and chronic obstructive pulmonary disease.

Second, one disease may have several different risk factors. Even though smoking is a strong risk factor for chronic obstructive pulmonary disease, it may be only one of several contributing factors in a given case. Other factors may include occupational exposure to dusts (e.g., coal dust or silicon) and genetic factors (e.g., alpha$_1$-antitrypsin deficiency). Similarly, the risk of myocardial infarction is influenced not only by a patient's genes, diet, exercise, and smoking but also by other conditions such as high blood pressure and diabetes. One of the tasks of epidemiologists, therefore, is to determine the relative amount that each risk factor contributes to a disease. This contribution, called the attributable risk, is discussed in Chapter 6.

The possibility of confounding and effect modification makes the interpretation of epidemiologic studies more difficult. Age may be a confounder because it has a direct effect on the risk of death and of many diseases, so that its impact must be removed before the causal impact of other variables can be known. But advancing age also can be an effect modifier, when it changes the magnitude of the risk of other variables (Jacobsen et al. 1992). For example, the risk of myocardial infarction increases both with age and with increasing levels of cholesterol and blood pressure. But both cholesterol levels and blood pressure also increase with age. To determine whether there is an association between cholesterol levels and myocardial infarction, the effects of both age and blood pressure must be controlled. Likewise, to determine the association of blood pressure and myocardial infarction, the effects of age and cholesterol levels must be controlled. Although controlling sometimes can be done by research design and sample selection (e.g., by selecting study subjects in a narrow range of age and blood pressure), usually this is accomplished in the statistical analysis (see Chapter 13).

■ SUMMARY

Epidemiologists are concerned with discovering the causes of disease in the environment, nutrition, life-style, and genes of individuals and populations—that is, the causes or factors that when removed or modified will be followed by a reduction in the disease burden. Research to determine causation is complicated, particularly because epidemiologists usually do not have experimental control and must rely on observational methods.

Several criteria must be met to establish a causal relationship between a factor and a disease. First, a statistical association must be shown between the factor and the disease. The association is more impressive if it is strong and consistent. Second, the factor must precede the disease. Third, there should be no alternative explanations that fit the data equally well. Demonstrating that these criteria are met is complicated by the hazards of bias, random error, confounding, synergism, and effect modification.

■ QUESTIONS

Directions (Items 1–11). The set of matching questions in this section consists of a list of lettered options followed by several numbered items. For each numbered item, select the ONE lettered option that is most closely associated with it. To avoid spending too much time on matching sets with large numbers of options, it is generally advisable to begin each set by reading the list of options. Then, for each item in the set, try to generate the correct answer and locate it in the option list, rather than evaluating each option individually. Each lettered option may be selected once, more than once, or not at all. Correct answers and explanations are given at the end of the chapter.

Items 1–11

(A) Biologic plausibility
(B) Confounder
(C) Effect modifier
(D) External validity
(E) Internal validity
(F) Intervening variable
(G) Measurement bias
(H) Necessary cause
(I) Recall bias
(J) Sufficient cause
(K) Synergism

The parameters listed are related to the assessment of causality. For each of the following descriptions, select the corresponding parameter.

1. This must be associated with both the exposure and the outcome.
2. This alters the nature of a true relationship between an exposure and an outcome.
3. This is a systematic distortion of study data; an example is weighing the subjects in a study while they are fully dressed.
4. This is a multiplicative effect of one exposure variable on another.
5. This is present when the study population resembles the larger population from which it was drawn.
6. This is present if it is possible to understand a mechanism by which the apparent cause could induce the apparent effect.
7. This is a means or the means by which the causal factor leads to the outcome.
8. This is required for a disease to occur; an example is exposure to the human immunodeficiency virus (HIV) prior to the development of acquired immunodeficiency syndrome (AIDS).
9. This is a systematic distortion in retrospective studies; it is eliminated by a prospective design.
10. This is the sole requirement for a disease to occur; an example is homozygosity for the sickle cell gene.
11. This is present when study results are obtained in an unbiased manner.

■ ANSWERS AND EXPLANATIONS

1. **The answer is B: confounder.** A confounder is a third variable that is associated with both the exposure variable and the outcome variable in question. For example, cigarette smoking is a confounder of the relationship between alcohol and lung cancer. Cigarette smoking is associated both with the outcome, lung cancer, and with the exposure, alcohol consumption (Bartecchi, MacKenzie, and Schrier 1994). If an investigator were to assess the relationship between alcohol and lung cancer and not take smoking into account, alcohol would be found to increase the risk of lung cancer. When the study has controls in place for smoking (i.e., when varying degrees

of alcohol consumption are compared in subjects with comparable cigarette consumption), the association between alcohol and lung cancer disappears. All of the increased risk that appeared to be attributable to alcohol is actually attributable to cigarettes. This is confounding. Note that if cigarettes were causally related to lung cancer but cigarette consumption did not vary with alcohol exposure, there would be no confounding.

2. **The answer is C: effect modifier.** Unlike a confounder, an effect modifier does not obscure the nature of a relationship between two other variables; rather, it changes the relationship. For example, consider the effect of age on the pharmacologic action of the drug methylphenidate. In children, the drug is used to treat hyperactivity and attention deficit disorder, both of which are conditions in which there is too much activity. In adults, the same drug is used to treat narcolepsy, a condition characterized by extreme daytime somnolence and, in essence, a paucity of energy and activity. There is a true and measurable effect of methylphenidate on energy and activity levels both in children and in adults. This effect is not confounded by age but is altered by it. This is effect modification. In contrast to confounders, which must be controlled, effect modifiers should not be controlled. Instead, effect modifiers should be analyzed to enhance understanding of the causal relationship in question.

3. **The answer is G: measurement bias.** Unlike random error, measurement bias is a systematic distortion of study data. Random error will produce some measurements that are too large, some that are too small, and perhaps some that are correct. Such error will contribute to variability within groups, thereby limiting an investigator's ability to detect a significant difference between groups. Random error therefore reduces the power of a study to demonstrate a true difference in outcome (see Chapters 10 and 11). When error is systematic, rather than random, statistical power may be preserved, but the study's validity (i.e., its most critical attribute) is threatened. Imagine a study of weight loss in which the control subjects and the intervention subjects were weighed fully clothed and with shoes on at enrollment. Then, following a weight loss intervention, the control subjects were again weighed fully dressed, but the intervention subjects were weighed after disrobing. This would clearly be a biased and invalid measure of the intervention and resultant weight loss. Bias may threaten internal validity, external validity, or both.

4. **The answer is K: synergism.** When the combined effect of two or more variables on an outcome is greater than the sum of the separate effects of the variables, their interaction is called synergy or synergism. For example, cigarette smoking and asbestos exposure have a synergistic effect on the risk of lung cancer (Harvey and Beattie 1993). If the relative risk or risk ratio (RR) for lung cancer in smokers is X and if the RR for lung cancer in asbestos workers is Y, then the RR in those with both exposures is XY.

5. **The answer is D: external validity.** The external validity of a study is determined by the resemblance of the study population to the larger population from which it was drawn. In a well-designed study of antihypertensive therapy in the prevention of stroke in middle-class white men, the validity of the findings for middle-class white women and for men and women of other socioeconomic and ethnic groups is uncertain. While internal validity defines whether a study's results may be trusted, external validity defines the degree to which the results may be considered relevant to individuals other than the study subjects themselves.

6. **The answer is A: biologic plausibility.** In affluent countries such as the USA, there is a relatively high incidence of cardiovascular disease. This is thought to be largely due to dietary factors and the lack of exercise, even though many other factors distinguish the USA from less affluent countries. For instance, there are more television sets per capita in the USA than in most developing countries. However, before an abundance of an exposure and an abundance of an outcome may be considered related, they must meet the test of biologic plausibility (i.e., the relationship must make sense). There is no plausible way that the presence of a television set in a home could produce heart disease (unless one considers a resultant state of "couch-potatohood" to be an intervening variable). While plausibility is required before a causal relationship can be established, an open mind is essential. What is implausible today may become plausible as the science of medicine advances. This can be seen, for example, with respect to the etiology of peptic ulcer disease. Long thought to be attributable to hypersecretion of gastric acid, this disease is now known to be caused in many cases by infection with *Helicobacter pylori* (Fennerty 1994).

7. **The answer is F: intervening variable.** An intervening variable often represents an important mechanism by which an initial causal variable leads ultimately to a particular outcome. For example, a sedentary life-style is causally related to an increased risk of cardiovascular disease. However, the connection between the two is not direct. Inactivity contributes to weight gain and obesity, as well as to deconditioning. Obesity in turn may lead to hypertension, dyslipidemia, and possibly diabetes. Each of these represents an in-

tervening variable on the causal chain from sedentariness to heart disease.

8. **The answer is H: necessary cause.** A necessary cause is a factor that is required for a disease to occur. A necessary cause will not invariably lead to the disease, but the disease will certainly not occur unless the necessary cause is present. In the case of an infectious disease, exposure to a pathogen is always a necessary cause. However, some people exposed to the pathogen may fail to acquire the disease because of robust immunity, limited exposure, or other factors.

9. **The answer is I: recall bias.** Recall bias is a systematic distortion found in retrospective studies. In a case-control study of congenital anomalies, for example, there is a risk that the study subjects' knowledge of their own or their family members' current health status will influence their recall of exposures in the past. For example, the mothers of children born with any sort of congenital anomaly might be more likely to recall being exposed during pregnancy to toxic substances (e.g., medications) than would the mothers of children born without congenital anomalies. In a prospective study, exposure is established at enrollment, before the subjects are distinguished on the basis of outcome. Therefore, recall bias is eliminated in a prospective study.

10. **The answer is J: sufficient cause.** A sufficient cause is one that, if present, will invariably cause a particular disease or condition. For example, sickle cell anemia will occur in individuals who are homozygous for the sickle cell gene. Therefore, homozygosity is a sufficient cause of the disease. Sufficient causes are rare; even highly pathogenic microbes fail to cause disease in some exposed individuals.

11. **The answer is E: internal validity.** The most important criterion upon which a study is judged is its internal validity. If study results are obtained in an unbiased manner, the study is said to have internal validity. If the study is biased, it lacks internal validity and its results are therefore unreliable and meaningless. Say, hypothetically, that in a study of prostate cancer, the outcome in men treated with orchiectomy (surgical removal of the testes) is found to be worse than the outcome in men treated with orange juice. If men debilitated by illness had been assigned to orchiectomy, while men with no overt signs of illness had been assigned to orange juice therapy, the better outcome seen with orange juice therapy would be invalid because of the biased design of the study. Internal validity can be present only if bias is eliminated. However, even if results are internally valid, it may not be possible to derive generalizations from them. To derive generalizations, the investigator must have externally valid results, as discussed in the answer to question 5 (see above).

References Cited

Anderson, G., M. Arnstein, and M. R. Lester. Chapter 17 in Communicable Disease Control, 4th ed. New York, Macmillan Company, 1962.

Bartecchi, C. E., T. D. MacKenzie, and R. W. Schrier. The human costs of tobacco use. New England Journal of Medicine 330:907–912, 1994.

Bauman, K. E. Research Methods for Community Health and Welfare. New York, Oxford University Press, 1980.

Belongia, E. A., et al. An investigation of the cause of the eosinophilia-myalgia syndrome associated with tryptophan use. New England Journal of Medicine 323:357–365, 1990.

Danesh, J., R. Collins, and R. Peto. Chronic infections and coronary heart disease: is there a link? Lancet 350:430–436, 1997.

Doll, R., and A. B. Hill. Lung cancer and other causes of death in relation to smoking. British Medical Journal 2:1071, 1956.

Doll, R., and R. Peto. The Causes of Cancer. Oxford, Oxford University Press, 1981.

Fabricant, C. G., et al. Virus-induced atherosclerosis. Journal of Experimental Medicine 148:335–340, 1978.

Fennerty, M. B. Helicobacter pylori. Archives of Internal Medicine 154:721–727, 1994.

Francis, T., Jr., et al. An evaluation of the 1954 poliomyelitis vaccine trials. American Journal of Public Health, April supplement, 1955.

Garrell, M., and J. F. Jekel. A comparison of quality of care on teaching and non-teaching services in a university-affiliated community hospital. Connecticut Medicine 43:659–663, 1979.

Geser, A., G. Brubaker, and C. C. Draper. Effect of a malaria suppression program on the incidence of African Burkitt's lymphoma. American Journal of Epidemiology 129:740–752, 1989.

Gurfinkel, E., et al. Randomized trial of roxithromycin in non–Q-wave coronary syndromes: ROXIS pilot study. Lancet 350:404–407, 1997.

Hammond, E. C., I. J. Selikoff, and H. Seidman. Asbestos exposure, cigarette smoking, and death rates. Annals of the New York Academy of Sciences 330:473–490, 1979.

Harvey, J. C., and E. J. Beattie. Lung cancer. Clinical Symposia 45:2–32, 1993.

Jacobsen, S. J., et al. Cholesterol and coronary artery disease: age as an effect modifier. Journal of Clinical Epidemiology 45:1053–1059, 1992.

Kelsey, J. L., et al. Chapter 9 in Methods in Observational Epidemiology, 2nd ed. New York, Oxford University Press, 1996.

Klerman, L. V., and J. F. Jekel. School-Age Mothers: Problems, Programs, and Policy. Hamden, Conn., Linnet Books, 1973.

Lam, J. A., S. Hartwell, and J. F Jekel. "I prayed real hard, so I know I'll get in": living with randomization in social research. New Directions in Program Evaluation 63:55–66, 1994.

Langmuir, A. D. Epidemiology of airborne infection. Bacteriological Reviews 24:173–181, 1961.

Mill, J. S. A System of Logic (1856). Summarized in J. M. Last. A Dictionary of Epidemiology, 2nd ed. New York, Oxford University Press, 1988.

Miller, H. C., and J. F. Jekel. Incidence of low birth weight infants born to mothers with multiple risk factors. Yale Journal of Biology and Medicine 60:397–404, 1987.

National Center for Health Statistics. Health Promotion and Disease Prevention: United States, 1990. Vital and Health Statistics, Series 10, No. 185. Atlanta, Centers for Disease Control and Prevention, April 1993.

Philen, R. M., et al. Tryptophan contaminants associated with eosinophilia-myalgia syndrome. American Journal of Epidemiology 138:154–159, 1993.

Physicians' Health Study Steering Committee. Final report on the aspirin component of the ongoing Physicians' Health Study. New England Journal of Medicine 321:129–135, 1989.

Salonen, J. T., et al. High stored iron levels are associated with excess risk of myocardial infarction in Eastern Finnish men. Circulation 86:803–811, 1992.

Slutsker, L., et al. Eosinophilia-myalgia syndrome associated with exposure to tryptophan from a single manufacturer. Journal of the American Medical Association 264:213–217, 1990.

Sullivan, J. L. Iron and the sex difference in heart disease risk. Lancet 1:1293–1294, 1981.

Susser, M. Causal Thinking in the Health Sciences. New York, Oxford University Press, 1973.

US Surgeon General. Smoking and Health. Public Health Service publication No. 1103. Washington, D. C., US Government Printing Office, 1964.

Selected Readings

Greenland, S., ed. Issues in causal inference. Part I *in* Evolution of Epidemiologic Ideas. Chestnut Hill, Mass., Epidemiology Resources, 1987.

Rothman, K. J. Causal Inference. Chestnut Hill, Mass., Epidemiology Resources, 1988.

Rothman, K. J. Chapter 2 *in* Modern Epidemiology. Boston, Little, Brown and Company, 1987.

Susser, M. Causal Thinking in the Health Sciences. New York, Oxford University Press, 1973.

5 Common Research Designs Used in Epidemiology

■ FUNCTIONS OF RESEARCH DESIGN

The basic function of most epidemiologic research designs is to permit a fair, unbiased comparison to be made between a group with and a group without a risk factor or intervention. In a case-control study, the contrast is between the frequency of the risk factor among the cases and the frequency of the risk factor among the controls.

A good research design should perform the following functions: (1) enable a comparison of a variable (such as disease frequency) between two or more groups at one point in time or, in some cases, between one group before and after receiving an intervention or being exposed to a risk factor; (2) allow the comparison to be quantified either in absolute terms (as with a risk difference or rate difference) or in relative terms (as with a relative risk or odds ratio), as discussed in detail in Chapter 6; (3) permit the investigators to determine when the risk factor and the disease occurred, in order to determine the temporal sequence; and (4) minimize biases, confounding, and other problems that would complicate interpretation of the data.

The research designs discussed in this chapter are the primary ones used in epidemiologic research. Cross-sectional surveys and ecologic studies are useful for developing hypotheses; cohort studies and case-control studies can be used both to develop hypotheses and to test them, although the hypothesis development and hypothesis testing must always be done on different data sets; and randomized clinical trials or field trials are usually the best for testing new treatments or preventive measures.

Hypothesis development is a critical step in the scientific process. Hypotheses are used to make predictions, which are then tested by further research. If the test results are consistent with the hypothesis, the likelihood of the hypothesis being true is strengthened. If the results are not consistent with the hypothesis, it needs modification.

■ TYPES OF RESEARCH DESIGN

Because some research questions can be answered by more than one type of research design, the choice of design depends on a variety of considerations, including speed, cost, and availability of data. Each type of research design has advantages and disadvantages, as discussed below and summarized in Table 5–1.

Observational Designs for Generating Hypotheses
Cross-Sectional Surveys

A cross-sectional survey is a survey of a population at a single point in time. Among the examples are an **interview survey** and a **mass screening program.** Interview surveys may be performed by trained interviewers in people's homes, by telephone surveys using random digit dialing, or by mailed questionnaires. The telephone surveys are often the quickest and usually the least costly, but they have many nonresponders and refusals, and some people do not have telephones. Mailed surveys are also relatively inexpensive, but they usually have poor response rates (except in the case of the US census).

Cross-sectional surveys have the advantages of being fairly quick and easy to perform. They are useful for determining the prevalence of risk factors and the frequency of prevalent cases of disease for a defined population. They are also useful for measuring current health status and planning for some health services, including setting priorities for disease control. For example, many surveys have been undertaken to determine the knowledge, attitudes, and health prac-

TABLE 5–1   Advantages and Disadvantages of Common Types of Studies Used in Epidemiology

Studies	Advantages	Disadvantages
Cross-sectional surveys	Are fairly quick and easy to perform; are useful for hypothesis generation.	Do not offer evidence of a temporal relationship between risk factors and disease; are subject to late look bias; are not good for hypothesis testing.
Ecologic studies	Are fairly quick and easy to perform; are useful for hypothesis generation.	Do not allow for causal conclusions to be drawn, since the data are not associated with individual persons; are subject to ecologic fallacy; are not good for hypothesis testing.
Cohort studies	Can be performed retrospectively or prospectively; can be used to obtain a true (absolute) measure of risk; can study many disease outcomes; are good for studying rare risk factors.	Are time-consuming and costly (especially prospective studies); can study only those risk factors measured at the beginning; can be used only for common diseases; may have losses to follow-up.
Case-control studies	Are fairly quick and easy to perform; can study many risk factors; are good for studying rare diseases.	Can obtain only a relative measure of risk; are subject to recall bias; selection of controls may be difficult; temporal relationships may be unclear; can study only one disease outcome at a time.
Randomized controlled trials	Are the "gold standard" for evaluating treatment interventions (clinical trials) or preventive interventions (field trials); allow investigator to have extensive control over research process.	Are time-consuming and usually costly; can study only interventions or exposures that are controlled by investigator; may have problems related to therapy changes and dropouts; may be limited in generalizability; are often unethical to perform at all.

tices of various populations regarding the human immunodeficiency virus (HIV) and acquired immunodeficiency syndrome (AIDS).

A major disadvantage of using a cross-sectional survey is that data about both the exposure to risk factors and the presence or absence of disease are collected simultaneously. This creates problems in determining the temporal relationship of a presumed cause and effect. Another disadvantage is that a cross-sectional survey selects for longer-lasting and more indolent diseases. These diseases are more likely to be found by a survey, because people live longer with them, enabling the affected individuals to be interviewed, whereas severe diseases that tend to be rapidly fatal are less likely to be found by a survey. This phenomenon is called **Neyman bias.** It is called **late look bias** if it results in selecting fewer individuals with severe disease because they died before detection. It is called **length bias** in screening programs, which tend to find (and therefore select) less aggressive cases for treatment.

Repeated cross-sectional surveys may be used to determine changes in risk factors and changes in disease frequency in populations over time (but not the nature of their association). The data derived from these surveys also can be examined for associations in order to generate hypotheses, but they are not good for testing the effectiveness of interventions. For example, in a cross-sectional survey, investigators might find that subjects who indicated that they had been immunized against a disease had fewer cases of the disease. However, the investigators would not know whether this finding was due to the fact that those who sought immunization were more concerned about their health and less likely to expose themselves to the disease. If the investigators randomized the subjects into two groups and immu-

nized only one of the groups, this would exclude self-selection as a possible explanation for the association.

Cross-sectional surveys are of particular value in infectious disease epidemiology, where the prevalence of antibodies against infectious agents, when analyzed by age or other variables, may provide evidence about when and in whom infection has occurred. Proof of a recent acute infection can be obtained by two serum surveys separated by a short interval. The first serum samples, called the **acute sera,** are collected soon after symptoms of an infectious disease appear. The second serum samples, called the **convalescent sera,** are collected 10–20 days later. A significant increase in the serum titer of antibody to a particular infectious agent is taken as proof of recent infection.

Even if two serum samples are not taken, important inferences can be drawn on the basis of titers of IgG and IgM, two immunoglobulin classes, in a single serum sample. A high IgG titer without an IgM titer of antibody to a particular infectious agent suggests that the study subject had been infected but that the infection occurred in the distant past. A high IgM titer with a low IgG titer suggests a current or very recent infection. An elevated IgM titer in the presence of a high IgG titer suggests that the infection occurred in the fairly recent past.

Cross-Sectional Ecologic Studies

Cross-sectional ecologic studies relate the frequency with which some characteristic (e.g., smoking) and some outcome of interest (e.g., lung cancer) occur in the same geographic area. These studies are often useful for suggesting hypotheses, but they cannot be used to draw causal conclusions, because there is no

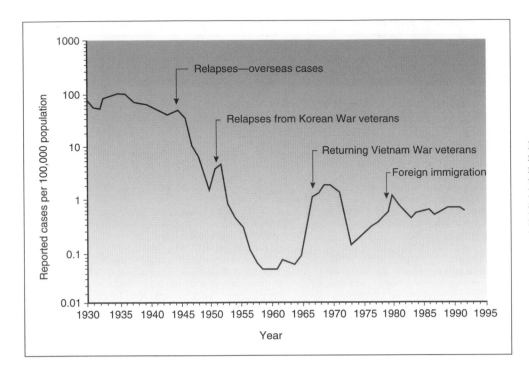

FIGURE 5–1   Incidence rates of malaria in the USA, by year of report, 1930–1992. (Source: Centers for Disease Control and Prevention. Summary of notifiable diseases, United States, 1992. Morbidity and Mortality Weekly Report 41:38, 1992.)

information as to whether the people who smoked are the same people who got the lung cancer. This problem with ecologic studies is often referred to as the **ecologic fallacy.**

Concerned citizens sometimes are unaware of the problem of ecologic fallacy and use the findings in surveys to make statements such as the following: "There are high levels of both toxic pollution and cancer in northern New Jersey, so the toxins are causing the cancer." This conclusion may or may not be correct. Remember that statistical association does not prove causation (see Chapter 4). Are the data adjusted for age? Has it been established that the cause came before the effect? And have all other explanations for the association been eliminated?

There are, of course, cases in which important hypotheses initially suggested by cross-sectional ecologic studies were later proved correct by other types of studies. For example, the rate of dental caries in children was found to be much higher in areas with low levels of natural fluoridation in the water than in areas with high levels of natural fluoridation (Arnim, Aberle, and Pitney 1937). Subsequent research established that this association was causal, and the introduction of water fluoridation and fluoride treatment of teeth has been followed by striking reductions in the rate of dental caries (see Centers for Disease Control and Prevention 1999).

Longitudinal Ecologic Studies

Longitudinal ecologic studies use ongoing surveillance or frequent cross-sectional studies to measure trends in disease rates over many years in a defined population. By comparing the trends in disease rates with other changes in the society (such as wars, immigration, or the introduction of a vaccine or antibiotics), epidemiologists attempt to determine the impact of these changes on the disease rates.

For example, as discussed in Chapter 3 and illustrated in Fig. 3–9, the introduction of the inactivated (Salk) polio vaccine and, subsequently, of the oral (Sabin) polio vaccine resulted in a precipitous drop in the rate of paralytic poliomyelitis in the US population. In this case, because of the large number of people involved in the immunization program and the relatively slow rate of change of other factors in the population, longitudinal ecologic studies were useful for determining the impact of the public health intervention. Nevertheless, confounding with other factors can distort the conclusions drawn from ecologic studies in circumstances like this, so if time is available (i.e., it is not an epidemic situation), investigators should perform field studies, such as randomized controlled field trials, before pursuing a large-scale, new public health intervention.

Another example of longitudinal ecologic research is the study of the rates of malaria in the US population since 1930. As shown in Fig. 5–1, the peaks in malaria rates can be readily related to social events such as wars and immigration. (The use of a logarithmic scale in the figure visually minimizes the relative drop in disease frequency, making it less impressive to the eye, but enables the reader to see in detail the changes occurring when the rates are low.)

Important causal associations have been suggested by longitudinal ecologic studies. For example, about 20 years after there was an increase in the smoking rates in men, the lung cancer rate in the male population began rising rapidly. Similarly, about 20 years after women began to smoke in large numbers, the lung cancer rate in the female population began to rise. The studies in this case were longitudinal ecologic studies in the sense that they used only national data on smoking and lung cancer rates, which did not relate the individual cases of lung cancer to individual smokers; the task of establishing a causal relationship was left to cohort and case-control studies.

Observational Designs for Generating or Testing Hypotheses

Cohort Studies

A cohort is a clearly identified group to be studied. In cohort studies, investigators begin by assembling one or more cohorts, either by choosing persons specifically because they were and were not exposed to one or more risk factors to be studied or else by taking a random sample of a population. After the cohort of study subjects is selected, the subjects are followed over time to determine whether or not they develop the diseases of interest and whether the risk factors that were measured at the beginning of the study predict the diseases that occur.

There are two general types of cohort study, the prospective type and the retrospective type. The time relationships of the two are shown in Fig. 5–2.

Prospective Cohort Studies. In a prospective cohort study, the investigator assembles the study groups in the present time, collects baseline data on them, and continues to collect data for a period that can last anywhere from hours to many years.

There are several advantages of performing prospective studies. The first is that the investigator is able to control the data collection as the study progresses and can check the outcome events (e.g., diseases and death) carefully when they occur, thereby making sure that they are correctly classified. The second advantage is that the estimates of risk obtained from prospective cohort studies are true (absolute) risks for the groups studied. The third advantage is that many different disease outcomes can be studied, including some that were not anticipated at the beginning of the study.

Cohort studies have disadvantages, however. In a cohort study, only those risk factors defined and measured at the beginning of the study can be used. Other disadvantages of cohort studies are their high costs and the long wait until their results are obtained.

The classic cohort study is the Framingham Heart Study, which was begun in 1950 (see Dawber, Meadors, and Moore 1951) and still continues today. Table 5–2 shows the 8-year risk of heart disease as calculated from the Framingham Study's equations (Breslow 1978). Although the risk ratios are not based on the most recent data from the study, the length of follow-up and clarity of the message still make them useful for sharing with patients.

Retrospective Cohort Studies. Some of the time and cost limitations of the prospective cohort study can be mitigated by doing a retrospective cohort study. In this approach, the investigator goes back into history to define a risk group (e.g., those exposed to the Hiroshima atomic bomb in August 1945) and follows the group members up to the present to see what outcomes (e.g., cancer and death) have occurred.

A retrospective cohort study was done by MacMahon (1962), who was interested in investigat-

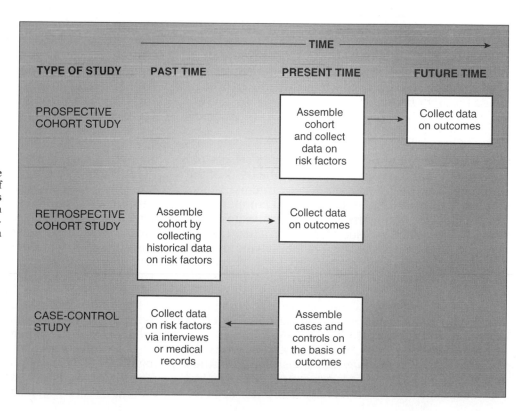

FIGURE 5–2   Illustration of the relationship between the time of assembling the study subjects and the time of data collection in a prospective cohort study, a retrospective cohort study, and a case-control study.

TABLE 5–2 The Risk That a 45-Year-Old Man Will Have Cardiovascular Disease Within 8 Years

Risk Group	Characteristics of Risk Group	Risk	Risk Ratio
Lowest	All of the following factors: -Nonsmoker -No glucose intolerance -No hypertrophy of left ventricle -Low systolic blood pressure (≤105 mm Hg) -Low cholesterol level (≤185 mg/dL)	2.2%	—
Highest	All of the factors listed below	77.8%	35.4
Intermediate	One of the following factors:		
	-Smoker	3.8%	1.7
	-Glucose intolerance	3.9%	1.8
	-Hypertrophy of left ventricle	6.0%	2.7
	-Severe hypertension (systolic blood pressure ≥195 mm Hg)	8.4%	3.8
	-High cholesterol level (≥335 mg/dL)	8.5%	3.8

Sources of data: (1) Pearson, T., and D. Becker. Cardiovascular risk. Computer program for IBM-compatible systems, using the Framingham Study 8-year risk equations. Developed at Johns Hopkins University on a Parke-Davis Educational Grant. (2) Breslow, L. Risk factor intervention for health maintenance. Science 200:908–912, 1978.

ing the effects of prenatal x-ray exposure. In the past, radiographs were often used to measure the size of the pelvic outlet of pregnant women, and this exposed their fetuses to x-rays in utero. MacMahon identified one group of subjects who had been exposed in utero and another group who had not. He followed these subjects to see how many from each group had gotten cancer during childhood or early adulthood (up to the time he did the study). He found that those who had been exposed to x-rays in utero had a 40% increase in the risk of childhood cancers (i.e., a risk ratio of 1.4) after adjustments had been made for other factors.

Case-Control Studies

The investigator in a case-control study selects the case group and the control group on the basis of the outcome (i.e., having the disease of interest versus not having the disease of interest) and compares the groups in terms of their frequency of past exposure to possible risk factors (see Fig. 5–2). This can be thought of as comparing the "risk of having the risk factor" in the two groups. The actual risk of the outcome cannot be determined from case-control studies, because the underlying population is not known. However, an estimate of the relative risk of the outcome, called the odds ratio, can be determined in case-control studies.

In this kind of study, the cases and controls are assembled and then they are questioned (or their relatives or medical records are consulted) regarding past exposure to risk factors. In past decades,

case-control studies were often called retrospective studies for this reason. The time relationships in a case-control study are similar to those in a cross-sectional study in that the investigator learns simultaneously about the current disease state and any risk factors that may have existed in the past. In terms of assembling the subjects, however, a case-control study differs from a cross-sectional study in that the sample for the case-control study is chosen specifically from groups with and without the disease of interest. Often, all the people with the disease of interest in a geographic area and time period can be selected as cases. This avoids bias in case selection.

Case-control studies are especially useful when a study must be done quickly and inexpensively or when the disease being studied is rare (e.g., has a prevalence of less than 1%). In a cohort study, a huge number of study subjects would have to be followed to find even a few cases of a rare disease, and the search might take a long time even if the funds were available. Although in case-control studies only one outcome (one disease) can be considered per study, many risk factors may be considered, and this makes case-control studies useful for generating hypotheses concerning the causes of a disease. Methodologic standards have been developed so that the quality of information obtained from case-control studies can approximate that obtained from the much more difficult, costly, and time-consuming randomized clinical trials (Imperiale and Horwitz 1989).

Despite these advantages, there are several disadvantages to the use of case-control studies. In determining the risk factors, a major problem is the potential for recall bias, a pitfall discussed in Chapter 4. Moreover, it is not easy to know what is the correct control group for the cases. The controls are usually matched individually to cases on the basis of age, sex, and often race. If possible, the investigator obtains controls from the same setting in which the cases were found, in order to avoid potential bias (e.g., having the disease more likely to be detected in one group than in another). For example, if the controls were taken from the same hospital and were examined for a disease of the same organ system (e.g., pulmonary disease), presumably a similar workup (including a chest x-ray and spirometry) would be done, so that cases of the disease would be less likely to be missed and classified as controls. Similarly, if a study concerns birth defects, the control subject for each case might be the next infant who was born at the same hospital, was of the same sex and race, and had a mother of similar age and from the same town. This would control for season, location, sex, race, and age of mother and infant. Given the difficulties of selecting a control group with no bias, the investigator often assembles two or more control groups, one of which is from the general population.

Case-control studies were used to clarify the etiology of the 1989 epidemic of eosinophilia-myalgia syndrome (EMS), which was associated with over-the-counter dietary supplements of L-tryptophan (see

Chapter 4). Investigators initially thought that the L-tryptophan itself was responsible for EMS, but additional investigation suggested that the problem was linked with pills produced by a particular manufacturer, the Showa-Denka Company. Two case-control studies were done to test this hypothesis and determine the odds that the source of the pills made a difference. If the source made no difference, the expected odds ratio would be 1. When Slutsker et al. (1990) compared the use of pills from Showa-Denka Company versus the use of pills from all other manufacturers, their data permitted calculation of an odds ratio of 57.5, as shown in Table 5–3. When Belongia et al. (1990) undertook a similar case-control study, they found an odds ratio of 19.3. Thus, in both studies, the odds ratio for the association of EMS with the Showa-Denka Company's L-tryptophan was strongly elevated.

Nested Case-Control Studies

A relatively new design for clinical research consists of a cohort study with a nested case-control study. In this design, a cohort of patients is defined, and the baseline characteristics of the patients are obtained by interview, physical examination, and pertinent laboratory or imaging studies. The patients are then followed to determine the outcome. Those patients who develop the condition of interest become cases in a case-control study, and those who do not develop the condition become eligible for the control group of a study. Next, the cases and a representative (or matched) sample of controls are studied, and data from the two groups are compared using analytic methods appropriate for case-control studies.

This nested design was used, for example, by Hasbun, Aoun, and Quagliarello in studies to shed light on two different questions about meningitis. (1) In cases of suspected meningitis, under what circumstances would patients be unlikely to benefit from undergoing computed tomography (CT) scans before antibiotic therapy is initiated? (2) Does the use of nonsteroidal anti-inflammatory drugs (NSAIDs) increase the risk of nonbacterial meningitis? The first question was important because CT scans are generally used to make sure that patients with sus-

pected meningitis have no contraindications to receiving a diagnostic spinal tap. However, CT scans are costly and time-consuming, and reports indicate that the long-term complications of meningitis are higher among patients in whom the initiation of antibiotics is delayed (Aronin, Peduzzi, and Quagliarello 1998). To answer the first question, Hasbun and Quagliarello (1999) determined that their cohort of patients would consist of individuals who were taken to the emergency room, were suspected of having meningitis, and were scheduled to undergo CT scanning. Based on the results that they found in this prospective cohort study, the investigators were later able to create a prediction algorithm to identify patients for whom CT scans of the head were unnecessary. Next, using patients from the same cohort, Aoun and Quagliarello (1999) designed and performed a nested case-control study. In this study, the cases consisted of all of the patients in whom nonbacterial meningitis was diagnosed, while the controls consisted of a sample of patients in whom meningitis was not diagnosed. The goal was to determine whether there was an association between the prior use of NSAIDs and the frequency of nonbacterial meningitis.

As this example shows, the nested research design has several advantages. First, investigators are able to test new hypotheses with data that were collected at baseline. Second, because the baseline data were collected before the outcome occurred, it is often possible to know the direction of causation. Third, for the data collected at baseline, recall bias should not be a problem, because the condition itself would not have influenced recall. Fourth, the design saves both time and money. If there is expensive baseline blood work whose results are needed only for the subsequent case-control study, baseline serum samples can be saved and the expensive laboratory work performed only on the samples taken from persons who eventually participate in the case-control study.

Experimental Designs for Testing Hypotheses

Two types of randomized controlled trials are discussed below: randomized controlled clinical trials (RCCTs) and randomized controlled field trials (RCFTs). While both types follow the same series of steps shown in Fig. 5–3 and have many of the same advantages and disadvantages, the major difference between the two is that clinical trials are usually used to test therapeutic interventions in ill persons, while field trials are usually done to test preventive interventions in well persons.

Randomized Controlled Clinical Trials

In a randomized controlled clinical trial (RCCT), patients are enrolled in a study and then randomly assigned to one of the following groups: (1) the intervention group, which will receive the experimental treatment, or (2) the control group, which will receive the nonexperimental treatment, consisting either of a

TABLE 5–3 Data from a Case-Control Study Showing the Source of L-Tryptophan Used by Subjects with Eosinophilia-Myalgia Syndrome (Cases) and the Source of L-Tryptophan Used by Subjects Without Eosinophilia-Myalgia Syndrome (Controls)

Source of L-Tryptophan	Cases	Controls	Calculation of Odds Ratio
Showa-Denka Company	45	18	$\frac{45 \times 23}{18 \times 1} = 57.5$
Other manufacturers	1	23	
Total	46	41	

Source of data: Slutsker, L., et al. Eosinophilia-myalgia syndrome associated with exposure to tryptophan from a single manufacturer. Journal of the American Medical Association 264:213–217, 1990.

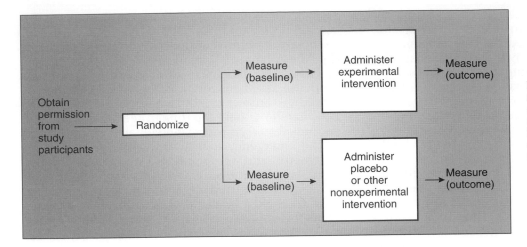

FIGURE 5–3 Illustration of the relationship between the time of assembling the study subjects and the time of data collection in a randomized controlled clinical trial (RCCT) or a randomized controlled field trial (RCFT).

placebo (inert substance) or of a standard method of treatment.

RCCTs are considered the "gold standard" for studying interventions, because of their ability to minimize bias in the information obtained from the study subjects. Nevertheless, they do not entirely eliminate bias, and they pose some challenges and ethical dilemmas for investigators.

To be enrolled in an RCCT, the patients must agree to participate without knowing whether they will be given the experimental or nonexperimental treatment. If possible, the observers who collect the data are also prevented from knowing which type of treatment each patient is given. When this is done, the trial is said to be a **double-blind study.** Blinding is needed to equalize any **placebo effect** (i.e., any bene-

fit from treatment with an inert substance). To have true blinding, the nonexperimental treatment must appear identical (in size, shape, color, taste, etc.) to the experimental treatment. Fig. 5–4 shows the pill packet from a trial of two preventive measures from the Physicians' Health Study (see Chapter 4). The round tablets were either aspirin or a placebo, but the study subjects could not tell which. The elongated capsules were either beta-carotene or a placebo, but the study subjects could not tell which.

It is usually impossible as well as unethical to have patients participate blindly in a study involving a surgical intervention, because blinding would require a sham operation. But in studies involving nonsurgical interventions, investigators can usually develop an effective placebo. For example, when Rubin

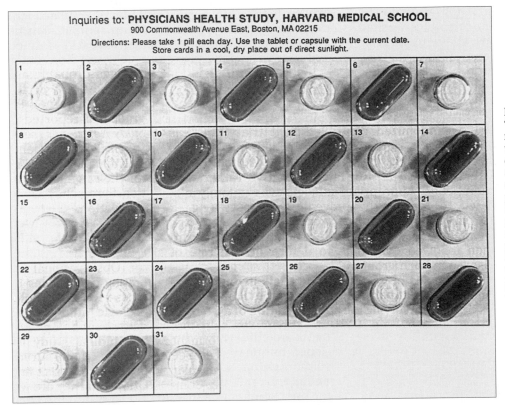

FIGURE 5–4 Photograph of the "bubble" pill packet provided monthly to the 22,000 physicians in the Physicians' Health Study, which consisted of a simultaneous trial of aspirin to reduce cardiovascular disease and of beta-carotene to prevent cancer. The round white tablets contained either aspirin or a placebo, and the elongated capsules contained either beta-carotene or a placebo. The participants did not know which substances they were taking. (Courtesy of Dr. Charles Hennekens, Director, Physicians' Health Study, Boston.)

et al. (1986) designed a computer game to teach asthmatic children how to care for themselves with the goal of reducing hospitalizations, they distributed similar-looking computer games to the children in both the intervention group and the control group, but the games for the control group were without asthma content.

Undertaking an RCCT would be unethical if the intervention is strongly believed to be the best available, whether or not that has been established scientifically by carefully designed and controlled studies. There have been no RCCTs to compare prenatal care versus no prenatal care, so there is no conclusive proof that prenatal care is valuable, and questions about this are raised from time to time. However, because prenatal care is strongly thought to be of value, it would be unethical to undertake an RCCT in which some pregnant women were deprived of prenatal care by being randomized to receive no prenatal care.

In RCCTs, many biases still are possible, even though some biases have been minimized by the randomized, prospective design and by double-blinding. For example, in the two groups being compared, there may be different rates at which patients drop out of the study or become lost to follow-up, and this could produce a greater change in the characteristics of the remaining study subjects in one group than in the other.

Therapy changes and dropouts are special problems in RCCTs involving severe diseases, such as advanced cancer. The patients receiving the new treatment may continue to fail to respond, and either they or their physicians may decide to try a different treatment, which they must be allowed to do. Patients may also leave a study if the new treatment has unpleasant side effects, even though the treatment may be effective. For example, some medications for hypertension reduce male potency, and many men will discontinue their medication when this happens, regardless of its beneficial effect on their hypertension.

Randomized Controlled Field Trials

A randomized controlled field trial (RCFT) is similar to a randomized controlled clinical trial (RCCT) (see Fig. 5–3), except that ordinarily the intervention in an RCFT is preventive rather than therapeutic. Appropriate subjects are randomly allocated to receive the preventive measure (e.g., a vaccine or oral drug) or to receive the placebo (e.g., an injection of sterile saline or an inert pill). They are then followed over time to determine the rate of disease in each group.

Examples of RCFTs include trials involving vaccines to prevent paralytic poliomyelitis (Francis et al. 1955); trials involving the administration of a 6-month course of isoniazid (INH) to tuberculin skin test converters to prevent the reactivation of dormant infections with *Mycobacterium tuberculosis* (Ferebee 1963); and trials of aspirin to reduce cardiovascular disease (see Physicians' Health Study Steering Committee 1989).

RCFTs and RCCTs have similar advantages and disadvantages. One disadvantage is that results may take a long time to obtain. The Physicians' Health Study (see above and Chapter 4) illustrates this problem. This trial of the preventive benefits of aspirin was begun in 1982. The final report on the aspirin component of the trial was released 7 years later.

Another disadvantage of RCFTs and RCCTs has to do with **external validity,** which is the ability to generalize the findings to other groups in the population (as opposed to **internal validity,** which concerns the validity of results for the persons in the study). After the study subjects for a randomized trial have been assembled and various potential subjects have been excluded according to the study's exclusion criteria, it may not be clear whom the remaining people in the trial actually represent. Therefore, it may not be clear who might benefit from the intervention tested.

Techniques for Data Summary and Analysis

Although meta-analysis, decision analysis, and cost-effectiveness analysis are not formal research designs, they are among the most important techniques used to examine and make use of data collected in clinical research. **Meta-analysis** is used to summarize the information obtained in many single studies on one topic. **Decision analysis** and **cost-effectiveness analysis** are used to summarize data and show how they can inform clinical or policy decisions. All three techniques are discussed in more detail in Chapter 8.

■ SUMMARY

Observational research designs suitable for generating hypotheses include cross-sectional surveys, cross-sectional ecologic studies, and longitudinal ecologic studies. A cross-sectional study collects data about a population at one point in time, while a longitudinal study is done over a period of time. Cross-sectional surveys are useful in determining the prevalence of risk factors and diseases in the population, but they are weak in determining the temporal relationship between variables. In ecologic studies, both the rate of a disease and the frequency of exposure to a risk factor are obtained for an entire population, but the unit of study is the population and not individuals within it, so the exposure and the disease cannot be linked in individual persons.

Observational research designs suitable for generating or testing hypotheses include prospective cohort studies, retrospective cohort studies, and case-control studies. For cohort studies, one group consists of persons exposed to risk factors, while another group consists of persons not exposed. The groups are studied to determine and compare their rates of disease. Fig. 5–2 illustrates the difference between a prospective and a retrospective cohort study. For case-control studies, the case group consists of persons who have a particular disease, and the control group consists of persons who do not have the disease but are matched individually to the cases (e.g., in terms of age, sex, and type of medical workup). Each group is studied to determine the frequency of past exposure to possible risk factors. Based on this information, the relative odds that a disease is linked with a particular risk factor (the odds ratio) can be calculated. The use of a cohort study with a nested case-control design may enable some hypotheses to be tested quickly and cheaply.

The experimental designs suitable for testing hypotheses are randomized controlled clinical trials and randomized controlled field trials. Both types of trials follow the steps shown in Fig. 5–3. The major difference between the two types is that clinical trials are generally used to test therapeutic interventions, while field trials are usually done to test preventive interventions. A trial is called a double-blind study if neither the subjects who participate in it nor the observers who collect the data know which type of intervention each participant is given.

■ QUESTIONS

Directions (Items 1–10). Each of the numbered items or incomplete statements in this section is followed by answers or by completions of the statement. Select the ONE lettered answer or completion that is BEST in each case. Correct answers and explanations are given at the end of the chapter.

1. The basic goal of epidemiologic research is to
   - (A) compare two groups that differ in terms of exposure or outcome
   - (B) eliminate all bias
   - (C) establish causality
   - (D) maximize external validity
   - (E) reject the null hypothesis

2. Studies may be conducted to generate or test hypotheses. The best design for testing a hypothesis is a
   - (A) case-control study
   - (B) cross-sectional survey
   - (C) longitudinal ecologic study
   - (D) randomized controlled field trial
   - (E) retrospective cohort study

3. The members of a public health team have a continuing interest in controlling measles infection through vaccination. To estimate the level of immunity in a particular population and derive data useful for generating vaccination policy, what type of study should they conduct?
   - (A) A case-control study of measles infection
   - (B) A cross-sectional survey of vaccination status
   - (C) A randomized trial of measles vaccination
   - (D) A retrospective cohort study of measles vaccination
   - (E) An ecologic study of measles in the population

4. A study published in the *Annals of Internal Medicine* purported to show that a variety of symptoms were more common in subjects with a history of suboptimally treated Lyme disease than in controls. The data were obtained largely by a survey of the participants. To which of the following distortions is the study most likely subject?
   - (A) Ecologic fallacy
   - (B) Intervention bias
   - (C) Late look bias, measurement bias, and length bias
   - (D) Lead-time bias
   - (E) Selection bias, recall bias, and random error

5. Cross-sectional surveys are subject to the Neyman bias, or late look bias. This may be explained as the tendency to
   - (A) detect only the late stages of a disease, when manifestations are more severe
   - (B) detect only those cases of a disease that are asymptomatic
   - (C) find more disease in older cohorts
   - (D) preferentially detect fatal illness
   - (E) preferentially detect the more indolent cases of a disease

6. A screening program analogue to the late look bias is
   - (A) length bias, because cases lasting longer are more apt to be detected
   - (B) recall bias, because only severe illness is recalled
   - (C) selection bias, because the program selects out asymptomatic illness
   - (D) selection bias, because the program selects out severe cases
   - (E) spectrum bias, because the cases are clustered at one end of the disease spectrum

7. In assessing the extent of a population's exposure to an infectious agent, the measurement of both IgG and IgM titers
   - (A) is of limited usefulness because the titers decline with time
   - (B) is useful for distinguishing cell-mediated from humoral immunity
   - (C) is useful for distinguishing remote from recent exposure
   - (D) is useful for distinguishing vaccination from infection
   - (E) is useful for establishing the degree of immunity

8. Which of the following is a measure of the risk of having a risk factor?
   - (A) Kappa
   - (B) The odds ratio
   - (C) The *p* value
   - (D) The relative risk
   - (E) The risk ratio

9. A case-control study may have a particular ad-

vantage over a cohort study when the disease in question is

(A) fatal
(B) indolent
(C) infectious
(D) rare
(E) virulent

10. In a case-control study that is being planned, patients with myocardial infarction will serve as the cases. Which of the following would be a poor choice to serve as the controls?

(A) Subjects who have no history of myocardial infarction
(B) Subjects who were admitted to the hospital for noncardiac diseases
(C) Subjects whose age distribution is similar to that of the cases
(D) Subjects whose cardiac risk factors are similar to those of the cases
(E) Subjects whose sociodemographic characteristics are similar to those of the cases

■ ANSWERS AND EXPLANATIONS

1. **The answer is A: compare two groups that differ in terms of exposure or outcome.** Virtually all epidemiologic research involves the study of two or more groups of subjects that differ in terms of their exposure to risk factors or their outcome. The basic goal of the research is to compare the frequency of a hypothetically associated outcome or exposure in one group with the frequency in other groups. For the study to be valid, bias and confounding must be minimized.

2. **The answer is D: randomized controlled field trial.** Randomized controlled trials (including randomized controlled field trials and randomized controlled clinical trials) represent the "gold standard" for hypothesis testing. However, these studies are costly in both time and money. Therefore, they are best reserved for testing hypotheses that are already supported by the results of prior studies of less rigorous design. Often, the randomized controlled trial is the final hurdle before a hypothesis is sufficiently supported to become incorporated into clinical practice. Cross-sectional surveys and longitudinal ecologic studies are among the designs that are appropriate only for hypothesis generation. Case-control studies and retrospective cohort studies are appropriate for hypothesis generation or for hypothesis testing. Recall, however, that it is not appropriate to generate and test hypotheses with the same set of data.

3. **The answer is B: a cross-sectional survey of vaccination status.** The research question is the foundation for study design. In this example, the study should answer the following questions: Is there adequate immunity to measles in the population? If immunity is not adequate, how should vaccination policy be directed to optimize protection of the community? These questions are themselves founded on the answers to other questions, such as whether there is an effective vaccine to prevent measles. There is a measles vaccine that is effective when it is administered according to guidelines (see Centers for Disease Control 1997). A cross-sectional survey of vaccination status (or antibody titers, or both) of community members would be the most expedient, cost-effective means to obtain answers to questions concerning the allocation of public health resources to prevent the spread of measles through vaccination. Cross-sectional surveys are often useful in setting disease control priorities.

4. **The answer is E: selection bias, recall bias, and random error.** In a sense, bias is important to science, because belief, which is similar to bias, is required for a hypothesis to be formulated. In the testing of the hypothesis, however, bias must be diligently avoided. Although subjects can be randomized in a prospective study, they cannot be randomized in a retrospective study, such as the study on Lyme disease described in the question (Shadick et al. 1994). This means that in almost any retrospective study, there is a risk of selection bias. In the quantification of symptoms, many of which are subjective, measurement bias is possible. Additionally, in any retrospective study in which subjects are surveyed, the category that defines their role in the study may influence their recall of relevant events. In the study described, for example, the subjects with a history of Lyme disease might be more likely to recall symptoms suggestive of the disease or its late complications than would the controls, who have no history of disease and might either dismiss or fail to remember episodes of minor joint pain. Recall bias is one of the most important limitations of case-control studies. Random error is possible in any study and is, in fact, never completely avoided. Any form of bias, inadequately addressed, can virtually invalidate the findings in a study. Lead-time bias is only germane to screening programs and the study of the time course of a disease, such as the time between the diagnosis and the outcome (e.g., death). Lead-time bias is the tendency for early detection to increase the interval between detection and the outcome without actually altering the natural history of the disease. Length bias refers to the tendency to preferentially detect more indolent cases of disease in a population screening program; it is therefore not germane to the study in question. The ecologic fallacy refers to the tendency to presume that an association found in a population (such as the frequency of an exposure and the frequency of a disease) is operative in individuals. Because the study in question is a

study of individuals, the ecologic fallacy is not relevant.

5. **The answer is E: preferentially detect the more indolent cases of a disease.** At any given moment, the prevalence of disease in a population is influenced by both the incidence of disease (the frequency with which new cases arise) and the duration. Diseases of long duration are more apt to accumulate in a population than are diseases that run a short course and result in either recovery or death. Even within the categories of a particular illness, such as prostate cancer, the prevalence of the more indolent cases (i.e., the slowly progressive cases) is likely to be higher than the prevalence of the aggressive cases. This is because the indolent cases accumulate, while the aggressive cases result in a rapid demise. A cross-sectional survey will preferentially detect the indolent cases that tend to accumulate and will miss the cases that have recently occurred but already resulted in death. This is the late look bias: one is looking too late to find aggressive cases that have already led to death.

6. **The answer is A: length bias, because cases lasting longer are more apt to be detected.** Length bias, the tendency to preferentially detect long-lasting cases of subclinical illness whenever screening is conducted, is analogous to late look bias. Length bias occurs for the same reasons as late look bias (see the answer to question 5, above). A screening program will usually be prospective and therefore will not be subject to recall bias. The intent of any disease screening program is to detect asymptomatic and unrecognized cases. Selection bias refers to the selection of individuals to participate, and screening programs may be subject to selection bias. This would limit external validity but is not a comparable effect to the late look bias. Spectrum bias is said to occur if the clinical spectrum (variety) of the patients used to measure the sensitivity and specificity of a diagnostic test differs from the clinical spectrum of the patients to whom the test will be applied, so that the values obtained are inaccurate in the test's actual use (see Lachs et al. 1992).

7. **The answer is C: is useful for distinguishing remote from recent exposure.** The timing of a person's exposure to an infectious agent may be determined by obtaining and testing serum samples on two occasions from the same person (i.e., by measuring acute and convalescent serum titers). Alternatively, it may be determined by obtaining one serum sample from the person and measuring the titers for both IgG and IgM antibodies. IgM antibody titers rise early after infection and then decline fairly rapidly (within weeks to months). In contrast, IgG antibody titers rise more slowly and then decline gradually (within

years). It is precisely because antibody titers decline over time that their measurement is useful in determining the time of exposure. Antibody titers are a measure of humoral immunity only, so they cannot be used to distinguish cell-mediated immunity from humoral immunity. The degree of immunity is determined to a limited extent by the IgG titer and does not require that the IgM titer be measured.

8. **The answer is B: the odds ratio.** The odds ratio, derived from a case-control study, indicates the relative frequency of a particular risk factor in the cases (i.e., the subjects with the outcome in question) and in the controls (i.e., the subjects without the outcome in question). The outcome has already occurred; the risk for developing the outcome therefore cannot be measured directly. What is measured is exposure, which is presumably the exposure that preceded the outcome and represented a risk factor for it. The odds ratio may be considered the risk of having been exposed in the past, given the presence or absence of the outcome now. Therefore, the odds ratio may be considered the risk of having the risk factor. The odds ratio approximates the risk ratio when the disease in question is rare. The relative risk and the risk ratio are the same measurement (the terms are interchangeable).

9. **The answer is D: rare.** The groups in a case-control study are assembled on the basis of the outcome. If the outcome is rare, this design is particularly advantageous. Risk factors in a defined group with the rare outcome can be assessed and compared with risk factors in a group without the outcome. There are two potential problems of conducting a cohort study for a disease that is rare. One is that too few cases will arise to permit meaningful interpretation of the data. The other is that a very large sample size will be required, resulting in great (often prohibitive) expense.

10. **The answer is D: subjects whose cardiac risk factors are similar to those of the cases.** The goal of a case-control study is to determine differences in the risk factors seen in the subjects with a particular outcome (which in this example is myocardial infarction) and the subjects without the outcome. If the two groups of subjects were matched on the basis of risk factors for the outcome, differences in these factors would be eliminated by design. Matching on the basis of known (established) risk factors to isolate differences in unknown (as yet unrecognized) risk factors is often appropriate. However, if the cases and controls resemble one another too closely, there is a risk of overmatching, with the result that no differences are detectable and the study becomes useless.

References Cited

Aoun, L., and V. J. Quagliarello [Yale University School of Medicine, New Haven, Conn.] Personal communication, 1999.

Arnim, S., S. Aberle, and E. Pitney. A study of dental changes in a group of Pueblo Indian children. Journal of the American Dental Association 24:478, 1937.

Aronin, S. I., P. Peduzzi, and V. J. Quagliarello. Community-acquired bacterial meningitis: risk stratification for adverse clinical outcome and effect of antibiotic timing. Annals of Internal Medicine 129:862–870, 1998.

Belongia, E. A., et al. An investigation of the cause of the eosinophilia-myalgia syndrome associated with tryptophan use. New England Journal of Medicine 323:357–365, 1990.

Breslow, L. Risk factor intervention for health maintenance. Science 200:908–912, 1978.

Centers for Disease Control and Prevention. Achievements in public health, 1900–1999: fluoridation of drinking water to prevent dental caries. Morbidity and Mortality Weekly Report 48:933–940, 1999.

Centers for Disease Control and Prevention. CDC Prevention Guidelines: A Guide to Action. Baltimore, Williams and Wilkins Company, 1997.

Dawber, T. R., G. F. Meadors, and F. E. Moore, Jr. Epidemiologic approaches to heart disease: the Framingham Study. American Journal of Public Health 41:279–286, 1951.

Ferebee, S. United States Public Health Service trials of isoniazid prophylaxis. In Proceedings of the XVIIth International Tuberculosis Conference. International Congress Series No. 69, Rome, 1963.

Francis, T., Jr., et al. An evaluation of the 1954 poliomyelitis vaccine trials. American Journal of Public Health, April supplement, 1955.

Hasbun, R., and V. J. Quagliarello [Yale University School of Medicine, New Haven, Conn.] Personal communication, 1999.

Imperiale, T. R., and R. I. Horwitz. Scientific standards and the design of case-control research. Biomedicine and Pharmacotherapy 43:187–196, 1989.

Lachs, M. S., et al. Spectrum bias in the evaluation of diagnostic tests: lessons from the rapid dipstick test for urinary tract infection. Annals of Internal Medicine 117:135–140, 1992.

MacMahon, B. Prenatal x-ray exposure and childhood cancer. Journal of the National Cancer Institute 28:1173, 1962.

Physicians' Health Study Steering Committee. Final report on the aspirin component of the ongoing Physicians' Health Study. New England Journal of Medicine 321:129–135, 1989.

Rubin, D. H., et al. Educational intervention by computer in childhood asthma. Pediatrics 77:1–10, 1986.

Shadick, N. A., et al. The long-term clinical outcomes of Lyme disease: a population-based retrospective cohort study. Annals of Internal Medicine 121:560–567, 1994.

Slutsker, L., et al. Eosinophilia-myalgia syndrome associated with exposure to tryptophan from a single manufacturer. Journal of the American Medical Association 264:213–217, 1990.

Selected Readings

Feinstein, A. R. Clinical Epidemiology. Philadelphia, W. B. Saunders Company, 1985.

Friedman, L. M., C. D. Furbang, and D. L. DeMets. Fundamentals of Clinical Trials, 3rd ed. St. Louis, Mosby, 1995.

Gerstman, B. B. Epidemiology Kept Simple. New York, Wiley-Liss, 1998.

Gordis, L. Epidemiology. Philadelphia, W. B. Saunders Company, 1996.

Hennekens, C. H., and J. E. Buring. Epidemiology in Medicine. Boston, Little, Brown, and Company, 1987.

Hulley, S. B., and S. R. Cummings. Designing Clinical Research. Baltimore, Williams and Wilkins Company, 1988.

Kelsey, J. L., et al. Methods in Observational Epidemiology, 2nd ed. New York, Oxford University Press, 1996.

Morgenstern, H. Uses of ecologic analysis in epidemiologic research. American Journal of Public Health 72:1336–1344, 1982.

Schlesselman, J. J. Case-Control Studies: Design, Conduct, Analysis. New York, Oxford University Press, 1982.

6 Assessment of Risk and Benefit in Epidemiologic Studies

Causal research in epidemiology requires that two fundamental distinctions be made. The first distinction is between those who do have and those who do not have the risk factor being studied (the **independent variable**), while the second distinction is between those who do have and those who do not have the disease being studied (the **dependent variable**). These distinctions are seldom simple, and they are subject to both random errors and biases.

In addition, epidemiologic research may be complicated by other requirements. There may be a need to analyze several independent (possibly causal) variables at the same time, including how they interact. For example, the frequency of hypertension is related to age and gender, and these variables interact in the following manner: before the age of about 50, men are more likely to be hypertensive; but after the age of 50, women are more likely to be hypertensive. Another complication involves the need to measure different degrees of strength of exposure to the risk factor, duration of exposure to the risk factor, or both. Investigators study strength and duration in combination, for example, when they measure exposure to cigarettes in terms of pack-years, which is the average

number of packs smoked per day times the number of years of smoking. Depending on the risk factor, it may be difficult to determine the time of onset of exposure. This is true, for example, for risk factors such as sedentary life-style and excess intake of fat in the diet. The last complication of analysis is the need to measure different levels of disease severity.

Despite these complexities, much epidemiologic research still relies on the dichotomies of exposed/unexposed and diseased/nondiseased, which are commonly presented in the form of a **standard 2 × 2 table,** as shown in Table 6–1.

■ DEFINITION OF STUDY GROUPS

Causal research depends on the measurement of differences. In cohort studies, the difference is between the frequency of disease in **persons exposed** to a risk factor and the frequency of disease in **persons not exposed** to the same risk factor. In case-control studies, the difference is between the frequency of the risk factor in **case subjects** (those with the disease) and the frequency of the risk factor in **control subjects** (those without the disease).

The exposure may be to a nutritional factor (e.g., a high-fat diet), an environmental factor (radiation following the Chernobyl disaster), a behavioral factor (cigarette smoking), a physiologic characteristic (a high total cholesterol level in the blood), a medical intervention (an antibiotic), or a public health intervention (a vaccine). This list is far from exhaustive.

■ COMPARISON OF RISKS IN DIFFERENT STUDY GROUPS

Although differences in risk can be measured either in absolute terms or in relative terms, the method used will depend on the type of study performed. For reasons discussed in Chapter 5, case-control studies allow investigators to obtain only a relative measure of risk, while cohort studies and randomized controlled trials allow them to obtain both absolute and relative measures of risk. Whenever possible, it is important to examine both absolute and relative risks, because they provide different information.

After the differences in risk are calculated by the methods outlined in detail below, the level of statistical significance must be determined to ensure that the observed difference is probably real—i.e., not due

TABLE 6–1   Standard 2 × 2 Table for Demonstrating the Association Between a Risk Factor and a Disease

		DISEASE STATUS		
		Present	Absent	Total
RISK FACTOR STATUS	Present	a	b	$a + b$
	Absent	c	d	$c + d$
	Total	$a + c$	$b + d$	$a + b + c + d$

Interpretation of the cells:

a = subjects with both the risk factor and the disease
b = subjects with the risk factor but not the disease
c = subjects with the disease but not the risk factor
d = subjects with neither the risk factor nor the disease

$a + b$ = all subjects with the risk factor
$c + d$ = all subjects without the risk factor
$a + c$ = all subjects with the disease
$b + d$ = all subjects without the disease

$a + b + c + d$ = all study subjects

to chance. (Significance testing is discussed in detail in Chapter 10.) When the difference is statistically significant but not clinically important, it is real but trivial. When the difference appears to be clinically important but is not statistically significant, it may be a false-negative (beta) error if the sample size is small (see Chapter 12), or it may be a chance finding.

Absolute Differences in Risk

Disease frequency usually is measured as a risk in cohort studies and clinical trials and as a rate when the disease and death data come from population-based reporting systems.

Absolute differences in risks or rates can be expressed as a risk difference or as a rate difference. The **risk difference** is the risk in the exposed group minus the risk in the unexposed group. The **rate difference** is the rate in the exposed group minus the rate in the unexposed group. The discussion here will focus on risks, which are used more often than rates in cohort studies.

When the level of risk in the exposed group is the same as the level of risk in the unexposed group, the risk difference is 0, and the conclusion is that the exposure makes no difference to that disease risk. If an exposure is harmful (as in the case of cigarette smoking), the risk difference is expected to be greater than 0. If an exposure is protective (as in the case of a vaccine), the risk difference will be less than 0 (i.e., a negative number, which in this case indicates a reduction in disease risk in the group exposed to the vaccine). The risk difference is also known as the **attributable risk** because it is an estimate of the amount of risk that is attributable to the risk factor.

In Table 6–1, the risk of disease in the exposed individuals is $a/(a + b)$, and the risk of disease in the unexposed individuals is $c/(c + d)$. Thus, when these symbols are used, the attributable risk (AR) can be expressed as the difference between the two:

$$AR = \text{Risk}_{(\text{exposed})} - \text{Risk}_{(\text{unexposed})}$$
$$= [a/(a + b)] - [c/(c + d)]$$

Fig. 6–1 provides data on age-adjusted death rates for lung cancer among adult male smokers and nonsmokers in the US population in 1986 (see Centers for Disease Control 1989 for a report of the 1986 data) and in the UK population (Doll and Hill 1956). For the USA in 1986, the lung cancer death rate in smokers was 191 per 100,000 population per year, while the rate in nonsmokers was 8.7 per 100,000 per year. Because the death rates for lung cancer in the population were low (under 1% per year) in the year for which data are shown, the rate and the risk for lung cancer death would be essentially the same. Therefore, the risk difference (attributable risk) in the USA can be calculated as follows: 191/100,000 minus 8.7/100,000 equals 182.3/100,000. Similarly, the attributable risk in the UK can be calculated as follows: 166/100,000 minus 7/100,000 equals 159/100,000.

Relative Differences in Risk

Relative risk can be expressed in terms of a risk ratio or in terms of an odds ratio.

The Relative Risk (Risk Ratio)

The relative risk, which is also known as the risk ratio (both being abbreviated as RR), is the ratio of the risk in the exposed group to the risk in the unexposed group. If the risks in the exposed group and unexposed group are the same, the RR will equal 1. If the

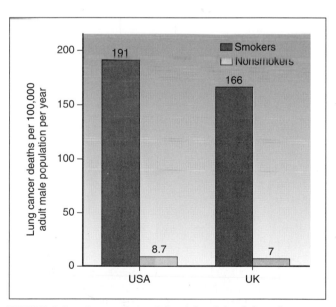

FIGURE 6–1   Comparison of the risks of death from lung cancer per 100,000 adult male population per year for smokers and nonsmokers in the USA and UK. (Source of US data: Centers for Disease Control. Chronic disease reports: deaths from lung cancer—United States, 1986. Morbidity and Mortality Weekly Report 38:501–505, 1989. Source of UK data: Doll, R., and A. B. Hill. Lung cancer and other causes of death in relation to smoking. British Medical Journal 2:1071, 1956.)

risks in the two groups are not the same, calculating the RR will provide a straightforward way of showing in relative terms how much different (greater or smaller) the risks in the exposed group are compared with the risks in the unexposed group. Remember that the risk for the disease in the exposed group will be greater if an exposure is harmful (as in the case of cigarette smoking) or will be smaller if an exposure is protective (as in the case of a vaccine).

In terms of the groups and symbols defined in Table 6–1, relative risk (RR) would be calculated as follows:

$$RR = Risk_{(exposed)}/Risk_{(unexposed)}$$
$$= [a/(a + b)]/[c/(c + d)]$$

Earlier, the data on lung cancer deaths in Fig. 6–1 were used to determine the attributable risk, or AR. This time, the same data can be used to calculate the RR. For adult males in the USA, 191/100,000 divided by 8.7/100,000 gives an RR of 22. The conversion from absolute to relative risks can be seen in Fig. 6–2. Absolute risk is shown on the left axis, and relative risk is on the right axis. Note that in relative risk terms, the value of the risk for lung cancer death in the unexposed group is 1. Compared to that, the risk for lung cancer death in the exposed group is 22 times as great, and the attributable risk is the difference, which is 182.3/100,000 in absolute risk terms and 21 in relative risk terms.

For the data in the UK study on lung cancer deaths, 166/100,000 divided by 7/100,000 gives an RR of 23.7, indicating that smokers were almost 24 times as likely to die of lung cancer as were nonsmokers.

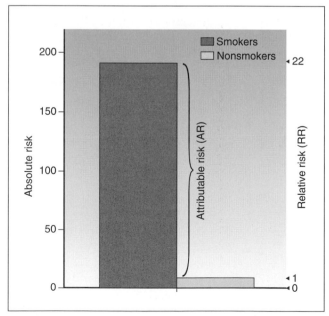

FIGURE 6–2 Diagram showing the risks of death from lung cancer per 100,000 adult male population per year for smokers and nonsmokers in the USA, expressed both in absolute terms (left axis) and in relative terms (right axis). (Source of data: Centers for Disease Control. Chronic disease reports: deaths from lung cancer—United States, 1986. Morbidity and Mortality Weekly Report 38:501–505, 1989.)

This estimate is very similar to the estimate from the US study, in which the RR was 22.

It is important to consider the number of people to whom the relative risk applies. A large relative risk that applies to a small number of people may actually produce few excess deaths or cases of disease, whereas a small relative risk that applies to a large number of people may produce many excess deaths or cases of disease.

The Odds Ratio

People who do not bet may be unfamiliar with the concept of odds and with the difference between the concepts of risk and odds. Based on the symbols used in Table 6–1, the **risk** of disease in the exposed group is $a/(a + b)$, whereas the **odds** of disease in the exposed group is simply a/b. If a is small compared to b, the odds will be similar to the risk. For example, if a particular disease occurs in 1 person among a group of 100 persons in a given year, the risk of that disease is 1 in 100 (0.0100), and the odds of that disease are 1 to 99 (0.0101). If the risk of the disease is relatively large (say, more than 5%), the odds ratio is not a very good estimate of the risk ratio.

The odds ratio can be calculated by dividing the odds of exposure in the diseased group by the odds of exposure in the nondiseased group. In the terms used in Table 6–1, the formula for the odds ratio (OR) is as follows:

$$OR = (a/c)/(b/d)$$
$$= ad/bc$$

In mathematical terms, it would make no difference whether the odds ratio was calculated as $(a/c)/(b/d)$ or as $(a/b)/(c/d)$, because cross-multiplication in either case would yield ad/bc. In a case-control study, it makes no sense to use $(a/b)/(c/d)$, because cells a and b come from different study groups. However, the fact that the odds ratio is the same whether it is developed from a horizontal analysis of the table or from a vertical analysis proves to be valuable for analyzing data from case-control studies. Although a risk or a risk ratio cannot be calculated from a case-control study, an odds ratio can be calculated. Moreover, under most real world circumstances, the odds ratio from a carefully performed case-control study is a good estimate of the risk ratio that would have been obtained from a more costly and time-consuming prospective cohort study. Therefore, the odds ratio may be used as an estimate of the risk ratio if the risk of disease in the population is low. (It can certainly be used if the risk ratio is less than 1%, and it can probably be used if it is less than 5%.)

The odds ratio also is used in logistic methods of statistical analysis (logistic regression, log-linear models, Cox regression analyses), which are discussed briefly in Chapter 11.

Which Side Is Up in the Risk Ratio and Odds Ratio?

If the risk for a disease is the same in the group exposed to a particular risk factor or protective factor as it is in the group not exposed to the factor, the risk ratio is expressed simply as 1. Hypothetically, the risk ratio could be as low as 0 (i.e., if the individuals exposed to a protective factor have no risk and the unexposed individuals have some risk), or it may be as high as infinity (i.e., if the individuals exposed to a risk factor have some risk and the unexposed individuals have no risk). In practical terms, however, because there usually is some disease in every large group, these extremes of the risk ratio are rare.

When risk factors are discussed, placing the exposed group in the numerator is a convention that makes intuitive sense (because the number gets larger as the risk has a greater impact), and this convention is followed in the literature. However, one of the interesting properties of the risk ratio is that it can also be expressed with the exposed group in the denominator. Consider the case of cigarette smoking and myocardial infarction, where the risk of this disease for smokers is greater than that for nonsmokers. On the one hand, it is acceptable to put the smokers in the numerator and express the risk ratio as 2/1 (i.e., 2), meaning that the risk of myocardial infarction is about twice as high for smokers as for nonsmokers of otherwise similar age, sex, and health status. On the other hand, it is also acceptable to put the smokers in the denominator and express the risk ratio as 1/2 (i.e., 0.5), meaning that nonsmokers have half the risk of smokers.

Another risk factor might produce, say, 4 times the risk of a disease, in which case the ratio could be expressed either as 4 or as 1/4. When the risk ratio is plotted on a logarithmic scale, as shown in Fig. 6–3, it is easy to see that regardless of which way the ratio is expressed, the distance to the risk ratio of 1 is the same. Mathematically, it does not matter whether the risk for the exposed group or the unexposed group is in the numerator: either way the risk ratio is easily interpretable. However, almost always the risk of the exposed group is expressed in the numerator, so that the numbers make intuitive sense.

Although the equation for calculating the odds ratio differs from that for calculating the risk ratio, once the odds ratio is calculated, the same principle applies: the ratio is usually expressed with the exposed group in the numerator, but mathematically it can be interpreted equally well if the exposed group is placed in the denominator.

It is important to remember that when a difference is measured as the contrast between two risks or two rates, the condition of no difference (i.e., the risks or rates are equal) is represented by 0.0. However, when the contrast is described by a relative risk or an odds ratio, the condition of no difference is represented by 1.0, because the numerator and denominator are equal.

OTHER MEASURES OF THE IMPACT OF RISK FACTORS

One of the most useful applications of epidemiology is to estimate how much disease burden is caused by certain modifiable risk factors. This is useful for pol-

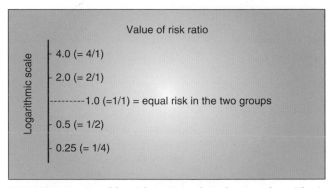

FIGURE 6–3 Possible risk ratios plotted on a logarithmic scale, showing that reciprocal risks are equidistant from the neutral point, where the risk ratio is equal to 1.0.

icy development, because the impact of risk factors or interventions to reduce risk factors can be compared to costs in cost-benefit and cost-effectiveness analyses. In addition, health education is often more effective when educators can demonstrate how big an impact a given risk factor has on individual risks.

In addition to the risk difference, relative risk, and odds ratio, the most common measures of the impact of exposures are (1) the attributable risk percent in the exposed, (2) the population attributable risk, and (3) the population attributable risk percent (Box 6–1). In the discussion of these measures, smoking and lung cancer will be used as the examples of risk factor and disease, and the calculations will be based on 1986 rates for the USA (see Fig. 6–1).

Attributable Risk Percent in the Exposed

If an investigator wanted to answer the question, "Among smokers, what percentage of the total risk for fatal lung cancer is due to smoking?" it would be necessary to calculate the attributable risk percent in the exposed, which is abbreviated as $AR\%_{(exposed)}$. There are two methods of calculation, one based on absolute differences in risk and the other based on relative differences in risk.

The following equation is based on absolute differences:

$$AR\%_{(exposed)} = \frac{Risk_{(exposed)} - Risk_{(unexposed)}}{Risk_{(exposed)}} \times 100$$

If the 1986 US data on the lung cancer death rates (expressed as deaths per 100,000 per year) in adult male smokers and nonsmokers are used, the calculation is as follows:

$$AR\%_{(exposed)} = \frac{(191 - 8.7)}{191} \times 100 = \frac{182.3}{191} \times 100 = 95.4\%$$

If the absolute risk is not known, the risk ratio (RR) can be used instead, with the following formula:

$$AR\%_{(exposed)} = \frac{RR - 1}{RR} \times 100$$

Earlier in this chapter, the RR for the US data was

BOX 6–1 Equations for Comparing Risks in Different Groups and Measuring the Impact of Risk Factors

(1) Risk difference
$$= \text{Attributable risk (AR)}$$
$$= \text{Risk}_{\text{(exposed)}} - \text{Risk}_{\text{(unexposed)}}$$
$$= [a/(a+b)] - [c/(c+d)]$$
where a represents subjects with both the risk factor and the disease; b represents subjects with the risk factor but not the disease; c represents subjects with the disease but not the risk factor; and d represents subjects with neither the risk factor nor the disease

(2) Relative risk
$$= \text{Risk ratio (RR)}$$
$$= \text{Risk}_{\text{(exposed)}}/\text{Risk}_{\text{(unexposed)}}$$
$$= [a/(a+b)]/[c/(c+d)]$$

(3) Odds ratio (OR)
$$= (a/b)/(c/d)$$
$$= (a/c)/(b/d)$$
$$= ad/bc$$

(4) Attributable risk percent in the exposed
$$= \text{AR\%}_{\text{(exposed)}}$$
$$= \frac{\text{Risk}_{\text{(exposed)}} - \text{Risk}_{\text{(unexposed)}}}{\text{Risk}_{\text{(exposed)}}} \times 100$$
$$= \frac{\text{RR} - 1}{\text{RR}} \times 100$$
$$\simeq \frac{\text{OR} - 1}{\text{OR}} \times 100$$

(5) Population attributable risk (PAR)
$$= \text{Risk}_{\text{(total)}} - \text{Risk}_{\text{(unexposed)}}$$

(6) Population attributable risk percent
$$= \text{PAR\%}$$
$$= \frac{\text{Risk}_{\text{(total)}} - \text{Risk}_{\text{(unexposed)}}}{\text{Risk}_{\text{(total)}}} \times 100$$
$$= \frac{(Pe)(\text{RR} - 1)}{1 + (Pe)(\text{RR} - 1)} \times 100$$
where Pe stands for the effective proportion of the population exposed to the risk factor

---

calculated as 22, so this figure can be used in the equation:

$$\text{AR\%}_{\text{(exposed)}} = \frac{(22 - 1)}{22} \times 100 = 95.5\%$$

Note that the percentage based on the formula using relative risk is the same as the percentage based on the formula using absolute risk (except for rounding errors). Why does this work? The important thing to remember is that the relative risk for the unexposed group is always 1, because that is the group to which the exposed group is compared. Therefore, the attributable risk, which is the amount of risk in excess of the risk in the unexposed group, is RR minus 1.

Because the odds ratio may be used to estimate the risk ratio if the risk of disease in the population is small, the AR%$_{\text{(exposed)}}$ also can be estimated by using odds ratios obtained from case-control studies and substituting them for the RR in the formula above.

Population Attributable Risk

The population attributable risk is defined as the risk in the total population minus the risk in the unexposed population. In the case of smoking and lung cancer, calculation of the population attributable risk allows an investigator to answer the question, "Among the general population, how much of the total risk for fatal lung cancer is due to smoking?" The answer to this question is not as useful to know for counseling patients, but it is of considerable importance to policy makers.

Using the US data for 1986, the investigator would subtract the risk in the adult male nonsmokers (8.7/ 100,000 per year) from the risk in the total adult male population (72.5/100,000 per year) to find the population attributable risk (63.8/100,000 per year). It can be presumed in this case that if there had never been any smokers or effects of second-hand smoke in the USA, the total US lung cancer death rate in adult males would be only 8.7/100,000 per year. Therefore, the excess over this figure—i.e., 63.8/100,000 per year—could be attributed to smoking.

Population Attributable Risk Percent

The population attributable risk percent (PAR%) answers the question, "Among the general population, what percentage of the total risk for fatal lung cancer is due to smoking?" As with the AR%$_{\text{(exposed)}}$, the PAR% can be calculated using either absolute or relative differences in risk.

The following equation is based on absolute differences:

$$\text{PAR\%} = \frac{\text{Risk}_{\text{(total)}} - \text{Risk}_{\text{(unexposed)}}}{\text{Risk}_{\text{(total)}}} \times 100$$

When the US data discussed above for males are used, the calculation is as follows:

$$\text{PAR\%} = \frac{(72.5 - 8.7)}{72.5} \times 100 = \frac{63.8}{72.5} \times 100 = 88\%$$

The PAR% could instead be calculated using the risk ratio (or the odds ratio if the data come from a case-control study). But first it is necessary to incorporate another measure into the formula—namely, the proportion exposed, which is abbreviated as *Pe* and is defined as the effective proportion of the population exposed to the risk factor. The equation is then as follows:

$$PAR\% = \frac{(Pe)(RR - 1)}{1 + (Pe)(RR - 1)} \times 100$$

In the case of smoking, the *Pe* would be the *effective* proportion of the adult population who smoked. This figure must be estimated, rather than being obtained directly, because of the long latent period from the start of smoking until the onset of lung cancer and occurrence of death. The proportion of smokers has

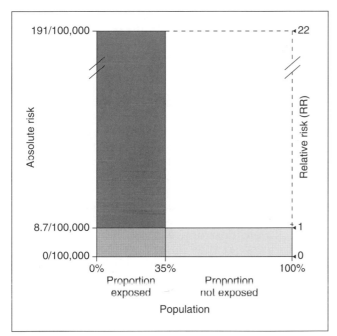

FIGURE 6–4   Diagram showing how the equation for population attributable risk percent (PAR%) works. The *x*-axis shows the population, divided into two groups: the 35% of the population representing the proportion exposed *(Pe)* to the risk factor (i.e., the effective population of smokers), and the remaining 65% of the population, who are nonsmokers. The right side of the *y*-axis shows the relative risk (RR) of lung cancer death. For reference, the left side of the *y*-axis shows the absolute risk of lung cancer death. Orange shading, gray shading, and a combination of the two are used to show the relationship between the risk factor (smoking) and the disease outcome (lung cancer death) in the smokers and nonsmokers. The purely orange part represents outcomes that are not attributable to the risk factor in nonsmokers. The purely gray part represents outcomes that are attributable to the risk factor in smokers. The overlapping gray and orange part represents outcomes that are not attributable to the risk factor in smokers (i.e., lung cancer deaths that are not attributable to smoking, even though they occurred in smokers). The equation is as follows:

$$PAR\% = \frac{(Pe)(RR - 1)}{1 + (Pe)(RR - 1)} \times 100$$

$$= \frac{(0.35)(22 - 1)}{1 + (0.35)(22 - 1)} \times 100$$

$$= \frac{7.35}{1 + 7.35} \times 100 = 88\%$$

been dropping over time (now down to about 25% of adults in the USA). Here, the *Pe* is assumed to be 0.35, or 35%.

As calculated earlier, the relative risk (RR) for lung cancer in the USA was 22. Thus, if this number is used, the calculation can be completed as follows:

$$PAR\% = \frac{(0.35)(22 - 1)}{1 + (0.35)(22 - 1)} \times 100 = \frac{7.35}{1 + 7.35} \times 100 = 88\%$$

Fig. 6–4 shows diagrammatically how the formula for PAR% works.

■ USES OF RISK ASSESSMENT DATA

After the various measures of the impact of smoking on lung cancer deaths have been calculated, the results can be used both in policy analysis and in counseling patients.

Application of Risk Data to Policy Analysis
Estimating the Benefit of Interventions in Populations

Population attributable risk (PAR) data can often be used to estimate the benefit of a proposed intervention, such as the number of lung cancer deaths that would be prevented by instituting a smoking reduction program in a large population.

For example, assume that in the USA the proportion of adult males who smoke has averaged about 25% for over 2 decades (as it did during much of the 1990s). Also assume that the amount of smoking has been constant among adult males who smoke and that the lung cancer death rate in this group remains constant (represented by the lung cancer death rate shown in Table 6–2, which is 191 per 100,000 per year for smokers versus 8.7 per 100,000 per year for nonsmokers).

Given these assumptions, the rate of lung cancer deaths in the total adult male population would be a weighted average of the rates in smokers and nonsmokers:

Rate per
100,000 male
population
per year $= (\text{Weight}_{smokers})(\text{Rate}_{smokers}) +$
$\qquad (\text{Weight}_{nonsmokers})(\text{Rate}_{nonsmokers})$

$\qquad = (0.25)(191) + (0.75)(8.7)$

$\qquad = 47.8 + 6.5 = 54.3$

Then the PAR, also expressed as a rate per 100,000 male population, would be calculated as follows:

$$PAR = 54.3 - 8.7 = 45.6$$

If a major smoking reduction program (possibly financed by the tobacco settlement money) were to reduce the proportion of adult male smokers from 25% to 20% for an extended period of time and if the

TABLE 6–2 Measures of Smoking and Lung Cancer Deaths in Adult Males in the USA, 1986

Measure	Amount
*Lung cancer deaths among smokers	191 per 100,000 per year
*Lung cancer deaths among nonsmokers	8.7 per 100,000 per year
Proportion exposed (Pe) to the risk factor (effective population of smokers, averaged over time)	35%, or 0.35
†Population risk of lung cancer death	72.5 per 100,000 per year
†Relative risk, or RR	22 [191/8.7 = 22]
†Attributable risk, or AR	182.3 per 100,000 per year [191 − 8.7 = 182.3]
†Attributable risk percent in the exposed, or AR%$_{(exposed)}$	95.4% [182.3/191 × 100 = 95.4]
†Population attributable risk, or PAR	63.8 per 100,000 per year [72.5 − 8.7 = 63.8]
†Population attributable risk percent, or PAR%	88% [63.8/72.5 × 100 = 88]

*The source of data for measures shown with an asterisk is as follows: Centers for Disease Control. Chronic disease reports: deaths from lung cancer—United States, 1986. Morbidity and Mortality Weekly Report 38: 501–505, 1989.
†These rates were calculated from the data marked with an asterisk.

lung cancer death rates for smokers and nonsmokers remained constant, the revised rate of lung cancer deaths in the total adult male population would be calculated as follows:

$$\begin{aligned}
\text{Rate per } & \\
\text{100,000 male} & \\
\text{population} & \\
\text{per year} &= (\text{Weight}_{smokers})(\text{Rate}_{smokers}) + \\
& \quad (\text{Weight}_{nonsmokers})(\text{Rate}_{nonsmokers}) \\
&= (0.20)(191) + (0.80)(8.7) \\
&= 38.2 + 7.0 = 45.2
\end{aligned}$$

Under these conditions,

$$PAR = 45.2 - 8.7 = 36.5$$

The difference between the first PAR (45.6) and the second PAR (36.5) is 9.1. This means that a smoking reduction program that was able to reduce the proportion of adult male smokers from 25% to 20% would eventually be expected to prevent about 9 lung cancer deaths per 100,000 adult males per year. If there were 100 million adult males, then the intervention would be responsible for preventing 9100 deaths per year. If there were a similar number of adult females and they had a similar reduction in smoking rate and lung cancer death rate, then 9100 deaths per year would be prevented in adult females, bringing the total to 18,200 deaths prevented in the adult population per year.

Cost-Effectiveness Analysis

In cost-effectiveness analysis, investigators estimate the costs of an intervention and compare them with the effects of that intervention. For health interventions, the effects are commonly measured in terms of the number of injuries, illnesses, or deaths prevented. Although external factors may complicate the calculation of both the costs and the effects, it is generally more difficult to measure effects, partly because many costs are known quickly, whereas effects may take a long time to measure.

In the above example of a smoking reduction program, if the costs of the program were $1 billion per year and if 18,200 lung cancer deaths were prevented per year, it would have cost about $54,945 to prevent each death. If the costs of the program were assigned to the 200 million adults in the population, instead of to the deaths that the program prevented, it would have cost $5 per adult per year. If the costs of the program were assigned to the adults who quit smoking (5%), it would have cost about $100 per "quitter" per year.

These amounts may seem high, but it is important to keep in mind that the cost estimates here are fictitious and that the adult population size estimates are crude. It is also important to remember that in addition to preventing lung cancer deaths, a smoking reduction program would offer other benefits. These would include reductions in the rates of various illnesses among smokers, as well as reductions in the numbers of deaths from heart attacks, chronic obstructive pulmonary disease, and other cancers, such as nasopharyngeal, esophageal, and bladder cancer. If the assumptions were accurate and if all of the positive effects of smoking cessation were included in the analysis, the costs per health benefit would be much less than that shown above.

Cost-Benefit Analysis

In cost-benefit analysis, both the costs and the benefits are measured in dollars. To calculate the benefits of a smoking reduction program, investigators would have to convert the positive effects (e.g., the reduction in lung cancer deaths) into dollar amounts before the comparison with costs is made. In their calculation of benefits, they would consider a variety of factors, including savings in medical care and the increased productivity from the added years of life. This would require them to estimate the average costs of care for one case of lung cancer; the dollar value (in terms of productivity) of adding 1 year of life; and the average number of productive years of life gained by preventing lung cancer. Investigators would also include the time value of money in their analysis by discounting benefits that would occur only in the future. For more details on cost-effectiveness analysis, cost-benefit analysis, cost-utility analysis, and discounting, see Chapter 14.

Other Ways of Describing the Value of Interventions

The anticipated value of an intervention—whether it is a vaccine, a type of treatment, or a change in nutrition or behavior—is frequently expressed in absolute terms (the absolute risk reduction), in relative terms (the relative risk reduction), or as the reduction in incidence density (e.g., the reduction in risk per 100 person-years). These epidemiologic expressions, however, may not give patients or their physicians a good sense of how much impact a particular intervention may have. Each method will tend to communicate different things, so a variety of measures are needed (Box 6–2).

Absolute and Relative Risk Reduction. The **absolute risk reduction** (ARR) and the **relative risk reduction** (RRR) are descriptive measures that are easy to calculate and understand (Sackett et al. 1991). Say that the yearly risk of a certain disease is 0.010 in the presence of the risk factor and 0.004 in the absence of the risk factor. The ARR and RRR would be calculated as follows:

$$ARR = Risk_{(exposed)} - Risk_{(unexposed)} = 0.010 - 0.004$$
$$= 0.006$$

$$RRR = \frac{Risk_{(exposed)} - Risk_{(unexposed)}}{Risk_{(exposed)}} = \frac{0.010 - 0.004}{0.010}$$
$$= \frac{0.006}{0.010} = 0.6 = 60\%$$

In this example, an intervention that removed the risk factor would reduce the risk of disease by 0.006 in absolute terms (ARR) or produce a 60% reduction of risk in relative terms (RRR). When the RRR is applied to the effectiveness of vaccines, it is called the **vaccine effectiveness or the protective efficacy** (see Chapter 16).

Reduction in Incidence Density. In estimating the effects of treatment methods used to eradicate or prevent a disease, it is important to incorporate the length of time that treatment is needed to obtain one **unit of benefit,** which is usually defined as the eradication or prevention of disease in one person (Laupacius, Sackett, and Roberts 1988). The easiest way to incorporate time is to use incidence density, expressed in terms of the **number of person-years** of treatment. For example, when warfarin treatment is given on a long-term basis to prevent strokes in patients who have atrial fibrillation, its benefits can be reported in terms of the reduction in strokes per 100 patient-years. When Baker (1997) reviewed five studies of warfarin versus placebo treatment in patients with atrial fibrillation, he found that the average number of strokes that occurred per 100 patient-years was 1.8 in those treated with warfarin and 5.1 in those treated with placebo. As shown in Box 6–2, the risk difference between these groups is 3.3 per 100 patient-years; the ARR is 0.033 per patient-year; and the RRR is 65%.

Number Needed to Treat or Harm. An increasingly popular measure used to describe the practical value of treatment is called the **number needed to treat** (NNT), meaning the number of patients who would need to receive a specific type of treatment in order for one patient to benefit from the treatment (Laupacius, Sackett, and Roberts 1988; Sackett et al. 1991). The NNT is calculated as the number 1 divided by the **absolute risk reduction** (ARR). In its simplest form, this is expressed as a proportion: NNT = 1/ARR. Say, for example, that a course of hyperbaric oxygen therapy healed the leg ulcers in one-third of patients whose ulcers were resistant to all other forms of treatment. The ARR would be 0.333, and the NNT would be 1/0.333 = 3. These results suggest that, on average, it would be necessary to give hyperbaric oxygen therapy to three patients with resistant leg ulcers to benefit one patient. The NNT is helpful for making comparisons of the effectiveness of different types of interventions (Kumana, Cheung, and Lauder 1999; Woolf 1999).

The idea behind the **number needed to harm** (NNH) is similar to that of the NNT, but it is applied to the negative effects of treatment. The fundamental item of data is the **absolute risk increase** (ARI), which is analogous to the absolute risk reduction (ARR) in the NNT. The NNH formula is similar to that of the NNT: NNH = 1/ARI. Results of a clinical trial by Oski et al. (1980) can be used as an example for calculating the NNH. In this trial, some infants were given iron-fortified formula, other infants were given formula without iron (regular formula), and the mothers of all of the infants were asked to report whether the infants had symptoms of colic. The mothers reported the occurrence of colic in 56.8% of infants receiving iron-fortified formula and in 40.8% of infants receiving regular formula. In this case, the ARI = 0.568 − 0.408 = 0.16. The NNH = 1/0.16 = 6.25. This suggests that one of every six or seven infants given iron-fortified formula would develop colic because of the formula (and another two or three infants would have had colic even without iron in the formula).

Although the NNT and NNH are helpful for describing the effects of treatment, several points about their use should be emphasized. First, Altman (1998) notes that a complete analysis of NNT and NNH should provide confidence intervals for the estimates, and he offers an appropriate formula. (For an introduction to confidence intervals, see Chapter 10.) Second, it is important to incorporate the length of time that treatment is needed to obtain a unit of benefit (see the discussion of incidence density, above). Third, the net benefit from an intervention should in some way be reduced to account for any harm done. The analysis becomes complicated if done with maximum precision, because the investigator needs to calculate the proportion of treated patients who derive benefit only, the proportion who derive harm only, and the proportion who derive both benefit and harm (Mancini and Schulzer 1999).

BOX 6–2   Calculation of Risk Reduction and Other Measures to Describe the Practical Value of Treatment

Part 1   Beginning data and assumptions

(a) Treatment-derived benefit

Various studies have shown that the risk of stroke in patients with atrial fibrillation can be prevented by long-term treatment with warfarin, an anticoagulant. Baker (1997) reviewed the results of five of these studies and reported the following:

$$\text{Average number of strokes without warfarin treatment} = 5.1 \text{ per 100 patient-years}$$
$$= 0.051 \text{ patients for 1 year each}$$
$$\text{Average number of strokes with warfarin treatment} = 1.8 \text{ per 100 patient-years}$$
$$= 0.018 \text{ patients for 1 year each}$$

(b) Treatment-induced harm

Patients who are treated with drugs are always at some risk of harm. Averages are not available for serious adverse events, such as cerebral and gastrointestinal hemorrhage, in the five studies analyzed by Baker. Assume here that the average number of serious adverse events in atrial fibrillation patients treated with warfarin is 1 per 100 patient-years = 0.01 patients for 1 year each (fictitious data).

Part 2   Measures of treatment-derived benefit

$$\text{Risk difference} = \text{Risk}_{(exposed)} - \text{Risk}_{(unexposed)}$$
$$= 5.1 - 1.8 = 3.3 \text{ per 100 patient-years}$$

$$\text{Absolute risk reduction (ARR)} = \text{Risk}_{(exposed)} - \text{Risk}_{(unexposed)}$$
$$= 0.051 - 0.018 = 0.033$$

$$\text{Relative risk reduction (RRR)} = \frac{\text{Risk}_{(exposed)} - \text{Risk}_{(unexposed)}}{\text{Risk}_{(exposed)}}$$
$$= \frac{0.051 - 0.018}{0.051} = \frac{0.033}{0.051} = 0.65 = 65\%$$

Part 3   Measures of treatment-induced harm (fictitious data)

$$\text{Absolute risk increase (ARI)} = \text{Risk}_{(exposed)} - \text{Risk}_{(unexposed)} = 0.01$$

Part 4   Calculation of number needed to treat (NNT) and number needed to harm (NNH)

(a) NNT is the number of patients with atrial fibrillation who would need to be treated with warfarin for 1 year each to prevent one stroke.

$$\text{NNT} = 1/\text{ARR} = 1/0.033 = 30.3 = \text{about 31 patients}$$

(b) NNH is the number of patients with atrial fibrillation who would need to be treated with warfarin for 1 year each to cause serious harm.

$$\text{NNH} = 1/\text{ARI} = 1/0.01 = 100 \text{ patients}$$

(c) Whenever the ARR is larger than the ARI (i.e., the NNH is larger than the NNT), more patients will be helped than will be harmed by the treatment. The ratio can be calculated in two different ways:

$$\text{ARR/ARI} = 0.033/0.01 = 3.3$$

$$\text{NNH/NNT} = 100/30.3 = 3.3$$

This means that the number of patients who will be helped is 3 times as large as the number who will be harmed. However, this result and the calculations on which it is based may be oversimplifications, because the amount of benefit may be quantitatively different from the amount of harm derived from a treatment.

Source of data for the average number of strokes with and without warfarin treatment: Baker, D. Anticoagulation for atrial fibrillation. The Health Failure Quality Improvement Newsletter, issue 4, Kerr L. White Institute for Health Services Research, Sept. 15, 1997.

Application of Risk Measures to the Counseling of Patients

Suppose a physician's patient is resistant to the idea of quitting smoking but is willing to be convinced. Or suppose the physician has been asked to give a short talk summarizing the effect of smoking on the lung cancer death rates, which is roughly equivalent to talking about the incidence of lung cancer, because most lung cancer patients die of their disease. Using the measures of risk discussed here and summarized in Table 6–2, the physician could make the following estimates of the impact of smoking (although the data come from studies in males, they apply reasonably well to females also): (1) Smokers are about 22 times as likely as nonsmokers to die of lung cancer. (2) About 95 out of every 100 lung cancer deaths in people who smoke can be attributed to the fact that they smoke. (3) There are about 158,000 deaths from respiratory tract cancer in the USA, and because about 88% can be attributed to smoking, this means that smoking is responsible for about 139,000 respiratory tract cancer deaths per year.

■ SUMMARY

Epidemiologic research is usually designed to permit one or more primary contrasts in risk, rate, or odds of disease or exposure. The most straightforward of these measures are the risk difference (the attributable risk) and the rate difference, which show in absolute terms how much the risk of one group (usually the group that is exposed to a risk factor or a preventive factor) differs from that of another group. This contrast can also be expressed as a ratio of risks, rates, or odds; the greater this ratio, the greater the difference the exposure makes.

The impact of the risk factor on the total disease burden can be measured in terms of an attributable risk percent for the exposed group or for the population in general. If it is known by how much a preventive program can reduce the risk ratio and in whom, the total benefit of the program, including its cost-effectiveness, can be calculated.

Measures such as the relative risk reduction, the number needed to treat, and the number needed to harm are also commonly used to determine the effect of intervention.

■ QUESTIONS

Directions (Items 1–15). Each of the numbered items or incomplete statements in this section is followed by answers or by completions of the statement. Select the ONE lettered answer or completion that is BEST in each case. Correct answers and explanations are given at the end of the chapter.

1. A team of researchers hypothesize that watching "Barney" might lead to epilepsy in childhood. Children with and without epilepsy are compared on the basis of hours spent watching "Barney." Which of the following statements best characterizes the assessment of data in a study such as this?

    (A) Absolute and relative measures of risk can be derived
    (B) Risk factor status is the basis for comparison
    (C) The risk ratio cannot be calculated directly
    (D) The temporal association between exposure and outcome can be established with certainty
    (E) The use of healthy controls ensures external validity

2. The researchers in question 1 do not find statistically significant evidence that "Barney" produces epilepsy in childhood. Unwilling, however, to relinquish their line of reasoning, they hypothesize that the parents of children who watch "Barney" are more likely to develop migraine headaches. They assemble two groups of parents: one with children who watch "Barney" and one with children who destroy furniture instead of watching "Barney." Which of the following is a characteristic of a study such as this?

    (A) Additional risk factors cannot be assessed as the study progresses
    (B) Internal validity is independent of confounders
    (C) Risk factor status does not serve as the basis for comparison
    (D) The relative risk cannot be calculated directly
    (E) The temporal association between exposure and outcome is uncertain

3. The risk of acquiring infection beta is 312 per 1000 among the unvaccinated and 7.2 per 1000 among the vaccinated. Approximately 80% of the population is exposed to the pathogen every year. Which of the following actions taken to develop policy would be incompatible with the above information?

    (A) Consideration of the clinical significance (severity) of infection
    (B) Consideration of the cost of universal vaccination
    (C) Consideration of the side effects of vaccination
    (D) Reporting a risk reduction of 304.8 per 1000 attributable to vaccination
    (E) Reporting that the population attributable risk percent (PAR%) is 27

Items 4–8

A study is conducted to determine the effects of drinking Mountain Dew on a teenager's willingness to bungee jump from frightful heights. A total of 500 teenagers are assembled on the basis of bungee-jumping status: 250 are jumpers, and 250 are not. Of the 250 jumpers, 150 report drinking Mountain Dew. Of the 250 nonjumpers, 50 report drinking Mountain Dew. A majority of the nonjumpers report a preference for warm milk.

4. Which of the following statements is true?

(A) Jumpers and nonjumpers should be matched for beverage consumption
(B) The absolute and relative risk of bungee jumping can be determined from this study
(C) This is a cohort study
(D) This study can be used to calculate an odds ratio
(E) Unanticipated outcomes can be assessed in this study

5. What is the absolute difference in the risk of jumping?

(A) It cannot be calculated, because jumping is the dependent variable
(B) It cannot be calculated, because this is a case-control study
(C) It is 3:1
(D) It is 100
(E) It is 150

6. The odds ratio calculated from this study will give the odds of

(A) drinking among jumpers to drinking among nonjumpers
(B) drinking among nonjumpers to drinking among jumpers
(C) drinking Mountain Dew to jumping
(D) jumping among drinkers to drinking among jumpers
(E) nonjumping among drinkers to nondrinking among jumpers

7. The odds ratio in this study is

(A) 0.2
(B) 0.6
(C) 2
(D) 5
(E) 6

8. The results of this study indicate that

(A) bungee jumping and beverage choice are associated
(B) bungee jumping and beverage choice are causally related
(C) bungee jumping influences a person's choice of beverage
(D) the choice of beverage influences a person's tendency to bungee jump
(E) there is no association between warm milk and bungee jumping

Items 9–10

Having obtained your master's degree in public health, not to mention a lifetime supply of Mountain Dew and your own initialized bungee cord, from con-

ducting the study described in items 4–8 (above), you decide to pursue a PhD, with further investigation of this provocative subject. Once again, your study involves a total of 500 teenagers, with 250 in each group. This time, however, you assemble the groups on the basis of their past history of Mountain Dew consumption, and you prospectively determine the incidence rate of bungee jumping. You exclude subjects with a prior history of jumping. Over a 5-year period, 135 of the exposed group and 38 of the unexposed group engage in jumping.

9. The relative risk of bungee jumping among the exposed is

(A) 2.12
(B) 3.6
(C) 4.8
(D) 6
(E) 115

10. Among bungee jumpers, what percentage of the total risk for jumping is due to consumption of Mountain Dew?

(A) 0%
(B) 0.36%
(C) 2.6%
(D) 36%
(E) 72%

Items 11–13

Assume that the risk of death in patients with untreated pneumonia is 15%, while the risk of death in patients with antibiotic-treated pneumonia is 2%. Assume as well that the risk of anaphylaxis with antibiotic treatment is 1%, while the risk without treatment is essentially 0%.

11. What is the number needed to treat (NNT) in this scenario?

(A) 2
(B) 5.4
(C) 7.7
(D) 8.7
(E) 100

12. What is the number needed to harm (NNH) in this scenario?

(A) 5.4
(B) 8.7
(C) 12.1
(D) 25
(E) 100

13. What will be the net result of intervention in this scenario?

(A) 7 patients harmed for each patient saved
(B) 7 patients saved for each patient harmed
(C) 12.1 patients harmed for each patient saved
(D) 13 patients saved for each patient harmed
(E) 100 patients saved for each patient harmed

Items 14–15

You randomly assign subjects to 4 years of medical school (intervention) or 4 years as understudies on "Baywatch" (control), and then you test for evidence of mental health (outcome). Of 100 subjects assigned to each condition, you find evidence of mental health in 12 in the medical school group and 92 in the "Baywatch" group.

14. An appropriate measure of association in this study is
    (A) incidence density
    (B) power
    (C) the likelihood ratio
    (D) the odds ratio
    (E) the risk ratio

15. The value of the measure identified in question 14 is
    (A) 0.08
    (B) 0.13
    (C) 1.3
    (D) 8.1
    (E) 13.1

■ ANSWERS AND EXPLANATIONS

1. **The answer is C: the risk ratio cannot be calculated directly.** This is a case-control study. The cases are children who have epilepsy, and the controls are (or should be) children who do not have epilepsy but whose characteristics are otherwise similar to those of the cases. The use of healthy controls does not ensure that the results will pertain to the general population, so external validity remains uncertain. The difference in the rate of exposure to a putative risk factor ("Barney") is the basis for comparison. In a case-control study, the risk ratio cannot be calculated directly but must be estimated from the odds ratio. The temporal relationship between exposure and outcome is usually not known with certainty in this type of study; both exposure and disease have already occurred at the time of enrollment. Only relative measures of risk can be calculated based on a case-control study. A cohort study is required to obtain absolute risk.

2. **The answer is A: additional risk factors cannot be assessed as the study progresses.** This is a cohort study. The two groups are assembled on the basis of exposure status (i.e., risk factor status), and they are then followed for and compared on the basis of disease status. Only the risk factors, or exposures, identified at study entry can be assessed as the study progresses. The development of migraine headaches in this case is the disease. The temporal association between exposure and outcome should be established to prevent bias; in a cohort study, subjects are generally free of the outcome (disease) at the time of enrollment.

The inclusion of subjects who developed migraine headaches prior to the defined exposure would bias the study, so these subjects should be excluded. In all epidemiologic studies, a thorough attempt must be made to control confounders, because confounding compromises internal validity. The relative risk (of migraine headaches, in this case) can be calculated directly in a cohort study.

3. **The answer is E: reporting that the population attributable risk percent (PAR%) is 27.** Option E is the only option that is incompatible with the information provided. As discussed in the text, one of two formulas can be used to determine the PAR%. The first is as follows:

$$PAR\% = \frac{Risk_{(total)} - Risk_{(unexposed)}}{Risk_{(total)}} \times 100$$

This is equivalent to:

$$PAR\% = \frac{(Pe)(RR - 1)}{1 + (Pe)(RR - 1)} \times 100$$

where Pe is the proportion of the population exposed and RR is the relative risk. In the case described in the question, it is impossible to calculate the PAR%, because we have not been told the proportion of the population exposed (i.e., vaccinated) and therefore do not know the Pe for the second formula. To determine the $Risk_{(total)}$ for the first formula, we again need to know the proportion of the population vaccinated (in whom the risk of infection is 7.2 per 1000) and the proportion unvaccinated (in whom the risk is 312 per 1000). With exposure to a preventive measure, such as a vaccine in this case, risk is reduced among the exposed. The risk of the outcome is therefore less among the exposed than among the unexposed, so the population attributable risk would be negative. The clinical significance (option A) of the infection for which vaccination is considered is always important; any risks of vaccination may not be justified if the infection is trivial. Just such a consideration generated controversy regarding the development and use of the vaccine against varicella, or chickenpox (Halloran et al. 1994). The costs (option B) and potential adverse effects (option C) are always essential considerations in vaccine use. If a vaccine is associated with a high rate of adverse effects, it may be ill-advised even if effective. Cost and cost-effectiveness are pertinent considerations in any population-based intervention. Option D (reporting a risk reduction of 304.8 per 1000 attributable to vaccination) is correct, although the attributable risk (AR) is of limited utility by itself in policy development because it fails to take into consideration the level of exposure in the population. The AR is as follows:

$$AR = Risk_{(exposed)} - Risk_{(unexposed)}$$

$$= (7.2/1000) - (312/1000)$$

$$= -304.8/1000$$

4. The answer is D: this study can be used to calculate an odds ratio. The study described is a case-control study. The cases are teenagers who have a history of bungee jumping, and the controls are (or should be) teenagers who have no history of bungee jumping but whose characteristics are otherwise similar to those of the cases. The cases and controls should not be matched for beverage consumption, since this is the exposure of interest. Overmatching is the result when cases and controls are matched on the basis of some characteristic or behavior that is highly correlated with the exposure of interest. Overmatching precludes the detection of a difference in exposure, even if one truly exists. The odds ratio is calculated from a case-control study and is used to estimate relative risk. Absolute risk cannot be determined from a case-control study. In this type of study, the outcome defines the group at study entry; while unanticipated risk factors can be assessed, only the outcome variables chosen as the basis for subject selection can be evaluated.

5. The answer is B: it cannot be calculated, because this is a case-control study. Risk can only be estimated from a case-control study; it cannot be calculated directly. In particular, relative risk can be estimated by the odds ratio; absolute risk cannot be determined from a case-control study, because the groups do not represent the population from which they were drawn. In this study, bungee jumping is the independent variable (not the dependent variable), since the groups were assembled on the basis of their jumping status. The odds to be calculated are the odds of drinking Mountain Dew, given an individual's history of jumping or not jumping.

6. The answer is A: drinking among jumpers to drinking among nonjumpers. The odds ratio in a case-control study is the odds of the exposure in cases relative to controls. The exposure in this study is drinking (specifically, drinking Mountain Dew). Cases are those who bungee jump, while controls are those who do not. The odds of drinking Mountain Dew among cases relative to controls is the outcome of interest. As noted in the text, the odds ratio is essentially a measure of the "risk of having the risk factor."

7. The answer is E: 6. As described in the text, the formula for the odds ratio (OR) is $(a/c)/(b/d)$. This is algebraically equivalent to ad/bc, where a represents cases with the exposure, b represents controls with the exposure, c represents cases without the exposure, and d represents controls without the exposure. Displaying the data from the study in a 2×2 table is helpful:

		BUNGEE JUMPING	
		Positive	Negative
MOUNTAIN DEW DRINKING	Positive	150 (a)	50 (b)
	Negative	100 (c)	200 (d)

Note that cells c and d had to be calculated so that the total in each column would be 250. For this study,

$$OR = (150/100)/(50/200)$$

$$= (150 \times 200)/(50 \times 100)$$

$$= 30,000/5000 = 6$$

By convention, the OR is expressed with the exposure rate among cases in the numerator. If the investigators were interested in reporting the odds of drinking Mountain Dew in nonjumpers relative to jumpers, the OR could be expressed as 1/6, or 0.17.

8. The answer is A: bungee jumping and beverage choice are associated. The odds of drinking Mountain Dew are 6 times as great in cases as they are in controls in this study. Therefore, there is an apparent association between beverage choice and tendency to jump. There may in fact be no true causal relationship if the findings are due to chance (i.e., not statistically significant), if the study is biased (e.g., if cases are interviewed more thoroughly or differently than controls with regard to drinking history), or if the apparent association is confounded by an unmeasured variable (e.g., alcohol consumption). If the apparent association is true, the investigators still cannot be certain whether bungee jumping predisposes to Mountain Dew consumption or vice versa, because the temporal sequence of exposure and outcome in a case-control study is uncertain. An association between Mountain Dew and bungee jumping is demonstrated in this study; to reach further conclusions regarding the association would require further study.

9. The answer is B: 3.6. The formula for relative risk (RR) is

$$RR = [a/(a + b)]/[c/(c + d)]$$

where a, b, c, and d are as defined in the explanation of item 7 (above) and in Table 6–1. The 2×2 table for this study is as follows:

		BUNGEE JUMPING	
		Positive	Negative
MOUNTAIN DEW DRINKING	Positive	135 (a)	115 (b)
	Negative	38 (c)	212 (d)

Note that cells *b* and *d* had to be calculated so that the total in each row would be 250. The risk ratio, or relative risk, is

$$RR = [135/(135 + 115)]/[38/(38 + 212)]$$

$$= (135/250)/(38/250)$$

$$= 0.54/0.152 = 3.55 = 3.6$$

10. **The answer is E: 72%.** The percentage of total risk due to an exposure among those with the exposure is the attributable risk percent in the exposed, or AR%$_{(exposed)}$. This can be calculated using the risk ratio (RR), which in this case is 3.6. Therefore,

$$AR\%_{(exposed)} = \frac{RR - 1}{RR} \times 100$$

$$= \frac{3.6 - 1}{3.6} \times 100 = 72.2\%$$

This indicates that among those who drink Mountain Dew, nearly three-fourths of the total risk for bungee jumping is attributable to the beverage. (N.B. These data are fictitious. But then again . . .)

11. **The answer is C: 7.7.** The number needed to treat (NNT) is calculated as 1 divided by the absolute risk reduction associated with an intervention. In the scenario described, the intervention (antibiotic treatment) reduces the risk of death from 15% to 2%, so the absolute risk reduction is 13%, or 0.13. Dividing 0.13 into 1 yields 7.7. This implies that one life is saved, on average, for every 7.7 patients treated.

12. **The answer is E: 100.** When an intervention increases (rather than decreases) the risk of a particular adverse outcome, the number of patients treated before, on average, one patient suffers the adverse outcome is the number needed to harm (NNH). To calculate the NNH, the absolute risk increase associated with the intervention is divided into 1. In the scenario described, there is a 1% risk of anaphylaxis (the adverse outcome) when antibiotic treatment (the intervention) is used and a 0% risk of anaphylaxis when antibiotic treatment is not used. Therefore, antibiotic treatment increases the risk of anaphylaxis by an absolute 1% (0.01). The NNH is 1/0.01, or 100. On average, 100 patients would need to be treated before one patient was harmed by the intervention.

13. **The answer is D: 13 patients saved for each patient harmed.** If the number needed to treat (NNT) is greater than the number needed to harm (NNH), the intervention will harm more patients than it helps. Ignoring the issue that the kind and degree of "harm" and "help" may differ, if the NNH is greater than the NNT, the

intervention in question will help more patients than it harms. In the scenario described, the NNH (100) is greater than the NNT (7.7); therefore, the procedure provides net benefit, because fewer patients need to be treated before one is "helped" than need to be treated before one is "harmed." The number of patients benefiting for each one harmed is calculated as follows:

$$NNH/NNT = 100/7.7 = 13$$

This represents 13 lives saved for every case of anaphylaxis induced by the antibiotic treatment. This same conclusion could have been reached by using the absolute risk reduction (ARR) and absolute risk increase (ARI) figures. In this case, dividing the ARR (13%) by the ARI (1%) again yields 13 as the number helped for each one harmed. When the ARR is greater than the ARI, there will be net benefit, with more than one patient helped for each one harmed. By the same reasoning, when the ARI exceeds the ARR, there will be net harm, with more than one patient harmed for each one helped. (The actual numbers in this case are fictitious and used for illustration purposes only.)

14. **The answer is E: the risk ratio.** The study described is a cohort study, in which subjects are assembled on the basis of exposure status and followed for outcome. The risk ratio is the outcome measure of a cohort study with a dichotomous outcome. The odds ratio is used in case-control studies, rather than cohort studies, and is in essence the "risk of having the risk factor." The likelihood ratio is used to evaluate the utility of a diagnostic test. Incidence density is an outcome measure of events per subject per unit of time (e.g., per 100 person-years) and is particularly useful when events may recur in individual subjects. Power is used to assess the capacity of a study to detect an outcome difference when there truly is one, given a particular sample size. As discussed in Chapter 12, for example, power is used to avoid beta error (type II or false-negative error).

15. **The answer is B: 0.13.** To calculate the risk ratio (relative risk), the risk of the outcome in the exposed is divided by the risk of the outcome in the unexposed. In the study described, the outcome is mental health; the exposure is medical school; the risk of the outcome in the exposed is 12/100, or 0.12; and the risk of the outcome in the unexposed is 92/100, or 0.92. Dividing 0.12 by 0.92 yields 0.13. This implies that the "risk" of mental health in those exposed to medical school was 0.13 times the risk of that outcome in the control group. Note that an "exposure" can raise or reduce risk. Note also that the outcome in question need not be an adverse outcome, despite the implications of the term "risk."

References Cited

Altman, D. G. Confidence intervals for the number needed to treat. British Medical Journal 317:1309–1312, 1998.

Baker, D. Anticoagulation for atrial fibrillation. The Health Failure Quality Improvement Newsletter, issue 4, Kerr L. White Institute for Health Services Research, Sept. 15, 1997.

Centers for Disease Control. Chronic disease reports: deaths from lung cancer—United States, 1986. Morbidity and Mortality Weekly Report 38:501–505, 1989.

Doll, R., and A. B. Hill. Lung cancer and other causes of death in relation to smoking. British Medical Journal 2:1071, 1956.

Halloran, M. E., et al. Theoretical epidemiologic and morbidity effects of routine varicella immunization of preschool children in the United States. American Journal of Epidemiology 140:81–104, 1994.

Kumana, C. R., B. M. Cheung, and I. J. Lauder. Gauging the impact of statins using number needed to treat. Journal of the American Medical Association 282:1899–1901, 1999.

Laupacius, A., D. L. Sackett, and R. S. Roberts. An assessment of clinically useful measures of the consequences of treatment. New England Journal of Medicine 318:1728–1733, 1988.

Mancini, G. B., and J. M. Schulzer. Reporting risks and benefits of therapy by use of the concepts of unqualified success and unmitigated failure. Circulation 99:377–383, 1999.

Oski, F., et al. Iron-fortified formulas and gastrointestinal symptoms in infants: a controlled study. Pediatrics 66:168–170, 1980.

Sackett, D. L., et al. Clinical Epidemiology: A Basic Science for Clinical Medicine, 2nd ed. Boston, Little, Brown, and Company, 1991.

Woolf, S. H. The need for perspective in evidence-based medicine. Journal of the American Medical Association 282:2358–2365, 1999.

Selected Readings

Gold, M., et al., eds. Cost-Effectiveness in Health and Medicine. New York, Oxford University Press, 1966.

Gordis, L. Epidemiology. Philadelphia, W. B. Saunders Company, 1996.

Kelsey, J. L., et al. Methods in Observational Epidemiology, 2nd ed. New York, Oxford University Press, 1996.

Kleinbaum, D. G., L. L. Kupper, and H. Morgenstern. Epidemiologic Research: Principles and Quantitative Methods. London, Lifetime Learning Publications, 1982.

Rothman, K. J. Modern Epidemiology. Boston, Little, Brown and Company, 1986.

Sackett, D. L., et al. Clinical Epidemiology: A Basic Science for Clinical Medicine, 2nd ed. Boston, Little, Brown, and Company, 1991.

■ GOALS OF DATA COLLECTION AND ANALYSIS

It may not be comforting to talk about errors in medicine, but they occur and are difficult to eliminate. This was emphasized in *To Err Is Human: Building a Safer Health System,* a report that was issued in the year 2000 by the Institute of Medicine and caused quite a stir both within and outside the medical community (see Kohn, Corrigan, and Donaldson 2000; Brennan 2000). In the field of medicine, quantitative methods are used to accomplish numerous goals, including the following: to measure and explain overall variation, some of which is due to errors; to distinguish between random and meaningful variation; and to facilitate interpretations of data needed for medical diagnosis, prognosis, and treatment.

Promoting Accuracy and Precision

Two distinct but related goals of data collection and analysis are accuracy and precision. **Accuracy** refers to the ability of a measurement to be correct on the average. If a measure is not accurate, it is biased. **Precision,** sometimes known as **reproducibility** or **reliability,** is the ability of a measurement to give the same result or a very similar result with repeated measurements of the same thing. Random error alone, if large, will result in lack of precision.

To ask whether accuracy or precision is more important in data collection and analysis would be somewhat like asking which wing of an airplane is more important. As shown in Figs. 7-1 and 7-2, unless both qualities are present, the data would be generally useless. The accuracy of Fig. 7-1A is reflected in the fact that the mean is the true value (correct value), while the precision (reliability) of Fig. 7-1A is evident in the fact that all values are close to the true value. Fig. 7-1B shows a measure that is accurate but not precise, meaning that it gives the correct answer only on the average. Such a measure might be useful for some kinds of research, but even so it would not be reassuring to the investigator. Moreover, for an individual patient, there is no value in something being correct on the average if it is wrong for that patient. To guide diagnosis and treatment, each observation must be correct. Fig. 7-1C shows data that are precise but are biased, rather than being accurate, and are therefore misleading. Fig. 7-1D shows data that are neither accurate nor precise and are obviously of no value. Finally, Fig. 7-2 uses a target and bullet holes to demonstrate the same concepts.

Reducing Differential and Nondifferential Errors

As discussed in Chapter 4, there are several types of errors to avoid in the collection and analysis of data. **Bias** is a **differential error**—that is, a nonrandom, systematic, or consistent error in which the values tend to be inaccurate in a particular direction. Bias results, for example, from measuring the heights of patients with their shoes on or from measuring blood pressures with an arm cuff that reads too high or too low. Statistical analysis cannot correct for bias unless the amount of bias in each individual measurement is known. In the example of the patients' height measurements, bias could be corrected only if the height of each patient's heel was known and subtracted from that patient's reported measurement.

While measuring patients in their bare feet could eliminate bias, it would not necessarily eliminate **random errors,** or **nondifferential errors.** When data have only random errors, some observations will be too high and some will be too low. It is possible for random errors to produce biased results (Dosemeci, Wacholder, and Lubin 1990). However, if there are

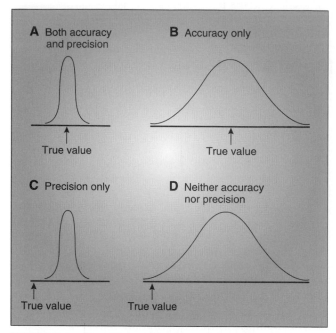

FIGURE 7–1 Possible combinations of accuracy and precision in describing a continuous variable. The *x*-axis is a range of values, with the arrow indicating the true value. The curves are the probability distributions of observed values.

enough observations, data with random errors may produce a correct estimate of the mean.

Reducing Intraobserver and Interobserver Variability

If the same physician takes successive measurements of the blood pressure or height of the same person or if the same physician examines the same x-ray several times without knowing that it is the same x-ray, there will usually be some differences in the mea-

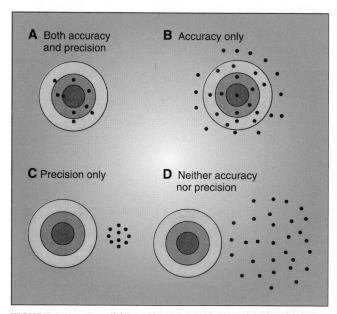

FIGURE 7–2 Possible combinations of accuracy and precision in describing a continuous variable, using a target and bullet holes to demonstrate the concepts.

surements or interpretations obtained. This is known as **intraobserver variability.** If two different physicians measure the same blood pressure or examine the same x-ray independently, there will usually be some differences. This is called **interobserver variability.** A goal of data collection and analysis is to reduce the amount of intraobserver (within observer) and interobserver (between observers) variability.

■ STUDYING THE ACCURACY AND USEFULNESS OF SCREENING AND DIAGNOSTIC TESTS

One way to judge the usefulness of a screening or diagnostic test for a particular disease is to evaluate how often its results are correct in two groups: (1) a group of persons in whom the disease is known to be present and therefore in whom the test results should be positive and (2) a group of persons in whom the disease is known to be absent and therefore in whom the test results should be negative. This kind of research is not as easy as it might initially appear, because several factors influence whether the results for an individual subject will be accurate and whether the test in general will be useful in diagnosing or screening for a particular disease. Among these factors are the stage of the disease and the spectrum of disease in the study population. As emphasized by Ransohoff and Feinstein (1978), the population in which the diagnostic or screening test is evaluated should have characteristics similar to those of the populations in which the test will be used. For example, data derived from evaluating tests in men or young people may not be applicable to women or older people.

False-Positive and False-Negative Results

In science, if something is said to be true when it is false, that is variously called a **type I error,** a **false-positive error,** or an **alpha error.** If something is said to be false when it is true, that is called a **type II error,** a **false-negative error,** or a **beta error.** Therefore, the finding of a positive result in a patient in whom the disease is absent is called a **false-positive result,** and the finding of a negative result in a patient in whom the disease is present is called a **false-negative result.**

The **stage of disease** often influences the test results. For example, tests for infectious diseases, such as the blood test for the human immunodeficiency virus (HIV) and the tuberculin skin test for tuberculosis, may be more accurate during the middle of the period of infection than they are early in the infection. Weeks or months may be required for detectable blood antibodies to appear in persons infected with the HIV virus, and weeks may be required following infection with the tuberculosis organism for the infected person to develop sufficient cell-mediated immunity to produce a positive skin reaction to the tuberculin antigen. Therefore, early in the course of either infection, an individual may not have immunologic evidence of infection, and tests done during this time may yield false-negative results.

Moreover, false-negative results may occur late in infections such as tuberculosis, when the disease is severe and the immune system is overwhelmed and unable to produce a positive skin test result. This inadequate immune system response is called **anergy** (from Greek, meaning "not working") and can develop with any illness or stress severe enough to cause depression of the immune system (Brooks et al. 1991). Advanced age can be a cause of anergy as well. Anergy is often seen in patients with acquired immunodeficiency syndrome (AIDS) when the level of T cells is lowered sufficiently. To determine whether anergy exists in a patient with immunodeficiency, an "anergy panel" of skin tests to common antigens may be applied. As exposure to the antigens in the panel (e.g., *Candida*, mumps virus, and *Trichophyton*) is virtually universal, if none of these evokes a hypersensitivity response in the skin, anergy is demonstrated.

The **spectrum of disease** in the study population is important in evaluating a test's potential usefulness in the real world. Both false-negative and false-positive results can be more of a problem than anticipated. In the case of the tuberculin skin test, for example, false-positive results used to be found in persons from the southeastern USA. Exposure to atypical mycobacteria in the soil is common in this region, and because there is some cross-reactivity between the atypical bacteria and the bacteria tested in the tuberculin skin test, equivocal and even false-positive test results were fairly common among this population until the standards were tightened. To accomplish this, the use of an antigen called old tuberculin (OT) was replaced by the use of a purified protein derivative (PPD) of mycobacteria at a standardized strength of 5 tuberculin units (5 TU). Moreover, the diameter of skin induration needed for a positive test result was increased from 5 mm to 10 mm. These tightened criteria worked satisfactorily for decades, until the appearance of AIDS. Now, because of the possibility of anergy in HIV-infected persons, it has been recommended that a smaller diameter of induration in the tuberculin skin test be considered positive for them (Rose, Schechter, and Adler 1995). Lowering the critical diameter also increases the frequency of false-positive results among those who have been immunized with bacille Calmette-Guérin (BCG) vaccine.

False-positive and false-negative results are not limited to tests of infectious diseases, as is illustrated in the following discussion concerning the use of serum calcium values to rule out parathyroid disease, particularly hyperparathyroidism, in new patients seen at an endocrinology clinic. Hyperparathyroidism is a disease of calcium metabolism. In an affected patient, the serum level of calcium is often elevated but will vary from time to time. When the level of calcium is not elevated in a patient who has hyperparathyroidism, the result would be considered falsely negative. Conversely, when the level of calcium is elevated in a patient who does not have hyperparathyroidism (but instead has cancer, sarcoidosis, multiple myeloma, milk-alkali syndrome, or another condition that can also cause a rise in the calcium level), the result would be considered falsely positive for hyperparathyroidism, even though it revealed a different problem.

Fig. 7–3 shows two anticipated frequency distributions of serum calcium values, one in a population of healthy people without parathyroid disease and the other in a population of patients with hyperparathyroidism. If the level of calcium was sufficiently low (say, below point A in Fig. 7–3), the patient would be unlikely to have hyperparathyroidism. If the level of calcium was sufficiently high (say, above point B in Fig. 7–3), the patient would be likely to have an abnormality of calcium metabolism, possibly hyperparathyroidism. However, if the level of calcium was in the intermediate range (between point A and point B) in a single calcium test, although the patient probably would not have a disease of calcium metabolism, this possibility could not be ruled out, and if such disease was suspected, serial calcium values should be obtained.

Laboratories usually provide a range of "normal" values for substances that they measure, such as calcium. A calcium value above the "normal" range will require further diagnostic tests. For many laboratories, the upper limit of normal for serum calcium is stated to be 11 mg/dL. If the **cutoff point** for the upper limit of normal is set too low, considerable time and money would be wasted following up on false-positive results; but if it is set too high, persons with the disease might be missed. As discussed be-

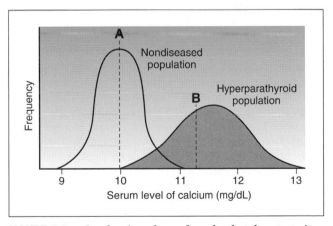

FIGURE 7–3   Overlap in values of randomly taken tests in a population where most of the people are healthy (curve on the left) but some of the people are diseased (curve on the right). A person with a level of calcium below point A would be unlikely to have hyperparathyroidism. A person with a level of calcium above point B would be likely to have an abnormality of calcium metabolism, possibly hyperparathyroidism. A person with a level of calcium between point A and point B may or may not have an abnormality of calcium metabolism. (Note: The normal range of calcium depends on the method used in a specific laboratory. In some laboratories, the range is from 8.5 to 10.5 mg/dL. In others, as in this illustration, it is from 9 to 11 mg/dL.)

low, determining the sensitivity, specificity, and predictive values of a test at different cutoff points will help investigators choose the best cutoff point for that test. It would be nice if there were no overlaps between the test results in diseased and nondiseased persons; if this were true, the only errors would be in the performance of the tests. Unfortunately, the distribution of test values in nondiseased persons often overlaps with the distribution of values in diseased persons.

It is easier to visualize the idea of a false-positive error where there is a clear distinction between diseased and nondiseased states, as in the evaluation of a spot on a mammogram. The area in question either does or does not represent cancer. Even here, however, the situation is not always simple. There may be an abnormality (e.g., fibrocystic disease) without the presence of cancer. If only fibrocystic disease was present, a radiologist's diagnosis of cancer would be falsely positive for cancer (the big concern), but it would be correct about the presence of an abnormality. In contrast, a radiologist's diagnosis of normal breast tissue would be a true-negative for cancer but a false-negative for fibrocystic disease. Radiologists frequently indicate uncertainty by reporting the results as "abnormality present—probably not cancer" and recommending that the mammogram be repeated after a defined number of months. Such readings really are analogous to laboratory values in the indeterminate range, and they are even more difficult to study than results from laboratory analysis (Elmore et al. 1994, 1998).

Sensitivity and Specificity

Sensitivity and specificity are two important measures of test function. To calculate these measures, the data concerning the subjects studied and the test results can be put in a 2 × 2 table of the type shown in Table 7–1. Note that the cells in this table are labeled *a, b, c,* and *d,* as in Table 6–1, but the measures to be calculated are different.

The first column in Table 7–1 represents all of the diseased subjects, consisting of those with **true-positive results** *(a)* and those with **false-negative results** *(c)*. The second column represents all of the nondiseased subjects, consisting of those with **false-positive results** *(b)* and those with **true-negative results** *(d)*. When the total in the first column is divided by the total of all of the subjects studied, the result represents the **prevalence rate** (proportion) of the disease in the study population.

Sensitivity, which refers to the ability of a test to detect a disease when it is present, is calculated as $a/(a+c)$. If a test is *not* sensitive, it will fail to detect disease in some of the diseased subjects, and these subjects will appear in cell *c*. The rate at which this occurs is called the **false-negative error rate** and is calculated as $c/(a+c)$. The correct denominator for the false-negative error rate is all of those who are diseased, because only those who are diseased can *falsely* be called nondiseased. The sensitivity and the false-negative error rate add up to 1.0 (100%).

TABLE 7–1   Standard 2 × 2 Table Comparing the Test Results and the True Disease Status of the Subjects Tested

		TRUE DISEASE STATUS		
		Diseased	Nondiseased	Total
TEST RESULT	Positive	*a*	*b*	*a + b*
	Negative	*c*	*d*	*c + d*
	Total	*a + c*	*b + d*	*a + b + c + d*

Interpretation of the cells is as follows:

> *a* = subjects with a true-positive test result
> *b* = subjects with a false-positive test result
> *c* = subjects with a false-negative test result
> *d* = subjects with a true-negative test result

> *a + b* = all subjects with a positive test result
> *c + d* = all subjects with a negative test result
> *a + c* = all subjects with the disease
> *b + d* = all subjects without the disease

> *a + b + c + d* = all study subjects

Formulas are as follows:

> $a/(a+c)$ = sensitivity

> $d/(b+d)$ = specificity

> $b/(b+d)$ = false-positive error rate (alpha error rate, type I rate)

> $c/(a+c)$ = false-negative error rate (beta error rate, type II rate)

> $a/(a+b)$ = positive predictive value

> $d/(c+d)$ = negative predictive value

> $[a/(a+c)]/[b/(b+d)] = (a/b)/[(a+c)/(b+d)]$ = likelihood ratio positive (LR+)

> $[c/(a+c)]/[d/(b+d)] = (c/d)/[(a+c)/(b+d)]$ = likelihood ratio negative (LR−)

> $(a+c)/(a+b+c+d)$ = prevalence

Specificity, which refers to the ability of a test to indicate nondisease when no disease is present, is calculated as $d/(b+d)$. If a test is *not* specific, it will falsely indicate the presence of disease in nondiseased subjects, and these subjects will appear in cell *b*. The rate at which this occurs is called the **false-positive error rate.** Since only nondiseased subjects are at risk for *falsely* being called diseased, this rate is calculated as $b/(b+d)$. The specificity and the false-positive error rate add up to 1.0 (100%).

First, suppose that 80 consecutive persons entering an endocrine clinic have their serum level of calcium checked and also have a hyperparathyroidism workup to determine whether they have the disease or not. Second, assume that the upper cutoff point for "normal" serum calcium is 11 mg/dL, so that levels above 11 mg/dL are presumptively "test positive" and levels of 11 mg/dL or less are "test negative." Third, assume that the results are as shown in Table 7–2. The following observations could be made. Of the 80 persons tested, 20 were ultimately shown to have hyperparathyroidism. Of these 20 persons, 12 had an elevated level of calcium in initial calcium testing. Thus, the sensitivity of the initial test was

60%, and the false-negative error rate was 40% (8/20). This is consistent with the fact that persons with hyperparathyroidism may have serum calcium levels that alternate between the high normal range and definite elevation, so that more than one calcium test is needed to make the diagnosis. The specificity in Table 7–2 was higher than the sensitivity, with normal levels correctly identified in 57 of 60 nondiseased persons, indicating 95% specificity. The false-positive error rate, therefore, was 5% (3/60).

Predictive Values

Sensitivity and specificity are interesting and are somewhat helpful in themselves, but they do not directly answer two important clinical questions: If a patient's test result is positive, what is the probability that he or she has the disease under investigation? If the result is negative, what is the probability that the patient does not have the disease? These questions, which are influenced by sensitivity, specificity, and prevalence, can be answered by doing a horizontal analysis, rather than a vertical analysis, in Table 7–1.

In Table 7–1, the formula $a/(a + b)$ is used to calculate the **positive predictive value.** In a study population, this measure indicates what proportion of the subjects who had positive test results had the disease. Likewise, the formula $d/(c + d)$ is used to calculate the **negative predictive value,** which indicates what proportion of the subjects who had negative test results were free of the disease.

In Table 7–2, the positive predictive value is 80% (12/15), and the negative predictive value is 88% (57/65). Based on these numbers, the physician could not be fully confident in either a positive or a negative test result. Why have the predictive values not fulfilled their promise? The predictive values would have been 100% correct if there were no false-positive or false-negative errors. Unfortunately, errors are present in almost any test, and this makes predictive values difficult to interpret, because in the presence of errors the predictive values are influenced profoundly by the prevalence of the condition being sought (Jekel, Greenberg, and Drake 1969).

As shown in Table 7–1, the prevalence is the total number of diseased persons $(a + c)$ divided by the total number of persons studied $(a + b + c + d)$. If, for example, there is a 1% prevalence of the condition (and most conditions are relatively rare), at most there could be an average of 1 true-positive test result out of each 100 persons examined. However, if there is a 5% false-positive rate (not unusual for many tests), 5% of 99 nondiseased persons would have false-positive test results. This would mean 5 false-positive results out of each 100 tests. Therefore, in this example, 5 out of every 6 positive test results could be expected to be falsely positive. It almost seems as though probability is conspiring against the use of screening and diagnostic tests in clinical medicine.

Whenever physicians are testing for *rare* conditions, whether in routine clinical examinations or in large community screening programs, they must be prepared for most of the positive test results to be falsely positive. Moreover, they must be prepared to follow up with additional testing in persons who have positive results to determine if the disease is really present. This does not mean that screening tests should be avoided for conditions that have a low prevalence. It still may be worthwhile to do a screening program, because the persons who need follow-up diagnostic tests will represent a small percentage of the total population. A crucial point to remember is that one test does not make a diagnosis, unless it is a **pathognomonic test**—that is, a test that elicits a reaction that is synonymous with having the disease (a "gold standard"). Box 7–1 summarizes principles concerning **screening tests** and **confirmatory tests.**

Likelihood Ratios, Odds Ratios, and Cutoff Points

Unlike predictive values, likelihood ratios are not influenced by the prevalence of the disease.

The **likelihood ratio positive** (LR+) is the ratio of the sensitivity of a test to the false-positive error rate of the test. As shown in Table 7–1, the equation is as follows: $[a/(a + c)]$ divided by $[b/(b + d)]$. Since the LR+ is the ratio of something that clinicians *do* want in a test (sensitivity) divided by something they do *not* want (false-positive error rate), the higher the ratio, the better the test. For a test to be a good one, the ratio should be much larger than 1. Note that both the sensitivity and the false-positive error rate are independent of the prevalence of the disease. Therefore, the ratio is also independent of the prevalence.

TABLE 7–2   The Serum Level of Calcium and the True Disease Status of 80 Subjects Tested (Fictitious Data)

		TRUE DISEASE STATUS		
		Diseased	Nondiseased	Total
SERUM LEVEL OF CALCIUM	High	12	3	15
	Normal	8	57	65
	Total	20	60	80

Calculations based on formulas in Table 7–1:

$12/20 = 60\% =$ sensitivity

$57/60 = 95\% =$ specificity

$3/60 = 5\% =$ false-positive error rate (alpha error rate, type I rate)

$8/20 = 40\% =$ false-negative error rate (beta error rate, type II rate)

$12/15 = 80\% =$ positive predictive value

$57/65 = 88\% =$ negative predictive value

$(12/20)/(3/60) = 12.0 =$ likelihood ratio positive (LR+)

$(8/20)/(57/60) = 0.42 =$ likelihood ratio negative (LR–)

$12.0/0.42 = 28.6 =$ ratio of LR+ to LR– = odds ratio

$20/80 = 25\% =$ prevalence of disease

When a patient presents with complaints of chest pain, the physician begins by obtaining a history, performing a physical examination, and developing a list of diagnoses that might explain the chest pain. The possible diagnoses have the logical status of hypotheses, and the physician must order various tests to screen or **"rule out"** (discard) the false hypotheses. These tests, which include laboratory analyses and imaging procedures, should be highly sensitive tests. Tests with a high degree of sensitivity have a low false-negative error rate, so they ensure that not many true cases of the disease are missed. Although the physician does not want false-positive results, they are tolerable at this stage, because they can be dealt with by more tests.

After most of the hypothesized diagnoses have been eliminated, the physician begins to consider tests that will **"rule in"** (confirm) the true diagnosis. These tests should be highly specific. Tests with a high degree of specificity have a small false-positive error rate, so they ensure that not many patients are misdiagnosed as having a particular disease when in fact they have another disease. The physician does not want to treat patients for diseases they do not have, whether the treatment is surgical or medical.

The principles of testing can therefore be summarized as follows: (1) A **screening test,** which is used to rule out a diagnosis, should have a high degree of **sensitivity.** (2) A **confirmatory test,** which is used to rule in a diagnosis, should have a high degree of **specificity.**

In a similar manner, the **likelihood ratio negative** (LR–) is the ratio of the false-negative error rate divided by the specificity, or $[c/(a+c)]$ divided by $[d/(b+d)]$. In this case, since the LR– is the ratio of something clinicians do *not* want (false-negative error rate) divided by something they *do* want (specificity), the smaller the LR– (i.e., the closer to 0 the ratio is), the better the test. In summary, if the LR+ of a test is large and the LR– is small, it is probably a good test.

The LR+ can be calculated from the hypothetical data in Table 7–2. The sensitivity is 12/20, or 60%. The false-positive error rate (1 – specificity) is 3/60, or 5%. The ratio of these is the LR+, which equals 0.60/0.05, or 12.0. Although this looks pretty good, the sensitivity data indicate that, on the average, 40% of the diseased persons would be missed. The LR– here would be 8/20 divided by 57/60, or 0.421, which is much larger than desirable.

Experts in test analysis sometimes calculate the **ratio of LR+ to LR–** to obtain a measure of separation between the positive and the negative test. In this example, LR+/LR– would be 12.0/0.421, which is equal to 28.5, a number not as large as desirable (a desirable number being somewhere around 50 or more). If the data are from a 2 × 2 table, the same result could have been obtained more simply by calculating the **odds ratio** (ad/bc), which here equals

$[(12)(57)]/[(3)(8)]$, or 28.5. For a discussion of the concepts of proportions and odds, see Box 7–2.

The LR+ will look better if a high (more stringent) **cutoff point** is used (e.g., a serum calcium level ≥13 mg/dL for hyperparathyroidism), even though choosing a high cutoff also lowers the sensitivity. This improvement in the LR+ occurs because as the cutoff point is raised, true-positive results are eliminated at a slower rate than are false-positive results. Moreover, the ratio of LR+ to LR– increases, despite the fact that more of the diseased individuals will be missed. The high LR+ means that when clinicians do happen to find a high level of calcium in an individual they are testing, they can be reasonably certain that hyperparathyroidism or some other disease of calcium metabolism is present. Similarly, if an extremely low cutoff point is used, when clinicians find a low level in an individual, they can be reasonably certain that the disease is absent.

Although these principles can be used to create value ranges that allow clinicians to be pretty certain about the results in the highest and lowest group, the results in the middle group are problematic. This situation is not necessarily bad, because now clinicians need to pursue additional testing only for those whose values fall in the middle. The same issues ap-

Most people are familiar with proportions (percentages), which take the form $a/(a+b)$. Those who have never gambled are probably less familiar with the idea of an odds, which is simply a/b. In a mathematical sense, a proportion is less pure, because the term a is in both the numerator and the denominator of a proportion, and that is not true of an odds. The odds is the probability that something will occur divided by the probability that it will not occur (or the number of times it occurs divided by the number of times it does not occur). Odds can only describe a variable that is dichotomous (i.e., has only two possible outcomes, such as success and failure).

The odds of a particular outcome (outcome X) can be converted to the probability of that outcome and vice versa, using the following formula:

$$\text{Probability of outcome } X = \frac{\text{Odds of outcome } X}{1 + \text{Odds of outcome } X}$$

Suppose, for example, that the proportion of successful at-bats of a baseball player on a certain night equals 1/3 (a batting average of 0.333). That means there was one success (X) and two failures (Y). The odds of success (number of successes to number of failures) is therefore 1:2, or 0.5. To convert back to a proportion from the odds, put the odds of 0.5 into the equation above, giving 0.5/(1 + 0.5) = 0.5/1.5 = 0.333.

If the player goes 1 for 4 another night, the proportion of success is 1/4 (a batting average of 0.250), and the odds of success is 1:3, or 0.333. The formula above converts the odds (0.333) back into a proportion: 0.333/(1 + 0.333) = 0.333/1.333 = 0.250.

TABLE 7–3   Calculation of Likelihood Ratios in Analyzing the Performance of a Serum Test with Multiple Cutoff Points (Multiple Ranges of Results)

Serum Creatine Kinase Value*	Diagnosis of Myocardial Infarction (MI)		Likelihood Ratio
	MI Present	MI Absent	
≥280 IU/L	97	1	$(97/1)/(230/130) = 54.8$
80–279 IU/L	118	15	$(118/15)/(230/130) = 4.45$
40–79 IU/L	13	26	$(13/26)/(230/130) = 0.28$
0–39 IU/L	2	88	$(2/88)/(230/130) = 0.013$
	230	130	

Source of data: Smith, A. F. Diagnostic value of serum creatine kinase in a coronary care unit. Lancet 2:178, 1967.
*The methods of determining creatine kinase values have changed since the time of this report, so these values cannot be directly applied to patient care today.

ply, for example, when interpreting a ventilation-perfusion scan (V/Q scan), the results of which are reported as normal, low probability, indeterminate, or high probability (Stein 1996).

Three or more ranges can be used to categorize the values of any test whose results occur along a continuum. In Table 7–3, the results of a serum test are divided into four ranges (Smith 1967). Here, 360 patients who had symptoms suggestive of myocardial infarction had an initial blood sample drawn to determine the level of creatine kinase (CK), an enzyme released into the blood of patients with myocardial infarction. After the final diagnoses were made, the initial CK values were compared with these diagnoses. In this case, the four levels are too many to measure the sensitivity and specificity in a 2×2 table (as was done in Tables 7–1 and 7–2), but likelihood ratios still can be calculated.

Likelihood ratios can be applied to multiple levels of a test because of a unique characteristic of odds: the result is the same regardless of whether the analysis in a table is done vertically or horizontally. The LR+ is the ratio of two probabilities: the ratio of sensitivity to (1 – specificity). This can also be expressed as $[a/(a + c)]$ divided by $[b/(b + d)]$. When this equation is rearranged algebraically, it can be rewritten as follows:

$$LR+ = (a/b)/[(a + c)/(b + d)]$$

which is the odds of disease among those in whom the test yielded positive results divided by the odds of disease in the entire population. The LR+, therefore, indicates how much the odds of disease was *increased* if the test result was positive.

Similarly, the LR– is the ratio of two probabilities: the ratio of (1 – sensitivity) to specificity. Alternatively, this can be expressed as $[c/(a + c)]$ divided by $[d/(b + d)]$, and the formula can be rearranged algebraically as follows:

$$LR– = (c/d)/[(a + c)/(b + d)]$$

which is the odds of missed disease among those in whom the test yielded negative results divided by the odds of disease in the entire population. The LR–, therefore, shows how much the odds of disease was *decreased* if the test result was negative.

Does this new way of calculating the LR really

work? Compare Table 7–2, where the LR+ can be calculated as follows and will yield exactly the same result as obtained before:

$$LR+ = (12/3)/[(12 + 8)/(3 + 57)]$$

$$= (12/3)/(20/60)$$

$$= 4/0.333 = 12.0$$

Likewise, the LR– can be calculated as follows and will yield the same result as before:

$$LR– = (8/57)/[(12 + 8)/(3 + 57)]$$

$$= (8/57)/(20/60)$$

$$= 0.140/0.333 = 0.42$$

Therefore, the likelihood ratio (without specifying positive or negative) can be described as the odds of disease given a specified test value divided by the odds of disease in the study population. This general definition of the likelihood ratio can be used for any number of test ranges. In Table 7–3, it is demonstrated for the four ranges of CK results. If the CK value was 280 IU/L or more, the LR was very large (54.8), making it highly probable that the patient had a myocardial infarction. If the CK was 39 IU/L or less, the LR was very small (0.013), meaning that myocardial infarction was probably absent. The LRs for the two middle ranges of CK values, however, do not elicit as much confidence in the test, so additional tests would be needed to make a diagnosis in patients whose CK values were between 40 and 279 IU/L.

Both in Table 7–2 and in Table 7–3, the **posttest odds** of disease (a/b) equals the **pretest odds** multiplied by the LRs. In Table 7–2, for example, the pretest odds of disease was 20/60, or 0.333; that is all that was known about the distribution of disease in the study population before the test was given. The LR+, as calculated above, turned out to be 12.0. When 0.333 is multiplied by 12.0, the result is 4. This is the same as the posttest odds, which was found to be 12/3, or 4. (See also Bayes' theorem in Chapter 8.)

Receiver Operating Characteristic (ROC) Curves

In clinical tests used to measure a continuous variable, such as serum calcium, blood glucose, or blood pressure, the choice of a good cutoff point is often difficult. As discussed above, there will be few false-positive results and many false-negative results if the cutoff point is very high, and the reverse will occur if the cutoff point is very low. Moreover, since calcium, glucose, blood pressure, and other values can fluctuate in any individual, whether healthy or diseased, there will be some overlap of values in the "normal" population and values in the diseased population, as shown in Fig. 7–3.

In order to decide on a good cutoff point, investigators could construct a receiver operating characteristic (ROC) curve. Beginning with either new or previously published data that showed both the test results and the true status for every person tested in a study, the investigators could calculate the sensitivity and false-positive error rate for several possible cutoff points and then plot the points on a square graph.

ROC curves are being seen increasingly in the medical literature. Legend has it that the term originated in England during the Battle of Britain, when the performance of radar receiver operators was evaluated on the following basis: a true-positive consisted of a correct early warning of German planes coming over the English Channel; a false-positive occurred when a receiver operator sent out an alarm but no enemy planes appeared; and a false-negative occurred when German planes appeared without previous warning from the radar operators.

An example of an ROC curve for blood pressure screening is shown in Fig. 7–4. The *y*-axis shows the **sensitivity** of a test, and the *x*-axis shows the **false-positive error rate** (1 – specificity). Since the LR+ of a test is defined as the sensitivity divided by the false-positive error rate, the ROC curve can be considered a kind of graph of the LR+.

If a group of investigators wanted to determine the best cutoff for a blood pressure screening program, they might begin by taking a single initial blood pressure measurement in a large number of persons and then performing a workup for persistent hypertension; therefore, each person would have a screening blood pressure value and a diagnosis concerning the presence or absence of hypertension. Based on this information, an ROC curve could be constructed. If the cutoff were set at 0 mm Hg (an extreme example used here to help illustrate the procedure), *all* study subjects would be included in the group suspected of having hypertension. This means that all of the persons with hypertension would be detected, and the sensitivity would be 100%. However, all of the normal persons would also screen positive for hypertension, so the false-positive error rate would be 100% and the point would be placed in the upper right (100%–100%) corner of the graph. By similar reasoning, if an extremely high blood pressure, such as 500 mm Hg, was taken as the cutoff, nobody would be detected with hypertension, so sensitivity would be 0%; however, there would be no false-positive results either, so the false-positive error rate would also be 0%. This point would be placed in the lower left (0%–0%) corner of the graph.

Next, the investigators would analyze the data for the lowest reasonable cutoff point—for example, a systolic blood pressure of 120 mm Hg—and plot the corresponding sensitivity and false-positive error rate on the graph. Then they could use 130 mm Hg as the cutoff, determine the new sensitivity and false-positive error rate, and plot the data point on the graph. This would be repeated for 140 mm Hg and for higher values. It is unlikely that the cutoff point for hypertension would be a systolic blood pressure of less than 120 mm Hg or higher than 150 mm Hg. When all of the points are in place, they can be connected to look like Fig. 7–4. Ordinarily, the best cutoff point would be the point closest to the upper left corner (the corner representing a sensitivity of 100% and a false-positive error rate of 0%).

The ideal ROC curve for a test would rise almost vertically from the lower left corner and then move horizontally almost along the upper line, as is shown in the uppermost ROC curve in Fig. 7–5 (the curve labeled "excellent"). If the sensitivity always equaled the false-positive error rate, the result would be a diagonal straight line from the lower left to the upper right corner, as shown in the bottom ROC curve in Fig. 7–5 (the curve labeled "no benefit"). The ROC curve for most clinical tests is somewhere between these two extremes—that is, similar to the curve labeled "good" or "fair" in Fig. 7–5.

The ROC curve in Fig. 7–6 shows the sensitivity and false-positive error rates found by Kinder (1994) in a study of patients with follicular thyroid neoplasms. Kinder sought to use the diameter of the neoplasms as measured at surgery to determine the probability of malignancy. Initially, when the ROC curve was plotted using the neoplasm diameters of patients of all ages, the curve was disappointing. But

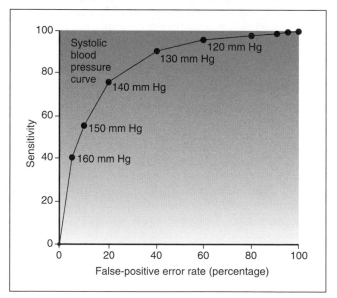

FIGURE 7–4   Receiver operating characteristic (ROC) curve from a study to determine the best cutoff point for a blood pressure screening program (fictitious data). Numbers beside the points on the curve are the cutoffs of systolic blood pressure that gave the corresponding sensitivity and false-positive error rate.

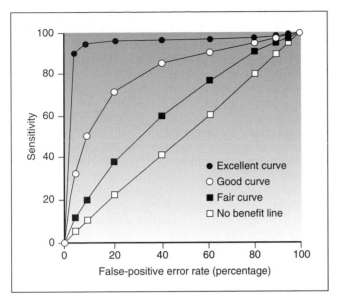

FIGURE 7–5 Examples of receiver operating characteristic (ROC) curves for four tests. The uppermost curve is the best of the four.

when the patients were divided into two age groups—those under 50 years and those 50 years or older—the diameter of the neoplasms was found to be strongly predictive of cancer in the older group but not in the younger one (see Fig. 7–6). It is unusual for the curve to hug the axes as it does for the older group in Fig. 7–6, but that was due to the relatively small number of patients involved (96 patients). In

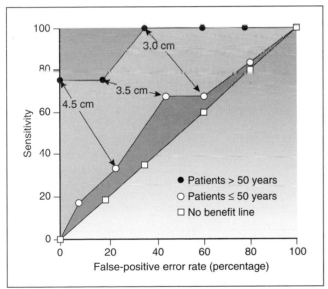

FIGURE 7–6 Receiver operating characteristic (ROC) curves for a test to determine the malignancy status of a follicular thyroid neoplasm on the basis of the diameter of the neoplasm. The upper curve plots the results in patients 50 years or older; the middle curve plots the results in patients under 50 years old; and the bottom curve represents the line of no benefit from the test. Numbers beside the points on the curves are the neoplasm diameters that gave the corresponding sensitivity and false-positive error rate. (Data courtesy of Dr. Barbara Kinder, Department of Surgery, Yale University School of Medicine, New Haven, Conn.)

Fig. 7–6, the curve for the older age group can be compared with that for the younger age group. For example, at a false-positive error rate of approximately 20%, the sensitivity is about 30% for the younger group and 75% for the older group. At a sensitivity of 75%, the false-positive error rate is almost 70% for the younger group and is between 0% and 20% for the older group (depending on whether the cutoff point chosen is a diameter of 3.5 cm or above).

Analysis of ROC curves is becoming more sophisticated and popular in certain fields, such as radiology. One method of comparing different tests is to determine the area under the ROC curve for each test and then to use a statistical test of significance to decide if the area under one curve differs significantly from the area under the other curve. The higher the percentage of area under the curve, the better the test.

■ MEASURING AGREEMENT

An important question both in clinical medicine and in research is the extent to which different observations of the same phenomenon differ. If there is intraobserver agreement or interobserver agreement, as defined at the beginning of this chapter, the data in a study are considered highly reliable and will elicit more confidence. However, reliability is not proof of validity; two observers can report the same readings (i.e., show reliability) but can both be wrong.

It is not unusual to find imperfect agreement between observers, nor is it unusual to find that the same individual looking at the same data (e.g., an x-ray or a pathology slide) often disagrees with his or her own reading done on a previous occasion. For example, in a study involving the interpretation of a series of chest x-ray films to diagnose the progression of tuberculosis, Yerushalmy et al. (1950) found that two different readers disagreed frequently and that the same person in two independent readings of the same x-ray disagreed with his or her own previous reading almost as frequently.

Overall Percent Agreement

If a test uses a dichotomous variable (i.e., two categories of results, such as positive and negative), the results can be placed in a standard 2×2 table, as shown in Table 7–4, so that observer agreement can be calculated. Cells a and d represent agreement, whereas cells b and c represent disagreement.

A common way to measure agreement is to calculate the overall percent agreement. Thus, if 90% of the observations are in cells a and d, the overall percent agreement would be 90%. Nevertheless, merely reporting the overall percent agreement is considered inadequate for a number of reasons. First, the overall percent agreement does not tell the prevalence of the finding in the subjects studied. Second, it does not tell how the disagreements occurred: were the positive and negative results evenly distributed between the two observers, or did one observer consistently find more positive results than the other? Third, con-

TABLE 7–4   Standard 2 × 2 Table Comparing the Test Results Reported by Two Observers

		OBSERVER NO. 1		
		Positive	Negative	Total
OBSERVER NO. 2	Positive	a	b	$a + b$
	Negative	c	d	$c + d$
	Total	$a + c$	$b + d$	$a + b + c + d$

Interpretation of the cells is as follows:

  a = positive/positive observer agreement

  b = negative/positive observer disagreement

  c = positive/negative observer disagreement

  d = negative/negative observer agreement

Formulas are as follows:

  $a + d$ = observed agreement (A_o)

  $a + b + c + d$ = maximum possible agreement (N)

  $(a + d)/(a + b + c + d)$ = overall percent agreement

  $[(a + b)(a + c)]/(a + b + c + d)$ = cell a agreement expected by chance

  $[(c + d)(b + d)]/(a + b + c + d)$ = cell d agreement expected by chance

  cell a agreement expected by chance + cell d agreement expected by chance = total agreement expected by chance (A_c)

  $(A_o - A_c)/(N - A_c)$ = kappa

siderable agreement would be expected by chance alone, and the overall percent agreement does not tell the extent to which the agreement improves on chance.

Kappa Test Ratio

Suppose two physicians examined the same 100 patients during the same hour and recorded the presence or absence of a heart murmur in each patient. Next, suppose that for 7 patients, the first physician reported the absence and the second physician reported the presence of a murmur; for 3 patients, the second physician reported the absence and the first physician reported the presence of a murmur; for 30 patients, the physicians agreed that a murmur was present; and for 60 patients, the physicians agreed that a murmur was absent. These results could be arranged in a 2 × 2 table as shown in Table 7–5. Then in addition to calculating the overall percent agreement, the **kappa test** could be performed to determine the extent to which the agreement between the two physicians improved on chance agreement alone. Even if the two physicians only guessed about the presence or absence of a murmur, they would agree sometimes by chance.

As shown in Tables 7–4 and 7–5, the **observed agreement** (A_o) is the sum of the actual number of observations in cells a and d. The **maximum possible agreement** is the total number of observations (N). The **agreement expected by chance** (A_c) is the sum

of the expected number of observations in cells a and d. The method used to calculate the expected agreement for the kappa test is the same method used for the chi-square test (see Chapter 11). For a given cell—for example, cell a—the cell's row total is multiplied by the cell's column total, and the product is then divided by the grand total. Thus, for cell a, the agreement expected by chance is calculated as $[(a + b)(a + c)]$ divided by $(a + b + c + d)$.

Kappa is a ratio: the numerator is the observed improvement over chance agreement (i.e., A_o minus A_c), and the denominator is the maximum possible improvement over chance agreement (i.e., N minus A_c). Thus, the kappa ratio is a proportion that can go from –1 (indicating perfect disagreement) through 0 (representing the agreement expected by chance) to +1 (indicating perfect agreement). Frequently, the results of the kappa test are expressed as a percentage. The following arbitrary divisions for interpreting the results are usually used: under 20% is negligible; from 20% to 40% is minimal; from 40% to 60% is fair; from 60% to 80% is good; and over 80% is excellent. In the example of cardiac murmurs, the kappa test yielded a result of 0.78, or 78%, indicating that the physician ratings were a "good" improvement on the chance expectation.

Although the kappa test described here provides valuable data on observer agreement, two important points should be noted. First, while many studies of observer variability involve **dichotomous (binary) data** (in which there are two categories of results, such as positive and negative), some studies involve **ordinal data** (in which there are three or more categories of results, such as negative, suspicious, and probable). If the data are ordinal, a **weighted kappa**

TABLE 7–5   Clinical Agreement Between Two Physicians Regarding the Presence or Absence of Cardiac Murmur on Physical Examination of 100 Patients (Fictitious Data)

		PHYSICIAN NO. 1		
		Murmur Present	Murmur Absent	Total
PHYSICIAN NO. 2	Murmur Present	30	7	37
	Murmur Absent	3	60	63
	Total	33	67	100

Calculations based on formulas in Table 7–4:

  $30 + 60 = 90$ = observed agreement (A_o)

  $30 + 7 + 3 + 60 = 100$ = maximum possible agreement (N)

  $(30 + 60)/(30 + 7 + 3 + 60) = 90/100 = 90\%$ = overall percent agreement

  $[(30 + 7)(30 + 3)]/100 = [(37)(33)]/100 = 12.2$ = cell a agreement expected by chance

  $[(3 + 60)(7 + 60)]/100 = [(63)(67)]/100 = 42.2$ = cell d agreement expected by chance

  $12.2 + 42.2 = 54.4$ = total agreement expected by chance (A_c)

  $(90 - 54.4)/(100 - 54.4) = 35.6/45.6 = 0.78 = 78\%$ = kappa

test must be used. The weighted test is similar in principle to the unweighted test described here but is somewhat more complex (see Cicchetti, Sharma, and Cotlier 1982). The weighted test gives partial credit for agreement that is close but not perfect. Second, in the evaluation of the accuracy and usefulness of a laboratory assay, imaging procedure, or any other clinical test, comparing the findings of one observer with those of another observer is not as useful as comparing the findings of an observer with the true status of disease in the patients being tested. The true disease status, which is used to determine the sensitivity and specificity of tests, is considered to be the "gold standard," and its use is preferable whenever data concerning the true status are available. Unfortunately, "gold standards" seldom exist in clinical medicine, and even a small error in the "gold standard" can create the incorrect appearance of considerable error in a test (Greenberg and Jekel 1969). Not only are careful studies of the errors of new diagnostic tests urgently needed, but additional studies of many of the older tests that have not been adequately analyzed are also needed in the field of clinical medicine.

■ SUMMARY

Three important goals of data collection and analysis are the promotion of accuracy and precision (see Figs. 7–1 and 7–2); the reduction of differential and nondifferential errors (that is, nonrandom and random errors); and the reduction in interobserver and intraobserver variability (that is, variability between the findings of two observers or between the findings of one observer on two different occasions).

Various statistical methods are available to study the accuracy and usefulness of screening tests and diagnostic (confirmatory) tests in clinical medicine. In general, tests with a high degree of sensitivity and a corresponding low false-negative error rate are helpful for screening patients, while tests with a high degree of specificity and a corresponding low false-positive error rate are useful for confirming the diagnosis in patients suspected of having a particular disease. Tables 7–1, 7–2, and 7–3 provide definitions of and formulas for calculating sensitivity, specificity, and error rates, as well as predictive values and likelihood ratios. Similarly, Tables 7–4 and 7–5 define measures concerning interobserver agreement and provide formulas for calculating the overall percent agreement and the kappa test ratio.

■ QUESTIONS

Directions (Items 1–10). The set of matching questions in this section consists of a list of lettered options followed by several numbered items. For each numbered item, select the ONE lettered option that is most closely associated with it. To avoid spending too much time on matching sets with large numbers of options, begin each set by reading the list of options. Then, for each item in the set, try to generate the correct answer and locate it in the option list, rather than evaluating each option individually. Each lettered option may be selected once, more than once, or not at all. Correct answers and explanations are given at the end of the chapter.

Items 1–10

(A) Accuracy
(B) Alpha error
(C) Beta error
(D) Bias
(E) Cutoff point
(F) False-negative error rate
(G) False-positive error rate
(H) Positive predictive value
(I) Precision
(J) Random error
(K) Sensitivity
(L) Specificity

Match each of the operating characteristics of an epidemiologic study or a diagnostic test with the appropriate description.

1. This is calculated as $c/(a + c)$.
2. This is the ability of a test to detect a disease when it is present.
3. This is type I error.
4. This defines normal and abnormal test results.
5. This is the tendency of a measure to be correct on average.
6. This is calculated as $a/(a + c)$.
7. This is the ability of a test to exclude a disease when it is absent.
8. This is nondifferential error.
9. The closer this is to the upper left corner of a receiver operating characteristic (ROC) curve, the better it is.
10. This is differential error.

Directions (Items 11–15). Each of the numbered items or incomplete statements in this section is followed by answers or by completions of the statement. Select the ONE lettered answer or completion that is BEST in each case.

11. The likelihood ratio associated with the use of creatine kinase levels for the diagnosis of myocardial infarction will vary with the

    (A) cutoff point
    (B) degrees of freedom
    (C) posterior probability
    (D) value of alpha
    (E) value of beta

12. As the sensitivity of a test rises, which of the following generally occurs?

    (A) The cutoff point falls
    (B) The false-negative error rate rises
    (C) The false-positive error rate rises
    (D) The specificity rises
    (E) The statistical power falls

13. Two radiologists interpret 100 mammograms. They agree that the results are normal in 70 and abnormal in 12 mammograms. In the remaining 18 cases, the first radiologist thinks that results are normal in 6 and abnormal in 12 mammograms, while the second radiologist thinks just the opposite. The value of an appropriate measurement of their agreement is

    (A) 6%
    (B) 16%
    (C) 26%
    (D) 46%
    (E) 86%

Items 14–15

The physicians in a primary care clinic do not know the prevalence of *Chlamydia trachomatis* infection in their community. In screening patients for this infection, they plan to use a test that performed with a sensitivity of 75% and a specificity of 75% in clinical trials.

14. When the physicians use the test to screen patients for *C. trachomatis* in their own community, which of the following could they use to interpret a positive test result?

    (A) Kappa
    (B) Phi
    (C) The likelihood ratio positive (LR+)
    (D) The odds ratio (OR)
    (E) The risk ratio (RR)

15. What is the value for the measure specified in question 14?

    (A) 2.6
    (B) 3
    (C) 5
    (D) 8.4
    (E) 16

■ ANSWERS AND EXPLANATIONS

1. **The answer is F: false-negative error rate.** The false-negative error rate is equal to $c/(a+c)$. In a 2×2 table, cell c represents the number of subjects who have a false-negative test result (subjects in whom the disease of interest is actually present but the test result is negative). Cell a represents the number of subjects who have a true-positive test result. The sum of cells a and c represents all subjects who have the disease; this is the denominator (population) from which false-negative results are derived. The false-negative error rate is the ratio of subjects who have false-negative results to all subjects who have the disease, including both those detected and those missed by the diagnostic test.

2. **The answer is K: sensitivity.** Sensitivity is defined as the ability of a test to detect true cases of a disease. Sensitivity is calculated as the number of true cases of the disease detected by the test (cell a in a 2×2 table) divided by all true cases (cell a plus cell c).

3. **The answer is B: alpha error.** False-positive error is also known as type I error or alpha error. These interchangeable designations refer to situations in which the data indicate that a particular finding (a test result or a study hypothesis) is true when it actually is not true. Typically, results attributable to chance or random error account for alpha error, although alpha error may result from bias as well. The value of alpha used in hypothesis testing specifies the level at which statistical significance is defined and thereby specifies the cutoff for p values (and the results to which they pertain, which are reported as positive or negative). Under most circumstances, the conventional level of alpha employed is 0.05 (see Chapter 10). The more stringent the value assigned to alpha (i.e., the smaller alpha is), the less likely that a false-positive result will occur. The clinical situation often dictates basic criteria for setting the value of alpha. For example, a false-positive error may be more tolerable in a study involving new therapies that are desperately sought for severely ill patients than in a study involving a preventive intervention to be applied to a healthy population.

4. **The answer is E: cutoff point.** In clinical medicine, there are relatively few pathognomonic findings (i.e., findings that are considered definitive of a particular disease and are expressed in dichotomous terms as the presence or absence of the disease). Most tests produce results that do not indicate the presence or absence of disease with absolute certainty. The cutoff point indicates the value beyond which a test result is considered abnormal, either leading to a diagnosis or suggesting the need for further testing. The cutoff point chosen is influenced by the situational priorities. An initial screening test, for example, should be highly sensitive, so the cutoff point for the upper limit of normal values should be set low. A follow-up test should be highly specific, so the cutoff point for the upper limit of normal values should be set high.

5. **The answer is A: accuracy.** Accuracy is the ability to obtain a test result or study result that is close to the true value. Accuracy is to be distinguished from precision, which is the ability to obtain consistent or reproducible results. An accurate result may not be precise. For example, repeated blood pressure measurements in a group of patients might lead to a correct value of the mean for the group, even if poor technique caused wide variation to occur in individual measurements. A precise result may not be accurate. The same mean weight might be obtained for a group of subjects on consecutive days, but if each measure were

obtained with the subjects clothed, all of the results would be erroneously high. Both accuracy and precision are desirable traits in research and diagnostic studies.

6. **The answer is K: sensitivity.** Refer to the explanation for question 2 (above).

7. **The answer is L: specificity.** Specificity is the capacity of a test to show positive results only in subjects who actually have the disease in question. Alternatively stated, specificity is the ability of a test to exclude a disease when it is absent. A test that is highly specific is a good "rule-in test," since it reliably indicates the presence of the disease when the result is positive. Specificity is calculated as the number of subjects with true-negative test results (cell d in a 2×2 table) divided by the total number of subjects who do not have the disease (cell b plus cell d).

8. **The answer is J: random error.** Random error is nondifferential error, because it does not distort data consistently in any one direction. Random error may produce some measurements that are too high and others that are too low. The mean may or may not be distorted by random error. Bias is differential error, because it produces measurements that are consistently too high or too low.

9. **The answer is E: cutoff point.** A cutoff point is used to distinguish normal from abnormal test results. If an upper limit cutoff point is set too high, the normal range will include many subjects with disease. If the upper limit cutoff point is set too low, many normal subjects will be said to have abnormal test results. The optimal cutoff point, where all cases of disease are detected with no false-positive results, is represented by the upper left corner of the receiver operating characteristic (ROC) curve. Such a point virtually never exists and is at best approximated. The closer the cutoff point is to the upper left corner of an ROC curve, the greater the sensitivity is and the lower the false-positive error rate is for a given test.

10. **The answer is D: bias.** Bias is differential error, since it distorts data in a particular direction. Examples of bias in measurement include weighing subjects after a meal, taking blood pressure readings after caffeine ingestion or exercise, and performing psychometric testing after alcohol ingestion. Unlike bias, random error is nondifferential error, since random error is equally likely to produce spuriously high or spuriously low results.

11. **The answer is A: cutoff point.** The likelihood ratio, or likelihood ratio positive (LR+), for a test is calculated as the test's sensitivity divided by its false-positive error rate (1 – specificity). In the case described, the diagnosis of myocardial infarction is based on testing the creatine kinase (CK) level. If the cutoff point for the CK level is set extremely high, then sensitivity will be low and specificity will be high. Lowering the cutoff point will generally raise the sensitivity and lower the specificity. Thus, the LR+ will vary with the cutoff point. The term "degrees of freedom" refers to a concept that is important in hypothesis testing (particularly when the chi-square test is used) but is not germane to the LR+. The values of alpha and beta are important in the interpretation of a study result but are not germane to the LR+. The posterior probability is a value that refers to the probability of disease after a test is performed; the value is distinct from the LR+.

12. **The answer is C: the false-positive error rate rises.** Sensitivity is the capacity of a test to identify the presence of disease in diseased individuals. The more sensitive a test is, the more likely it is to yield positive results (whether or not disease is actually present) and the less likely it is to yield negative results. This is why a rise in sensitivity is typically accompanied by an increase in the false-positive error rate, and it is also why a negative result in a highly sensitive test is more likely to be a true-negative. As a test's sensitivity rises, its specificity often falls. Specificity is the capacity of a test to identify the absence of disease in nondiseased individuals. The more specific a test is, the more readily it will yield negative results (whether or not the disease is actually absent). This is why a rise in specificity is accompanied by a rise in the false-negative error rate, and it is also why a positive result in a highly specific test is more likely to be a true-positive. The cutoff point will influence sensitivity and specificity and is generally chosen to strike the "optimal" balance between the two, with optimal being dependent on the context. Statistical power is related to research, rather than clinical diagnosis.

13. **The answer is D: 46%.** To assess the measure of agreement, kappa, the investigator should begin by setting up a 2×2 table and placing the number of "abnormal" (positive) results and "normal" (negative) results in cells a, b, c, and d:

		RADIOLOGIST NO. 1	
		Positive	Negative
RADIOLOGIST NO. 2	Positive	12 (a)	6 (b)
	Negative	12 (c)	70 (d)

The equation for kappa is as follows:

$$\text{kappa} = (A_o - A_c)/(N - A_c)$$

where N is the sample size; A_o is the observed agreement; and A_c is the total agreement attributable to chance, which is equal to the sum of cell a agreement expected by chance plus cell d agreement expected by chance.

N is given as 100. A_o is calculated as $a + d$, so here it is $12 + 70 = 82$. The agreement expected by chance is calculated as follows:

for cell $a = [(a + b)(a + c)]/(a + b + c + d)$

$$= [(12 + 6)(12 + 12)]/(12 + 6 + 12 + 70)$$

$$= (18)(24)/100 = 432/100 = 4.32$$

for cell $d = [(c + d)(b + d)]/(a + b + c + d)$

$$= [(12 + 70)(6 + 70)]/(12 + 6 + 12 + 70)$$

$$= (82)(76)/100 = 6232/100 = 62.32$$

Based on the above numbers, the A_c and kappa can now be calculated as follows:

$$A_c = 4.32 + 62.32 = 66.64$$

$$\text{kappa} = (82 - 66.64)/(100 - 66.64)$$

$$= 15.36/33.36 = 0.46 = 46\%$$

14. **The answer is C: the likelihood ratio positive (LR+).** As discussed in the answer to question 11 (above), the LR+ for a test is calculated as the test's sensitivity divided by its false-positive error rate (1 – specificity). The LR+ can be used to estimate the reliability of a positive test result when the prevalence of disease is not known. It is useful in this context because the components of the LR+ are contained within the columns of a contingency table and are therefore independent of disease prevalence. The odds ratio is used to evaluate the outcome of a case-control study. The risk ratio is used to evaluate the outcome of a cohort study. Kappa measures agreement, and phi measures the strength of association of a chi-square value.

15. **The answer is B: 3. The sensitivity of the test is 75%, or 0.75.** The specificity is also 0.75, so the false-positive error rate (1 – specificity) is 0.25. The likelihood ratio positive (LR+) is therefore 0.75/0.25, or 3.

References Cited

Brennan, T. The Institute of Medicine report on medical errors: could it do harm? New England Journal of Medicine 342:1123–1125, 2000.

Brooks, G. F., et al. Medical Microbiology, 19th ed. Norwalk, Conn., Appleton and Lange, 1991.

Cicchetti, D. V., Y. Sharma, and E. Cotlier. Assessment of observer variability in the classification of human cataracts. Yale Journal of Biology and Medicine 55:81–88, 1982.

Dosemeci, M., S. Wacholder, and J. H. Lubin. Does nondifferential misclassification of exposure always bias a true effect toward the null value? American Journal of Epidemiology 132:746–748, 1990.

Elmore, J. G., et al. Ten-year risk of false-positive screening mammograms and clinical breast examinations. New England Journal of Medicine 338:1089–1096, 1998.

Elmore, J. G., et al. Variability in radiologists' interpretations of mammograms. New England Journal of Medicine 331:1493–1499, 1994.

Greenberg, R. A., and J. F. Jekel. Some problems in the determination of the false positive and false negative rates of tuberculin tests. American Review of Respiratory Disease 100:645–650, 1969.

Jekel, J. F., R. A. Greenberg, and B. M. Drake. Influence of the prevalence of infection on tuberculin skin testing programs. Public Health Reports 84:883–886, 1969.

Kinder, B. [Professor of Surgery, Yale University School of Medicine, New Haven, Conn.] Personal communication, 1994.

Kohn, L. T., J. M. Corrigan, and M. S. Donaldson, eds. To Err Is Human: Building a Safer Health System. Report of the Institute of Medicine. Washington, D. C., National Academy Press, 2000.

Ransohoff, D. F., and A. R. Feinstein. Problems of spectrum and bias in evaluating the efficacy of diagnostic tests. New England Journal of Medicine 299:926–930, 1978.

Rose, D. N., C. B. Schechter, and J. J. Adler. Interpretation of the tuberculin skin test. Journal of General Internal Medicine 10:635–642, 1995.

Smith, A. F. Diagnostic value of serum creatine kinase in a coronary care unit. Lancet 2:178, 1967.

Stein, P. D. Diagnosis of pulmonary embolism. Current Opinion in Pulmonary Medicine 2:295–299, 1996.

Yerushalmy, J., et al. The role of dual reading in mass radiography. American Review of Respiratory Disease 61:443–464, 1950.

Selected Readings

Ransohoff, D. F., and A. R. Feinstein. Problems of spectrum and bias in evaluating the efficacy of diagnostic tests. New England Journal of Medicine 299:926–930, 1978. [The use of diagnostic tests to rule in and rule out a disease.]

Sackett, D. L. et al. Clinical Epidemiology: A Basic Science for Clinical Medicine, 2nd ed. Boston, Little, Brown, and Company, 1991. [Likelihood ratios, pretest odds, and posttest odds.]

8

Improving Decisions in Clinical Medicine

There is a steadily increasing demand for clinical decisions to be based on the best available clinical research. In the 1990s, this approach to clinical practice came to be widely referred to as **evidence-based medicine.** Since early in the 20th century, medical decisions have been based on a combination of clinical experience and knowledge gained from the literature. More recently, with the rapid increase in the accessibility of the literature through Internet searches and with the steady improvements in the methods of clinical epidemiology and biostatistics, it has become possible to base more diagnostic and therapeutic decisions on quantitative information provided by clinical research. Some have referred to this trend as a "paradigm shift" (see Evidence-Based Medicine Working Group 1992), but that term implies a more sudden shift in approach than the evolutionary changes in clinical science over the last century seem to justify.

Evidence-based medicine requires that clinicians (1) access the most relevant research data; (2) decide which studies are most trustworthy and applicable to the clinical question under consideration; and (3) use the best methods available to weigh the diagnostic, therapeutic, and prognostic probabilities of each course of action. Many methods described in this text—but especially some of the tools discussed in this chapter, such as Bayes' theorem, clinical decision analysis, and meta-analysis—may be considered tools for the practice of evidence-based medicine.

There is no controversy about the need to improve clinical decision making. There is, however, some difference of opinion regarding the extent to which the tools discussed in this chapter are likely to help in actual clinical decision making. Some individuals and medical centers already use these tools to guide the care of individual patients. Others acknowledge that the tools can help to formulate policy and analyze the cost-effectiveness of medical interventions such as immunizations (see, for example, Koplan et al. 1979; Bloom et al. 1993), but they may not use them for making decisions about individual patients. Regardless of one's philosophic approach to using these tools, they can help physicians and other health care workers understand the quantitative basis for making clinical decisions in the increasingly complex field of medicine.

■ BAYES' THEOREM

It is useful to know the sensitivity and specificity of a test, but as noted in Chapter 7, once a physician decides to use a certain test, two important clinical questions require answers: If the test results are positive, what is the probability that the patient has the disease? If the test results are negative, what is the probability that the patient does not have the disease? Bayes' theorem provides a way to answer these questions.

Bayes' theorem, which was first described centuries ago by the English clergyman after whom it is named, is one of the most imposing statistical formulas in medicine. Put in symbols more meaningful in medicine, the formula is as follows:

$$p(D+ \mid T+) = \frac{p(T+ \mid D+)p(D+)}{[p(T+ \mid D+)p(D+)] + [p(T+ \mid D-)p(D-)]}$$

where p denotes probability; D+ means that the patient has the disease in question; D− means that the patient does not have the disease; T+ means that a certain diagnostic test for the disease is positive; T− means that the test is negative; and the vertical line (|) means "conditional upon" what immediately follows.

Many clinicians, even those who can deal with

sensitivity, specificity, and predictive values, throw in the towel when it comes to Bayes' theorem. This is odd, because a close look at the above equation reveals that Bayes' theorem is merely the formula for the **positive predictive value,** a value discussed in Chapter 7 and illustrated there in a standard 2×2 table (Table 7–1).

The **numerator of Bayes' theorem** merely describes **cell *a*** (the true-positive results) in Table 7–1. The probability of being in cell *a* is equal to the prevalence times the sensitivity, where $p(\text{D+})$ is the prevalence (expressed as the probability of being in the diseased column) and where $p(\text{T+} \mid \text{D+})$ is the sensitivity (the probability of being in the top, test-positive, row, *given the fact of being in the diseased column*). The **denominator of Bayes' theorem** consists of two terms, the first of which once again describes **cell *a*** (the true-positive results) and the second of which describes **cell *b*** (the false-positive results) in Table 7–1. In this second term of the denominator, the probability of the false-positive error rate, or $p(\text{T+} \mid \text{D–})$, is multiplied by the prevalence of nondiseased persons, or $p(\text{D–})$. As outlined in Chapter 7, the true-positive results *(a)* divided by the true-positive plus false-positive results $(a + b)$ gives $a/(a + b)$, which is the positive predictive value.

In genetics, an even simpler-appearing formula for Bayes' theorem is sometimes used. The numerator is the same, but the denominator is merely $p(\text{T+})$. This makes sense because the denominator in $a/(a + b)$ is equal to all of those who have positive test results, whether they are true-positive or false-positive results.

Now that Bayes' theorem has been demystified, its uses in community screening and in individual patient care can be discussed.

Bayes' Theorem and Community Screening Programs

In a population with a low prevalence of a particular disease, it is likely that most of the positive results in a screening program for that disease would be falsely positive (see Chapter 7). Although this fact does not automatically invalidate a screening program, it raises some concerns about cost-effectiveness, and these can be explored using Bayes' theorem.

A program employing the tuberculin tine test to screen children for tuberculosis will be discussed as an example. This test uses small amounts of tuberculin antigen on the tips of tiny prongs called tines. The tines pierce the skin on the forearm and leave some antigen behind. The skin is examined 48 hours later, and the presence of an inflammatory reaction in the area where the tines entered is considered a positive result. If the sensitivity and specificity of the test and the prevalence of tuberculosis in the community are known, Bayes' theorem can be used to predict what proportion of the children with positive test results will have true-positive results (actually be infected with mycobacteria).

Box 8–1 shows how the calculations are made. If the test has a sensitivity of 96% and a specificity of 94% and if the prevalence of tuberculosis in the community is 1%, only 13.9% of those with a positive test result are predicted actually to be infected (Jekel, Greenberg, and Drake 1969). Those involved in community health programs can quickly develop a table that lists different levels of test sensitivity, test specificity, and disease prevalence and shows how these levels affect the proportion of positive results that are likely to be true-positive results. Although this calculation is fairly straightforward and is extremely useful, it has seldom been used in the early stages of planning for screening programs.

If the primary concern is to determine the overall value of a test, the use of likelihood ratios is recommended when the prevalence is unknown (see Chapter 7). However, before a new test is used, particularly for screening a large population, it is best to apply the test's sensitivity and specificity to the anticipated prevalence of the condition in the population. This will help avoid awkward surprises and will be useful in the planning of appropriate follow-up for test-positive individuals.

Another important point to keep in mind when planning community screening programs is that the first time a previously unscreened population is screened, a considerable number of cases of disease may be found, but repeating the screening program soon afterward may result in finding relatively few cases of new disease. This is because the first screening will detect cases that had their onset during a period of many years **(prevalent cases),** while the second screening will primarily detect cases that had their onset during the interval since the last screening **(incident cases).**

Bayes' Theorem and Individual Patient Care

Suppose a clinician is uncertain about a patient's diagnosis and obtains a positive test result for a certain disease. Even if the clinician knows the sensitivity and specificity of the test, that does not solve the problem, because to calculate the positive predictive value, whether using Bayes' theorem or a table like Table 7–1, it is necessary to know the prevalence of the particular disease that the test is designed to detect. In a clinical setting, the prevalence is thought of as the expected prevalence in the population from which the patient comes. The actual prevalence is usually not known, but often a reasonable estimate can be made.

Say, for example, a physician in a general medical clinic sees a male patient who complains of easy fatigability and has a history of kidney stones but has no other symptoms or signs of parathyroid disease on physical examination. The physician considers the probability of hyperparathyroidism and decides that it is low, perhaps 2% (reflecting that in 100 similar patients, probably only 2 of them would have the disease). This probability is called the **prior probability,** reflecting the fact that it is estimated prior to the performance of laboratory tests and is based on the estimated prevalence of a particular disease among pa-

BOX 8–1 Use of Bayes' Theorem or a 2 × 2 Table to Determine the Positive Predictive Value of a Hypothetical Tuberculin Screening Program

Part 1 Beginning data

Sensitivity of tuberculin tine test	= 96% = 0.96
False-negative error rate of the test	= 4% = 0.04
Specificity of the test	= 94% = 0.94
False-positive error rate of the test	= 6% = 0.06
Prevalence of tuberculosis in the community	= 1% = 0.01

Part 2 Use of Bayes' theorem

$$p(D+ \mid T+) = \frac{p(T+ \mid D+)p(D+)}{[p(T+ \mid D+)p(D+)] + [p(T+ \mid D-)p(D-)]}$$

$$= \frac{(Sensitivity)(Prevalence)}{[(Sensitivity)(Prevalence)] + [(False\text{-}positive\ error\ rate)(1 - Prevalence)]}$$

$$= \frac{(0.96)(0.01)}{[(0.96)(0.01)] + [(0.06)(0.99)]} = \frac{0.0096}{0.0096 + 0.0594} = \frac{0.0096}{0.0690} = 0.139 = \mathbf{13.9\%}$$

Part 3 Use of a 2 × 2 table, with numbers based on the assumption that 10,000 persons are in the study

		TRUE DISEASE STATUS					
		Diseased		Nondiseased		Total	
		Number	(Percentage)	Number	(Percentage)	Number	(Percentage)
TEST RESULT	Positive	96	(96)	594	(6)	690	(7)
	Negative	4	(4)	9,306	(94)	9,310	(93)
	Total	100	(100)	9,900	(100)	10,000	(100)

Positive predictive value = 96 / 690 = 0.139 = **13.9%**

Source of data: Jekel, J.F., R.A Greenberg, and B.M. Drake. Influence of prevalence of infection on tuberculin skin testing programs. Public Health Reports 84:883–886, 1969.

tients with similar signs and symptoms. Although the physician believes that the probability of hyperparathyroidism is low, she orders a serum calcium test to "rule out" the diagnosis. Somewhat to her surprise, the results of the test come back positive, with an elevated level of 12.2 mg/dL. She could order more tests for parathyroid disease, but even here, some test results might come back positive and some negative.

Under the circumstances, Bayes' theorem could be used to make a second estimate of probability, which is called the **posterior probability,** reflecting the fact that it is made after the test results are known. Calculation of the posterior probability is based on the sensitivity and specificity of the test that was performed, which in this case was the serum calcium test, and on the prior probability, which in this case was 2%. If the serum calcium test had a 90% sensitivity and a 95% specificity, that means it had a false-positive error rate of 5% (specificity plus the false-positive error rate equals 100%). When this information is used in the Bayes' equation, as shown in Box 8–2, the result is a posterior probability of 27%. This means that the patient is now in a group of pa-

tients with a substantial possibility of parathyroid disease. In Box 8–2, note that the result is the same (i.e., 27%) when a 2 × 2 table is used. This is true because, as discussed above, the probability based on the Bayes' theorem is identical to the positive predictive value.

In light of the 27% posterior probability, the physician decides to order a parathyroid hormone radioimmunoassay with simultaneous measurement of serum calcium, even though this test is expensive. If the radioimmunoassay had a sensitivity of 95% and a specificity of 98% and the results turned out to be positive, the Bayes' theorem could again be used to calculate the probability of parathyroid disease. This time, however, the posterior probability for the first test (27%) would be used as the prior probability for the second test. The result of the calculation, as shown in Box 8–3, is a new probability of 94%. Thus, the patient in all probability does have hyperparathyroidism.

Why did the posterior probability increase so much the second time? One reason was that the prior probability was considerably higher in the second calculation than in the first (27% versus 2%), based

---

BOX 8–2 Use of Bayes' Theorem or a 2 × 2 Table to Determine the Posterior Probability and the Positive Predictive Value in a Clinical Setting

Part 1 Beginning data (before performing the first test)

Sensitivity of the first test   = 90% = 0.90
Specificity of the first test   = 95% = 0.95
Prior probability of disease   = 2% = 0.02

Part 2 Use of Bayes' theorem to calculate the first posterior probability

$$p(D+ \mid T+) = \frac{p(T+ \mid D+)p(D+)}{[p(T+ \mid D+)p(D+)] + [p(T+ \mid D-)p(D-)]}$$

$$= \frac{(0.90)(0.02)}{[(0.90)(0.02)] + [(0.05)(0.98)]}$$

$$= \frac{0.018}{0.018 + 0.049} = \frac{0.018}{0.067} = 0.269 = \mathbf{27\%}$$

Part 3 Use of a 2 × 2 table to calculate the first positive predictive value

		TRUE DISEASE STATUS						
		Diseased		Nondiseased		Total	
		Number	(Percentage)	Number	(Percentage)	Number	(Percentage)
TEST RESULT	Positive	18	(90)	49	(5)	67	(6.7)
	Negative	2	(10)	931	(95)	933	(93.3)
	Total	20	(100)	980	(100)	1000	(100.0)

Positive predictive value = 18 / 67 = 0.269 = **27%**

---

on the fact that the first test yielded positive results. Another reason was that the specificity of the second test was quite high (98%), which markedly reduced the false-positive error rate and therefore increased the positive predictive value.

Influence of the Order of Testing

When a patient requires multiple diagnostic tests, one issue confronting the clinician is whether to do the tests simultaneously or sequentially.

As outlined in Chapter 7 (see Box 7–1), tests used to "rule out" a diagnosis should have a high degree of sensitivity, whereas tests used to "rule in" a diagnosis should have a high degree of specificity. Therefore, the sequential approach is best done by (1) starting with the most sensitive test, (2) continuing with increasingly specific tests if the previous test yields positive results, and (3) stopping when a test yields negative results. In comparison with the simultaneous approach, the sequential approach to testing is more conservative and is more economical in the care of outpatients. However, the sequential approach may increase the length of stay for a hospitalized patient, so the cost implications may not be clear.

The sequence of testing may have implications for the overall sensitivity and specificity of the testing process. If multiple diagnostic tests are performed at the same time, the natural tendency is to ignore the

negative results while seriously considering the positive results. However, this approach to establishing a diagnosis may not be ideal. Even if the tests are performed simultaneously, it is probably best to first consider the results of the most sensitive test. If a negative result is reported for that test, the result is probably a true-negative one (i.e., the patient probably does not have the disease). Simultaneous testing may produce many conflicting results, but a careful consideration of each test's result in light of the test's sensitivity and specificity should improve the likelihood of making the correct diagnosis.

■ DECISION ANALYSIS

A decision-making tool that has come into the medical literature from management science is called decision analysis. Its purpose is to improve decision making under conditions of uncertainty. In clinical medicine, decision analysis can be used for an individual patient or for a general class of patients. As a technique, decision analysis is somewhat more popular clinically than Bayes' theorem, and it is being used with increasing frequency in the literature, particularly to make judgments about a class of patients or clinical problems.

The benefit of decision analysis is to help health care workers understand (1) the kinds of data that must go into a clinical decision, (2) the sequence in which decisions have to be made, and (3) the personal values of the patients that must be considered before major decisions are made. As a general rule, decision analysis is more important as a tool to help health care workers take a disciplined approach to decision making than as a tool for making the actual clinical decisions. Nevertheless, as computer programs for using decision analysis become more available, some clinicians are using decision analysis regularly in their clinical work.

Steps in Creating a Decision Tree

There are four logical steps to be taken when setting up a decision tree (see Weinstein and Fineberg 1980): (1) identify and set limits to the problem, (2) diagram the options, (3) obtain information concerning each option, and (4) compare the utility values and perform sensitivity analysis.

Identify the Problem

In identifying the problem, the clinician must determine the possible alternative clinical decisions, the sequence in which the decisions must be made, and the possible patient outcomes of each decision.

Diagram the Options

Fig. 8–1 provides a simple example of how to diagram the options. The beginning point of a decision tree is the patient's current clinical status. **Decision nodes,** defined as points where clinicians have to make decisions, are represented by squares. **Chance nodes,** defined as points where clinicians have to wait to see the outcomes, are represented by circles. Time goes from left to right, so the first decision is at the left and subsequent decisions are progressively to the right. In Fig. 8–1, the beginning point is the presence of asymptomatic gallstones, and the primary decision at the decision node is whether to operate immediately or to wait (Rose and Wiesel 1983).

Obtain Information Concerning Each Option

First, the **probability of each possible outcome** must either be obtained from published studies or be estimated on the basis of clinical experience. For example, in Fig. 8–1, if the physician waits rather than operating, the probability is 81.5% (0.815) that the patient will remain asymptomatic, 15% that the patient will have occasional biliary pain, 3% that the patient will develop complications such as acute cholecystitis or common duct obstruction from gall-

---

BOX 8–3   Use of Bayes' Theorem or a 2 × 2 Table to Determine the Second Posterior Probability and the Second Positive Predictive Value in a Clinical Setting

Part 1   Beginning data (before performing the second test)

Sensitivity of the second test	= 95% = 0.95
Specificity of the second test	= 98% = 0.98
Prior probability of disease (see Box 8–2)	= 27% = 0.27

Part 2   Use of Bayes' theorem to calculate the second posterior probability

$$p(D+ \mid T+) = \frac{p(T+ \mid D+)p(D+)}{[p(T+ \mid D+)p(D+)] + [p(T+ \mid D-)p(D-)]}$$

$$= \frac{(0.95)(0.27)}{[(0.95)(0.27)] + [(0.02)(0.73)]}$$

$$= \frac{0.257}{0.257 + 0.0146} = \frac{0.257}{0.272} = 0.9449^* = \mathbf{94\%}$$

Part 3   Use of a 2 × 2 table to calculate the second positive predictive value

		TRUE DISEASE STATUS					
		Diseased		Nondiseased		Total	
		Number	(Percentage)	Number	(Percentage)	Number	(Percentage)
TEST RESULT	Positive	256	(95)	15	(2)	271	(27.1)
	Negative	13	(5)	716	(98)	729	(72.9)
	Total	269	(100)	731	(100)	1000	(100.0)

Positive predictive value = 256 / 271 = 0.9446* = **94%**

---

*The slight difference in the results for the two approaches is due to rounding errors. It is not important clinically.

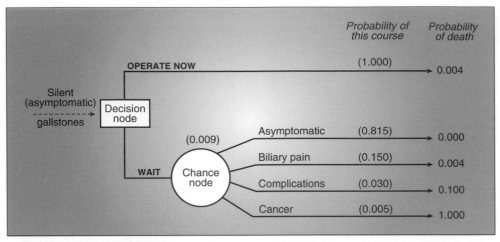

FIGURE 8–1   A decision tree concerning treatment for silent (asymptomatic) gallstones. The decision node, defined as a point where the clinician has to make a decision, is represented by a square. The chance node, defined as a point where the clinician must wait to see the outcome, is represented by a circle. If the clinician decides to operate now, the probability of surgery is 100% (1.000), and the probability of death (the negative utility value) from complications of surgery is 0.04% (0.004, or 1 out of every 250 patients undergoing surgery). If, instead, the clinician decides to wait, there are four possible outcomes, each with a different probability and negative utility value: (1) There is an 81.5% (0.815) probability of remaining asymptomatic, in which case the probability of dying from gallstones would be 0% (0.000). (2) There is a 15% (0.150) probability of developing biliary pain, which would lead to surgery and a 0.4% (0.004) risk of death. (3) There is a 3% (0.030) probability of biliary complications (such as acute cholecystitis or common duct obstruction), with a 10% (0.100) risk of death. (4) There is a 0.5% (0.005) probability of gallbladder cancer, with a 100% (1.000) risk of death. The probabilities of the possible outcomes at the chance node add up to 1 (here, 0.815 + 0.150 + 0.030 + 0.005 = 1.000). (From Rose, D. N., and J. Wiesel. Letter to the editor. New England Journal of Medicine 308:221–222, 1983. Copyright © 1983, Massachusetts Medical Society. All rights reserved. Adapted with permission in 1996 and 1999.)

stones, and 0.5% that the patient eventually will develop cancer of the gallbladder. Note that the probabilities of the possible outcomes for a chance node must add up to 100%, as they do in this case.

Second, the **utility of each final outcome** must be obtained. In decision analysis, the term "utility" is used to mean the value of a chosen course of action. Utility may be expressed as a **desirable outcome** (e.g., years of disease-free survival), in which case larger values have greater utility; or it may be expressed as an **undesirable outcome** (e.g., death, illness, or high cost), in which case smaller values have greater utility. Clinical decision analysis seeks to show which clinical decision would maximize utility. In Fig. 8–1, each final outcome is expressed in terms of a negative utility (i.e., probability of death). If surgery is performed now, the probability of death is 0.4% (0.004). If the surgeon waits and the patient remains asymptomatic, however, the probability of a gallbladder-related death is 0%. The probabilities of death for biliary pain, complications, and cancer are 0.4%, 10%, and 100%, respectively. For many patients, however, other considerations—such as the timing of death and the quality of life in the interim—are of equal or greater importance than the quantity of life. For example, a person who wanted to finish writing a book while he or she was still in relatively good health might prefer a nonaggressive approach to disease treatment. Someone else who was willing to risk everything for the sake of a cure might express a preference for the most aggressive treatment possible.

Compare the Utility Values and Perform a Sensitivity Analysis

The decision tree can show how a given set of probabilities and utilities will turn out. If the decision tree shows that one or another choice is clearly preferable to any other, that would be strong evidence in favor of that choice. Often, however, the decision analysis will give two or more outcomes with similar utilities, which means either that better data are needed or that there really are options at that decision node. In addition to comparing the utility values, it is sometimes helpful to perform a **sensitivity analysis,** which consists of varying the estimated probabilities of occurrence of a particular outcome at various points in the decision tree (one at a time) to see how the overall outcomes and clinical decisions would be affected by these changes. This helps both clinician and patient to see which assumptions and decisions have the largest impact on the outcomes through a reasonable range of values. Fig. 8–1 can be used to demonstrate how to compare utility values and to discuss the rationale for performing a sensitivity analysis.

On the decision tree shown in Fig. 8–1, there are two branches from the decision node, one labeled "operate now" and the other labeled "wait." As discussed earlier, the probability of death from operating immediately is 0.004, whereas there are four different probabilities of death from waiting, depending on what happens during the waiting period (patient remains asymptomatic or patient develops pain, complications, or cancer). Before the utility of operating now versus waiting can be compared, it is necessary to **"average out"** the data associated with waiting. First, the probability of each outcome of waiting is multiplied by the probability that death will ensue following that particular outcome. Next, the four products are summed. In Fig. 8–1, the calculation for averaging out is $(0.815 \times 0.000) + (0.150 \times 0.004) + (0.030 \times 0.100) + (0.005 \times 1.000) = 0.0086 = 0.009$, or a little over twice the risk of operating now.

Based on the above calculations, the best option would seem to be to operate now. However, because these two outcome probabilities are fairly close to each other (0.004 versus 0.009 is only a difference of 0.005, or 0.5%), even modest errors in the data estimate, if corrected, might lead to a different conclusion. Therefore, in the absence of better data on the risk of clinical states and the probabilities of death, it would be a good idea to perform a sensitivity analysis on these data, to see which estimates are the most crucial for stability of the decision tree.

The majority of the deaths that occur if surgery is not performed immediately are deaths caused by cancer of the gallbladder. It is not fair to make a direct comparison of deaths resulting from surgery and deaths caused by gallbladder cancer, however, because surgical deaths would occur immediately, whereas most of the cancer deaths would occur many years hence. Given the option, many people would choose to avoid immediate surgery (because they are feeling well, have family responsibilities, and so forth), preferring simply to deal with complications if and when they arise.

Although this was a simple example, other decision trees have multiple decision nodes that involve complicated issues and factors such as the passage of time and reevaluation. In these more complex decision analyses, the objective is to find decisions that are clearly less satisfactory than others and to cut off or "prune" these branches, because they are not rational alternatives. The process of choosing the best branch at each decision node, working backward from the right to the left, is called **"folding back."**

Applications of Decision Trees

Decision trees can be used in the clinical setting, as discussed above in the case of patients with asymptomatic gallstones, but they are also increasingly being applied to public health problems.

Although a safe and effective hepatitis B vaccine became available in 1981, the incidence of hepatitis B in the USA increased by 37% from 1981 to 1991 (Schaffner, Gardner, and Gross 1993). In considering what strategy would be most cost-effective in reversing this trend, Bloom et al. (1993) turned to the use of a decision tree and analyzed data concerning several

possible options: no routine hepatitis B vaccination; a screening program followed by hepatitis B vaccination for persons meeting certain criteria; and hepatitis B vaccination for specific populations (newborns, 10-year-olds, high-risk adults, or the general adult population in the USA). Included in the decision tree were the effects of compliance with recommendations.

■ META-ANALYSIS

Meta-analysis (meaning "analysis among") is being used increasingly in medicine to try to obtain a qualitative or quantitative synthesis of the research literature on a particular issue. The technique is usually (but not always) applied to the synthesis of several randomized clinical trials.

The technique of meta-analysis is in its early stages, and it has many critics. For example, Shapiro (1994) referred to it as "meta-analysis/shmeta-analysis," and Feinstein (1995) called it "statistical alchemy for the 21st century." Their skepticism is reinforced by significant discrepancies between some meta-analyses and large randomized controlled trials examining the same questions (see Borzak and Kidker 1995; LeLorier et al. 1997; Bailar 1997). Nevertheless, methodologic work on the technique of meta-analysis continues, and the use of meta-analyses is growing, so readers of medical literature today must be aware of the strengths and weaknesses of this technique.

Selection of the Studies to Be Analyzed

The issue of study selection is perhaps the most troublesome issue for those doing meta-analysis. Several questions need to be addressed.

(1) Should studies in a meta-analysis be limited to those that are published? It is well known that negative studies (studies that report little or no benefit from following a particular course of action) are less likely to be published than are positive studies. Therefore, the published literature may be biased toward studies with positive results, and a synthesis of these studies would give a biased estimate of the impact of pursuing some courses of action. Unpublished studies, however, often are of lower quality than are published studies, and poor research methods often produce an underestimate of impact. Moreover, the unpublished studies are often difficult to find. Some maintain that meta-analysis should be performed on raw data from many studies, rather than on published summaries of data.

(2) Should studies be limited to those that appear in peer-reviewed publications? Peer review is considered the primary method for quality control in medical publishing. Some investigators recommend that only those studies that are published in peer-reviewed publications be considered in meta-analysis. Although this may seem an attractive option, it might also contribute to selection bias in the studies chosen.

(3) Should studies be limited to those that meet additional quality-control criteria? If investigators impose additional criteria (such as random allocation and double-blinding) before including a study in meta-analysis, this may further improve the average quality of the studies used, but it introduces still greater concerns about selection bias. Moreover, different investigators studying the same topic might use different criteria for a "good" study and therefore select different studies for meta-analysis.

(4) Should studies be limited to randomized controlled trials, or is it acceptable to do meta-analyses of observational epidemiologic studies? This is a variant of the above question concerning quality control. At one time, standards for high-quality research were more likely to be met by randomized controlled trials than by case-control studies. However, case-control methods have subsequently been improved by applying the scientific principles employed in randomized controlled trials (see Horwitz and Feinstein 1981). Case-control methods are particularly valuable when the outcome event is relatively rare (see Chapter 5). For example, they have been used to evaluate vaccines for uncommon diseases, because they are less costly and provide results more quickly (see Shapiro et al. 1991).

(5) Should studies be limited to those using identical methods, treatment dosages, patient characteristics, or durations of follow-up? For practical purposes, this would mean using only separately published studies from multicenter trials, for which the methods were the same for all and the similarity of methods was monitored. This criterion is very difficult to achieve.

Types of Meta-Analysis
Pooled (Quantitative) Analysis

Usually, the main purpose of meta-analysis is quantitative. The goal is to develop better overall estimates of the amount of benefit achieved by particular medical interventions, based on the combining (pooling) of estimates found in the existing studies of the interventions. This type of meta-analysis is sometimes called a pooled analysis (Gerbarg and Horwitz 1988) because the analysts pool the observations of many studies and then calculate parameters such as risk ratios or odds ratios from the pooled data.

Because of the many decisions regarding inclusion or exclusion of studies, different meta-analyses might reach very different conclusions on the same topic. Even after the studies are chosen, there are many other methodologic issues in choosing how to combine means and variances from the different studies (e.g., what weighting methods should be used). Pooled analyses should report both relative risks and risk reductions as well as absolute risks and risk reductions (Sinclair and Bracken 1994).

There is a philosophic debate regarding the most appropriate way to pool data from the various studies into a single meta-analysis. Say, for example, that a meta-analysis is being done to determine the effect of treatment with a particular antihypertensive drug. Proponents of the **fixed-effects model** assume that there is only one true mean value for the effect and that all of the study means represent estimates of this true mean. These assumptions permit the pooling of values from all patients in the several studies being considered. In contrast, proponents of the **random-effects model** assume that each study measures its own (unique) mean value for the effect and that a more complex statistical approach is required to estimate the main or general effect of treatment (DerSimonian and Laird 1986).

Methodologic (Qualitative) Analysis

Sometimes the question to be answered is not how much benefit is derived from the use of a particular intervention but whether there is any benefit at all. In this case, a qualitative meta-analysis may be done, in which the quality of the research concerning the intervention is scored according to a list of objective criteria. The meta-analyst then examines the methodologically superior studies to determine whether or not the question of benefits is answered consistently by them. This qualitative approach has been called methodologic analysis (Gerbarg and Horwitz 1988) or quality scores analysis (Greenland 1994).

In some cases, the methodologically strongest studies agree with one another and disagree with the weaker studies, which may or may not be consistent with one another. An example was provided by a meta-analysis showing that of the eight major controlled trials of the bacillus Calmette-Guérin (BCG) vaccine against tuberculosis, only three trials met all or almost all of the methodologic criteria for a good study and had precise statistical estimates (Clemens, Chuong, and Feinstein 1983). These three trials agreed that BCG vaccine afforded a high level of protection against tuberculosis. The remaining five studies were methodologically weaker and had large confidence intervals (see Chapter 10). Their conclusions varied from showing a weak protective efficacy to actual harm from the vaccine. It should be noted that not everyone believes that this type of methodologic analysis is generally useful (Greenland 1994).

■ SUMMARY

Although there is general agreement about the need to improve clinical decision making, there is controversy about the methods to be used to achieve this goal. Among the tools available for decision analysis are Bayes' theorem and decision trees. These tools can be applied to individual patient care as well as to community health programs. Bayes' theorem can be used to calculate positive predictive values and posterior probabilities (see Boxes 8–1, 8–2, and 8–3). Decision trees can help health care workers pursue a logical, step-by-step approach to exploring the possible alternative clinical decisions, the sequence in which these decisions must be made, and the probabilities and utilities of each possible outcome (see Fig. 8–1).

Another tool used increasingly in medicine is meta-analysis, a technique to obtain either a quantitative or a qualitative synthesis of the research literature on a specific topic or question. In exploring the question of benefits derived from a particular treatment or vaccine, for example, either pooled analysis or methodologic analysis might be performed. Pooled analysis would focus on providing a quantitative estimate of benefits, based on data derived from many studies. In contrast, methodologic analysis would pursue the issue of whether methodologically superior studies found that the treatment or vaccine provided any benefit at all.

■ QUESTIONS

Directions (Items 1–16). Each of the numbered items or incomplete statements in this section is followed by answers or by completions of the statement. Select the ONE lettered answer or completion that is BEST in each case. Correct answers and explanations are given at the end of the chapter.

1. In Bayes' theorem, the numerator represents
   (A) false-negative results
   (B) incidence
   (C) prevalence
   (D) sensitivity
   (E) true-positive results

2. In a screening program, Bayes' theorem may be used to determine
   (A) cost-effectiveness
   (B) disease prevalence
   (C) false-negative results
   (D) positive predictive value
   (E) test sensitivity

3. When applying Bayes' theorem to the care of an individual patient, the prior probability is analogous to
   (A) prevalence
   (B) sensitivity
   (C) specificity
   (D) the likelihood ratio
   (E) the odds ratio

4. The application of Bayes' theorem to patient care will generally result in
   (A) greater sensitivity
   (B) greater specificity
   (C) higher costs
   (D) improved selection of diagnostic studies
   (E) more diagnostic testing

5. A young man complains of reduced auditory acuity on the left side. You take his medical history and perform a physical examination. Before you begin diagnostic testing, you estimate a 74%

chance that the patient has a large yellow fruit in his left ear. This estimate is the
   (A) likelihood ratio
   (B) odds ratio
   (C) posterior probability
   (D) prevalence
   (E) prior probability

6. To apply Bayes' theorem to a screening program, which of the following information must be known?
   (A) Prevalence, sensitivity, and prior probability
   (B) Prevalence, sensitivity, and specificity
   (C) Prevalence, specificity, and posterior probability
   (D) Prior probability and the false-positive error rate
   (E) The false-positive error rate and the false-negative error rate

Items 7–8

A 62-year-old woman complains that during the past several months she has been experiencing intermittent left-sided chest pain when she exercises. Her medical records indicate that she has a history of mild hyperlipidemia (with a high-density lipoprotein cholesterol level of 38 mg/dL and a total cholesterol level of 232 mg/dL), and she says that she has a family history of heart disease in male relatives only. Her current blood pressure is 132/68 mm Hg, and her heart rate is 72 beats per minute. On cardiac examination, you detect a physiologically split second heart sound (S2) and a faint midsystolic click without any appreciable murmur. The point of maximal impulse is nondisplaced, and the remainder of the examination is unremarkable. You are concerned that the patient's chest pain may represent angina pectoris and decide to initiate a workup. You estimate that the odds of the pain being angina are 1 in 3. You order an electrocardiogram (ECG), which reveals nonspecific abnormalities in the ST segments and T waves across the precordial leads. You decide to order a perfusion stress test, the sensitivity of which is 98% and the specificity of which is 85%. The stress test results are positive, demonstrating reversible ischemia in the distribution of the circumflex artery on perfusion imaging, with compatible ECG changes.

7. The prior probability of angina pectoris is
   (A) 25%
   (B) 33%
   (C) 66%
   (D) 75%
   (E) unknown

8. The posterior probability of angina pectoris following the stress test is

   (A) 10%
   (B) 33%
   (C) 67%
   (D) 76%
   (E) unchanged

Items 9–10

Based on the above findings, you decide to treat the patient for angina pectoris. You prescribe aspirin and a long-acting β-adrenergic receptor antagonist (atenolol) to be taken on a daily basis, and you prescribe sublingual nitroglycerin tablets to be used if pain recurs. Pain does recur, with increasing frequency and severity, despite treatment. After you consult a cardiologist (or maybe you are the cardiologist), you recommend cardiac catheterization. Assume that the sensitivity of cardiac catheterization for coronary disease is 96% and that the specificity is 99%. When the procedure is performed, it yields negative results.

9. At this stage of the workup, the prior probability of angina pectoris is

   (A) 15%
   (B) 33%
   (C) 67%
   (D) 76%
   (E) unknown

10. Based on the results of cardiac catheterization, the probability of coronary disease is

    (A) 11%
    (B) 20%
    (C) 33%
    (D) 76%
    (E) unknown

Items 11–12

A pregnancy test is applied to a population of 10,000 women. Based on prior evaluation, the test's sensitivity is known to be 98%, and its specificity is known to be 99%. Assume that the percentage of subjects who are actually pregnant is 0.1%.

11. The probability of pregnancy given a positive test result is

    (A) 0.1
    (B) 8.9%
    (C) 47%
    (D) 50%
    (E) 89%

12. For women found to have a positive pregnancy test result, an ultrasound examination is performed to confirm the diagnosis. The sensitivity of this examination is 90%, and the specificity is

95%. The probability of pregnancy given a positive ultrasound result is

    (A) 0.1
    (B) 6.4%
    (C) 20%
    (D) 64%
    (E) 75%

Items 13–15

A 75-year-old man is scheduled to undergo open reduction and internal fixation of a left hip fracture, an injury sustained while he was bungee jumping from a helicopter. Although the helicopter pilot was unaware that the patient had stowed away, the patient has already initiated litigation against the pilot, the helicopter owner, the helicopter manufacturer, the steel company that produced the metal used to construct the helicopter, the mine used to extract the iron used in making the steel used in making the helicopter, the gasoline company responsible for the fuel used to run the helicopter, the United Arab Emirates for exporting the fuel in the first place, and the Federal Aviation Administration for failing to adequately control the use of airspace. Be that as it may, the patient undergoes surgery, and there are no immediate complications. Fourteen hours later, the patient suddenly develops dyspnea, tachypnea, and tachycardia. His oxygen saturation falls to 80%, and an electrocardiogram reveals a right heart strain pattern. You are quite convinced that the patient has suffered a pulmonary embolism. You estimate the likelihood of pulmonary embolism at 90%. You order a ventilation-perfusion scan, which has a sensitivity of 80% and a specificity of 60%. The results of the scan are positive, meaning there is a high probability of pulmonary embolism.

13. The probability of pulmonary embolism is now

    (A) 10%
    (B) 75%
    (C) 90%
    (D) 95%
    (E) 99%

14. If the results of the ventilation-perfusion scan had been negative, given the operating characteristics described above, the posterior probability of pulmonary embolism would be

    (A) 1%
    (B) 75%
    (C) 90%
    (D) 95%
    (E) 99%

15. What is the most appropriate way to manage patients such as the one described above?

    (A) Begin definitive therapy immediately
    (B) Perform additional tests if the ventilation-perfusion scan yields negative results

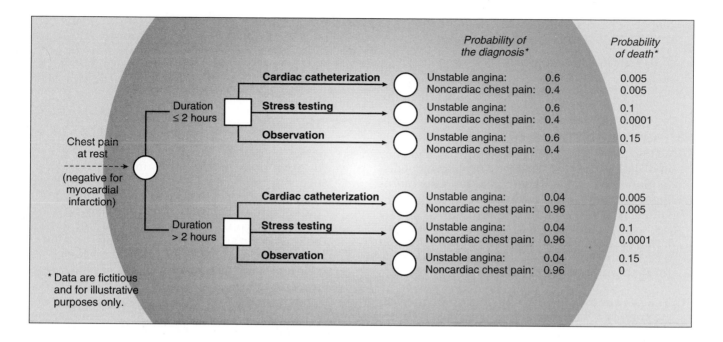

* Data are fictitious and for illustrative purposes only.

(C)   Treat for pulmonary embolism only if the ventilation-perfusion scan yields positive results

(D)   Treat for pulmonary embolism regardless of the ventilation-perfusion scan results

(E)   Treat for pulmonary embolism without ordering a ventilation-perfusion scan

Item 16

16. Two patients present with complaints of chest pain at rest. Neither patient has suffered a myocardial infarction. The duration of pain is less than 2 hours in one patient (patient A) but is greater than 2 hours in the other (patient B). Based on the decision tree shown in the accompanying figure, which of the following courses of action is most appropriate?

(A)   Cardiac catheterization for patient A and stress testing for patient B

(B)   Cardiac catheterization for patients A and B

(C)   Observation for patients A and B

(D)   Stress testing for patient A and cardiac catheterization for patient B

(E)   Stress testing for patients A and B

■ ANSWERS AND EXPLANATIONS

1. **The answer is E: true-positive results.** Bayes' theorem is essentially an expression of the positive predictive value. Given a particular estimate of the prior probability of disease (the probability of a given disease before testing), the theorem adjusts the estimate based on the results of testing. The numerator of the formula represents true-positive test results; the denominator, as in the formula for the positive predictive value, represents all positive test results (i.e., true-positive and false-positive results). The proportion of all positive test results that are true-positive results provides an estimate of the likelihood of disease if a test is positive (i.e., the positive predictive value).

2. **The answer is D: positive predictive value.** It is necessary to know how likely disease is when the results of testing are positive in a screening program. Bayes' theorem is used to establish the positive predictive value of a screening test, based on an estimate of the underlying population prevalence of the disease under investigation. Disease prevalence must be known or estimated to use Bayes' theorem; the theorem is not used to determine prevalence. The test sensitivity is an intrinsic property of the test when applied to a population with given characteristics; it is unaffected by prevalence and is not determined by use of Bayes' theorem. The cost-effectiveness of a screening program is an important consideration but is distinct from the predictive value of the test. Bayes' theorem is based on the proportion of true-positive results to all positive results (both true-positive and false-positive results). False-negative results are irrelevant to use of the theorem.

3. **The answer is A: prevalence.** Conceptually, Bayes' theorem states that the probability of a disease in an individual is partly dependent on the prevalence of that disease in the population of which the individual is a member. For a child with fever in New Haven, Connecticut, the probability of malaria is low. The probability (prior probability) is low in this child because the prev-

alence of malaria is so low in the population. For a child with fever in a refugee population in Zaire, the probability (prior probability) of malaria might be high because malaria is prevalent in the population. The prior probability of a disease in an individual is an estimate based on the prevalence of that disease in a population of similar persons.

To emphasize this point, one more example will be given. The prior probability of pregnancy in a male patient presenting with abdominal distention and complaining of nausea in the morning is 0. It is not 0 because the status of the individual is known with certainty; rather, it is 0 because the prevalence of pregnancy in a population of males is 0. When the prior probability of a condition is either 0 or 100%, no further testing for that condition is indicated.

4. **The answer is D: improved selection of diagnostic studies.** When Bayes' theorem is used appropriately in planning patient care, the result is more careful selection and refined use of diagnostic testing. Even when the theorem is used qualitatively, it suggests that if the prior probability of disease is high enough, no further testing is required. At other times, when successive tests fail to establish a posterior probability that is sufficiently high for decisive action to be taken, the theorem will compel the clinician to continue testing. Neither sensitivity nor specificity is enhanced by use of the theorem, because both depend in part on the choice of particular diagnostic modalities. Therefore, using Bayes' theorem in planning patient care should result in better use of diagnostic tests—sometimes more frequent use, sometimes less frequent use. The overall cost will vary accordingly.

Say, for example, that a 52-year-old woman visits your office because she has a cough. You quickly learn that the cough is productive and associated with pleuritic chest pain, fever, and mild dyspnea (breathlessness) on exertion. She has smoked a pack of cigarettes daily for many years. You examine her and find that her temperature is 38.2° C (100.8° F) and her respiratory rate is normal at rest. Auscultation of her lungs reveals rhonchi and wheezes but not rales. In a patient with these findings, you estimate that the prior probability of bronchitis is 95%. By reflex—the type of reflex acquired only in medical school—you might order some blood tests and a chest x-ray. But if you pause and think, you may realize that you have already made up your mind to treat this condition with antibiotics and perhaps corticosteroids and a β-agonist inhaler. When the prior probability is sufficiently high, further diagnostic testing will not, and should not, alter your course of action and is therefore not indicated. Conversely, it may be inappropriate to take immediate action when you have a considerable amount of uncertainty about what to do next for your patient and further diagnostic studies would help reduce the uncertainty. If you apply the concept of Bayes' theorem to your clinical care planning, without even using the actual formula, the standards of your practice are likely to improve.

5. **The answer is E: prior probability.** The prior probability is an estimate of the probability of a given condition in a given patient at a given point in time, prior to further testing. In actual practice, prior and posterior probabilities flow freely into one another. For example, estimating the probability of sinusitis after interviewing a patient gives you the prior probability of disease before you examine the patient. The revision in your estimate after the examination is the posterior probability, but this revision is also the prior probability before any diagnostic testing, such as sinus x-rays, that you may be considering.

6. **The answer is B: prevalence, sensitivity, and specificity.** The only choice that includes everything that must be known to use Bayes' theorem, in terms appropriate for a screening program, is choice B. The numerator for Bayes' theorem is the sensitivity of the test being used, multiplied by the prevalence. Therefore, both the prevalence and the sensitivity must be known before the theorem can be used. The denominator contains the numerator term plus a term that is the false-positive error rate, or $(1 - \text{specificity})$, multiplied by $(1 - \text{prevalence})$. Note that the numerator of Bayes' theorem describes cell a in a 2×2 table (see Box 8–1), and the denominator includes the term from the numerator (cell a, or the true-positive results) and adds to it the term for the false-positive results (cell b from a 2×2 table). Thus, Bayes' theorem can be rewritten as $a/(a + b)$, which is the formula for the positive predictive value. This is what the theorem is used to determine, so it is not necessary to know the predictive value before using the theorem. Choice D (prior probability and the false-positive error rate) is incorrect because the prior probability generally pertains to an individual patient (while prevalence is the more appropriate term for population screening) and because neither sensitivity nor specificity is provided. However, with the false-positive error rate, the specificity is easily derived. Choice E (the false-positive error rate and the false-negative error rate) is incorrect because no measure of prevalence is provided; both sensitivity and specificity are easily derived from false-negative and false-positive error rates, respectively.

7. **The answer is B: 33%.** Prior probability is analogous to prevalence and represents an estimate of the likelihood of disease in a patient. In this case, the prior probability is your estimate of the likelihood of angina pectoris prior to any testing. This

was stated as odds of 1 in 3 and therefore represents a 33% prior probability.

8. **The answer is D: 76%.** Either Bayes' theorem or a 2×2 table can be used to calculate the posterior probability.

   Use of Bayes' theorem: The sensitivity is provided in the vignette as 98%, or 0.98. The prior probability estimate is substituted for the prevalence and is 33%, or 0.33. The false-positive error rate is (1 – specificity). The specificity is provided as 85%, so the false-positive error rate is 15%, or 0.15. In this case, (1 – prevalence) is the same as (1 – prior probability) and is therefore (1 – 0.33), or 0.67.

$$p(\text{D+} \mid \text{T+}) = \frac{p(\text{T+} \mid \text{D+})p(\text{D+})}{[p(\text{T+} \mid \text{D+})p(\text{D+})] + [p(\text{T+} \mid \text{D-})p(\text{D-})]}$$

$$= \frac{(\text{Sensitivity})(\text{Prevalence})}{[(\text{Sensitivity})(\text{Prevalence})] + [(\text{False-positive error rate})(1 - \text{Prevalence})]}$$

$$= \frac{(0.98)(0.33)}{[(0.98)(0.33)] + [(0.15)(0.67)]}$$

$$= \frac{0.32}{(0.32 + 0.10)} = \frac{0.32}{0.42} = 0.76 = 76\%$$

   Use of a 2×2 table: To use this method, an arbitrary "sample size" must be chosen. Assuming that the sample size is 100, the following is true: Cell a is the true-positive results, or sensitivity multiplied by prevalence. The prior probability becomes the prevalence. Therefore, cell a is $(0.98)(33) = 32.3$ (rounded to 32). Cells a plus c must sum to 33, so cell c is 0.7 (rounded to 1). Cell d is the true-negative results, which is specificity multiplied by (1 – prevalence), or $(0.85)(67) = 57$. Cells b plus d must sum to 67, so cell b is 10.

		DISEASE	
		Positive	Negative
TEST RESULT	Positive	32	10
	Negative	1	57

Once the 2×2 table is established, the formula for positive predictive value, which is $a/(a + b)$, can be used to calculate the posterior probability, which is as follows:

$$a/(a + b) = 32/(32 + 10) = 32/42 = 0.76 = 76\%$$

9. **The answer is D: 76%.** As discussed in the explanation for question 5 (above), prior and posterior probabilities may flow freely into one another. At any given stage in a workup, the best estimate of disease probability is the posterior probability after the last examination or test, and it is also the prior probability before the next test that is to be done. For this reason, the answer to question 9 is the same as the answer to question 8. Following the stress test, the posterior probability of angina is 76%. This is also the probability of angina prior to any further diagnostic studies and is therefore the prior probability at this stage of the workup.

10. **The answer is A: 11%.** To calculate the posterior probability after a negative test result, the formula for negative predictive value, which is $d/(c + d)$, can be used. To use this formula, a 2×2 table must first be set up. Assume a sample size of 100. The prior probability, 76%, becomes the prevalence. Cell a is the sensitivity multiplied by the prevalence, or $(0.96)(76) = 73$. Cells a plus c sum to the prevalence, so cell c is 3. Cell d is the specificity multiplied by (1 – prevalence), or $(0.99)(24) = 23.8$. Cells b plus d sum to (1 – prevalence), so cell b is 0.2.

		DISEASE	
		Positive	Negative
TEST RESULT	Positive	73	0.2
	Negative	3	23.8

The negative predictive value is the probability that coronary disease is truly absent given a negative cardiac catheterization result. The formula and calculation are as follows:

$$d/(c + d) = 23.8/(3 + 23.8) = 23.8/26.8 = 89\%$$

The probability that the patient does not have coronary disease is now 89%. However, you are interested in knowing how likely it is, given the prior probability of 76% and the negative results of the catheterization, that your patient does have coronary disease. This is (1 – negative predictive value), or $(1 - 0.89) = (100\% - 89\%) = 11\%$.

11. **The answer is B: 8.9%.** Either Bayes' theorem or a 2×2 table can be used to calculate the positive predictive value.

   Use of Bayes' theorem: The sensitivity is 0.98. The specificity is 0.99. The prevalence is 0.1%, or 0.001. The false-positive error rate is (1 – specificity), or 0.01. The (1 – prevalence) is 0.999.

$$p(\text{D+} \mid \text{T+}) = \frac{p(\text{T+} \mid \text{D+})p(\text{D+})}{[p(\text{T+} \mid \text{D+})p(\text{D+})] + [p(\text{T+} \mid \text{D-})p(\text{D-})]}$$

$$= \frac{(\text{Sensitivity})(\text{Prevalence})}{[(\text{Sensitivity})(\text{Prevalence})] + [(\text{False-positive error rate})(1 - \text{Prevalence})]}$$

$$= \frac{(0.98)(0.001)}{[(0.98)(0.001)] + [(0.01)(0.999)]}$$

$$= \frac{0.00098}{(0.00098 + 0.00999)} = \frac{0.00098}{0.01097} = 0.089 = 8.9\%$$

Use of a 2 × 2 table: Cell *a* is the true-positive results, which is sensitivity multiplied by prevalence, or (0.98)(0.001) = 0.00098. Cells *c* plus *a* must sum to the prevalence, so cell *c* is 0.00002. Cell *d* is the true-negative results, which is specificity multiplied by (1 – prevalence), or (0.99)(0.999) = 0.989. Cells *b* plus *d* must sum to (1 – prevalence), so cell *b* is 0.01. In a population of 10,000, the contigency table is as follows:

| TEST RESULT | PREGNANCY STATUS | |
	Positive	Negative
Positive	9.8	100
Negative	0.2	9890

The posterior probability is derived by calculating the positive predictive value as follows:

$$a/(a+b) = \frac{9.8}{(9.8+100)} = \frac{9.8}{109.8} = 0.089 = 8.9\%$$

Note: Despite the use of a highly accurate pregnancy test, the probability of pregnancy in a woman from this population (perhaps a population of women who are being followed after having tubal ligation), given a positive test result, is only 8.9%. This is due to the extremely low prevalence of pregnancy in the cohort, and it demonstrates the fundamental concept on which Bayes' theorem is based: the likelihood of any condition in an individual depends largely on the prevalence of that condition in the population of which the individual is representative.

The false-positive error rate is worth noting. This term, as described in Chapter 7, is calculated as follows:

$$b/(b+d) = \frac{100}{(100+9890)} = \frac{100}{9990} = 0.01$$

Therefore, the results of 1 out of every 100 tests performed on women who are *not* pregnant will be positive (false-positive). In this population of 10,000 women, the prevalence of pregnancy is 0.001; this means that there are approximately 10 pregnant women in the entire population. The remaining 9990 women are not pregnant and are therefore candidates for a false-positive test result. (Recall that only true-negative cases may yield false-positive results.) Of the 9990 pregnancy tests in nonpregnant women, 1 per 100, or 99.9, will yield false-positive results. Therefore, because of the low prevalence of pregnancy in this group, there will be nearly 10 false-positive results for every true-positive result.

One other issue to consider is that sensitivity and specificity represent the performance characteristics of a test in a particular population or populations. These values may vary as the test is brought into wider use and applied to populations of differing composition.

12. **The answer is D: 64%.** Either Bayes' theorem or a 2 × 2 table can be used to make the calculation.

Use of Bayes' theorem: The sensitivity is 0.90. The specificity is 0.95. The prevalence is the prior probability of pregnancy, or 8.9% (0.089). The false-positive error rate is (1 – specificity), or 0.05. The (1 – prevalence) is 0.911.

$$p(D+ \mid T+) = \frac{p(T+ \mid D+)p(D+)}{[p(T+ \mid D+)p(D+)] + [p(T+ \mid D-)p(D-)]}$$

$$= \frac{(\text{Sensitivity})(\text{Prevalence})}{[(\text{Sensitivity})(\text{Prevalence})] + [(\text{False-positive error rate})(1 - \text{Prevalence})]}$$

$$= \frac{(0.90)(0.089)}{[(0.90)(0.089)] + [(0.05)(0.911)]}$$

$$= \frac{0.0801}{(0.0801 + 0.0456)} = \frac{0.0801}{0.1257} = 0.64 = 64\%$$

Use of a 2 × 2 table: Cell *a* is the true-positive results, which is sensitivity multiplied by prevalence, or (0.90)(0.089) = 0.0801. Cells *c* plus *a* must sum to the prevalence, so cell *c* is 0.0089. Cell *d* is the true-negative results, which is specificity multiplied by (1 – prevalence), or (0.95)(0.911) = 0.865. Cells *b* plus *d* must sum to (1 – prevalence), so cell *b* is 0.046. In a population of 10,000, the contigency table is as follows:

| TEST RESULT | PREGNANCY STATUS | |
	Positive	Negative
Positive	801	460
Negative	89	8650

The posterior probability is the positive predictive value, which is calculated as follows:

$$a/(a+b) = \frac{801}{(801+460)} = \frac{801}{1261} = 0.635 = 64\%$$

Note: Although the ultrasound study is a less accurate test than the initial pregnancy test (as described here), the probability of pregnancy is much higher following a positive ultrasound result than a positive pregnancy test result. This is because the ultrasound study is applied to a population with a much higher prevalence of pregnancy (i.e., only those women who initially tested positive).

13. **The answer is D: 95%.** Either Bayes' theorem or a 2 × 2 table can be used to make the calculation.

Use of Bayes' theorem: The sensitivity is 0.80. The specificity is 0.60. The prevalence (prior probability) is 0.90. The false-positive error rate is (1 – specificity), or 0.40. The (1 – prevalence) is 0.10.

$$p(D+ \mid T+) = \frac{p(T+ \mid D+)p(D+)}{[p(T+ \mid D+)p(D+)] + [p(T+ \mid D-)p(D-)]}$$

$$= \frac{\text{(Sensitivity)(Prevalence)}}{\begin{array}{c}[\text{(Sensitivity)(Prevalence)}] + \\ [\text{(False-positive error rate)}(1 - \text{Prevalence})]\end{array}}$$

$$= \frac{(0.80)(0.90)}{[(0.80)(0.90)] + [(0.40)(0.10)]}$$

$$= \frac{0.72}{(0.72 + 0.04)} = \frac{0.72}{0.76} = 0.947 = 95\%$$

Use of a 2 × 2 table: Cell *a* is the true-positive results, which is sensitivity multiplied by prevalence, or (0.80)(0.90) = 0.72. Cells *c* plus *a* must sum to the prevalence, so cell *c* is 0.18. Cell *d* is the true-negative results, which is specificity multiplied by (1 – prevalence), or (0.60)(0.10) = 0.06. Cells *b* plus *d* must sum to (1 – prevalence), so cell *b* is 0.04. In a population of 100, the contingency table is as follows:

		PULMONARY EMBOLISM	
		Positive	Negative
TEST RESULT	Positive	72	4
	Negative	18	6

The posterior probability of pulmonary embolism is the positive predictive value, which is calculated as follows:

$$a/(a + b) = \frac{72}{(72 + 4)} = \frac{72}{76} = 0.947 = 95\%$$

14. The answer is B: 75%. The question asks for the probability of disease given a negative test result. The negative predictive value provides the probability of nondisease given a negative result. Therefore, calculating the (1 – negative predictive value) will provide the answer. This can be done by using the 2 × 2 table in the explanation for question 13 (above).

$$d/(c + d) = \frac{6}{(18 + 6)} = \frac{6}{24} = 0.25$$

The posterior probability of pulmonary embolism is (1 – negative predictive value), or (1 – 0.25) = 0.75 = 75%. The take-home message here is that the probability of disease remains high after a negative test result if the prior probability of disease was very high. Certainty in medicine is elusive at best and unattainable at worst. You will need to decide whether to take therapeutic action based on the prior probability of disease or whether additional testing is truly required to inform such a decision.

15. The answer is B: perform additional tests if the ventilation-perfusion scan yields negative results. The patient is very likely to have pulmonary embolism. The incidence of deep venous thrombosis and pulmonary embolism following internal fixation of a hip fracture is high, and the clinical description is classic for pulmonary embolism (see Goldhaber and Morpurgo 1992). However, the use of intravenous heparin, essential in the treatment of pulmonary embolism, is hazardous so soon after major surgery. Therefore, before this therapy is used, diagnostic certainty must be quite high. Alternative diagnoses, such as right ventricular infarction, pulmonary atelectasis, or even acute bronchospasm, might produce a similar clinical picture, but each would call for a different treatment. A clinician might treat for pulmonary embolism without first obtaining confirmatory test results in this case, but most clinicians would attempt to confirm the diagnosis with a ventilation-perfusion scan. When ordering a test, however, the clinician must consider all of the possible outcomes; if only one outcome were possible, the test would be unnecessary. Therefore, a test ordered to confirm a diagnostic impression might, in fact, refute that impression when results defy expectation. In such situations, further diagnostic testing is often obtained to resolve the discrepancy. The pursuit of certainty in clinical practice is often frustrating, with unanticipated test results frequently generating the need for further testing. The best course through this labyrinth, in answering this question and in general, is to anticipate all of the possible results of any tests that are ordered and the action indicated by each. Inaction must be considered among the available courses of action. The challenge is to minimize risk to the patient and maximize benefit, despite the constant burden of uncertainty.

16. The answer is A: cardiac catheterization for patient A and stress testing for patient B. In a decision tree, a square represents a decision node, and a circle represents a chance node. Once a decision is made, the probability of that decision is 1 (100%), so that the chance occurrences beyond each decision node must add to 100%. This is because they must represent all of the possible outcomes of that decision. In this tree, there are two categories of patients who have chest pain at rest: those whose chest pain has a duration of 2 hours or less (the group in which patient A is included) and those whose chest pain has a duration of more than 2 hours (the group in which patient B is included). Both groups are negative for myocardial infarction. The decision to be made is whether patients A and B should undergo cardiac catheterization, stress testing, or observation. The tree provides the probability that a patient has unstable angina or noncardiac chest pain, based on the duration of the pain. (The idea behind this is that if the pain is caused by ischemia and is of long duration, it should

...ad to signs of infarction; but if the pain does not produce infarction after so protracted a period, it is unlikely to be ischemic pain.) The probability of death associated with each intervention is the product of the probability that the pain is unstable angina or noncardiac chest pain, multiplied by the probability of death for each intervention given that diagnosis. For example, the probability of death due to cardiac catheterization in a patient with chest pain for less than 2 hours' duration is calculated by multiplying the probability that the pain is unstable angina (0.6) by the risk of death in similar patients (0.005). The answer is 0.003. To this answer must be added the risk of death from cardiac catheterization in similar patients who turn out to have noncardiac chest pain, which is (0.4)(0.005) = 0.002. Thus, the total risk of death associated with cardiac catheterization in all patients with chest pain of less than 2 hours' duration is 0.003 + 0.002 = 0.005. By a similar means, the risk associated with each possible intervention can be calculated. The risks of death derived are as follows:

Duration of Pain	Procedure	Risk of Death
≤ 2 hours	Catheterization	0.005
	Stress testing	0.06
	Observation	0.09
> 2 hours	Catheterization	0.005
	Stress testing	0.0041
	Observation	0.006

The risk of the particular adverse outcome of interest (in this case, death) associated with each decision node is determined in a process called "averaging out." The probabilities of death associated with the different interventions following a particular decision node are summed to give the aggregate risk of death associated with the decision to be made. Then, in a process called "folding back," those branches of the decision tree that have unacceptably high attendant risks can be eliminated, or "pruned." Only options within a range of acceptable risk are thus left to consider. In this case, the risk of death is minimized in the patient (or group of patients) with chest pain of short duration by performing cardiac catheterization, and it is minimized in the group with chest pain of longer duration by stress testing. These interventions represent the preferred interventions, so cardiac catheterization is indicated for patient A and stress testing is indicated for patient B. (Note that the data used here and in the accompanying figure are fictitious and are provided for illustrative purposes only.)

References Cited

Bailar, J. C., III. The promise and problems of meta-analysis. New England Journal of Medicine 337:559–560, 1997.

Bloom, B. S., et al. A reappraisal of hepatitis B virus vaccination strategies using cost-effectiveness analysis. Annals of Internal Medicine 118:298–306, 1993.

Borzak, S., and P. M. Kidker. Discordance between meta-analyses and large-scale randomized controlled trials: examples from the management of acute myocardial infarction. Annals of Internal Medicine 123:873–877, 1995.

Clemens, J. D., J. J. Chuong, and A. R. Feinstein. The BCG controversy: a methodological and statistical reappraisal. Journal of the American Medical Association 249:2362–2369, 1983.

DerSimonian, R., and N. Laird. Meta-analysis in clinical trials. Controlled Clinical Trials 7:177–188, 1986.

Evidence-Based Medicine Working Group. Evidence-based medicine: a new approach to teaching the practice of medicine. Journal of the American Medical Association 268:2420–2425, 1992.

Feinstein, A. R. Meta-analysis: statistical alchemy for the 21st century. Journal of Clinical Epidemiology 48:71–79, 1995.

Gerberg, Z. B., and R. I. Horwitz. Resolving conflicting clinical trials: guidelines for meta-analysis. Journal of Clinical Epidemiology 41:503–509, 1988.

Goldhaber, S. Z., and M. Morpurgo, eds. Report of the World Health Organization/International Society and Federation of Cardiology Task Force on Pulmonary Embolism: diagnosis, treatment, and prevention of pulmonary embolism. Journal of the American Medical Association 268:1727–1733, 1992.

Greenland, S. Invited commentary: a critical look at some popular meta-analytic methods. American Journal of Epidemiology 140:290–296, 1994.

Horwitz, R. I., and A. R. Feinstein. The application of therapeutic-trial principles to improve the design of epidemiologic research: a case-control study suggesting that anticoagulants reduce mortality in patients with myocardial infarction. Journal of Chronic Disease 34:575–583, 1981.

Jekel, J. F., R. A. Greenberg, and B. M. Drake. Influence of prevalence of infection on tuberculin skin testing programs. Public Health Reports 84:883–886, 1969.

Koplan, J. P., et al. Pertussis vaccine: an analysis of benefits, risks, and costs. New England Journal of Medicine 301:906–911, 1979.

LeLorier, J., et al. Discrepancies between meta-analyses and subsequent large randomized, controlled trials. New England Journal of Medicine 337:536–542, 1997.

Rose, D. N., and J. Wiesel. Letter to the editor. New England Journal of Medicine 308:221–222, 1983.

Schaffner, W., P. Gardner, and P. A. Gross. Hepatitis B immunization strategies: expanding the target. Annals of Internal Medicine 118:308–309, 1993.

Shapiro, E. D., et al. The protective efficacy of polyvalent pneumococcal polysaccharide vaccine. New England Journal of Medicine 325:1453–1460, 1991.

Shapiro, S. Meta-analysis/shmeta-analysis. American Journal of Epidemiology 140:771–778, 1994.

Sinclair, J. C., and M. B. Bracken. Clinically useful measures of effect in binary analyses of randomized trials. Journal of Clinical Epidemiology 47:881–889, 1994.

Weinstein, M. C., and H. V. Fineberg. Clinical Decision Analysis. Philadelphia, W. B. Saunders Company, 1980.

Selected Readings

Blettner, M., et al. Traditional reviews, meta-analysis, and pooled analyses in epidemiology. International Journal of Epidemiology 28:1–9, 1999.

Fletcher, R. H., S. W. Fletcher, and E. H. Wagner. Clinical Epidemiology: The Essentials, 3rd ed. Baltimore, Williams and Wilkins, 1996.

Friedland, D. J., ed. Evidence-Based Medicine: A Framework for Clinical Practice. Stamford, Conn., Appleton and Lange, 1998.

Petitti, D. B. Meta-Analysis, Decision Analysis, and Cost-Effectiveness Analysis: Methods for Quantitative Synthesis in Medicine. New York, Oxford University Press, 1994.

Sackett, D. L., et al. Evidence-Based Medicine: How to Practice and Teach EBM. Edinburgh, Churchill Livingstone, 1997.

Weinstein, M. C., and H. V. Fineberg. Clinical Decision Analysis. Philadelphia, W. B. Saunders Company, 1980.

BIOSTATISTICS

9

Describing Variation in Data

Variation is evident in almost every characteristic of patients, including their physiologic measurements, diseases, diets, environments, and life-styles. A measure of a single characteristic is called a **variable.** Statistics enables investigators to (1) describe the patterns of variation in single variables, as discussed in this chapter; (2) determine when observed differences are likely to be real differences, as discussed in Chapters 10 and 11; and (3) determine the patterns and strength of association between variables, as discussed in Chapters 11 and 13.

■ SOURCES OF VARIATION IN MEDICINE

While variation in clinical medicine may be due to biologic differences or the presence or absence of disease, it may also be due to differences in measurement techniques and conditions, errors in measurement, and random variation.

Biologic differences include factors such as differences in genes, nutrition, and environmental exposures. Height provides a good example. Tall parents usually have tall children. Extremely short people may have specific genetic conditions (such as achondroplasia) or a deficiency of growth hormone. While poor nutrition will slow growth and starvation may stop growth altogether, good nutrition allows the full genetic growth potential to be achieved. A polluted environment may cause many infections in children, and this in turn can retard growth.

Variation is seen not only in the **presence or absence of disease** but also in the **stages of disease.** For example, cancer of the cervix may be in situ, localized, invasive, or metastatic. In some cases, multiple diseases (comorbidity) may be present. Insulin-dependent diabetes mellitus, for instance, may be accompanied by coronary artery disease or renal disease.

Different conditions of measurement often account for the variations observed in medical data and include factors such as time of day, ambient temperature or noise, and the presence of fatigue or anxiety in the patient. Differences in measurement caused by different environments and conditions are not errors of measurement, but standardizing the conditions under which the data are obtained is important to ensure that observed variation is due to factors of interest.

Different methods of measurement can produce different results. For example, a blood pressure measurement derived from the use of an intra-arterial catheter may differ from that derived from the use of an arm cuff. This may be due to differences in the measurement site (e.g., a central or distal arterial site), the thickness of the arm (which influences the reading from the blood pressure cuff), the rigidity of the artery (reflecting the degree of atherosclerosis), and the different ways in which the blood pressure is measured.

Some variation is due to **measurement error.** Different blood pressure cuffs of the same size may give different measurements because of errors in some cuffs; different laboratory instruments or methods may produce different readings from the same sample; and different x-ray machines may produce films of different quality. When two different observers are examining the same patient or the same specimen (e.g., an x-ray), these observers may report different results. For example, one radiologist may read a mammogram as abnormal and recommend further tests such as a biopsy, while another radiologist may read the same mammogram as normal and not recommend any further workup (Elmore et al. 1994). One clinician may detect a problem such as a retinal hemorrhage or a heart murmur, and another clinician may fail to detect it. Two clinicians may both detect a heart murmur in the same patient but disagree on its characteristics. And if two clinicians are asked to characterize a dark skin lesion, one may call it a nevus, while the other diagnoses it as a malignant melanoma.

Determinists would probably say that if clinicians and investigators only knew enough and measured accurately enough, **random variation** would disappear. Perhaps, but unexplained variation seems to be a ubiquitous phenomenon in clinical medicine and research. Statistics helps investigators to interpret data despite random variation, but statistics cannot correct for errors in the observation or recording of data.

■ STATISTICS AND VARIABLES

Statistical methods help clinicians and investigators understand and explain the variation in medical data. The first step in understanding variation is to describe the variation. Therefore, this chapter focuses on how to describe variations in medical observations. Statistics can be thought of as a set of tools for working with data, just as brushes are tools used by an artist for painting. One reason for the choice of a specific tool over another is the kind of material on which the tool will be used. One kind of brush is needed for oil paints, another kind for tempera paints, and another kind for water colors. The artist must know the materials to be used in order to choose the correct tools. Similarly, a person who works with data must understand the different types of variables that exist in medicine.

Quantitative and Qualitative Data

The first question to answer before analyzing data is whether the data describe a quantitative or a qualitative characteristic. A **quantitative characteristic,** such as a systolic blood pressure or serum sodium level, can be characterized using a rigid, dimensional measurement scale. A **qualitative characteristic,** such as coloration of the skin, must be described in detail. For example, normal skin can vary in color from pinkish-white through tan to dark brown or black. Medical problems can cause changes in skin color, with white denoting pallor, as in anemia; red suggesting rash or a sunburn; blue denoting cyanosis, as in cardiac or lung failure; bluish-purple occurring when blood has been released subcutaneously, as in a bruise; and yellow suggesting the presence of jaundice, as in common bile duct obstruction or liver disease.

Examples of disease manifestations that have both quantitative and qualitative characteristics are heart murmurs and bowel sounds. Not only does the loudness of a heart murmur vary from patient to patient (and can be described on a 5-point scale), but the sound may vary from blowing to harsh or rasping in quality.

Information on any characteristic that can vary is called a variable. Thus, the qualitative information on colors just described could form a qualitative variable called skin color. The quantitative information on blood pressure could be contained in variables called systolic pressure and diastolic pressure.

Types of Variables

Variables can be classified as nominal variables, dichotomous (binary) variables, ordinal (ranked) variables, continuous (dimensional) variables, ratio variables, and risks and proportions.

Nominal Variables

Nominal variables are "naming" or categorical variables that have no measurement scales. Examples are blood groups (O, A, B, and AB), occupations, food groups, and skin color. If skin color is the variable being examined, a different number can be assigned to each color (for example, 1 is bluish-purple, 2 is black, 3 is white, 4 is blue, 5 is tan, and so forth) before the information is entered into a computer data system. Any number could be assigned to any color, and that would make no difference to the statistical analysis. This is because the number is merely a numerical name for a color, and the number given to a particular color has nothing to do with the quality, value, or rank of the color.

Dichotomous Variables (Binary Variables)

If all possible skin colors were included in one nominal variable (as was done just above), there is a problem: this variable does not distinguish between normal and abnormal skin color, which is usually the most important aspect of skin color for both clinical and research purposes. As discussed above, abnormal skin color (pallor, jaundice, cyanosis, etc.) may be a sign of any number of health problems (anemia, liver disease, cardiac failure, etc.). Therefore, researchers might choose to create a variable with only two levels: normal skin color (coded as a 1) and abnormal skin color (coded as a 2), for example. This variable, which has only two levels, is said to be dichotomous (from the Greek language, meaning "cut into two").

Some dichotomous variables—such as well/sick, living/dead, and normal/abnormal—have an implied qualitative direction, with the first option in the pair clearly preferred. Skin color as a dichotomous variable has a directional value, since having normal coloration is preferable to having abnormal coloration. Other dichotomous variables—such as female/male and treatment/placebo—have no a priori qualitative direction. Usually, it makes no difference to the statistical analysis whether or not the dichotomous variable has an implied direction, but the direction may be important for the conclusions drawn from the data.

Dichotomous variables, although common and important, often are not adequate by themselves. For example, in analyzing cancer therapy, not only is it important to know whether the patient survives or dies (a continuous variable), but it is also crucial to know how long the patient survives (time forms a continuous variable) and to know the quality of the patient's life (which may be an ordinal variable, as discussed below). A survival analysis or life table analysis, as described in Chapter 11, may therefore be done. Similarly, for a study of heart murmurs, various types of data may be needed, such as dichotomous data concerning a murmur's timing (systolic or diastolic); nominal data concerning its location (e.g., aortic valve area) and character (e.g., rough); and ordinal data concerning its loudness (e.g., grade III).

Dichotomous variables and nominal variables are sometimes called **discrete variables** because the different categories are completely separate from each other.

Ordinal Variables (Ranked Variables)

Many types of medical data can be characterized in terms of more than two values and have a clearly implied direction from better to worse, but the data are not measured on a measurement scale. These data form ordinal (i.e., ordered or ranked) variables.

There are many clinical examples of ordinal variables. The amount of swelling in a patient's legs is estimated by the clinician and is usually reported as "none" or 1+, 2+, 3+, or 4+ pitting edema (puffiness). A patient may have a systolic murmur ranging from 1+ to 6+. Respiratory distress is reported as being absent, mild, moderate, or severe. Although pain also may be reported as being absent, mild, moderate, or severe, in some cases patients are asked to describe their pain on a scale from 0 to 10, with 0 being no pain and 10 being the worst imaginable pain.

None of these variables is measured on an exact measurement scale, but more information is contained in them than in nominal variables. This is so because it is possible to see the relationship between ordinal categories and know whether one is more desirable, equally desirable, or less desirable than another. Because ordinal variables contain more information than nominal variables, the ordinal variables enable more informative conclusions to be drawn. As described in Chapter 11, ordinal variables often require special techniques of analysis.

Continuous Variables (Dimensional Variables)

Many types of medically important data are measured on continuous (dimensional) measurement scales. Patients' heights, weights, systolic and diastolic blood pressures, and serum glucose levels are all examples of data measured on continuous scales. Even more information is contained in continuous data than in ordinal data, because continuous data not only show the position of the different observations relative to each other but also show the extent to which one observation differs from another. Continuous data usually enable investigators to make more detailed inferences than do ordinal or nominal data.

Perhaps surprisingly, relationships between continuous variables are not always linear (in a straight line). For example, there is not a linear relationship between the birth weight and the probability of survival of newborns (Buehler et al. 1987). As shown in Fig. 9–1, infants weighing under 3000 g and infants weighing over 4500 g are both at greater risk for neonatal death than are infants weighing between 3000 and 4500 g (between about 6.6 and 9.9 pounds).

Ratio Variables

If a continuous scale has a true 0 point, the variables derived from it can be called ratio variables. The Kelvin temperature scale is a ratio scale, because 0 degrees on this scale is absolute 0. The centigrade temperature scale is a continuous scale but not a ratio scale, because 0 degrees on this scale does not mean the absence of heat. For descriptive purposes, it may be useful to know that 200 units of something is twice as big as 100 units. For most statistical analyses, including significance testing, the distinction between continuous and ratio variables is usually not important.

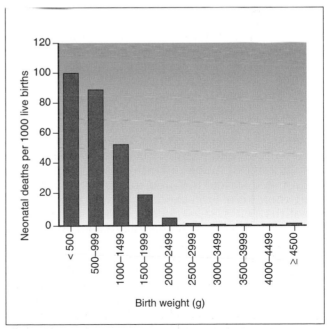

FIGURE 9–1 **Histogram showing the neonatal mortality rate by birth weight group, all races, USA, 1980.** (Source of data: Buehler, J. W., et al. Birth weight–specific infant mortality, United States, 1960 and 1980. Public Health Reports 102:151–161, 1987.)

TABLE 9–1   Standard 2 × 2 Table Showing the Gender of 71 Subjects and Whether the Serum Level of Total Cholesterol Was Checked

| | | CHOLESTEROL LEVEL | | | | | |
| | | Checked | | Not Checked | | Total | |
		Number	(Percentage)	Number	(Percentage)	Number	(Percentage)
GENDER	Female	17	(63)	10	(37)	27	(100)
	Male	25	(57)	19	(43)	44	(100)
	Total	42	(59)	29	(41)	71	(100)

Source of data: Unpublished findings in a sample of 71 professional persons in Connecticut.

Risks and Proportions as Variables

As discussed in Chapter 6, a risk is the conditional probability of an event (e.g., death or disease) in a defined population. Risks and proportions, which are two important types of variables in medicine, share some characteristics of a discrete variable and some characteristics of a continuous variable. Just as it makes no sense to say that a fraction of a death occurred, it makes no sense to say that a fraction of a person suffered an event. However, it does make sense to say that a discrete event (e.g., death) or a discrete characteristic (e.g., presence of a murmur) occurred in a fraction of a population. Risks and proportions are variables created by the ratio of discrete counts in the numerator to counts in the denominator. Depending on the circumstances, they may be analyzed as discrete variables or as continuous variables.

Counts and Units of Observation

The unit of observation is the person or thing from which the data came. Common examples of units of observation in medical studies are persons, animals, and cells. The same statistical principles apply in clinical research as in laboratory research. Units of observation may be arranged in a **frequency table,** with one characteristic on the *x*-axis, some other characteristic on the *y*-axis, and the appropriate counts in the cells of the table. Table 9–1, which provides an example of this type of 2 × 2 table, shows that among 71 young professional persons studied, 63% of females and 57% of males had previously had their cholesterol level checked. Using these data and a test that will be described in Chapter 11, analysts can determine whether the difference between the percentage of women and the percentage of men with cholesterol checks was likely to have been due to chance variation.

Combining Data

A continuous variable may be converted to an ordinal variable by grouping units with similar values together. For example, the individual birth weights of infants (a continuous variable) can be converted to ranges of birth weights (an ordinal variable), as shown in Fig. 9–1. When the data are presented as categories or ranges (less than 500 g, 500–999 g, 1000–1499 g, and so forth), information is lost, because the individual weights of infants are no longer apparent. However, the advantage is that now percentages can be created, and the relationship of birth weight to mortality is easier to show.

Three or more groups must be formed to convert a continuous variable to an ordinal variable. In the example of birth weight, the result of forming several groups is that it creates a ranked order that goes progressively from lightest to heaviest birth weight. By dividing the data into only two groups, it is possible to convert a continuous variable into a dichotomous variable. For example, dividing infants into two groups creates a dichotomous variable of those weighing less than 2500 g (low birth weight) and those weighing 2500 g or more (normal birth weight). However, more information is lost by forming only two groups than by forming more than two.

■ FREQUENCY DISTRIBUTIONS
Frequency Distributions of Continuous Variables

Observations on one variable may be shown visually by putting the value on one axis (usually the horizontal or *x*-axis) and putting the frequency with which that value appears on the other axis (usually the vertical or *y*-axis). This is known as a frequency distribution. For example, Table 9–2 and Fig. 9–2 both show the distribution of the levels of total cholesterol among 71 professional persons; the distribution is easier to see in the figure.

Range of a Variable

A frequency distribution can be described, albeit imperfectly, using only the lowest and highest numbers in the data set. For example, the cholesterol levels in Table 9–2 vary from a low value of 124 mg/dL to a high value of 264 mg/dL. The distance between the lowest and highest observations is called the range of the variable. Thus, the range of the total cholesterol values in Table 9–2 is the difference between 124 mg/dL and 264 mg/dL, or 140 mg/dL.

TABLE 9–2   Serum Levels of Total Cholesterol Reported in 71 Subjects*

Cholesterol Value (mg/dL)	Number of Observations	Cholesterol Value (mg/dL)	Number of Observations	Cholesterol Value (mg/dL)	Number of Observations
124	1	169	1	217	1
128	1	171	4	220	1
132	1	175	1	221	1
133	1	177	2	222	1
136	1	178	2	226	1
138	1	179	1	227	1
139	1	180	4	228	1
146	1	181	1	241	1
147	1	184	2	264	1
149	1	186	1		
151	1	188	2		
153	2	191	3		
158	3	192	2		
160	1	194	2		
161	1	196	2		
162	1	197	2		
163	2	206	1		
164	3	208	1		
165	1	209	1		
166	1	213	1		

Source of data: Unpublished findings in a sample of 71 professional persons in Connecticut.
*In this data set, the mean is 179.1 mg/dL, and the standard deviation is 28.2 mg/dL.

Real and Theoretical Frequency Distributions

Real frequency distributions are those obtained from actual data, and theoretical frequency distributions are calculated using certain assumptions. When theoretical distributions are used, they are assumed to describe the underlying populations from which data are obtained. The majority of measurements of continuous data in medicine and biology tend to approximate the theoretical distribution that is known as the **normal distribution** and is also called the **gaussian distribution** (named after Johann Karl Gauss, the person who best described it).

The normal (gaussian) distribution looks something like a bell seen from the side, as shown in Fig. 9–3. In statistical texts, smooth, bell-shaped curves are drawn to describe normal distributions. Real distributions, found by gathering real data, however, are seldom (if ever) perfectly smooth and bell-shaped. For example, the frequency distribution of total cholesterol values among the 71 young professionals shows peaks and valleys when the data are presented in the manner shown in Fig. 9–2. This should not cause concern, however, if partitioning the same data into reasonably narrow ranges results in a bell-shaped frequency distribution. For example, when the cholesterol levels from Table 9–2 and Fig. 9–2 are partitioned into seven groups with narrow ranges (ranges of 20 mg/dL width), the resulting frequency distribution appears almost perfectly normal (gaussian), as shown in Fig. 9–4. If the sample size had been much larger than 71, the distribution of raw data (see Fig. 9–2) would probably have looked much smoother.

In textbooks, the smooth, bell-shaped curves are often used to represent the **expected frequency of observations** (on the y-axis) according to their observed value on a measurement scale (on the x-axis) (see Fig. 9–3). When readers see a perfectly smooth, bell-shaped gaussian distribution, they should remember that the y-axis is really describing the frequency with which the corresponding values in the x-axis are expected to be found. With an intuitive feeling for the meaning of Fig. 9–3, it will be easier to understand the medical literature, advanced statistical textbooks, and problems presented on examinations.

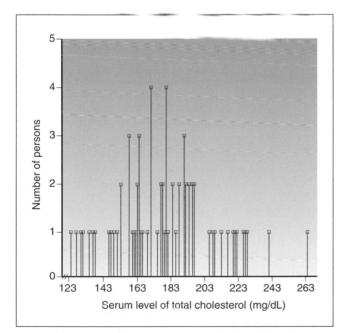

FIGURE 9–2   Histogram showing the frequency distribution of the serum levels of total cholesterol reported in a sample of 71 subjects. The data shown here are the same data listed in Table 9–2. (Source of data: Unpublished findings in a sample of 71 professional persons in Connecticut.)

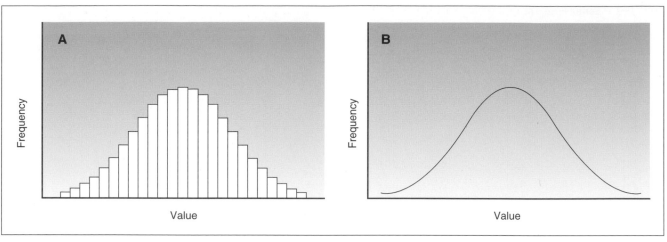

FIGURE 9–3   The normal (gaussian) distribution, with the value shown on the *x*-axis and with the frequency shown on the *y*-axis. Diagram A illustrates a probability distribution of actual data, plotted as a histogram with very narrow ranges, and diagram B illustrates the way this idea is represented, for simplicity, in textbooks, articles, and tests.

Although the term "normal" distribution is used in this book and is used frequently elsewhere in the literature, there is no implication that data which do not strictly follow this distribution are somehow abnormal. Even when data do not form perfectly normal distributions, it is possible to draw powerful inferences (tentative conclusions) about the data by using certain statistical tests that assume the observed data came from a normal (gaussian) distribution. If the sample size is sufficiently large, this assumption usually works well (see the discussion of the central limit theorem and tests of statistical significance in Chapter 10).

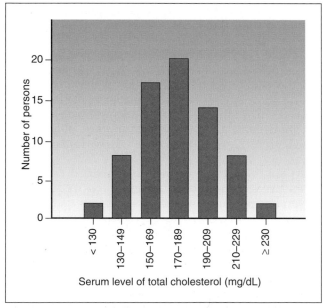

FIGURE 9–4   Histogram showing the frequency distribution of the serum levels of total cholesterol reported in a sample of 71 subjects, grouped in ranges of 20 mg/dL. Individual values for the 71 subjects are reported in Table 9–2 and Fig. 9–2. The mean is 179.1 mg/dL, and the median is 178 mg/dL.

Histograms, Frequency Polygons, and Line Graphs

There are several ways to illustrate the characteristics of the frequency distribution of a set of data. Usually, the best way is to create a **histogram,** which is a bar graph in which the number of units of observation (e.g., persons) is shown on the *y*-axis, the measurement values (e.g., cholesterol levels) are shown on the *x*-axis, and the frequency distribution is illustrated by a series of bars. In a histogram, the area of each bar represents the relative proportion of all observations that fall in the range represented by that bar. Fig. 9–2 is a histogram in which each bar represents a single number value for the cholesterol level. An extremely large number of observations would be needed to get a smooth curve for single values such as these.

A shorthand way of presenting a histogram is first to put a dot at the center of the top of each bar and then to connect these dots with a line. In this way, a graph called a **frequency polygon** is created. Fig. 9–5 shows a frequency polygon that was constructed from the histogram shown in Fig. 9–4. Although histograms generally are recommended for presenting frequency distributions, frequency polygons have two advantages. First, the shape of the distribution is more easily seen in a frequency polygram than in a histogram. Second, a linear dose-response relationship (discussed in Chapter 4 and illustrated in Fig. 4–1) is suggested more clearly by a frequency polygon than by a histogram.

Chapter 3 provides numerous examples of graphs depicting relationships between time and incident cases or between time and incidence rates. The **epidemic time curve** (illustrated in Figs. 3–11, 3–12, 3–13, 3–14, and 3–19) is a kind of histogram in which the *x*-axis is time and the *y*-axis is the *number of incident cases* in each time interval. When the *x*-axis represents time and the *y*-axis presents *rates,* a **line graph** is recommended.

Fig. 3–1, which shows the incidence rates of reported salmonellosis in the USA during several de-

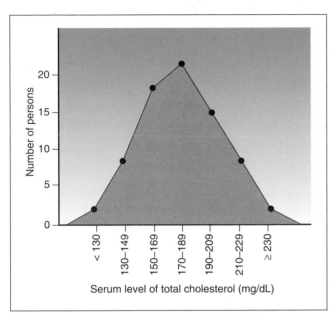

FIGURE 9–5   Frequency polygon showing the frequency distribution of the serum levels of total cholesterol reported in a sample of 71 subjects, grouped in ranges of 20 mg/dL. The data in this polygon are the same as the data in the histogram shown in Fig. 9–4. Individual values for the 71 subjects are reported in Table 9–2 and Fig. 9–2.

cades, is an example of an **arithmetic line graph,** meaning that both the x-axis and the y-axis use an arithmetic scale. Fig. 3–2, which illustrates the impact that diphtheria vaccine (and perhaps other factors) had on the incidence rates of disease and death during several decades, is an example of a **semilogarithmic line graph** in which the x-axis uses an arithmetic scale but the y-axis uses a logarithmic scale in order to amplify the lower end of the scale. Although semilogarithmic line graphs have the disadvantage of making the absolute magnitude of the changes that occurred look less dramatic, they have two advantages. First, they enable the detail of changes in very low rates of disease to be seen, which would be difficult on an arithmetic graph comparing current rates with those decades ago. Second, as shown in Fig. 3–2, they depict proportionately similar changes as parallel lines. The decline in diphtheria deaths was proportionately similar to the decline in reported cases of disease, so that the case fatality ratio remained fairly constant.

Parameters of a Frequency Distribution

Frequency distributions from continuous data are defined by two types of measures, or parameters: measures of central tendency and measures of dispersion. The **measures of central tendency** locate a scale of observations in space and are something like a street address for the variable. The **measures of dispersion** suggest how widely the observations are spread out and can be thought of as indicating the property lines for the variable. In the case of a perfectly normal (gaussian) distribution, the bell-shaped curve can be fully described using only the mean (a measure of central tendency) and the standard deviation (a measure of dispersion).

Measures of Central Tendency. The first step in examining a distribution is to look for the central tendency of the observations. Most types of medical data tend to clump in such a way that the density of observed values is greatest near the center of the distribution. In the case of the observed cholesterol values listed in Table 9–2 and depicted graphically in Fig. 9–2, there appears to be some tendency for the values to cluster near the center of the distribution, but this tendency is much clearer visually when the values from Table 9–2 and Fig. 9–2 are grouped in ranges of 20 mg/dL, as shown in Fig. 9–4.

The next step is to examine the distribution in greater detail and look for the mode, the median, and the mean, which are the three measures of central tendency.

(1) Mode. The most commonly observed value (that is, the value that occurs most frequently) in a data set is called the mode. The mode is of some clinical interest but seldom is of statistical value. It is not uncommon for a distribution to have a mode at more than one value. For example, in Fig. 9–2, the most commonly observed cholesterol values (each with 4 observations) are 171 mg/dL and 180 mg/dL. In this case, although technically the figure shows a **bimodal distribution,** the two modes are close enough together to be considered part of the same central cluster. In other cases, distributions may be truly bimodal, usually because the population contains two subgroups, each of which has a different distribution that peaks at a different point. More than one mode can also be produced artificially by what is known as **digit preference,** when observers tend to favor certain numbers over others. For example, persons who measure blood pressure values tend to favor even numbers, particularly those ending in 0 (e.g., 120 mm Hg).

(2) Median. The median is the middle observation when data have been arranged in order from the lowest to the highest value. The median value in Table 9–2 is 178 mg/dL. When there is an even number of observations, the median is considered to lie halfway between the two middle observations. For example, in Table 9–3, which shows the high-density lipoprotein (HDL) cholesterol values for 26 persons, the two middle observations are the 13th and 14th observations. The corresponding values for these are 57 and 58 mg/dL, so the median is 57.5 mg/dL.

The median HDL value is also called the 50th percentile observation, because 50% of the observations lie below it. Percentiles are frequently used in medicine to describe normal growth standards for children. They are also used to describe the LD_{50} for experimental animals, defined as the dose of an agent, such as a drug, which is lethal for 50% of the animals that are exposed to it. The median length of survival is more useful than the mean (average) length of survival, because it is not strongly influenced by a small number of study subjects with unusually short or unusually long survival periods. Therefore, the median gives a better sense of the survival of most study sub-

TABLE 9–3 **Raw Data and Results of Calculations in a Study Concerning Serum Levels of High-Density Lipoprotein (HDL) Cholesterol in 26 Subjects**

Parameter	Raw Data or Results of Calculation
Number of observations, or N	26
Initial HDL cholesterol values of the subjects	31, 41, 44, 46, 47, 47, 48, 48, 49, 52, 53, 54, 57, 58, 58, 60, 60, 62, 63, 64, 67, 69, 70, 77, 81, and 90 mg/dL
Highest value	90 mg/dL
Lowest value	31 mg/dL
Mode	47, 48, 58, and 60 mg/dL
Median	$(57 + 58)/2 = 57.5$ mg/dL
Sum of the values, or sum of x_i	1,496 mg/dL
Mean, or $\bar{x}$	$1,496/26 = 57.5$ mg/dL
Range	$90 - 31 = 59$ mg/dL
Interquartile range	$64 - 48 = 16$ mg/dL
Sum of $(x_i - \bar{x})^2$, or TSS	4,298.46 mg/dL squared*
Variance, or s^2	171.94 mg/dL†
Standard deviation, or s	$\sqrt{171.94} = 13.1$ mg/dL

*For a discussion and example of how statisticians measure the total sum of the squares (TSS), see Box 9–3.
†Here, the following formula is used:

$$\text{Variance} = s^2 = \frac{\sum(x_i^2) - \left[\frac{(\sum x_i)^2}{N}\right]}{N-1} = \frac{90,376 - \frac{2,238,016}{26}}{26-1}$$

$$= \frac{90,376 - 86,077.54}{25} = \frac{4,298.46}{25} = 171.94$$

jects. The median is seldom used to make complicated inferences from medical data, however, because it does not lend itself to the development of advanced statistics.

(3) Mean. The mean is the average value, or the sum (Σ) of all of the observed values (x_i) divided by the total number of observations (N):

$$\text{Mean} = \bar{x} = \frac{\sum(x_i)}{N}$$

Here, the subscript letter i means "for each individual observation." The mean ($\bar{x}$) has both practical and theoretical advantages as a measure of central tendency. It is simple to calculate, and the sum of the deviations of observations from the mean (expressed in terms of negative and positive numbers) should equal 0, which provides a simple check of the calculations. As listed in Box 9–1, the mean also has mathematical properties that enable the development of advanced statistics. Most descriptive analyses of continuous variables and even advanced statistical analyses use the mean as the measure of central tendency. Table 9–3 gives an example of the calculation of the mean.

Measures of Dispersion. After the central tendency of a frequency distribution is determined, the next step is to determine how spread out (dispersed) the numbers are. This can be done by calculating measures based on percentiles or measures based on the mean.

(1) Measures of dispersion based on percentiles. Percentiles, which are sometimes called **quantiles,** are the percentage of observations below the point indicated when all of the observations are ranked in descending order. The median, discussed above, is the 50th percentile. The 75th percentile is the point below which 75% of the observations lie, while the 25th percentile is the point below which 25% of the observations lie.

In Table 9–3, the **overall range** of HDL cholesterol values is 59 mg/dL, reflecting the distance between the highest value (90 mg/dL) and the lowest value (31 mg/dL) in the data set. In the same table, the 75th and 25th percentiles are 64 mg/dL and 48 mg/dL, respectively, and the distance between them is 16 mg/dL. This distance is called the **interquartile range** (sometimes abbreviated Q3 – Q1). Because of central clumping, the interquartile range is usually considerably smaller than half the size of the overall range of values.

The advantage of using percentiles is that they can be applied to any set of continuous data, even if the data do not form any known distribution. Percentiles are often used to describe the results of educational testing and to set ranges for growth standards for infants and children. Because few statistical tests of inference have been developed for use with medians and other percentiles, their use in medicine is mostly limited to description, but in this role, percentiles are often useful clinically.

(2) Measures of dispersion based on the mean. Mean deviation, variance, and standard deviation are three measures of dispersion based on the mean. Although mean deviation is seldom used, a discussion of it will provide a better understanding of the concept of dispersion.

(a) Mean deviation. Because the mean has many advantages, it might seem logical to measure dispersion by taking the "average deviation" from the mean. That proves to be useless, because the sum of the

---

BOX 9–1 Properties of the Mean

(1) The mean of a sample is an *unbiased estimator* of the mean of the population from which it came.
(2) The mean is the *mathematical expectation.* As such, it is different from the mode, which is the value observed most often.
(3) The sum of the squared deviations of the observations from the mean is *smaller* than the sum of the squared deviations from any other number.
(4) The sum of the squared deviations from the mean is *fixed* for a given set of observations. This property is not unique to the mean, but it is a necessary property of any good measure of central tendency.

deviations from the mean is 0. However, this inconvenience can easily be solved by computing the mean deviation, which is the average of the absolute value of the deviations from the mean, as shown in the following formula:

$$\text{Mean deviation} = \frac{\sum(|x_i - \bar{x}|)}{N}$$

Because the mean deviation does not have mathematical properties that enable many statistical tests to be based on it, the formula has not come into popular use. Instead, the variance has become the fundamental measure of dispersion in statistics that are based on the normal distribution.

(b) Variance. The variance for a set of observed data is the sum of the squared deviations from the mean, divided by the number of observations minus 1:

$$\text{Variance} = s^2 = \frac{\sum(x_i - \bar{x})^2}{N - 1}$$

The symbol for a variance calculated from observed data, or a sample variance, is s^2. In the above formula, the squaring solves the problem that the deviations from the mean add up to 0. Dividing by $N - 1$ (called the **degrees of freedom** and discussed in Chapter 10), instead of dividing by N, is necessary for the sample variance to be an unbiased estimator of the population variance.

The numerator of the variance (i.e., the sum of the squared deviations of the observations from the mean) is an extremely important entity in statistics. It is usually called either the **sum of squares** (abbreviated SS) or the **total sum of squares** (TSS). The TSS measures the total amount of variation in a set of observations. Box 9–2 lists the mathematical properties of variance that permit the development of statistical tests, and Box 9–3 explains how statisticians measure variation. Understanding what the concept of variation means in statistics will make much of the following discussion easier to grasp. Therefore, readers may wish to refer to these boxes now.

For simplicity of calculation, there is another (but algebraically equivalent) formula used to calculate the variance. It is the sum of the squared value of each observation, minus a correction factor (to correct for the fact that it is the absolute values, rather than the deviations from the mean, which are being squared), all divided by $N - 1$:

$$\text{Variance} = s^2 = \frac{\sum(x_i^2) - \left[\dfrac{(\sum x_i)^2}{N}\right]}{N - 1}$$

Table 9–3 illustrates the calculation of a variance using this second formula.

(c) Standard deviation. The variance tends to be a large and unwieldy number, and its value falls outside the range of observed values in a data set. Therefore, the standard deviation, which is the square root

---

BOX 9–2   **Properties of the Variance**
(1) When the denominator of the equation for variance is expressed as the number of observations minus 1 ($N - 1$), the variance of a random sample is an *unbiased estimator* of the variance of the population from which it was taken.
(2) The variance of the sum of two independently sampled variables is equal to the *sum* of the variances.
(3) The variance of the difference between two independently sampled variables is equal to the *sum* of their individual variances as well. (The importance of this will become clear when the *t*-test is considered in Chapter 10.)

of the variance, can be used to describe the amount of spread in the frequency distribution. The symbol for the standard deviation of an observed data set is s, and the formula is as follows:

$$\text{Standard deviation} = s = \sqrt{\frac{\sum(x_i - \bar{x})^2}{N - 1}}$$

In an observed data set, the term $\bar{x} \pm s$ represents 1 standard deviation above and below the mean, and the term $\bar{x} \pm 2s$ represents 2 standard deviations above and below the mean. One standard deviation falls well within the range of observed numbers in the data set and has a known relationship to the normal (gaussian) distribution, which is given in a table of the z distribution (see Appendix). This relationship often is useful in drawing inferences in statistics.

In a theoretical normal (gaussian) distribution, as shown in Fig. 9–6, the area under the curve represents all of the observations in the distribution. One standard deviation above and below the mean, represented in Fig. 9–6 by the distance from point A to point B, is equivalent to 68% of the area under the curve, and therefore 68% of the observations in a normal distribution fall within this range. Two standard deviations above and below the mean are equivalent to 95.4% of the area (i.e., 95.4% of the observations) in a normal distribution. Exactly 95.0% of the observations from a normal frequency distribution lie between 1.96 standard deviations below the mean and 1.96 standard deviations above the mean. The formula $\bar{x} \pm 1.96$ standard deviations is often used in medicine to show the extent of variation in clinical data.

Problems in Analyzing a Frequency Distribution

In a normal (gaussian) distribution, the following holds true: mean = median = mode. In an observed data set, there may be skewness, kurtosis, and extreme values, in which case the measures of central tendency may not follow this pattern.

Skewness and Kurtosis. A horizontal stretching of a frequency distribution to one side or the other, so

BOX 9–3 How Do Statisticians Measure Variation?

In statistics, variation is measured as the sum of the squared deviations of the individual observations from an expected value, such as the mean. The mean is the mathematical expectation or expected value of a continuous frequency distribution. The quantity of variation in a given set of observations, therefore, is simply the numerator of the variance, which is the sum of the squares. The sum of the squares (SS) of a dependent variable is sometimes called the total sum of the squares (TSS), which is the total amount of variation that needs to be explained.

For purposes of illustration, assume that the data set consists of the following six numbers: 1, 2, 4, 7, 10, and 12. Assume that x_i denotes the individual observations, $\bar{x}$ is the mean, N is the number of observations, s^2 is the variance, and s is the standard deviation.

Part 1 Tabular representation of the data

	x_i	$(x_i - \bar{x})$	$(x_i - \bar{x})^2$
	1	−5	25
	2	−4	16
	4	−2	4
	7	+1	1
	10	+4	16
	12	+6	36
Sum, or Σ	36	0	98

Part 2 Graphic representation of the data shown in the third column of the above table—that is, $(x_i - \bar{x})^2$ for each of the six observations

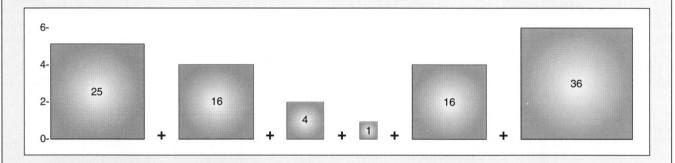

Part 3 Calculation of numbers that describe a distribution

$$\Sigma(x_i) = 36 \qquad \Sigma(x_i - \bar{x})^2 = \text{TSS} = 98$$

$$N = 6 \qquad s^2 = \text{TSS}/(N-1) = 98/5 = 19.6$$

$$\bar{x} = 6 \qquad s = \sqrt{19.6} = 4.43$$

that one tail of observations is longer and has more observations than the other tail, is called **skewness.** When a histogram or frequency polygon has a longer tail on the left side of the diagram, as in Fig. 9–7, the distribution is said to be skewed to the left. If a distribution is skewed, the mean moves farther in the direction of the long tail than does the median, because the mean is more heavily influenced by extreme values. A quick way to get an approximate idea of whether or not a frequency distribution is skewed is to compare the mean and the median. If these two measures are close to each other, the distribution is probably not skewed. For example, in the data from Table 9–2, the mean equals 179.1 mg/dL and the median equals 178 mg/dL. These two values are very

close, and as can be seen from Fig. 9–4, the distribution is not skewed very much either.

Kurtosis is characterized by a vertical stretching of the frequency distribution. As shown in Fig. 9–8, a kurtotic distribution could look more peaked or could look more flattened than the bell-shaped normal distribution.

Significant skewness or kurtosis can be detected by statistical tests that reveal that the observed data do not form a normal distribution. Many statistical tests require that the data they analyze be normally distributed, and the tests may not be valid if they are used to compare very abnormal distributions. On the other hand, the statistical tests discussed in this book are relatively robust, meaning

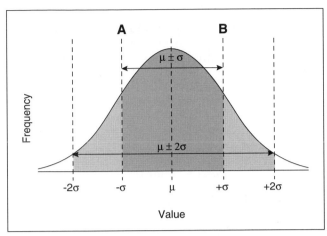

FIGURE 9–6 Theoretical normal (gaussian) distribution showing where 1 and 2 standard deviations above and below the mean would fall. The Greek letter mu (μ) stands for the mean in the theoretical distribution, and the Greek letter sigma (σ) stands for the standard deviation in the theoretical population. (The italic Roman letters $\bar{x}$ and s apply to an observed [sample] population.) In this figure, the area under the curve represents all of the observations in the distribution. One standard deviation above and below the mean, shown in dark orange and represented by the distance from point A to point B, is equivalent to 68% of the area under the curve, and therefore 68% of the observations in a normal distribution fall within this range. Two standard deviations above and below the mean, represented by the areas shown in dark and light orange, are equivalent to 95.4% of the area of the curve or 95.4% of the observations in a normal distribution.

that as long as the data are not too badly skewed or kurtotic, the results can be considered valid. Kurtosis is seldom discussed as a problem in the medical literature, although skewness is frequently observed and is treated as a problem.

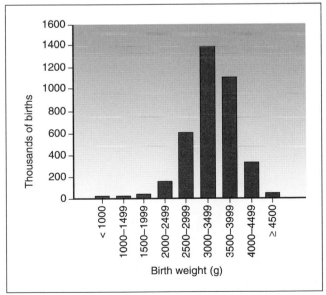

FIGURE 9–7 Histogram showing a skewed frequency distribution. Values are for thousands of births by birth weight group, USA, 1987. Note the long tail on the left. (Source of data: National Center for Health Statistics. Trends in Low Birth Weight: United States, 1975–85. Series 21, No. 48. Washington, D.C., Government Printing Office, 1989.)

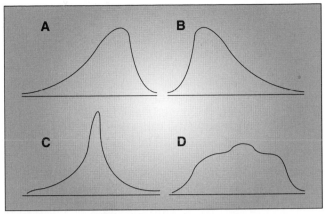

FIGURE 9–8 Examples of skewed and kurtotic frequency distributions. Distribution A is skewed to the left; distribution B is skewed to the right; distribution C is kurtotic, with abnormal peaking; and distribution D is kurtotic, with abnormal flattening in comparison to the normal distribution.

Extreme Values (Outliers). One of the most perplexing problems for the analysis of data is how to treat a value that is abnormally far above or below the mean. This problem is suggested in the data set of cholesterol values shown in Table 9–2 and Fig. 9–2. The standard deviation of the distribution in the data set is 28.2 mg/dL, so that if the distribution were normal, 95% of the cholesterol values would be expected to be between 123.8 mg/dL and 234.4 mg/dL—i.e., the mean plus or minus 1.96 standard deviations = 179.1 mg/dL plus or minus the product of 1.96 × 28.2. Moreover, 99% of the values would be expected to be found within the range of the mean plus or minus 2.58 standard deviations, which in this case would be between 106.3 mg/dL and 251.9 mg/dL.

When the data are observed visually in Fig. 9–2, everything looks normal below the mean; the lowest value is 124 mg/dL, which is within the 95% limits. The upper value, however, is 264 mg/dL, which is beyond the 99% limits of expectation and looks suspiciously far from the other values. Because many people have total cholesterol values this high and because the observation is almost within the 99% limits, there is probably no reason to be concerned that the value is erroneous (although there might be a reason to be clinically concerned with such a high cholesterol value in a young person). However, before analyzing the data set, the investigator would want to be sure that this item of data was legitimate and would check the original source of data. In this case, although the value is an outlier, it is what the laboratory reported and is probably correct.

Methods of Depicting a Frequency Distribution

In the medical literature, **histograms** and **line graphs** are commonly used to illustrate frequency distributions. These were introduced earlier in the chapter, along with **frequency polygons.** Among the other methods of visually displaying data are stem and leaf diagrams, quantiles, and boxplots—all of which are printed out by computer programs such as the Statistical Analysis System (SAS). Examples of these are shown in Fig. 9–9. In each example, the HDL cholesterol values for 26 young adults, as given in Table 9–3, are plotted.

Stem and Leaf Diagrams. As shown in Fig. 9–9, the stem and leaf diagram has three components. The **stem,** which is the vertical column of numbers on the left, represents the value of the left-hand digit (in this case, the 10s digit). The **leaf** is the set of numbers immediately to the right of the stem and is sometimes separated from the stem by a vertical line. Each of the numbers in the leaf represents the next digit in one of the 26 observations in the data set of HDL cholesterol values. Thus, the stem and leaf value shown on the top line of the diagram represents 90 mg/dL. The # **symbol** to the right of the leaf tells how many observations were seen in the range indicated (in this case, 1 observation of 90 mg/dL or greater).

Among the observations that can quickly be made from viewing the stem and leaf diagram in Fig. 9–9 are the following: (1) The highest value in the data set was 90 mg/dL. (2) The lowest value was 31 mg/dL. (3) There were 8 observations in the range of the 40s, consisting of 41, 44, 46, 47, 47, 48, 48, 49. (4) When the diagram is viewed with the left side turned to the bottom, the distribution looks fairly normal, although it has a long tail to the left (that is, it is skewed to the left).

Quantiles. Below the stem and leaf diagram in Fig. 9–9 is a display of the quantiles (percentiles). Among the data included are the maximum (100% of the values were at this level or below) and minimum (0% of the values were below this); the 99%, 95%, 90%, 10%, 5%, and 1% values; the range; the mode; and the interquartile range (from the 25th percentile to the 75th percentile, abbreviated Q3 – Q1).

Boxplots. The modified boxplot is shown to the right of the stem and leaf diagram in Fig. 9–9 and provides an even briefer way of summarizing the data. In the boxplot, the rectangle formed by four plus signs (+) and the horizontal dashes (----) depicts the interquartile range. The two asterisks (*) connected by dashes depict the median. The mean, shown by the smaller plus sign (+), is very close to the median. Outside of the rectangle, there are two vertical lines, called the "whiskers" of the boxplot. The whiskers extend 1.5 times the interquartile range above the 75th percentile and 1.5 times the interquartile range below the 25th percentile (but not below 0). They show the range where most of the values would be expected, given the median and interquartile range of the distribution. In Fig. 9–9, all of the observed data values except the value of 90 mg/dL might reasonably have been expected; this value, however, is considered an outlier observation, which status is indicated by the 0 near the top, just above the top of the upper whisker. Thus, it takes only a quick look at the boxplot to see how wide the distribution is, whether or not it is skewed, where the interquartile range falls, how close the median is to the mean, and how many (if any) observations might reasonably be considered outliers.

Use of Unit-Free (Normalized) Data

Data from a normal (gaussian) frequency distribution can be described completely by the **mean** and the **standard deviation.** However, even the same set of data will provide a different value for the mean and standard deviation depending on the choice of **units of measurement.** For example, the same person's height may be expressed as 66 inches or 167.6 cm, and an infant's birth weight may be recorded as 2500 g or 5.5 pounds. Here, the units of measurement

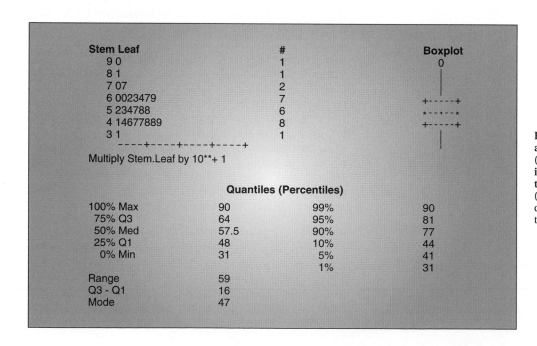

FIGURE 9–9 Stem and leaf diagram, boxplot, and quantiles (percentiles) for the data shown in Table 9–3, as printed out by the Statistical Analysis System (SAS). See the text for a detailed description of how to interpret the data shown here.

differ, even though the true height and weight are the same. To eliminate the effects produced by the choice of units, the data can be put into a unit-free form (normalized).

The first step in normalizing data is to calculate the mean and standard deviation. The second step is to set the mean equal to 0 by subtracting the mean from each observation in whatever units have been used. The third step is to measure each observation in terms of the number of standard deviations it is above or below the mean. As long as the same units are used to calculate the mean and the standard deviation, the same value (in terms of standard deviations) will be obtained for each observation, regardless of which unit of measurement was initially used. The normalized values obtained by this process are called z values, and the formula for creating individual z values (z_i) is as follows:

$$z_i = \frac{x_i - \bar{x}}{s}$$

where x_i represents individual observations, $\bar{x}$ represents the mean of the observations, and s is the standard deviation.

Suppose, for example, that the goal is to standardize blood pressure values for a group of patients whose systolic blood pressures were observed to have a mean of 120 mm Hg and a standard deviation of 10 mm Hg. If two of the values to be standardized were 140 mm Hg and 115 mm Hg, the calculations would be as follows:

$$\frac{140 - 120}{10} = +2.0 \qquad \frac{115 - 120}{10} = -0.5$$

A distribution of z values always has a mean of 0 and a standard deviation of 1. The z values here are called by various names, often **standard normal deviates.**

Clinically, z values are useful for determining how extreme an observed test result is. For example, in Table 9–2, the highest total cholesterol value observed among 71 persons was 264 mg/dL, 23 points higher than the next highest value. Is this cholesterol value suspect? When the formula above is used, the z value is $(264 - 179.1)/28.2 = +3.0$. This means that it is 3 standard deviations above the mean. Usually, about 1% of observed values are 2.58 standard deviations or more away from the mean, and this is the only one of the 71 observed values this far away; therefore, there is no strong reason to suppose it is an error.

Frequency Distributions of Dichotomous Data and Proportions

Dichotomous data can be thought of in terms of flipping a coin. If the coin is flipped in an unbiased manner, on the average it would be expected to land with the heads side up in half of the flips and with the tails side up in half of the flips, so the probability of heads would equal 0.5 and the probability of tails would

equal 0.5. The sum of all of the probabilities for all of the possible outcomes must equal 1.0. If a coin is flipped 10 times, the result would very rarely be 10 heads or 10 tails, would somewhat less rarely be a combination of 9 heads plus 1 tail, and would most frequently be a combination of 5 heads and 5 tails.

The probabilities of getting various combinations of heads and tails from flipping a coin can be calculated by **expanding the binomial formula,** $(a + b)^n$, as shown in Box 9–4. In this formula, a is the probability of heads, b is the probability of tails, and n is the number of coin tosses in a trial.

If n is large (say, hundreds of tosses of the coin) and if the coin is thrown in an unbiased manner, the distribution of the binomial toss would look much like a normal (gaussian) distribution. In fact, if n were infinite, a were 0.5, and b were 0.5, then the **binomial distribution** would be *identical* to the normal distribution. Therefore, a mean and standard deviation can be calculated for the binomial distribution.

If the probability of heads does not equal 0.5, the binomial distribution would look like a skewed distribution, and the previously mentioned cautions concerning statistical analysis would apply (see Problems in Analyzing a Frequency Distribution, above).

Because of the close relationship between the binomial and the normal distributions, binary data expressed as **proportions** can be analyzed using theory based on the normal distribution.

Frequency Distributions of Other Types of Data

Data from nominal (categorical) and ordinal (ranked) variables are not properly analyzed using theory and tests based on the normal (gaussian) distribution. These data should be analyzed using statistical methods that do not make any assumptions about an underlying frequency distribution. Because they are not based on either the normal or binomial distribution (for which parameters such as means and standard deviations can be calculated), statistical tests for nominal and ordinal variables are called **nonparametric tests.**

Of particular importance, the analysis of the counts in frequency tables (such as Table 9–1) depends on a different distribution, which is known as the chi-square distribution and is discussed in Chapter 11. The chi-square analysis, however, does not require that the data themselves follow any particular distribution, so it is a nonparametric test.

Ordinal data are sometimes analyzed in the medical literature as though they were continuous data, and means and standard deviations are reported. This is usually satisfactory for describing ordinal data, but it is generally not appropriate for significance testing. The preferred tests are discussed in Chapter 11 and include the Wilcoxon test, the Mann-Whitney U test, and other tests for ordinal data. These tests do not require that the data follow any particular distribution; they require only that the data be ordinal.

BOX 9–4   How to Determine Probabilities by Expanding the Binomial

The basic binomial formula is $(a + b)^n$. The probabilities of getting various combinations of heads and tails from flipping a coin can be calculated by expanding this formula. Although the example of head/tails is used here, the formula and concepts that are described can also be applied to the probabilities of life/death associated with particular diagnoses, success/failure in treatment, and other clinically relevant dichotomous data.

When the binomial formula is applied to flipping a coin in an unbiased manner, a is the probability of obtaining heads, b is the probability of obtaining tails, and n is the number of trials (coin tosses). The process of calculating the probabilities is called **expanding the binomial,** and the distribution of probabilities for each combination is the **binomial distribution.**

With one flip of the coin, there is a 0.5 (50%) chance of heads and a 0.5 (50%) chance of tails, with the sum of 1.0.

Two flips of the coin could produce the following outcomes: two heads; one head and one tail (in either the head/tail or tail/head order); or two tails. What are the probabilities of these possible outcomes? The answer is given by the above formula, with $n = 2$. It is $(a + b)$ times itself:

$$(a + b)^2 = a^2 + 2ab + b^2$$
$$= (0.5)(0.5) + (2)(0.5)(0.5) + (0.5)(0.5)$$
$$= 0.25 + 0.50 + 0.25$$

In other words, with two flips of a coin, the probabilities of the various possible outcomes are:

Two heads = 0.25
One head and one tail (in either order) = 0.25 + 0.25 = 0.50
Two tails = 0.25
The sum of the probabilities = 1.0

Three flips of a coin could produce the following outcomes: three heads; two heads and one tail; two tails and one head; or three tails. The probabilities, calculated by using the formula $(a + b)^3$, are:

Three heads = $a^3 = (0.5)^3 = 0.125$
Two heads and one tail = $3(a^2)(b) = (3)(0.25)(0.5) = 0.375$
One head and two tails = $3(a)(b^2) = (3)(0.5)(0.25) = 0.375$
Three tails = $b^3 = (0.5)^3 = 0.125$
The sum of the probabilities = 1.0

If a biased coin (say, $a = 0.4$ and $b = 0.6$) were tossed three times, the probabilities would be

Three heads = $a^3 = (0.4)^3 = 0.064$
Two heads and one tail = $3(a^2)(b) = (3)(0.16)(0.6) = 0.288$
One head and two tails = $3(a)(b^2) = (3)(0.4)(0.36) = 0.432$
Three tails = $b^3 = (0.6)^3 = 0.216$
The sum of the probabilities = 1.0

Note that the coefficients for expanding $(a + b)^n$ can be easily found using Pascal's triangle, in which each coefficient is the sum of the two above.

n Equals	Coefficients	Examples
1	1 1	$1a + 1b$
2	1 2 1	$1a^2 + 2ab + 1b^2$
3	1 3 3 1	$1a^3 + 3(a^2)(b) + 3(a)(b^2) + 1b^3$
4	1 4 6 4 1	$1a^4 + 4(a^3)(b) + 6(a^2)(b^2) + 4(a)(b^3) + 1b^4$
etc.	etc.	etc.

If the probabilities from tossing an unbiased coin are plotted as histograms, as the number of coin tosses becomes greater, the probabilities look more and more like a normal (gaussian) distribution.

■ SUMMARY

While variation in clinical medicine may be due to biologic differences or the presence or absence of disease, it may also be due to differences in measurement techniques and conditions, errors in measurement, and random variation. Statistics is an aid to describing and understanding the variation and minimizing errors.

Statistical analysis cannot correct for bias (see Chapter 4), and the analysis can only "adjust" for random error in the sense that it can estimate how much of the total variation is due to random error and how much is due to a particular factor being investigated.

Fundamental to any analysis of data is understanding the types of variables or data (including nominal, dichotomous, ordinal, continuous, and ratio data) as well as risks, rates, and proportions.

Continuous (measurement) data have a frequency distribution that can be described in terms of two types of parameters: the measures of central tendency (of which median and mean are the most important) and the measures of dispersion based on the mean (of which variance and standard deviation are the most important). The most common distribution is called the normal (gaussian) distribution and has the shape of a bell when viewed from the side.

In a normal distribution, the mean and the median coincide, and 95% of the observations are within 1.96 standard deviations above and below the mean. Frequently, the normal distribution appears pulled to one side or the other (appears to have a long tail), in which case it is called a skewed distribution. In a skewed distribution, the mean is farther in the direction of the long tail than is the median.

Data may be made unit-free by creating z values, in which the mean is subtracted from each value and the result is divided by the standard deviation. This expresses the value of each observation as the number of standard deviations it is above or below the mean.

The probability distribution for dichotomous data may be described by the binomial distribution. If the probability of success and failure are the same (i.e., 0.5 each) and if the number of trials is very large, the binomial distribution is identical to the normal distribution.

When an approximately normal (gaussian) distribution cannot be assumed, a separate group of statistics, called nonparametric statistics, can be used to study differences and associations between variables. These are discussed in Chapter 11.

■ QUESTIONS

Directions (Items 1–8). Each of the numbered items or incomplete statements in this section is followed by answers or by completions of the statement. Select the ONE lettered answer or completion that is BEST in each case. Correct answers and explanations are given at the end of the chapter.

1. A 62-year-old man is rushed to the emergency department by ambulance during an episode of chest pain. The initial evaluation is performed by a triage nurse, who reports to the emergency department attending physician that the patient's pain is probably angina and seems to be severe. This characterization is

    (A) dichotomous
    (B) nominal
    (C) ordinal
    (D) parametric
    (E) qualitative

2. When the patient described above is asked to evaluate his pain on a scale of 0 (no pain) to 10 (the worst pain), he reports to the evaluating physician that his pain is an 8. After the administration of sublingual nitroglycerin and high-flow oxygen, the patient reports that the pain is now a 4 on the same scale. After the administration of morphine sulfate, given as an intravenous push, the pain is gone. This commonly applied scale is a

    (A) continuous scale
    (B) dichotomous scale
    (C) nominal scale
    (D) ordinal scale
    (E) ratio scale

Items 3–8

Ten volunteers are weighed in a consistent manner before and after they have been consuming an experimental diet for 6 weeks. This diet consists of apple strudel, tomatilla salsa, and gummy bears. (N.B. Don't try this at home!) The weights are shown in the accompanying table.

Volunteer	Weight Before Diet (kg)	Weight After Diet (kg)
1	81	79
2	79	87
3	92	90
4	112	110
5	76	74
6	126	124
7	80	78
8	75	73
9	68	76
10	78	76

3. The mean weight before the intervention is

    (A) 76.8
    (B) 79
    (C) 80
    (D) 86.7
    (E) 91

4. The median weight after the intervention is

    (A) 71.8
    (B) 78.5
    (C) 81.7
    (D) 86.7
    (E) 89

5. The mode of the weights after the intervention is

    (A) 76
    (B) 78.5
    (C) 80
    (D) 86
    (E) 100

6. The standard deviation of the weights before the intervention is

    (A) 6.1
    (B) 18.3
    (C) 75.7
    (D) 330
    (E) 3026

7. To determine whether this diet is effective in promoting weight loss, you intend to perform a statistical test of significance on the differences in weights before and after the intervention. Unfortunately, you do not know how to do this until you get through Chapter 10. What you *do* know now is that, in order to use a parametric test of significance,

    (A)   the data in both data sets must be normally distributed

    (B)   the data must not be skewed

    (C)   the distribution of weight in the underlying population must be normal (gaussian)

    (D)   the means for the two data sets must be equal

    (E)   the variances for the two data sets must be equal

8. To determine whether this diet is effective in promoting weight loss, a statistical approach should

    (A)   avoid assumptions about parameters of the frequency distribution

    (B)   compensate for random error

    (C)   compensate for selection bias

    (D)   minimize variation due to factors other than the intervention

    (E)   produce a binary outcome variable

■ ANSWERS AND EXPLANATIONS

1. **The answer is E: qualitative.** A great deal of clinical information is purely descriptive and not specifically quantifiable. Such information is qualitative data. Magnitude is implied by the descriptive modifiers applied to qualitative data, such as "severe" in this case. While everyone may readily agree that "severe" is of greater magnitude than "mild," the actual measure of the discrepancy is subjective. Qualitative data need not be free of implied magnitude but are, by definition, devoid of any objective scale of measurement.

2. **The answer is E: ratio scale.** The scale described uses ratio data. A ratio scale is defined by a continuous variable and a true 0 point. The pain scale has a true 0, indicating the absence of pain. A score of 8 on the scale implies that the pain is twice as severe as pain having a score of 4. Of course, there is a subjective component to all human experience, even when a quantitative system is used in its description. One person's 4 on this scale is likely to be another's 7. While the exact meaning of "twice as much pain" may be unclear, it is also generally of little importance. For the practitioner attempting to alleviate a patient's pain, this scale provides the essential information—i.e., information about whether the pain is increasing or decreasing and by relatively how much.

3. **The answer is D: 86.7.** The mean is the sum of all of the observed values in a data set, divided by the number of observations. The sum of the 10 observed values (i.e., weights prior to the intervention) is 867. Dividing this figure by 10 (the number of observations) yields 86.7.

4. **The answer is B: 78.5.** The median is the middle observed value in a data set after the data have been arranged in ascending or descending order. The data provided here can be rewritten as 73, 74, 76, 76, 78, 79, 87, 90, 110, and 124. In a set of 10 observed values, the median is the average of the fifth and sixth data points. In this case, it is 78 (the fifth data point) plus 79 (the sixth data point) divided by 2, which is 78.5.

5. **The answer is A: 76.** The mode is the most frequently occurring value in a set of data. The value 76 occurs twice in this set, so it is the mode. The mode can occur anywhere in the range represented by a set of data. If more than one value in a data set occurs repeatedly with equal frequency, the set may have more than one mode.

6. **The answer is B: 18.3.** The standard deviation is the square root of the variance. The variance is $\Sigma(x_i - \bar{x})^2$ divided by the degrees of freedom, or $N - 1$. The mean is subtracted from the first observation, and the difference is squared. This is repeated for each observation in the set, and the values obtained are all added together. For this set of data, the result is 3026.1. This figure is divided by $N - 1$, or 9, to yield the variance, which is 336.2. The square root of 336.2 is 18.3.

7. **The answer is C: the distribution of weight in the underlying population must be normal (gaussian).** All so-called parametric tests of significance rely on assumptions about the parameters that define a frequency distribution—namely, the mean and the standard deviation. To employ parametric methods of statistical analysis, the data being analyzed need not be normally distributed, but the means of repeated samples from the underlying population from which the samples are drawn must be. Neither the means nor the variances of two data sets under comparison need to be equal to support the use of parametric methods. In this case, to employ a parametric test of significance, one needs to assume that the distribution of weight in the general population is normal. This assumption is reasonable.

8. **The answer is D: minimize variation due to factors other than the intervention.** There are many sources of variation in clinical data. The goal of statistical analysis in medical research is generally to measure the effect of a particular intervention. The effect of the intervention must therefore be isolated from other sources of varia-

tion in the data. For example, subjects may gain or lose weight for reasons having nothing to do with the particular diet under investigation. A statistical approach should be taken to minimize variation due to factors other than the intervention of interest. For this study, the optimal method of analysis would be to compare each subject with himself or herself, thereby eliminating a great deal of intersubject variability (see Chapter 10). Random error should be minimized by meticulous study design, because once this type of error is introduced, it cannot be corrected by statistical methods. An example of random error in this study would be inaccuracies in the measurement of weight. Selection bias (see Chapters 4 and 12) also cannot be corrected by statistical methods. Selection bias is introduced whenever the subjects in a study differ in some important way from the larger population that they are meant to represent; this compromises the study's external validity. Selection bias is also introduced if a nonrandom method of allocating subjects to study groups causes the groups to differ from each other; this compromises the study's internal validity. Assumptions about the parameters of the underlying frequency distribution—for example, the assumption that weight is normally distributed in the general population—are essential to the use of parametric methods, as discussed in the explanation of item 7 (see above). Although it is useful at times to convert a continuous variable into a binary variable, there is no advantage in it here, and considerable information would be lost.

References Cited

Buehler, J. W., et al. Birth weight–specific infant mortality, United States, 1960 and 1980. Public Health Reports 102:151–161, 1987.

Elmore, J. G., et al. Variability in radiologists' interpretations of mammograms. New England Journal of Medicine 331:1493–1499, 1994.

Selected Reading

Dawson-Saunders, B., and R. G. Trapp. Basic and Clinical Biostatistics, 2nd ed. Norwalk, Conn., Appleton and Lange, 1994.

10 Statistical Inference and Hypothesis Testing

■ THE NATURE AND PURPOSE OF STATISTICAL INFERENCE

Inference means the drawing of conclusions from data. Statistical inference can be defined as the drawing of conclusions from quantitative or qualitative information using the methods of statistics to describe and arrange the data and to test suitable hypotheses.

Differences Between Deductive Reasoning and Inductive Reasoning

Because data do not come with their own interpretation, the interpretation must be put into the data by **inductive reasoning** (from Latin, meaning "to lead into"). This approach to reasoning is less familiar to most people than is **deductive reasoning** (from Latin,

meaning "to lead out from"), which is learned from mathematics, particularly from geometry.

Deductive reasoning proceeds *from the general* (i.e., from assumptions, from propositions, and from formulas considered true) *to the specific* (i.e., to specific members belonging to the general category). Consider, for example, the following two propositions: (1) All Americans believe in democracy. (2) This person is an American. If both propositions are true, then the following deduction must be true: This person believes in democracy.

Deductive reasoning is of special use in science once hypotheses are formed. Using deductive reasoning, an investigator says, *If* the following hypothesis is true, *then* the following prediction or predictions also should be true. If a prediction can be tested empirically, the hypothesis may be rejected or not rejected on the basis of the findings.

If the data are inconsistent with the predictions from the hypothesis, they force a rejection or modification of the hypothesis. If the data are consistent with the hypothesis, they cannot prove that the hypothesis is true, although they do lend support to the hypothesis. To reiterate, even if the data are consistent with the hypothesis, they do not prove the hypothesis, as was discussed in Chapter 4 and demonstrated with regard to Fig. 4–3.

Physicians often proceed from formulas accepted as true and from observed data to determine the values that variables must have in a certain clinical situation. For example, if the amount of a medication that can be safely given per kilogram of body weight (a constant) is known, then it is simple to calculate how much of that medication can be given to a patient weighing 50 kg. This is deductive reasoning, because it proceeds from the general (a constant and a formula) to the specific (the patient).

Inductive reasoning, in contrast, seeks to find valid generalizations and general principles from data. Statistics, the quantitative aid to inductive reasoning, proceeds *from the specific* (that is, from data) *to the general* (that is, to formulas or conclusions about the data). For example, by sampling a population and determining both the age and the blood pressure of the persons in the sample (the specific data), an investigator using statistical methods can determine the general relationship between age and blood pressure (e.g., that, on the average, blood pressure increases with age).

Differences Between Mathematics and Statistics

The differences between mathematics and statistics can be illustrated by showing that they form the basis for very different approaches to the same basic equation:

$$y = mx + b$$

This equation is the formula for a straight line in analytic geometry. It is also the formula for simple regression analysis in statistics, although the letters used and their order customarily are different.

In the mathematical formula above, the b is a constant, and it stands for the y-intercept (i.e., the value of y when the variable x equals 0). The value m also is a constant, and it stands for the slope (the amount of change in y for a unit increase in the value of x). The important thing to note is that in mathematics, one of the variables (either x or y) is unknown (i.e., to be calculated), while the formula and the constants are known.

In statistics, however, just the reverse is true: the variables, x and y, are known for all observations, and the investigator usually wishes to determine whether or not there is a linear (straight line) relationship between x and y, by estimating the slope and the intercept. This can be done using the form of analysis called linear regression, which is discussed in Chapter 11.

As a general rule, what is known in statistics is unknown in mathematics, and vice versa. In statistics, the investigator starts from specific observations (data) to induce or estimate the general relationships between variables.

■ THE PROCESS OF TESTING HYPOTHESES

Hypotheses are predictions about what the examination of appropriate data will show. The following discussion introduces the basic concepts underlying the usual tests of statistical significance. These tests determine the probability that a finding (such as a difference between means or proportions) represents a true deviation from what was expected (i.e., from the model, which is often a null hypothesis that there will be no difference between the means or proportions). The discussion in this chapter focuses on the justification for and interpretation of the p value, which is designed to minimize false-positive error. False-negative error is discussed more fully in Chapter 12 under sample size.

False-Positive and False-Negative Errors

Science is based on the following set of principles: (1) previous experience serves as the basis for developing hypotheses; (2) hypotheses serve as the basis for developing predictions; (3) and predictions must be subjected to experimental or observational testing. In deciding whether data are consistent or inconsistent with the hypotheses, investigators are subject to two types of error. They could assert that the data support a hypothesis when in fact the hypothesis is false; this would be a **false-positive error,** which is also called an **alpha error** or a **type I error.** Conversely, they could assert that the data do not support the hypothesis when in fact the hypothesis is true; this would be a **false-negative error,** which is also called a **beta error** or a **type II error.**

Based on the knowledge that scientists become attached to their own hypotheses and based on the conviction that the proof in science, as in the courts, must be "beyond a reasonable doubt," investigators have historically been particularly careful to avoid the false-positive error. Probably this is best for theoretical science. In medicine, however, where a false-negative error in a diagnostic test may mean missing a disease until it is too late to institute therapy and where a false-negative error in the study of a medical intervention may mean overlooking an effective treatment, investigators cannot feel comfortable about false-negative errors either.

The Null Hypothesis and the Alternative Hypothesis

The process of significance testing involves three basic steps: (1) asserting the null hypothesis, (2) establishing the alpha level, and (3) rejecting or failing to reject the null hypothesis.

The first step consists of asserting the **null hypothesis,** which is the hypothesis that there is no real (true) difference between means or proportions of the groups being compared or that there is no real association between two continuous variables. For example, the null hypothesis for the data discussed in Chapter 9 and presented in Table 9–1 is that there is no real difference between the percentage of men and the percentage of women who had previously had their serum cholesterol levels checked. It may seem strange to begin the process by asserting that something is not true, but it is far easier to reject an assertion than to prove that something is true. (If the data are not consistent with a hypothesis, the hypothesis can be rejected. If the data are consistent with a hypothesis, this still does not prove the hypothesis, because other hypotheses may fit the data equally well.)

The second step is to determine the probability of being in error if the null hypothesis is rejected. This step requires that the investigator establish an alpha level, as described below.

If the p value is found to be greater than the alpha level, the investigator fails to reject the null hypothesis. If, however, the p value is found to be less than or equal to the alpha level, the next step is to reject the null hypothesis and to accept the **alternative hypothesis,** which is the hypothesis that there is in fact a real difference or association. Although it may seem awkward, this process is now standard in medical science and has yielded considerable scientific benefits.

As an example, consider a hypothetical clinical trial of a drug designed to lower high blood pressure among patients with essential hypertension (hypertension occurring without a discoverable organic cause). One group of patients would receive the experimental drug, and the other group (the control group) would receive a placebo. The null hypothesis might be that following the intervention, the average change in blood pressure in the treatment group will not differ from the average change in blood pressure in the control group. If a test of significance (such as a *t*-test on the average change in systolic blood pressure) forces rejection of the null hypothesis, then the alternative hypothesis—namely, the hypothesis that there was a true difference in the average change in blood pressure in the two groups—will be accepted.

The Alpha Level and *p* Value

Before doing any calculations to test the null hypothesis, the investigator must establish a criterion called the **alpha level,** which is the maximum probability of making a false-positive error that the investigator is willing to accept. By custom, the level of alpha is usually set at $p = 0.05$. This says that the investigator is willing to run a 5% risk (but no more) of being in error when asserting that the treatment and control groups truly differ. In choosing an alpha level, the investigator inserts value judgment into the process. However, when that is done before the data are collected, at least the post hoc bias of being tempted to adjust the alpha level to make the data show statistical significance is avoided.

The ***p*** **value** obtained by a statistical test (such as the *t*-test described later in this chapter) gives the probability that the observed difference could have been obtained by chance alone, given random variation and a single test of the null hypothesis. Usually, if the observed *p* value is ≤ 0.05, members of the scientific community who read about an investigation will accept the difference as being real. Although setting alpha at ≤ 0.05 is somewhat arbitrary, that level has become so customary that it is wise to provide explanations for choosing another alpha level or for choosing not to perform tests of significance at all, which may be the best approach in some descriptive studies.

Once the alpha level is established, the *p* value for the data can be obtained. In this process, the first step is to calculate a critical ratio (such as the *t, z, F,* or chi-square value) from the data, using a statistical test of significance. The second step is to consult a standard table of the possible values of *p* (see the Appendix). If the *p* value determined from the table is less than or equal to the preselected alpha level (in this example, $p \leq 0.05$), the null hypothesis is rejected and the alternative hypothesis is accepted. If the *p* value is greater than the alpha level (in this example, $p > 0.05$), the investigator fails to reject the null hypothesis.

Note that failing to reject the null hypothesis is *not* the same as accepting the null hypothesis as true. Rather, it is similar to a jury's finding that the evidence did not prove the guilt (or in the example here, did not prove the difference) beyond a reasonable doubt. In the USA, a court trial is not designed to prove innocence. The defendant's innocence is assumed and must be disproved beyond a reasonable doubt. Similarly, in statistics, a lack of difference is assumed, and it is up to the statistical analysis to demonstrate that this condition (the null hypothesis) is unlikely. The rationale for using this approach in medical research is similar to the rationale in the courts. While the courts are able to convict the guilty, the goal of exonerating the innocent is a higher priority. In medicine, confirming the benefit of a new treatment is important, but avoiding the use of ineffective therapies is an even higher priority ("first, do no harm").

An everyday analogy may help to simplify the logic of the level of alpha and the process of significance testing. Suppose that a young couple was given instructions to buy a silver bracelet for a friend during a trip if one could be bought for $50 or less. If a suitable bracelet is found, it would be bought only if it could be obtained for $50 or less. Any more would be too high a price to pay. Alpha is like the price limit in the analogy. Once it has been set (say, at $p \leq 0.05$, as opposed to $\leq$ $50), an investigator would "buy" the alternative hypothesis of a true difference or association if the cost (in terms of the probability of being wrong) were no greater than 1 in 20 (0.05). The alpha, therefore, is the price that an investigator is willing to pay in the probability of being wrong if he or she rejects the null hypothesis.

Variation in Individual Observations and in Multiple Samples

Most tests of significance relate to a difference between means or proportions. They help investigators decide whether an observed difference is real, which in statistical terms is defined as whether the difference is greater than would be expected by chance alone. In the example of the experimental drug to lower blood pressure in hypertensive patients, the experimenters would measure the blood pressures of the study subjects under experimental conditions both before and after the new drug or placebo is given. They would determine the average change seen in the treatment group and the average change seen in the control group and then pursue tests to determine whether the difference was large enough to be unlikely to have occurred by chance alone. Therefore, the fundamental process in this test of significance would be to see if the mean blood pressure changes in the two study groups were different from each other.

Why not just inspect the means to see if they were different? This is inadequate because it is not known whether the observed difference was unusual or whether a difference that large might have been found frequently if the experiment were repeated. Although the investigators examine the findings in particular patients, their real interest is determining whether the findings of the study could be generalized to other, similar hypertensive patients. To generalize beyond the particular subjects in the single study, the investigators must know the extent to which the differences discovered in the study are reliable. The estimate of reliability is given by the standard error, which is not the same as the standard deviation discussed in Chapter 9.

Standard Deviation and Standard Error

Chapter 9 focused on individual observations and the extent to which they differed from the mean. One of the assertions discussed in the chapter was that a normal (gaussian) distribution could be completely described by its mean and **standard deviation.** Fig. 9–6 demonstrated that 68% of observations fall within the range described as the mean plus or minus 1 standard deviation, 95.4% fall within the range of the mean plus or minus 2 standard deviations, and 95% fall within the range of the mean plus or minus 1.96 standard deviations. This information is useful in describing individual observations (raw data), but it is not useful in determining how close a sample mean from research data is to the mean for the underlying population (which is also called the true mean or the population mean). This determination must be made on the basis of the standard error.

The **standard error** is related to the standard deviation, but it differs from the standard deviation in important ways. Basically, the standard error is the standard deviation of a population of sample means, rather than of individual observations. Therefore, the standard error refers to the variability of means, rather than the variability of individual observations, so that it provides an idea of how variable a single estimate of the mean from one set of research data is likely to be.

The data shown in Table 10–1 can be used to explore the concept of standard error. The table lists the systolic and diastolic blood pressures of 26 young, healthy, adult subjects. To determine the range of expected variation in the estimate of the mean blood pressure obtained from the 26 subjects, the investigator would need an unbiased estimate of the variation in the underlying population. How can this be done with only one rather small sample? The solution requires a bit of statistical theory. Suppose instead of the single research sample, there were 100 different research samples, each consisting of 26 individuals, from the same underlying population. (This supposition is not as farfetched as it might seem; the same research is often funded in many different medical centers, using strictly comparable criteria.) Then 100 mean blood pressure values could be determined from the 100 different research samples.

The frequency distribution of the 100 different means could be plotted, treating each mean as a single observation. These sample means will form a truly normal (gaussian) frequency distribution, the mean of which would be very close to the true mean for the underlying population. More important for this discussion, the standard deviation of this distribution of sample means is an unbiased estimate of the standard deviation of the underlying population

TABLE 10–1 Systolic and Diastolic Blood Pressure Values of 26 Young, Healthy, Adult Subjects

Subject	Systolic (mm Hg)	Diastolic (mm Hg)	Sex
1	108	62	Female
2	134	74	Male
3	100	64	Female
4	108	68	Female
5	112	72	Male
6	112	64	Female
7	112	68	Female
8	122	70	Male
9	116	70	Male
10	116	70	Male
11	120	72	Male
12	108	70	Female
13	108	70	Female
14	96	64	Female
15	114	74	Male
16	108	68	Male
17	128	86	Male
18	114	68	Male
19	112	64	Male
20	124	70	Female
21	90	60	Female
22	102	64	Female
23	106	70	Male
24	124	74	Male
25	130	72	Male
26	116	70	Female

Source of data: Unpublished findings in a sample of 26 professional persons in Connecticut.

and is called the standard error of the distribution. (Technically, the variance is an unbiased estimator of the population variance, and the standard deviation, although not quite unbiased, is close enough to being unbiased that it works well.)

The standard error is a parameter that enables the investigator to do two things that are central to the function of statistics. One is to estimate the probable amount of error around a quantitative assertion. The other is to perform tests of statistical significance. If only the standard deviation and sample size of one research sample are known, however, the standard deviation can be converted to a standard error so that these functions can be pursued.

Although the proof will not be shown here, an unbiased estimate of the standard error can be obtained from the standard deviation of a single research sample if the standard deviation was originally calculated using the degrees of freedom ($N-1$) in the denominator (see Chapter 9). The formula for converting a standard deviation (SD) to a standard error (SE) is as follows:

$$\text{Standard error} = \text{SE} = \frac{\text{SD}}{\sqrt{N}}$$

The larger the sample size (N), the smaller the standard error, and the better the estimate of the population mean. At any given point on the x-axis, the height of the bell-shaped curve of the sample means represents the relative probability that a single sample mean would fall at that point. Most of the time, the sample mean would be near the true mean. Less often, it would be farther away.

In the medical literature, means or proportions are often reported either as the mean plus or minus 1 SD or as the mean plus or minus 1 SE. Reported data must be examined carefully to determine whether the SD or the SE is shown. Either is acceptable in theory, because an SD can be converted to an SE and vice versa if the sample size is known. However, many journals have a policy stating whether the SD or SE must be reported. The sample size should also be shown.

Confidence Intervals

Whereas the SD shows the variability of individual observations, the SE shows the variability of means. Whereas the mean plus or minus 1.96 SD estimates the range in which 95% of individual observations would be expected to fall, the mean plus or minus 1.96 SE estimates the range in which 95% of the means of repeated samples of the same size would be expected to fall. Moreover, if the value for the mean plus or minus 1.96 SE is known, it can be used to calculate the 95% confidence interval, which is the range of values in which the investigator can be 95% confident that the true mean of the underlying population falls. Other confidence intervals, such as the 99% confidence interval, can easily be determined as well.

Box 10–1 shows the calculation of the SE and the 95% confidence interval for the systolic blood pressure data in Table 10–1.

Confidence intervals alone can be used as a test to see whether a mean or proportion differs significantly from a **fixed value**. The most common situa-

tion for this is testing to see whether a risk ratio or an odds ratio differs significantly from the ratio of 1.0 (which means no difference). Thus, if a risk ratio of 1.7 had a 95% confidence interval between 0.92 and 2.70, it would not be significantly different from 1.0 if the alpha was chosen to be 0.05, because the confidence interval includes 1.0. However, if the same risk ratio had a 95% confidence interval between 1.02 and 2.60, it would be significantly different from a risk ratio of 1.0, because 1.0 does not fall within the 95% confidence interval shown.

■ TESTS OF STATISTICAL SIGNIFICANCE

The tests described below allow investigators to compare two parameters, such as means or proportions, and to determine whether the difference between them is statistically significant. The various **t-tests** (the one-tailed Student's t-test, the two-tailed Student's t-test, and the paired t-test) compare differences between **means,** while **z-tests** compare differences between **proportions.** All of these tests make comparisons possible by calculating the appropriate form of a ratio, which is called a **critical ratio** because it permits the investigator to make a decision. This is done by comparing the ratio obtained from whatever test is performed (e.g., a t-test) with the values in the appropriate statistical table (e.g., a table of t values) for the observed number of degrees of freedom. Before individual tests are discussed in detail, the concepts of critical ratios and degrees of freedom are defined. The statistical tables of t values and z values are included at the end of the book (see the Appendix).

Critical Ratios

Critical ratios are a class of tests of statistical significance that depend on dividing some parameter (such as a difference between means) by the standard error (SE) of that parameter. The general formula for tests of significance is as follows:

$$\text{Critical ratio} = \frac{\text{Parameter}}{\text{SE of that parameter}}$$

When applied to the Student's t-test, the formula becomes:

$$\text{Critical ratio} = t = \frac{\text{Difference between two means}}{\text{SE of the difference between two means}}$$

When applied to a z-test, the formula becomes:

$$\text{Critical ratio} = z = \frac{\text{Difference between two proportions}}{\text{SE of the difference between two proportions}}$$

The value of the critical ratio (e.g., t or z) is then looked up in the appropriate table (of t or z) to deter-

---

BOX 10–1   Calculation of the Standard Error and the 95% Confidence Interval for Systolic Blood Pressure Values of 26 Subjects

Part 1   Beginning data (see Table 10–1)

Number of observations, or $N = 26$
Mean, or $\bar{x}$ = 113.1 mm Hg
Standard deviation, or SD = 10.3 mm Hg

Part 2   Calculation of the standard error, or SE

$$SE = \frac{SD}{\sqrt{N}} = \frac{10.3}{\sqrt{26}} = \frac{10.3}{5.1} = 2.02 \text{ mm Hg}$$

Part 3   Calculation of the 95% confidence interval, or 95% CI

95% CI = mean ± 1.96 SE
= 113.1 ± (1.96)(2.02)
= 113.1 ± 3.96
= between 113.1 − 3.96 and 113.1 + 3.96
= **109.1, 117.1 mm Hg**

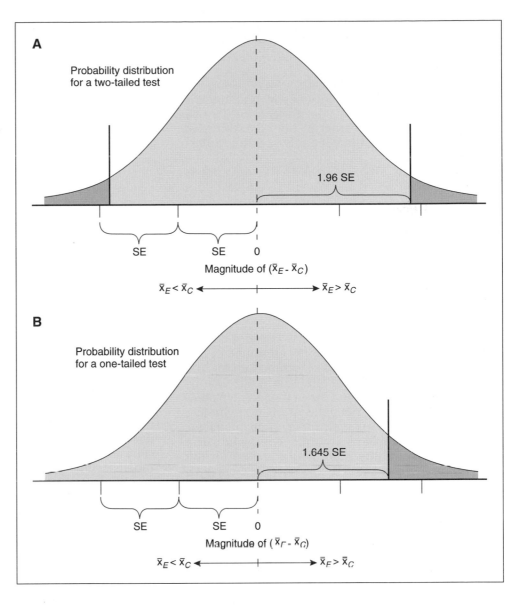

FIGURE 10–1 Probability distribution of the difference between two means when the null hypothesis is actually true (i.e., when there is no real difference between the two means). Dark orange indicates the zone for rejecting the null hypothesis, and light orange indicates the zone for failing to reject the null hypothesis. When a two-tailed test is used, there is a rejection zone on each side of the distribution. When a one-tailed test is used, there is a rejection zone on only one side. SE is the standard error, $\bar{x}_E$ is the mean for the experimental group, and $\bar{x}_C$ is the mean for the control group.

mine the corresponding value of *p*. For any critical ratio, the larger the ratio, the more likely that the difference between means or proportions is due to more than just random variation (i.e., the more likely it is that the difference can be considered statistically significant and, hence, real). Unless the total sample size is small (say, under 30), the finding of a critical ratio of greater than about 2 usually indicates that the difference is real and enables the investigator to reject the null hypothesis. The statistical tables adjust the critical ratios for the sample size by means of the degrees of freedom.

The reason that a critical ratio works is somewhat complex and can best be explained through the use of an illustration. Assume that an investigator conducted 1000 different clinical trials of the same *ineffective* antihypertensive drug and that each of the trials had the same large sample size. In each trial, assume that the investigator obtained an average value for the change in blood pressure in the experimental group $(\bar{x}_E)$ and an average value for the

change in blood pressure in the control group $(\bar{x}_C)$. Therefore, for each trial, there would be two means, and the difference between the means could be expressed as $\bar{x}_E$ minus $\bar{x}_C$. In this study, the null hypothesis would be that the difference between the means was not a real difference.

If the null hypothesis were true, chance variation would cause $\bar{x}_E$ to be greater than $\bar{x}_C$ about half the time, despite the drug's lack of effect. The reverse would be true, also by chance, about half the time. In a rare trial, $\bar{x}_E$ would exactly equal $\bar{x}_C$. On the average, however, the differences between the two means would be near 0, reflecting the drug's lack of effect.

If the values representing the difference between the two means in each of the 1000 clinical trials were plotted on a graph, the distribution curve would appear normal (i.e., gaussian), with an average difference of 0, as in Fig. 10–1A. Chance variation would cause 95% of the values to fall within the large central zone, which covers the area of 0 ± 1.96 standard errors and is colored light orange in Fig. 10–1A. This is the zone for *failing to reject* the null hypothesis. Outside of this zone is the zone for *rejecting* the null hypothesis, which consists of two areas colored in dark orange in Fig. 10–1A.

Therefore, if only one clinical trial was performed and if the ratio of the difference between the means of the two groups was outside the area of 0 ± 1.96 standard errors of the difference, either the study was a rare (i.e., ≤ 0.05) example of a false-positive difference or there was a true difference between the groups. By setting alpha at 0.05, the investigator is willing to take a 5% risk (i.e., a 1-in-20 risk) of a false-positive assertion but is not willing to take a higher risk. This implies that if alpha is set at 0.05 and if 20 data sets of two research samples that are *not* truly different are compared, one "statistically significant" difference would be expected by chance alone.

Degrees of Freedom

The term "degrees of freedom" refers to the number of observations that are free to vary. The idea behind this important statistical concept is presented in Box 10–2. For simplicity, the degrees of freedom for any test are considered to be the total sample size minus 1 degree of freedom for each mean that is calculated. In the Student's *t*-test, 2 degrees of freedom are lost because two means are calculated (one mean for each group whose means are to be compared). The general formula for the degrees of freedom for the Student's two-group *t*-test is $N_1 + N_2 - 2$, where N_1 is

---

BOX 10–2   The Idea Behind the Degrees of Freedom

The term "degrees of freedom" refers to the number of observations *(N)* that are free to vary. A degree of freedom is lost every time a mean is calculated. Why should this be?

Before putting on a pair of gloves, a person has the freedom to decide whether to begin with the left or right glove. However, once the person puts on the first glove, he or she loses the freedom to decide which glove to put on last. If centipedes put on shoes, they would have a choice to make for the first 99 shoes but not for the 100th shoe. Right at the end, the freedom to choose (vary) is restricted.

In statistics, if there are two observed values, only one estimate of the variation between them is possible. Something has to serve as the basis against which other observations are compared. The mean is the most "solid" estimate of the expected value of a variable, so it is assumed to be "fixed." This implies that the numerator of the mean (the sum of individual observations, or the sum of x_i), which is based on N observations, is also fixed. Once $N - 1$ observations (each of which was, presumably, free to vary) have been added up, the last observation is not free to vary, because the total values of the N observations must add up to the sum of x_i. For this reason, 1 degree of freedom is lost each time a mean is calculated. The proper average of a sum of squares when calculated from an observed sample, therefore, is the sum of squares divided by the degrees of freedom $(N - 1)$.

---

the sample size in the first group and N_2 is the sample size in the second group.

Use of *t*-Tests

In medical research, *t*-tests are among the three or four most commonly used statistical tests (Emerson and Colditz 1983). The purpose of a *t*-test is to compare the means of a continuous variable in two research samples in order to determine whether or not the difference between the two observed means exceeds the difference that would be expected by chance from random samples.

Sample Populations and Sizes

If the two research samples come from two different groups (e.g., a group of men and a group of women), the Student's *t*-test is used. If the two samples come from the same group (e.g., pretreatment and posttreatment values for the same study subjects), the paired *t*-test is used.

Both types of *t*-test depend on certain assumptions, including the assumption that the data in the continuous variable are normally distributed (i.e., have a bell-shaped distribution). Very seldom, however, will observed data be perfectly normally distributed. Does this invalidate the *t*-test? Fortunately, it does not. There is a convenient theorem, called the central limit theorem, that rescues the *t*-test (and much of statistics as well). The **central limit theorem** can be derived theoretically or observed by experimentation. According to the theorem, for reasonably large samples (say, 30 or more observations in each sample), the distribution of the means of many samples is normal (gaussian), even though the data in individual samples may have skewness, kurtosis, or unevenness. Because the critical theoretical requirement for the *t*-test is that the sample means be normally distributed, a *t*-test may be computed on almost any set of continuous data, if the observations can be considered a random sample and the sample size is reasonably large.

The *t* Distribution

The *t* distribution was described by William Gosset, who used the pseudonym "Student" when he wrote the description. (For one explanation of how the *t*-test received its name and for other humorous perspectives on statistics, see Smith 1993.)

The normal distribution is the *z* distribution. The *t* distribution looks similar to it, except that its tails are somewhat wider and its peak is slightly less high, depending on the sample size. The *t* distribution is necessary because when sample sizes are small, the observed estimates of the mean and variance are subject to considerable error. The larger the sample size is, the smaller the errors are, and the more the *t* distribution looks like the normal distribution. In the case of an infinite sample size, the two distributions are identical. For practical purposes, when the com-

---

BOX 10–3   The Formula for the Standard Error of the Difference Between Means

The standard error equals the standard deviation (σ) divided by the square root of the sample size (N). Alternatively, this can be expressed as the square root of the variance (σ²) divided by N:

$$\text{Standard error} = \frac{\sigma}{\sqrt{N}} = \sqrt{\frac{\sigma^2}{N}}$$

As mentioned in Chapter 9, Box 9–3, the variance of a difference is equal to the sum of the individual variances. Therefore, the variance of the difference between the mean of an experimental group (μ_E) and the mean of a control group (μ_C) could be expressed as follows: $\sigma_E^2 + \sigma_C^2$.

As shown above, a standard error can be written as the square root of the variance divided by the sample size, allowing the equation to be expressed as:

$$\text{Standard error of } \mu_E - \mu_C = \sqrt{\frac{\sigma_E^2}{N_E} + \frac{\sigma_C^2}{N_C}}$$

---

bined sample size of the two groups being compared is larger than 120, the difference between the normal distribution and the t distribution is negligible.

Student's *t*-Test

There are two types of Student's *t*-test: the one-tailed and the two-tailed type. The calculations are the same, but the interpretation of the resulting *t* differs somewhat. The common features will be discussed before the differences are outlined.

Calculation of the Value of t. In both types of Student's *t*-test, *t* is calculated by taking the observed difference between the means of the two groups (the numerator) and dividing this difference by the standard error of the difference between the means of the two groups (the denominator). Before *t* can be calculated, then, the **standard error of the difference between the means** (SED) must be determined. The basic formula for this is the square root of the sum of the respective population variances, each divided by its own sample size.

In theoretical terms, the correct equation for the SED would be as follows:

$$\text{SED of } \mu_E - \mu_C = \sqrt{\frac{\sigma_E^2}{N_E} + \frac{\sigma_C^2}{N_C}}$$

where the Greek symbol μ is the population mean, E is the experimental population, C is the control population, σ^2 is the variance of the population, and N is the number of observations in the population. The rationale behind this formula is discussed in Box 10–3.

The theoretical formula requires that the population variances be known, which usually is not true with experimental data. Nevertheless, if the sample sizes are large enough (e.g., if the total of the two

samples is 30 or greater), the above formula can be used with the sample variances substituted for the population variances. In this case, instead of using Greek letters in the formula, the italic Roman symbol $\bar{x}$ is used to indicate the mean of the sample and the italic Roman symbol s^2 is used to indicate the variance:

$$\text{Estimate of the SED of } \bar{x}_E - \bar{x}_C = \sqrt{\frac{s_E^2}{N_E} + \frac{s_C^2}{N_C}}$$

Because the *t*-test is usually used to test a null hypothesis of no difference between two means, the assumption is generally made that there is no difference between the variances either, so that a **pooled estimate of the SED** (SED$_p$) is used instead. In this case, if the sample sizes are approximately equal in the two groups and if the combined sample size is large enough (say, more than 30 in the combined sample), the above formula for the standard error of the difference becomes:

$$\text{SED}_p \text{ of } \bar{x}_E - \bar{x}_C = \sqrt{s_p^2 \left(\frac{1}{N_E} + \frac{1}{N_C}\right)}$$

$$= \sqrt{s_p^2 [(1/N_E) + (1/N_C)]}$$

The s_p^2, which is called the **pooled estimate of the variance,** is a weighted average of s_E^2 and s_C^2. The s_p^2 is calculated as the sum of the two sums of squares, divided by the combined degrees of freedom:

$$s_p^2 = \frac{\sum (x_E - \bar{x}_E)^2 + \sum (x_C - \bar{x}_C)^2}{N_E + N_C - 2}$$

If one sample size is much greater than the other or if the variance of one sample is much greater than the variance of the other, more complex formulas are needed (see Moore and McCabe 1993).

When the Student's *t*-test is used to test the null hypothesis in research involving an experimental group and a control group, it usually takes the general form of the following equation:

$$t = \frac{\bar{x}_E - \bar{x}_C - 0}{\sqrt{s_p^2 [(1/N_E) + (1/N_C)]}}$$

$$df = N_E + N_C - 2$$

The 0 in the numerator of the equation for *t* was added for correctness, because the *t*-test determines if the difference between the means is significantly different from 0. However, because the 0 does not affect the calculations in any way, it is usually omitted from *t*-test formulas.

The same formula, recast in terms to apply to any two independent samples (e.g., samples of men and women), is as follows:

$$t = \frac{\bar{x}_1 - \bar{x}_2 - 0}{\sqrt{s_p^2 [(1/N_1) + (1/N_2)]}}$$

$$df = N_1 + N_2 - 2$$

in which $\bar{x}_1$ is the mean of the first sample, $\bar{x}_2$ is the mean of the second sample, s_p^2 is the pooled estimate

BOX 10–4   Calculation of the Results of the Student's *t*-Test Comparing the Systolic Blood Pressure Values of 14 Male Subjects with Those of 12 Female Subjects

Part 1   Beginning data (see Table 10–1)

Number of observations, or N = 14 for males, or M
                                  12 for females, or F

Mean, or $\bar{x}$ =   118.3 mm Hg for males
                           107.0 mm Hg for females

Variance, or s^2 =   70.1 mm Hg for males
                           82.5 mm Hg for females

Sum of $(x_i - \bar{x})^2$, or TSS =   911.3 mm Hg for males
                           907.5 mm Hg for females

Alpha value for the *t*-test =   0.05

Part 2   Calculation of the *t* value based on the pooled variance ($s_p{}^2$) and the pooled standard error of the difference (SED$_p$)

$$s_p{}^2 = \frac{\text{TSS}_M + \text{TSS}_F}{N_M + N_F - 2} = \frac{911.3 + 907.5}{14 + 12 - 2} = \frac{1818.8}{24} = 75.78 \text{ mm Hg}$$

$$\text{SED}_p = \sqrt{s_p{}^2[(1/N_M) + (1/N_F)]}$$

$$= \sqrt{75.78(1/14 + 1/12)}$$

$$= \sqrt{75.78(0.1548)} = \sqrt{11.73} = 3.42 \text{ mm Hg}$$

$$t = \frac{\bar{x}_M - \bar{x}_F - 0}{\sqrt{s_p{}^2[(1/N_M) + (1/N_F)]}} = \frac{\bar{x}_M - \bar{x}_F - 0}{\text{SED}_p}$$

$$= \frac{118.3 - 107.0 - 0}{3.42} = \frac{11.30}{3.42} = 3.30$$

Part 3   Alternative calculation of the *t* value based on the SED equation using the observed variances for males and females, rather than on the SED$_p$ equation using the pooled variance

$$\text{SED} = \sqrt{\frac{s_M{}^2}{N_M} + \frac{s_F{}^2}{N_F}} = \sqrt{\frac{70.1}{14} + \frac{82.5}{12}}$$

$$= \sqrt{5.01 + 6.88} = \sqrt{11.89} = 3.45 \text{ mm Hg}$$

$$t = \frac{\bar{x}_M - \bar{x}_F - 0}{\text{SED}}$$

$$= \frac{118.3 - 107.0 - 0}{3.45} = \frac{11.30}{3.45} = 3.28$$

In comparison with the equation in Part 2, the equation in Part 3 is usually easier to remember and to calculate, and it adjusts for differences in the variances and the sample sizes. Note that the result here ($t = 3.28$) is almost identical to that above ($t = 3.30$), even though the sample size is small.

Part 4   Calculation of the degrees of freedom *(df)* for the *t*-test and interpretation of the *t* value

$$df = N_M + N_F - 2 = 14 + 12 - 2 = 24$$

For a *t* value of 3.30, with 24 degrees of freedom, *p* is less than 0.01, as indicated in the table of the values of *t* (see Appendix). This means that the male subjects have a significantly different (higher) systolic blood pressure than do the female subjects in this data set.

of the variance, N_1 is the size of the first sample, N_2 is the size of the second sample, and df is the degrees of freedom. The 0 in the numerator indicates that the null hypothesis states that the difference between the means will not be significantly different from 0. The df is needed to enable the investigator to refer to the correct line in the table of the values of t and their relationship to p (see the Appendix).

Box 10–4 shows the use of a t-test to compare the mean systolic blood pressures of the 14 men and 12 women whose data were given in Table 10–1. A different and more visual way of understanding the t-test is presented in Box 10–5.

The t-test is designed to help investigators distinguish "explained variation" from "unexplained variation" (random error, or chance). These concepts are similar to the concepts of "signal" and "background noise" in radio broadcast engineering. Listeners who are searching for a particular station on their radio dial will find background noise on almost every radio frequency. When they reach the station that they want to hear, they may not notice the background noise, since the signal is so much stronger than this noise. Because the radio can amplify a weak signal greatly, the critical factor is the ratio of the strength of the signal to the strength of the background noise. The greater the ratio, the clearer the station's sound. The closer the ratio is to 1.0 (i.e., the point at which the magnitude of the signal equals that of the noise), the less satisfactory will be the sound that the listener hears. In medical studies, the particular factor that is being investigated is similar to the radio signal, and random error is similar to background noise. Statistical analysis helps distinguish one from the other by comparing their strengths. If the variation caused by the factor of interest is considerably larger than the variation caused by random factors (i.e., if in the t-test the ratio is approximately 1.96), the effect of the factor of interest becomes detectable above the statistical "noise" of random factors.

Interpretation of the Results. If the value of t is large, the p value will be small, because it is unlikely that a large t ratio will be obtained by chance alone. If the p value is 0.05 or less, it is customary to assume that there is a real difference. Conceptually, the p value is the probability of being in error if the null hypothesis of no difference between the means is rejected and the alternative hypothesis of a true difference is accepted.

One-Tailed and Two-Tailed t-Tests. The conceptual diagram in Fig. 10–1 shows the theory behind the acceptance and rejection regions for the two different types of Student's t-test. These tests are sometimes called the one-sided test and the two-sided test.

In the two-tailed test, alpha is equally divided at the ends of the two tails of the distribution (see Fig. 10–1A). The two-tailed test is generally recommended, because differences in either direction are usually important to document. For example, it is obviously important to know if a new treatment is significantly better than a standard or placebo treatment, but it is also important to know if a

new treatment is significantly worse and should therefore be avoided. In this situation, the two-tailed test provides an accepted criterion for when a difference shows the new treatment to be either better or worse.

Sometimes, however, only a one-tailed test is needed. Suppose, for example, that a new therapy is known to cost much more than the currently used therapy. Obviously, it would not be used if it were worse than the current therapy, but it would also not be used if it were merely as good as the current therapy. It would be used only if it were significantly better than the current therapy. Under these circumstances, some investigators consider it acceptable to use a one-tailed test. When this occurs, the 5% rejection region for the null hypothesis is all put on one tail of the distribution (see Fig. 10–1B), instead of being evenly divided between the extremes of the two tails.

In the one-tailed test, the null hypothesis nonrejection region extends only to 1.645 standard errors above the "no difference" point of 0. In the two-tailed test, it extends to 1.96 standard errors above and below the "no difference" point. This makes the one-tailed test more robust—that is, more able to detect a significant difference, if it is in the expected direction. Many investigators dislike one-tailed tests, because they believe that if an intervention is significantly worse than the standard therapy, that should be documented scientifically. Most reviewers and editors require that the use of a one-tailed significance test be justified.

The implications of choosing a one-tailed or two-tailed test are further explored in Box 10–6.

Paired *t*-Test

In many medical studies, individuals are followed over time to see if there is a change in the value of some continuous variable. Typically, this occurs in a "before and after" experiment, such as one testing to see if there was a drop in average blood pressure following treatment or to see if there was a drop in weight following the use of a special diet. In this type of comparison, an individual patient serves as his or her own control. The appropriate statistical test for this kind of data is the paired t-test. The paired t-test is more robust than the Student's t-test because it considers the variation from only one group of people, whereas the Student's t-test considers variation from two groups. Any variation that is detected in the paired t-test is attributable to the intervention or to changes over time in the same person.

Calculation of the Value of t. To calculate a paired t-test, a new variable is created. This variable, called d, is the difference between the values before and after the intervention for each individual studied. The paired t-test is a test of the null hypothesis that, on the average, the difference is equal to 0, which is what would be expected if there were no change over time. Using the symbol $\bar{d}$ to indicate the mean observed

BOX 10–5   **Does the Eye Naturally Perform *t*-Tests?**

The paired diagrams below show three patterns of overlap between two frequency distributions (e.g., a treatment group and a control group). These distributions can be thought of as the frequency distributions of systolic blood pressure values among hypertensive patients following randomization and treatment either with the experimental drug or with a placebo. The treatment group's distribution is shown in gray, the control group's distribution is shown in orange, and the area of overlap is shown with gray and orange hatch marks. The means are indicated by the vertical dotted lines. The three different pairs show variation in the spread of systolic blood pressure values.

Examine the three diagrams. Then try to guess whether each pair was sampled from the *same* universe (i.e., was not significantly different) or was sampled from two *different* universes (i.e., was significantly different).

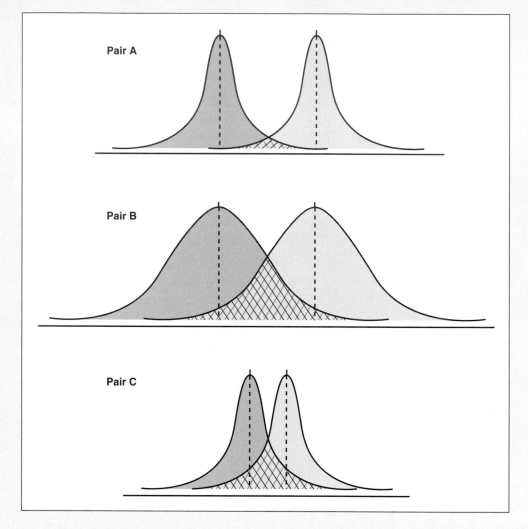

Most observers believe that the distributions in pair A look as though they were sampled from different universes. When asked why they think so, they usually state that there is little overlap between the two frequency distributions. Most observers are not convinced that the distributions in either pair B or pair C were sampled from different universes. They say that there is considerable overlap in each of these pairs, and this makes them doubt that there is a real difference. Their visual impressions are indeed correct.

It is not the absolute distance between the two means which leads most observers to say "different" for pair A and "not different" for pair B, because the distance between the means was drawn to be exactly the same in pairs A and B. Nor is it the absolute amount of dispersion that causes them to say "different" for pair A and "not different" for pair C,

because the dispersions were drawn to be the same in pairs A and C. Rather, the essential point, which the eye notices, is the ratio of the distance between the means to the variation around the means. The greater the distance between the means for a given amount of dispersion, the less likely it is that the samples were from the same universe. This ratio is exactly what the *t*-test calculates:

$$t = \frac{\text{Distance between the means}}{\text{Variation around the means}}$$

where the variation around the means is expressed as the standard error of the difference between the means. Therefore, the eye naturally does a *t*-test, although it does not quantify the relationship as precisely as does the *t*-test.

For students who are confused by the implications of choosing a one-tailed or two-tailed test, a football analogy may be helpful.

The coach of a football team wants to assess the skill of potential quarterbacks. He is unwilling to allow mere completion of a pass to serve as evidence of throwing accuracy, because he knows that a pass could be completed by chance, even if the football did not go where the quarterback intended. Because the coach is something of a Monday-morning statistician, he further infers that if the quarterback were to throw randomly, the ball would often land near the center of the field and would less often land way off toward one sideline or the other. The distribution of random throws on the 100-foot-wide field might even be gaussian (thinks the coach).

Therefore, the coach asks quarterback applicants to throw to a receiver along the sideline. The coach announces that each applicant has a choice: (1) he may pick one side ahead of time and complete a pass to that side within 5 feet of the sideline, or (2) he may throw to either side but then must complete the pass within 2.5 feet of the sideline. The coach's null hypothesis is simply that the quarterback will not be able to complete a pass within the specified zone. In either case, a complete pass outside the specified zone will be attributed to chance, since it is not what was intended.

Note that the coach does not give applicants the option of throwing to either side and completing the pass within 5 feet of the sideline. If the coach were to allow applicants to elect this option, the coach would "reject" his null hypothesis on the basis of chance 10% of the time, and he is unwilling to take so great a risk of selecting a lucky but unskillful quarterback.

Clearly, the quarterback has more room to work with if he prefers to throw to one side (one-tailed test) and can count on throwing in only that direction. If he is unsure in which direction he may wish to throw, he can get credit for a completed pass in either direction (two-tailed test) but has only a very narrow zone for which to aim.

lation and therefore can be omitted. Because the 0 in the above formula is a constant, it has no variance, and the only error in estimating the mean difference is its own standard error.

The formulas for the Student's t-test and the paired t-test are similar: the ratio of a difference to the variation around that difference (the standard error). In the Student's t-test, each of the two distributions to be compared contributes to the variation of the difference, and the two variances must be added. But in the paired t-test, there is only one frequency distribution, that of the before-after difference in each person. In the paired t-test, because only one mean is calculated $(\overline{d})$, only 1 degree of freedom is lost; therefore, the formula for the degrees of freedom is $N-1$.

Interpretation of the Results. The values of t and their relationship to p are shown in a statistical table in the Appendix. If the value of t is large, the p value will be small, because it is unlikely that a large t ratio will be obtained by chance alone. If the p value is 0.05 or less, it is customary to assume that there is a real difference (i.e., that the null hypothesis of no difference can be rejected).

Use of z-Tests

In contrast to t-tests, which compare differences between means, z-tests compare differences between proportions. In medicine, examples of proportions that are frequently studied are sensitivity, specificity, positive predictive value, risks, percentages of people with a given symptom, percentages of people who are ill, and percentages of ill people who survive their illness. Frequently, the goal of research is to see if the proportion of patients surviving in a treated group differs from that in an untreated group. This can be evaluated using a z-test for proportions.

Calculation of the Value of z. As discussed earlier in this chapter (see Critical Ratios), z is calculated by taking the observed difference between the two proportions (the numerator) and dividing it by the standard error of the difference between the two proportions (the denominator). For purposes of illustration, assume that research is being conducted to see if the proportion of patients surviving in a treated group is greater than that in an untreated group. For each group, if p is the proportion of successes (survivals), then $1-p$ is the proportion of failures (nonsurvivals). If N represents the size of the group on which the proportion is based, the parameters of the proportion could be calculated as follows:

$$\text{Variance (proportion)} = \frac{p(1-p)}{N}$$

$$\text{Standard error (proportion)} = \text{SE}_p = \sqrt{\frac{p(1-p)}{N}}$$

$$95\% \text{ Confidence interval} = 95\% \text{ CI} = p \pm 1.96\,\text{SE}_p$$

If there is a 0.60 (60%) survival rate following a given treatment, the calculations of SE_p and the 95%

difference between the before and after values, the formula for the paired t-test is as follows:

$$t_{\text{paired}} = t_p = \frac{\overline{d} - 0}{\text{Standard error of } \overline{d}}$$

$$= \frac{\overline{d} - 0}{\sqrt{\dfrac{s_d^{\,2}}{N}}}$$

$$df = N - 1$$

The numerator contains a 0 because the null hypothesis says that the observed difference will not differ from 0; however, the 0 does not enter into the calcu-

CI of the proportion, based on a sample of 100 study subjects, would be as follows:

$$SE_p = \sqrt{(0.6)(0.4)/100}$$
$$= \sqrt{0.24/100}$$
$$= 0.49/10$$
$$= 0.049$$
$$95\% \text{ CI} = 0.6 \pm (1.96)(0.049)$$
$$= 0.6 \pm 0.096$$
$$= \text{between } 0.6 - 0.096 \text{ and } 0.6 + 0.096$$
$$= 0.504, 0.696$$

The result of the CI calculation means that in 95% of cases, the "true" proportion surviving in the universe is between 50.4% and 69.6%.

Now that there is a way to obtain the standard error of a proportion, the **standard error of the difference between proportions** also can be obtained, and the equation for the z-test can be expressed as follows:

$$z = \frac{p_1 - p_2 - 0}{\sqrt{\overline{p}(1-\overline{p})[(1/N_1) + (1/N_2)]}}$$

in which p_1 is the proportion of the first sample, p_2 is the proportion of the second sample, N_1 is the size of the first sample, N_2 is the size of the second sample, and $\overline{p}$ is the mean proportion of successes in all observations combined. The 0 in the numerator indicates that the null hypothesis states that the difference between the proportions will not be significantly different from 0.

Interpretation of the Results. Note that the above formula for z is similar to the formula for t in the Student's t-test, as described earlier (see the pooled variance formula). However, because the variance and the standard error of the proportion are based on a theoretical distribution (the binomial approximation to the z distribution), the z distribution is used instead of the t distribution in determining whether the difference is statistically significant. When the z ratio is large (as when the t ratio is large), the difference is more likely to be real.

The computations for the z-test appear different from the computations for the chi-square test (see Chapter 11), but when the same data are set up as a 2×2 table, technically the computations for the two tests are identical. Most people find it easier to do a chi-square test than to do a z-test for proportions.

Use of Other Tests

Chapter 11 discusses other statistical significance tests used in the analysis of two variables (bivariate analysis), and Chapter 13 discusses tests used in the analysis of multiple independent variables (multivariable analysis).

■ SPECIAL CONSIDERATIONS

Variation Between Groups Versus Variation Within Groups

If the differences between two groups are found to be statistically significant, it is appropriate to wonder why the groups are different and how much of the total variation is explained by the variable defining the two groups. Here, a straightforward comparison of the heights of men and women can be used to illustrate the considerations involved in answering the following question: Why are men taller than women? While biologists might respond that genetic, hormonal, and perhaps nutritional factors explain the differences in height, a biostatistician would take a different approach. After first pointing out that individual men are not always taller than individual women but the average height of men is greater than that of women, the biostatistician would seek to determine the amount of the total variation in height that is explained by the gender difference and also determine whether or not the difference is more than would be expected by chance.

For purposes of this discussion, suppose that the heights of 200 randomly selected university students were measured, that 100 of these students were men and 100 were women, and that the unit of measure was centimeters. As discussed in Chapter 9, the **total variation** would be equal to the sum of the squared deviations, which is usually called the **total sum of squares** (TSS) but is sometimes referred to simply as the **sum of squares** (SS). In the total group of 200 students, suppose that the total SS was found to be 10,000 cm². This number is the total amount of variation to be "explained" in the data set. The biostatistician would begin by seeking to determine how much of this variation was actually due to gender and how much was due to other factors.

Fig. 10–2 shows a hypothetical frequency distribution of the heights of a sample of women (black marks) and a sample of men (orange marks), indicating the density of observations at the different heights. An approximate normal curve is drawn over each of the two distributions, and the overall mean (grand mean) is indicated, along with the mean height for women (a gender mean) and the mean height for men (a gender mean).

Although measuring the TSS from the grand mean yielded a result of 10,000 cm², measuring the SS from the gender means would yield a much smaller amount of unexplained variation—say, about 6,000 cm². This leaves 60% of the variation still to be explained. The other 40% of the variation is explained by the variable gender. Therefore, from a statistical perspective, "explaining variation" implies reducing the unexplained SS. If more explanatory variables (such as age, height of father, height of mother, and nutritional status) are analyzed, the unexplained SS may be reduced still further, and even more of the variation can be explained.

The following question is even more specific: Why is the shortest woman shorter than the tallest man?

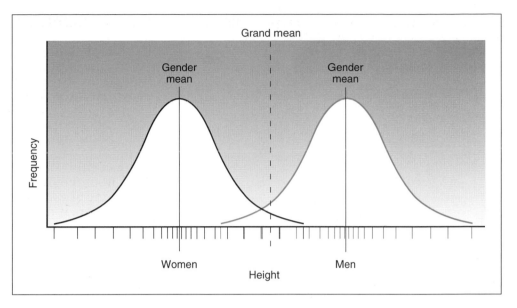

FIGURE 10–2   Hypothetical frequency distribution of the heights of a sample of women (black marks along the *x*-axis) and a sample of men (orange marks along the *x*-axis), indicating the density of observations at the different heights. An approximate normal curve is drawn over each of the two distributions, and the overall mean (grand mean) is indicated, along with the mean height for women (a gender mean) and the mean height for men (a gender mean).

Statistically, there are two parts to the explanation: (1) She is a member of the class (group) of individuals (women) who have a shorter mean height than that of men. (2) She is the shortest of her group of women, and the man selected is the tallest of the group of men, so they are at the opposite extremes of height within their respective groups.

The greater the distance between the means for men and women, the greater the proportion of the variation that is likely to be explained by **variation between groups.** The larger the standard deviations of heights of women and of men, the greater the proportion of the variation that is likely to be explained by **variation within groups.** The within-groups variation, however, might be reduced still further if other independent variables were added.

Suppose that all adult women were of equal height, that all adult men were of equal height, and that men were taller than women (Fig. 10–3A). What percentage of the variation in height would be explained by gender, and what percentage would be unexplained? The answer is that all of the variation would be due to gender (between-groups variation), and because there is no within-groups variation, no variation would be left unexplained.

Alternatively, suppose that women varied in height, that men varied in height, and that the mean heights of the men and women were the same (see Fig. 10–3B). Now what percentage of the variation in height would be explained by gender, and what percentage would be unexplained? None of the variation would be due to gender, and all of it would be left unexplained.

This simple example demonstrates what statistics ultimately tries to do: divide the total variation into a part that is explained by the independent variables (the model) and a part that is still unexplained. This activity is called **analyzing variation** or analyzing the TSS. A specific method for doing this under certain circumstances and testing hypotheses at the same time is called **analysis of variance,** or ANOVA (see Chapter 13).

Clinical Importance and External Validity Versus Statistical Significance

A frequent error made by investigators has been to find a statistically significant difference, reject the null hypothesis, and recommend the finding as being useful for determining disease etiology, making a clinical diagnosis, or treating disease, without considering whether the finding is really clinically important and whether it has external validity.

There is no doubt that testing for statistical significance is important, because it helps investigators reject assertions that are not true. But even if a finding is **statistically significant,** it may not be **clinically or scientifically important.** For example, with a very large sample size, it is possible to show that a 2 mm Hg average drop in blood pressure with a certain blood pressure medication is statistically significant, but such a small drop in blood pressure would not be of much clinical use and therefore is not clinically important.

In addition, before the findings of a study can be put to general clinical use, the issue of whether the study has **external validity,** or **generalizability,** must be addressed. For example, in a clinical trial of a new drug, whether the **sample** (the patients in the study) is representative of the **universe** (the patients for whom the new drug might eventually be used) depends on questions concerning the spectrum of disease and the spectrum of individual characteristics in the sample group.

Was the **spectrum of disease** in the sample of patients representative of the spectrum of disease in the universe of patients? Types, stages, and severity of disease can all vary. The spectrum must be clearly defined in terms of the criteria for including or ex-

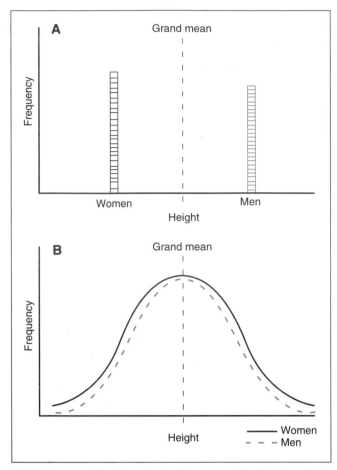

FIGURE 10–3   Two hypothetical frequency distributions of the heights of a sample of women (black lines) and a sample of men (orange lines). Diagram A shows how the distribution would appear if all women were of equal height, all men were of equal height, and men were taller than women. Diagram B shows how the distribution would appear if women varied in height, men varied in height, and the mean heights of the men and women were the same.

cluding patients, and these criteria must be reported when the findings are reported. For example, if patients with a severe form of the disease were excluded from the study, this **exclusion criterion** must be reported, since the results of the study would not be generalizable to those with severe disease (see the discussion of the Physicians' Health Study in Chapter 4).

Was the **spectrum of individual characteristics** in the sample of patients representative of the spectrum of individual characteristics in the universe of patients? Ages, genders, income levels, ethnic backgrounds, and a whole host of characteristics such as these can vary. An appropriate sampling technique (see Chapter 12) is needed for the selection of the individual study subjects. The sampling method should always be reported along with the findings, because the generalizability of results will depend on both the sampling techniques and the spectrum of characteristics in the sample of patients.

SUMMARY

Statistics is an aid to inductive reasoning, which is the effort to find generalizable relationships and differences in observed data. It is the reverse process from mathematics, which is the attempt to apply known formulas to specific data in order to predict an outcome.

Statistics helps investigators to make reasonable conclusions and estimations from observed data and to provide approximate limits to the probability of being in error when making conclusions and estimations from the data. Significance testing starts with the stating of a null hypothesis, such as the hypothesis that there is no real (true) difference between the mean found in an experimental group and the mean found in the control group. The test of statistical significance (a critical ratio) then provides a p value that gives the probability of being wrong if the null hypothesis is rejected. If the results of the significance test allow the investigator to reject the null hypothesis, then the investigator can accept the alternative hypothesis that a true difference exists.

The Student's t-test enables the investigator to compare the means of a continuous variable from two different groups of study subjects in order to determine whether the difference between the means is greater than would be expected by chance alone. The paired t-test enables the investigator to evaluate the average difference in score on a continuous variable in a group of study subjects before and after some intervention was given. Unlike t-tests, which compare the difference between means, z-tests compare the difference between proportions.

QUESTIONS

Directions (Items 1–10). Each of the numbered items or incomplete statements in this section is followed by answers or by completions of the statement. Select the ONE lettered answer or completion that is BEST in each case. Correct answers and explanations are given at the end of the chapter.

1. The first three interns you meet feel a lot better since they started to take a commonly prescribed antidepressant. You reluctantly draw the conclusion that internship is associated with depression. (You also strive to identify any talent you might have to pursue a nonmedical career.) This is an example of

    (A)   deductive reasoning
    (B)   hypothesis testing
    (C)   inductive reasoning
    (D)   interpolation
    (E)   transference

2. The formula for a straight line is $y = mx + b$. The conceptual approach to this formula is not the same in statistics as it is in mathematics. In statistics,

    (A)   only m is unknown
    (B)   this equation is irrelevant

(C)   *x* and *y* are known, and *m* and *b* are to be determined

(D)   *x, y,* and *m* are known, and *b* is to be determined

(E)   *y* is known, and *x* is to be determined

3. The basic goal of hypothesis testing is

(A)   to confirm the alternative hypothesis

(B)   to distinguish between random and meaningful differences in outcome

(C)   to enhance the predictive value of a particular study design

(D)   to establish the value of alpha

(E)   to establish the value of beta

4. The value of alpha serves as protection against

(A)   false-negative results

(B)   inadequate sample size

(C)   selection bias

(D)   type I error

(E)   type II error

5. Statistical significance is achieved when

(A)   alpha is greater than *p*

(B)   beta equals alpha

(C)   *p* is greater than alpha

(D)   *p* is greater than beta

(E)   the result is two-tailed

Items 6–10

Six volunteers have gone on a cholesterol-lowering diet for 3 months. The study diet is very strict: one-third teaspoon of diluted oat bran is sprinkled over the subjects' chocolate mousse every day. Gaunt and haggard from their ascetic experience, the subjects are recovering under the golden arches of the neighborhood dietary deprivation treatment center. You are left in the lab with a stale tuna sandwich and the data shown in the accompanying table.

Subject	Pretrial Cholesterol Level (mg/dL)	Posttrial Cholesterol Level (mg/dL)
1	180	182
2	225	220
3	243	241
4	150	140
5	212	222
6	218	216

6. The standard deviation of the pretrial cholesterol values is

(A)   12.5

(B)   33.8

(C)   42.6

(D)   100

(E)   210

7. The standard error of the pretrial cholesterol values is

(A)   7.4

(B)   13.8

(C)   27

(D)   33.6

(E)   33.8

8. The appropriate test of statistical significance for this trial is

(A)   the critical ratio

(B)   the odds ratio

(C)   the paired *t*-test

(D)   the Student's *t*-test

(E)   the *z*-test

9. By mere inspection of the data, what can you conclude about the difference in pretrial and posttrial cholesterol values?

(A)   Even if clinically meaningful, the difference is not statistically significant

(B)   Even if statistically significant, the difference cannot be clinically meaningful

(C)   If clinically meaningful, the difference must be statistically significant

(D)   If statistically significant, the difference must be clinically meaningful

(E)   The difference cannot be either clinically or statistically significant

10. Before concluding that a lack of statistical significance in this trial proves that oat bran does not lower cholesterol levels, you would want to consider

(A)   beta error

(B)   the alpha level

(C)   the critical ratio

(D)   the *p* value

(E)   type I error

■ ANSWERS AND EXPLANATIONS

1. **The answer is C: inductive reasoning.** As discussed at the beginning of this chapter, statistics is based on inductive reasoning, a logical progression from the specific to the general. In statistics, conclusions are drawn about general associations based on the available data. In this example, based on a sample of three interns, the general association between internship and depression is drawn. In contrast, mathematics is based on deductive reasoning, in which general associations are known but specific values are unknown.

2. **The answer is C: *x* and *y* are known, and *m* and *b* are to be determined.** Question 2, like question 1, highlights the distinction between mathematics and statistics. In mathematics, the formula for a linear (straight line) relationship between *x* and *y* is used to calculate the value of *y* for a given value of *x*. In statistics, however, the values of both *x* (the independent variable) and *y* (the dependent variable, or outcome variable) are known. What is to be established in statistics is

the nature of the relationship between x and y. If x and y are related in a linear fashion, then the specific goal of statistics is to estimate values of m (the slope) and b (the y-intercept).

3. **The answer is B: to distinguish between random and meaningful differences in outcome.** A medical study begins with a hypothesis or belief. The belief, for example, that a particular drug effectively lowers blood pressure must be tested before the belief can gain widespread acceptance. The fundamental goals of hypothesis testing are to observe differences in outcome between two groups and to determine whether such differences are the result of random variation or are large enough to be significant (i.e., not likely the result of random variation). Much of statistics is devoted to this one basic task. The values of alpha and beta should be established before hypothesis testing begins and should influence only the stringency of requirements for statistical significance. Predictive value, discussed in Chapter 7, is not related to hypothesis testing. While rejection of the null hypothesis (and, thus, acceptance of the alternative hypothesis) might result from hypothesis testing, it cannot be considered the basic goal; hypothesis testing might show a lack of statistical significance and indicate that the null hypothesis should not be rejected.

4. **The answer is D: type I error.** The value of alpha represents the probability of type I error (false-positive error). By convention, alpha is set at 0.05, indicating that a statistically significant result is one with no more than a 5% chance of occurring because of random variation. The smaller the value of alpha, the more difficult it becomes to achieve statistical significance and the less likely one is to make a type I error. However, to prevent an extreme type II error (false-negative error), some risk of type I error is unavoidable. Alpha, therefore, protects against type I error by setting a limit to its likelihood of occurrence.

5. **The answer is A: alpha is greater than p.** The value of p, as discussed in the chapter, is the likelihood that an observed outcome difference is due to random variation, or chance, alone. Alpha is the maximum risk one is willing to take that the observed outcome difference is due to chance when asserting the alternative hypothesis. Therefore, one rejects the null hypothesis and asserts the alternative hypothesis whenever p is less than or equal to the preselected value of alpha. By convention, $p \leq 0.05$ indicates statistical significance.

6. **The answer is B: 33.8.** As discussed in Chapter 9, the formula for the standard deviation is as follows:

$$\text{Standard deviation} = \sqrt{\frac{\sum(x_i - \overline{x})^2}{N - 1}}$$

The mean for the six pretrial observations is 204.67, rounded to 205. This value is subtracted from each of the observations, and the difference for each observation is squared. These values are then summed to yield 5712. This figure is divided by $(N - 1)$, or 5, to yield 1142.4. The square root of this figure, 33.8, is the standard deviation for the data set.

7. **The answer is B: 13.8.** As discussed in this chapter, the standard error is the standard deviation divided by the square root of the sample size, or $\text{SE} = \text{SD}/\sqrt{N}$. As calculated in question 6 (above), the standard deviation for the six pretrial values is 33.8. The standard error is therefore equal to 33.8 divided by the square root of 6. With rounding, the answer is 13.8. Note that the standard error is smaller than the standard deviation. This is to be expected, both conceptually and mathematically. Conceptually, while the standard deviation is a measure of dispersion (variation) among individual observations, the standard error is a measure of variation among means derived from repeated trials. One would expect that mean outcomes would vary less than their constituent observations. Mathematically, the standard error is the standard deviation divided by the square root of the sample size. Therefore, the larger the sample size, the smaller the standard error and the greater the difference between the standard deviation and the standard error.

8. **The answer is C: the paired t-test.** A t-test is appropriate whenever two means are being compared and the population data from which the observations are derived are normally distributed. When the two means are from distinct groups, a Student's t-test is appropriate, as discussed in this chapter. When the data represent pretrial and posttrial results for a single group of subjects (i.e., when subjects serve as their own controls), the paired t-test is appropriate. The calculations for the value of t in a paired t-test are provided in the chapter. The paired t-test is more apt to detect a statistically significant difference than the Student's t-test because the variation has been reduced to that from one group, rather than two groups.

9. **The answer is B: even if statistically significant, the difference cannot be clinically meaningful.** As discussed in the chapter, statistical significance and clinical significance are not synonymous. A clinically important intervention might fail to show statistical benefit over another intervention in a trial if the sample size is too small. A statistically significant difference in outcomes in a very large sample might be of no clinical impor-

tance. In the cholesterol-lowering diet described, mere inspection of the pretrial and posttrial data suggests that the data are unlikely to result in statistical significance, but one cannot be certain of this without formal hypothesis testing. However, the data clearly do not demonstrate a clinically meaningful effect, even if statistical significance is achieved (which it is not, by the way). Unlike statistical significance, which is purely numerical, clinical significance is the product of judgment.

10. **The answer is A: beta error.** A negative result in a trial may indicate that the null hypothesis is actually true, or it may be due to beta error (false-negative error). Beta error generally receives less attention in medicine than does alpha error. Consequently, the likelihood of a false-negative outcome is often unknown. A negative result can occur, for example, if the sample size is too small or if an inadequate dosage is administered. See Chapter 12 for further discussion of beta error and the related concept of power.

References Cited

Emerson, J. D., and G. A. Colditz. Use of statistical analysis. New England Journal of Medicine 309:709–713, 1983.

Moore, D. S., and G. P. McCabe. Introduction to the Practice of Statistics. New York, W. H. Freeman and Company, 1993.

Smith, R. P. Statistically speaking. Journal of Clinical Epidemiology 46:1293–1294, 1993.

Selected Readings

Dawson-Saunders, B., and R. G. Trapp. Basic and Clinical Biostatistics, 2nd ed. Norwalk, Conn., Appleton and Lange, 1994.

Inglefinger, J. A., et al. Biostatistics in Clinical Medicine, 2nd ed. New York, Macmillan Publishing Company, 1987.

11 Bivariate Analysis

A variety of statistical tests can be used to analyze the relationship between two or more variables. This chapter, like the previous chapter, focuses on **bivariate analysis,** which is the analysis of the relationship between one independent (possibly causal) variable and one dependent (outcome) variable. Chapter 13 will focus on **multivariable analysis,** or the analysis of the relationship of more than one independent variable to a single dependent variable. Statistical tests should be chosen only after the types of clinical data to be analyzed and the basic research design have been established. In general, the analytic approach should begin with a study of the individual variables, including their distributions and outliers, and with a search for errors. Then bivariate analysis can be done to test hypotheses and probe for relationships. Only after these procedures have been done carefully should multivariable analysis be attempted.

■ CHOOSING AN APPROPRIATE STATISTICAL TEST

Among the factors involved in choosing an appropriate statistical test are the goals and research design of the study and the type of data being gathered.

In some studies, the investigators are interested in descriptive information, such as the sensitivity or specificity of a laboratory assay, in which case there may be no reason to perform a test of statistical significance. In other studies, the investigators are interested in determining whether the difference between two means is real, in which case testing for statistical significance is appropriate.

As shown in Table 11–1, numerous tests of statistical significance are available for bivariate analysis. However, the types of variables and the research design set the limits to statistical analysis and determine which test or tests are appropriate. The four **types of variables** shown in the table are continuous data (e.g., levels of glucose in blood samples), ordinal data (e.g., rankings of very satisfied, satisfied, and unsatisfied), dichotomous data (e.g., alive versus dead), and nominal data (e.g., ethnic group). An investigator's knowledge of the types of variables and appropriate statistical tests is analogous to a painter's knowledge of the types of media (oils, tempera, water colors, and so forth) and the appropriate brushes and techniques to be used. If the **research design** involves before and after comparisons in the same study subjects or involves comparisons of matched pairs of study subjects, a paired test of statistical significance—such as the paired *t*-test, the Wilcoxon matched-pairs signed-ranks test, or the McNemar chi-square test—would be appropriate. Moreover, if the sampling procedure in a study is not random, statistical tests that assume random sampling, such as most of the parametric tests, may not be valid.

■ MAKING INFERENCES FROM CONTINUOUS (PARAMETRIC) DATA

Studies often involve one variable that is continuous and another variable that is not. As shown in Table 11–1, a *t*-test is appropriate for analyzing the relationship between one continuous and one dichotomous variable, while a one-way analysis of variance

TABLE 11–1   Choice of an Appropriate Statistical Significance Test to Be Used in Bivariate Analysis (Analysis of One Independent Variable and One Dependent Variable)

Variables to Be Tested			
First Variable	**Second Variable**	**Examples***	**Appropriate Test or Tests of Significance**
Continuous (C)	Continuous (C)	Age (C) and systolic blood pressure (C).	Pearson correlation coefficient *(r)*; linear regression.
Continuous (C)	Ordinal (O)	Age (C) and satisfaction (O).	Group the continuous variable and calculate Spearman correlation coefficient (rho); possibly use one-way analysis of variance (ANOVA, or *F*-test).
Continuous (C)	Dichotomous unpaired (DU)	Systolic blood pressure (C) and gender (DU).	Student's *t*-test.
Continuous (C)	Dichotomous paired (DP)	Difference in systolic blood pressure (C) before versus after treatment (DP).	Paired *t*-test.
Continuous (C)	Nominal (N)	Hemoglobin level (C) and blood type (N).	ANOVA (*F*-test).
Ordinal (O)	Ordinal (O)	Correlation of satisfaction with care (O) and severity of illness (O).	Spearman correlation coefficient (rho); Kendall correlation coefficient (tau).
Ordinal (O)	Dichotomous unpaired (DU)	Satisfaction (O) and gender (DU).	Mann-Whitney *U* test.
Ordinal (O)	Dichotomous paired (DP)	Difference in satisfaction (O) before versus after a program (DP).	Wilcoxon matched-pairs signed-ranks test.
Ordinal (O)	Nominal (N)	Satisfaction (O) and ethnicity (N).	Kruskal-Wallis test.
Dichotomous (D)	Dichotomous unpaired (DU)	Success/failure (D) in treated/untreated groups (DU).	Chi-square test; Fisher exact probability test.
Dichotomous (D)	Dichotomous paired (DP)	Change in success/failure (D) before versus after treatment (DP).	McNemar chi-square test.
Dichotomous (D)	Nominal (N)	Success/failure (D) and blood type (N).	Chi-square test.
Nominal (N)	Nominal (N)	Ethnicity (N) and blood type (N).	Chi-square test.

*The following is an example of satisfaction described by an ordinal scale: very satisfied, somewhat satisfied, neither satisfied nor dissatisfied, somewhat dissatisfied, and very dissatisfied.

(ANOVA) is appropriate for analyzing the relationship between one continuous and one nominal variable. Chapter 10 discusses the Student's and paired *t*-tests in detail (see the section entitled Use of *t*-Tests) and introduces the concept of ANOVA (see the section entitled Variation Between Groups Versus Variation Within Groups).

If a study involves two continuous variables, such as systolic blood pressure and diastolic blood pressure, the following questions may be answered: (1) Is there a real relationship between the variables or not? (2) If there is a real relationship, is it a positive or negative linear relationship (a straight line relationship), or is it more complex? (3) If there is a real relationship, how strong is it? (4) How likely is the relationship to be generalizable? The best way to answer these questions is first to plot the continuous data on a joint distribution graph and then to perform correlation analysis and simple linear regression analysis.

The Joint Distribution Graph

The raw data concerning the systolic and diastolic blood pressures of 26 young, healthy, adult subjects

were introduced in Chapter 10 and listed in Table 10–1. These same data can be plotted on a joint distribution graph, as shown in Fig. 11–1. The data do not form a perfectly straight line, but they do appear to lie along a straight line, going from the lower left to the upper right on the graph, and all of the observations but one are fairly close to the line.

As indicated in Fig. 11–2, the correlation between two variables, labeled *x* and *y*, can range from nonexistent to strong. If the value of *y* increases as *x* increases, the correlation is positive; if *y* decreases as *x* increases, the correlation is negative. It appears from the graph in Fig. 11–1 that the correlation between diastolic and systolic blood pressure is strong and is positive.

Therefore, based on Fig. 11–1, the answer to the first question above is that there is a real relationship between diastolic and systolic blood pressure. The graph, however, does not reveal the probability that such a relationship could have occurred by chance. The answer to the second question is that the relationship is positive and is linear. The graph does not provide quantitative information about how strong the association is (although it looks strong to the eye).

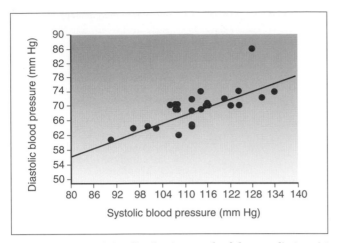

FIGURE 11–1   A joint distribution graph of the systolic (*x*-axis) and diastolic (*y*-axis) blood pressure values of 26 young, healthy, adult subjects. The raw data for these subjects are listed in Table 10–1. The correlation between the two variables is strong and is positive.

To answer these questions more precisely, it is necessary to use the techniques of correlation and simple linear regression. Neither the graph nor these techniques, however, can answer the question of how generalizable the findings are.

The Pearson Correlation Coefficient

Even without plotting the observations for two variables (variable *x* and variable *y*) on a graph, the extent of their linear relationship can be determined by calculating the **Pearson product-moment correlation**

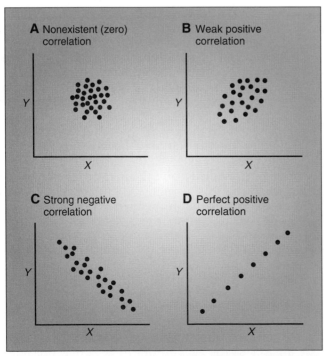

FIGURE 11–2   Four possible patterns in joint distribution graphs. As seen in these examples, the correlation between two continuous variables, labeled *x* and *y*, can range from nonexistent to perfect. If the value of *y* increases as *x* increases, the correlation is positive. If *y* decreases as *x* increases, the correlation is negative.

coefficient, which is given the symbol *r* and is referred to as the ***r* value.** This statistic varies from –1 to +1, going through 0. A finding of –1 indicates that the two variables have a perfect negative linear relationship; +1 indicates that they have a perfect positive linear relationship; and 0 indicates that the two variables are totally independent of each other. The *r* value is rarely found to be –1 or +1. Frequently, there is an imperfect correlation between the two variables, resulting in *r* values between 0 and 1 or between 0 and –1. Because the Pearson correlation coefficient is strongly influenced by extreme values, the value of *r* can only be trusted when the distribution of each of the two variables to be correlated is approximately normal (i.e., without severe skewness or extreme outlier values).

The formula for the correlation coefficient *r* is shown below. The numerator is the sum of the covariances. The **covariance** is the product of the deviation of an observation from the mean of the *x* variable multiplied by the same observation's deviation from the mean of the *y* variable. (When marked on a graph, this usually gives a rectangular area, in contrast to the sum of squares, in which the areas generated are squares of the deviation from the mean.) The denominator is the square root of the sum of the squared deviations from the mean of the *x* variable multiplied by the sum of the squared deviations from the mean of the *y* variable:

$$r = \frac{\sum (x_i - \bar{x})(y_i - \bar{y})}{\sqrt{\sum (x_i - \bar{x})^2 \sum (y_i - \bar{y})^2}}$$

Using statistical computer programs, investigators can determine whether the value of *r* is greater than would be expected by chance alone (i.e., whether the two variables are statistically associated). Most statistical programs provide the *p* value along with the correlation coefficient, but the *p* value of the correlation coefficient can easily be calculated. Its associated *t* can be calculated from the following formula, and then the *p* value can be determined from a table of *t* (Phillips 1978; Dawson-Saunders and Trapp 1994).

$$t = \frac{r\sqrt{N-2}}{\sqrt{1-r^2}}$$

$$df = N - 2$$

As is the case in every test of significance, for a fixed level of strength of association, the larger the sample size, the more likely it is to be statistically significant. A weak correlation in a large sample might be statistically significant, despite the fact that it was not etiologically or clinically important.

There is no perfect statistical way to estimate clinical importance, but with continuous variables a valuable concept is the **strength of the association,** measured by the square of the correlation coefficient, or r^2. The **r^2 value** is the proportion of variation in *y* explained by *x* (or vice versa). It is an important parameter in advanced statistics. Looking at the strength of association is analogous to looking at the

---

BOX 11–1   Analysis of the Relationship Between Height and Weight (Two Continuous Variables) in a Study of 8 Subjects

Part 1   Tabular and graphic representation of the data

Subject	Variable x (Height)	Variable y (Weight)
1	182.9 cm	78.5 kg
2	172.7 cm	60.8 kg
3	175.3 cm	68.0 kg
4	172.7 cm	65.8 kg
5	160.0 cm	52.2 kg
6	165.1 cm	54.4 kg
7	172.7 cm	60.3 kg
8	162.6 cm	52.2 kg

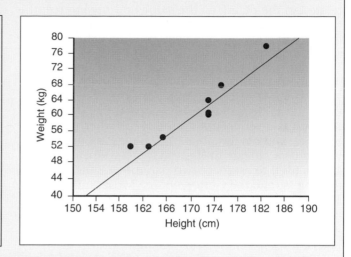

Part 2   Calculation of moments

$$\Sigma(x_i) = 1364.0 \text{ cm}$$

$$\Sigma(y_i) = 492.2 \text{ kg}$$

$$N = 8$$

$$\bar{x} = 1364.0/8 = 170.50 \text{ cm}$$

$$\bar{y} = 492.2/8 = 61.53 \text{ kg}$$

$$\Sigma(x_i - \bar{x})(y_i - \bar{y}) = 456.88$$

$$\Sigma(x_i - \bar{x})^2 = 393.1$$

$$\Sigma(y_i - \bar{y})^2 = 575.1$$

Note: Moments are various descriptors of a distribution, including the number of observations, the sum of their values, the mean, the variance, the standard deviation, and tests of normality.

Part 3   Calculation of the Pearson correlation coefficient (r) and the strength of the association of the variables (r²)

$$r = \frac{\sum (x_i - \bar{x})(y_i - \bar{y})}{\sqrt{\sum (x_i - \bar{x})^2 \sum (y_i - \bar{y})^2}}$$

$$= \frac{456.88}{\sqrt{(393.1)(575.1)}} = \frac{456.88}{\sqrt{226,071.8}} = \frac{456.88}{475.47} = 0.96$$

$$r^2 = (0.96)^2 = 0.92 = 92\%$$

Interpretation: The two variables are highly correlated. The association between the two variables is strong, with 92% of variation in weight (y) explained by variation in height (x).

Part 4   Calculation of the slope (b) for a regression of weight (y) on height (x)

$$b = \frac{\sum (x_i - \bar{x})(y_i - \bar{y})}{\sum (x_i - \bar{x})^2} = \frac{456.88}{393.1} = 1.16$$

Interpretation: There is a 1.16-kg increase in weight (y) for each 1-cm increase in height (x). The y-intercept, which indicates the value of x when y is 0, is not meaningful in the case of these two variables; therefore, it is not calculated here.

Source of data: Unpublished findings in a sample of 8 professional persons in Connecticut.

---

size and clinical importance of an observed difference, as discussed in Chapter 10.

For purposes of demonstrating the calculation of r and r^2, a small set of data is introduced in Box 11–1. The data, consisting of the observed heights (variable x) and weights (variable y) of 8 subjects, are presented first in tabular form and then in graph form. When r is calculated, the result is 0.96 (+0.96), which indicates a strong positive linear relationship and provides quantitative information to confirm what is visually apparent in the graph. Given that r is 0.96, then r^2 is $(0.96)^2$, or 0.92. A 0.92 strength of association means that 92% of the variation in weight is "explained" by height. Therefore, the remaining 8% of the variation is presumed to be due to factors other than height.

Linear Regression Analysis

Linear regression is related to correlation analysis, but it produces two parameters that can be directly related to the data (i.e., the slope and the intercept). Linear regression seeks to quantify the linear relationship that may exist between an independent variable x and a dependent variable y.

Recall that the formula for a straight line, as expressed in statistics, is $y = a + bx$ (see Chapter 10). The y is the value of an observation on the y-axis; x is the value of the same observation on the x-axis; a is the regression constant (the value of y when the value of x is 0); and b is the slope (the change in the value of y for a unit change in the value of x). Linear regression is used to estimate two parameters: the slope of the line (b) and the y-intercept (a). Most fundamental is the slope, which determines the strength of the impact of variable x on y. For example, the slope can tell how much weight will increase, on the average, for each additional centimeter of height.

When the usual statistical notation is used for a regression of y on x, the formulas for the slope (b) and y-intercept (a) are as follows:

$$b = \frac{\sum (x_i - \overline{x})(y_i - \overline{y})}{\sum (x_i - \overline{x})^2}$$

$$a = \overline{y} - b\overline{x}$$

Box 11–1 shows the calculation of the slope (b) for the observed heights and weights of 8 subjects. The graph in Box 11–1 shows the linear relationship between the height and weight data, with the regression line inserted. In these 8 subjects, the slope was 1.16, meaning that there was an average increase of 1.16 kg of weight for every 1 cm increase in height. Note that the slope does not appear greater than 45 degrees, as would be expected from a slope of 1.16, because the scale is compressed more tightly on the y-axis.

Linear regression analysis enables investigators to predict the value of y from the values that x takes. In other words, the formula for linear regression is a form of statistical modeling, and the adequacy of the model is determined by how closely the value of y can be predicted from the other data in the model. Just as it is possible to set confidence intervals around parameters such as means and proportions (see Chapter 10), it is possible to set confidence intervals around the slope and the intercept, using computations based on linear regression formulas. Most statistical computer programs perform these computations, and moderately advanced statistics books provide the formulas (see, for example, Kleinbaum and Kupper 1978).

Multiple linear regression and other methods involved in the analysis of more than two variables are discussed in Chapter 13.

■ MAKING INFERENCES FROM ORDINAL DATA

Many medical data are ordinal data, which are ranked from the lowest value to the highest value but are not measured on an exact scale. In some cases, investigators will assume that ordinal data meet the criteria for continuous (measurement) data and will treat the ordinal data as though they had been obtained from a measurement scale. For example, if the patients' satisfaction with the care in a given hospital were being studied, the investigators might assume that the conceptual distance between "very satisfied" (say, coded as a 3) and "fairly satisfied" (coded as a 2) is equal to the difference between "fairly satisfied" (coded as a 2) and "unsatisfied" (coded as a 1). If the investigators are willing to make these assumptions, the data can be analyzed using the parametric statistical methods discussed in this and the previous chapter, such as t-tests, analysis of variance, and analysis of the Pearson correlation coefficient. However, sometimes clinical investigators make this assumption when it is inappropriate, because the statistics are easier to obtain and are more likely to produce statistical significance.

If the investigator is unwilling to make such assumptions, statistics for discrete (nonparametric) data, such as a chi-square test (see below), can be used. However, analysis using chi-square would require discarding the information about the rank of each observation. Fortunately, there are a number of bivariate statistical tests for ordinal data that can be used. These tests are listed in Table 11–1 and described briefly below. For more details, see Dawson-Saunders and Trapp (1994) or Siegel (1956). Hand calculation of these tests for ordinal data is extremely tedious and invites errors. Therefore, no examples are given here, and the use of a computer for these calculations is strongly recommended.

The Mann-Whitney *U* Test

The test for ordinal data that is similar to the Student's t-test is the Mann-Whitney U test, also called the **Wilcoxon rank-sum test.** U, like t, designates a probability distribution. In the Mann-Whitney test, all of the observations in a study of two samples are ranked numerically from the smallest to the largest, without regard to whether the observations came from the first sample (e.g., the control group) or from the second sample (e.g., the experimental group). Next, the observations from the first sample are identified, the ranks in this sample are summed, and the average rank for the first sample and the variance of those ranks are determined. The process is repeated for the observations from the second sample. If the null hypothesis is true (i.e., if there is no real difference between the two samples), the average ranks of the two samples should be similar. If the average rank of one sample is considerably greater or considerably smaller than that of the other sample, the null hypothesis probably can be rejected, but a test of significance is needed to be sure. Because the U-test method for calculating t is tedious, a t-test can be done instead and will yield very similar results (Dawson-Saunders and Trapp 1994). The Student's t-test uses the raw ranked data and divides the difference between the two average ranks (which form the numerator) by the square root of the pooled variances of the two rank lists. The degrees of freedom equals the sum of the sample sizes of the two groups minus 2.

The Wilcoxon Matched-Pairs Signed-Ranks Test

The rank-order test that is comparable to the paired *t*-test is the Wilcoxon matched-pairs signed-ranks test. In this test, all of the observations in a study of two samples are ranked numerically from the largest to the smallest, without regard to whether the observations came from the first sample (e.g., the pretreatment sample) or from the second sample (e.g., the posttreatment sample). After pairs of data are identified (e.g., pretreatment and posttreatment samples are matched), the difference in rank is identified for each pair. If in a given pair the pretreatment observation scored 7 ranks higher than the posttreatment observation, the difference would be noted as −7. If in another pair the pretreatment observation scored 5 ranks lower than the posttreatment observation, the difference would be noted as +5. Each pair would be scored in this way. If the null hypothesis is true (i.e., if there is no real difference between the samples), the sum of the positive scores and negative scores should be close to 0. If the average difference is considerably different from 0, the null hypothesis can be rejected.

The Kruskal-Wallis Test

If the investigators in a study involving continuous data want to compare the means of three or more groups simultaneously, the appropriate test is a one-way analysis of variance (a one-way ANOVA), usually called an *F*-test. The comparable test for ordinal data is called the Kruskal-Wallis test or the **Kruskal-Wallis one-way ANOVA.** As in the Mann-Whitney *U* test (see above), in the Kruskal-Wallis test all of the data are ranked numerically, and the rank values are summed in each of the groups to be compared. The Kruskal-Wallis test seeks to determine if the average ranks from three or more groups differ from one another more than would be expected by chance alone.

The Spearman and the Kendall Correlation Coefficients

When relating two continuous variables to each other, investigators can use regression analysis or correlation analysis. For ordinal variables, there is no test comparable to regression, because it is difficult to see how a "slope" could be measured without assuming an underlying measurement scale. However, for ordinal data, there are several tests comparable to correlation, the two most common of which are briefly described here. The first is the **Spearman rank correlation coefficient,** which is symbolized by **rho** and is similar to *r*. The second is the **Kendall rank correlation coefficient,** which is symbolized by **tau.** The tests for rho and tau will usually give similar re-

sults, but the rho is usually used in the medical literature, perhaps because of its conceptual similarity to the Pearson *r*. The tau may give better results with small sample sizes.

The Sign Test

Sometimes an experimental intervention produces positive results in many areas, but few if any of the individual outcome variables show a statistically significant improvement. In this case, the sign test can be extremely helpful in comparing the results in the experimental group with those in the control group. If the null hypothesis is true (i.e., there is no real difference between the groups), then, by chance, for half of the outcome variables the experimental group should perform better, and for half of the outcome variables the control group should perform better.

The only data needed for the sign test are the record of whether, on the average, the experimental subjects or the control subjects scored "better" on each outcome variable (by what amount is not important). If the average score in the experimental group is better, the result is recorded as a plus sign (+); if the average score in the control group is better, the result is recorded as a minus sign (−); and if the average score in the two groups is exactly the same, no result is recorded and the variable is omitted from the analysis. For the sign test, "better" can be determined from a continuous variable, an ordinal variable, a dichotomous variable, a clinical score, or a component of a score. Because under the null hypothesis, the expected proportion of plus signs is 0.5 and of minus signs is 0.5, the test compares the observed proportion of successes with the expected value of 0.5.

■ MAKING INFERENCES FROM DICHOTOMOUS AND NOMINAL (NONPARAMETRIC) DATA

As indicated in Table 11–1, the chi-square test, the Fisher exact probability test, and the McNemar chi-square test can be used in the bivariate analysis of dichotomous nonparametric data. Usually, the data are first arranged in a 2 × 2 table, and the goal is to test the null hypothesis that the variables are independent.

The 2 × 2 Contingency Table

Data arranged as in Box 11–2 form what is known as a contingency table because it is used to determine whether the distribution of one variable is conditionally dependent (contingent) upon the other variable. More specifically, Box 11–2 provides an example of a 2 × 2 contingency table, meaning that it has two cells in each direction. In this case, the table shows the data for a study of 91 patients who had a myocardial infarction (Snow 1965). One variable is treatment

BOX 11–2 Chi-Square Analysis of the Relationship Between Treatment and Outcome (Two Nonparametric Variables, Unpaired) in a Study of 91 Subjects

Part 1 Beginning data, presented in a 2 × 2 contingency table, where *O* denotes observed counts and *E* denotes expected counts

			OUTCOME					
			Survival for at Least 28 Days		Death		Total	
			Number	(Percentage)	Number	(Percentage)	Number	(Percentage)
	Propranolol	*(O)*	38	(84)	7	(16)	45	(100)
	Propranolol	*(E)*	33.13		11.87		45	
TREATMENT								
	Placebo	*(O)*	29	(63)	17	(37)	46	(100)
	Placebo	*(E)*	33.87		12.13		46	
	Total		67	(74)	24	(26)	91	(100)

Part 2 Calculation of the chi-square (χ^2) value

$$\chi^2 = \sum \left[\frac{(O-E)^2}{E} \right]$$

$$= \frac{(38-33.13)^2}{33.13} + \frac{(7-11.87)^2}{11.87} + \frac{(29-33.87)^2}{33.87} + \frac{(17-12.13)^2}{12.13}$$

$$= \frac{(4.87)^2}{33.13} + \frac{(-4.87)^2}{11.87} + \frac{(-4.87)^2}{33.87} + \frac{(4.87)^2}{12.13}$$

$$= \frac{23.72}{33.13} + \frac{23.72}{11.87} + \frac{23.72}{33.87} + \frac{23.72}{12.13}$$

$$= 0.72 + 2.00 + 0.70 + 1.96 = \mathbf{5.38}$$

Part 3 Calculation of the degrees of freedom *(df)* for a contingency table, based on the number of rows *(R)* and columns *(C)*

$$df = (R-1)(C-1) = (2-1)(2-1) = 1$$

Part 4 Determination of the *p* value

Value from the chi-square table for 5.38 on 1 *df*: $0.01 < p < 0.025$ (statistically significant)

Exact *p* from a computer program: 0.0205 (statistically significant)

Interpretation: The results noted in this 2 × 2 table are statistically significant. That is, it is highly probable (only 1 chance in about 50 of being wrong) that the investigator can reject the null hypothesis of independence and accept the alternative hypothesis that propranolol does affect the outcome of myocardial infarction in a positive direction.

Source of data: Snow, P. J. Effect of propranolol in myocardial infarction. Lancet 2:551–553, 1965.

(propranolol versus a placebo), and the other is outcome (survival for at least 28 days versus death within 28 days).

In a contingency table, a **cell** is a specific location in the matrix created by the two variables whose relationship is being studied. Each cell shows the observed number, the expected number, and the percentage of study subjects in each treatment group who lived or died. For example, in Box 11–2, the top left cell indicates that 38 patients who were treated with propranolol survived the first 28 days of observation, that the 38 patients represented 84% of all patients who were treated with propranolol, and that 33.13 patients treated with propranolol were ex-

pected to survive the first 28 days of observation. The methods for calculating the percentages and expected counts are discussed below.

The other three cells indicate the same type of data (observed number, expected number, and percentage) for those who died after propranolol treatment, those who survived after placebo treatment, and those who died after placebo treatment. The bottom row shows the column totals, and the right-hand column shows the row totals.

If there are more than two cells in each direction of a contingency table, the table is called an *R* × *C* table, where *R* stands for the number of rows and *C* stands for the number of columns. Although the principles of the chi-square test are valid for $R \times C$ tables, the discussion below focuses on 2×2 tables.

The Chi-Square Test of Independence

After t-tests, the most basic and common form of statistical analysis in the medical literature is the chi-square test of the independence of two variables in a contingency table (Emerson and Colditz 1983). The chi-square test is an example of a common approach to statistical analysis known as **statistical modeling,** which seeks to develop a statistical expression (the model) that predicts the behavior of a dependent variable on the basis of knowledge of one or more independent variables. The process of comparing the **observed counts** with the **expected counts**—that is, of comparing O with E—is called a **goodness-of-fit test,** because the goal is to see how well the observed counts in a contingency table "fit" the counts expected on the basis of the model. Usually, the model in such a table is the null hypothesis that the two variables are independent of each other. If the chi-square value is small, the fit is good and the null hypothesis is not rejected. If, however, the chi-square value is large, the data do not fit the hypothesis well.

Box 11–2 will be used here to illustrate the steps and considerations involved both in constructing a 2×2 contingency table and in calculating the chi-square value. For the data presented in Box 11–2, the **null hypothesis** is that the method of treating the myocardial infarction patients did not influence the proportion of patients who survived for at least 28 days. The **alternative hypothesis** is that the outcome (survival or death) depended on the treatment, meaning that the outcome was the **dependent variable** and the treatment was the **independent variable.**

Calculation of Percentages

Each of the four cells of Box 11–2 shows an observed count (or O) and a percentage. The percentage in the first cell of the contingency table was calculated by dividing the number of propranolol-treated patients who survived (38) by the total number of propranolol-treated patients (45), with the result being 84%. Thus, the percentage was calculated as the frequency distribution of the dependent variable, which in this case was survival, reflecting the fact that survival was contingent (dependent) on treatment.

If treatment depended on survival, rather than vice versa, the percentage would be calculated by dividing the number of propranolol-treated patients who survived (38) by the total number of survivors (67). Although the way in which the percentages are calculated does not affect the chi-square test, it does affect the way in which people think about and interpret the data. Therefore, the appropriate way to calculate the percentages in a contingency table is to determine which of the variables is the dependent one and

then calculate the frequency distribution of that variable within each level of the independent variable.

Calculation of Expected Counts

In Box 11–2, the propranolol-treated group consists of 45 patients, the placebo-treated group consists of 46 patients, and the total for the study is therefore 91 patients. While the observed counts indicate how many of each group actually survived, the expected counts indicate how many of each group would be expected to survive if the method of treatment made no difference whatsoever (i.e., if survival were independent of treatment).

The general formula for calculating the expected count in the top left cell of a contingency table is as follows:

$$E_{1,1} = \frac{\text{Row}_1 \text{ total}}{\text{Study total}} \times \text{Column}_1 \text{ total}$$

where $E_{1,1}$ is defined as the cell in row_1, column_1.

In Box 11–2, for example, if survival were independent of the treatment group, 45/91 (or 49.45%) of the observations in each column would be expected to be in the top row, because that is the overall proportion of patients who received propranolol. It follows that 0.4945×67 (or 33.13) observations (the total in column_1) would be expected in the top left cell, while 0.4945×24 (or 11.87) observations (the total in column_2) would be expected in the top right cell. Note that the expected counts may include fractions and that the sum of the expected counts in a given row will equal the sum of the observed counts in that row ($33.13 + 11.87 = 45$). By the same logic, 50.55% of observations would be expected to be in the bottom row, with 33.87 in the left bottom cell and 12.13 in the right bottom cell, so that the row total equals the sum of the observed counts ($33.87 + 12.13 = 46$). Finally, as shown in Box 11–2, the column totals for expected counts should add up to the column totals for observed counts.

The expected counts in each cell of a 2×2 contingency table should equal five or more or the assumptions and approximations inherent in the chi-square test may break down. For a study involving a larger contingency table (an $R \times C$ table), the investigator can usually compromise on this slightly by allowing 20% of the expected counts to be less than five but at the same time making sure that none of the expected counts is less than two. If these conditions are not met and the table is a 2×2 table, the Fisher exact probability test (see below) should be used instead of the chi-square test. If the conditions are not met and the table is larger than a 2×2 table, the best solution is to combine (collapse) categories. For example, if the variable were "ethnic group" and it had seven categories, for many geographic areas of the USA there might be few persons other than African-Americans, Caucasians, or Hispanics. Under the circumstances, the Asians, Native Americans, Pacific Islanders, and members of other ethnic groups might be combined into one category called "other." This might give enough numbers in the revised "other" category that the expected counts would be large enough to use the chi-square test.

Calculation of the Chi-Square Value

Once the observed *(O)* and expected *(E)* counts are known, the chi-square (χ^2) value can be calculated. One of two methods can be used, depending on the size of the counts.

Method for Large Numbers. In Box 11–2, the investigators begin by calculating the chi-square value for each cell in the table, using the following formula:

$$\frac{(O-E)^2}{E}$$

Here, the numerator is the square of the deviation of the observed count in a given cell from the count that would be expected in that cell if the null hypothesis were true. This is similar to the numerator of the variance, which is expressed as $(x_i - \overline{x})^2$, where x_i represents the observed value and $\overline{x}$ (the mean) is the expected value (see Chapter 9). However, whereas the denominator for variance is the degrees of freedom $(N-1)$, the denominator for chi-square is the expected number *(E)*.

To obtain the total chi-square value for a 2×2 table, the investigators then add up the chi-square values for the four cells:

$$\chi^2 = \sum \left[\frac{(O-E)^2}{E} \right]$$

Thus, the basic statistical method for measuring the total amount of variation in a data set, the total sum of squares (TSS), is rewritten for the chi-square test as the sum of $(O-E)^2$.

Box 11–2 shows how chi-square is calculated for the study of 91 patients with myocardial infarction. Before the result (chi-square value = 5.38) can be interpreted, the degrees of freedom must be determined (see below).

Method for Small Numbers. Because the chi-square test is based on the normal approximation of the binomial distribution (which is discontinuous), many statisticians believe that a correction for continuity is needed in the equation for calculating chi-square, while others believe that this is unnecessary. The correction, originally described by F. Yates and called the **Yates correction for continuity,** makes little difference if the numbers in the table are large, but in tables with small numbers it probably is worth doing. The only change in the chi-square test formula given above is that in the continuity-corrected chi-square test, the number 0.5 is subtracted from the absolute value of the $(O - E)$ in each cell before squaring. The formula is as follows:

$$\text{Yates } \chi^2 = \sum \left[\frac{(|O-E| - 0.5)^2}{E} \right]$$

Clearly, the use of this formula reduces the size of the chi-square value somewhat and reduces the chance of finding a statistically significant difference, so that correction for continuity makes the test more conservative.

Determination of the Degrees of Freedom

As discussed in Chapter 10 and Box 10–2, the term "degrees of freedom" refers to the number of observations that can be considered to be free to vary. According to the null hypothesis, the best estimate of the expected distribution of counts in the cells of a contingency table is provided by the row and column totals. Therefore, the row and column totals are considered to be "fixed," as is the mean in caculating a variance (see Chapter 10). An observed count can be entered "freely" into one of the cells of a 2×2 table (e.g., the top left cell), but once that count is entered, none of the other three cells are free to vary. This means that a 2×2 table has only 1 degree of freedom.

Another look at Box 11–2 will help explain why there is only 1 degree of freedom in a table with two rows and two columns. If 38 is entered freely in the top left cell, the only possible number that can go in the cell immediately to the right of it is 7, because the two numbers in the top row must equal the fixed row total of 45. Similarly, the only possible number that can go in the cell below the one containing 38 is the number 29, because the column must add up to 67. Finally, the only possible number that can go in the remaining cell is 17, because the row total must equal 46 and the column total must equal 24.

The same principle applies to tables with more than two rows and columns. In $R \times C$ contingency tables, imagine that the right-hand column and the bottom row are never free to vary, because they must consist of the numbers that make the totals come out right. This is illustrated in Fig. 11–3, where the cells that are free to vary are shown in white, the cells that are not free to vary are shown in light orange, and the fixed row and column totals are shown in dark orange. Therefore, the formula for degrees of freedom in a contingency table of any size is as follows:

$$df = (R-1)(C-1)$$

where *df* denotes degrees of freedom, *R* is the number of rows, and *C* is the number of columns.

Interpretation of the Results

After the chi-square value and the degrees of freedom are known, a standard table of chi-square values (see the Appendix) can be consulted to determine the corresponding *p* value. The *p* value indicates the probability that a chi-square value that large would have resulted from chance alone. For data shown in Box 11–2, the chi-square value was 5.38 on 1 degree of freedom, and the *p* value listed in the standard table for a two-tailed test was between 0.01 and 0.025 $(0.01 < p < 0.025)$. Most computer programs will

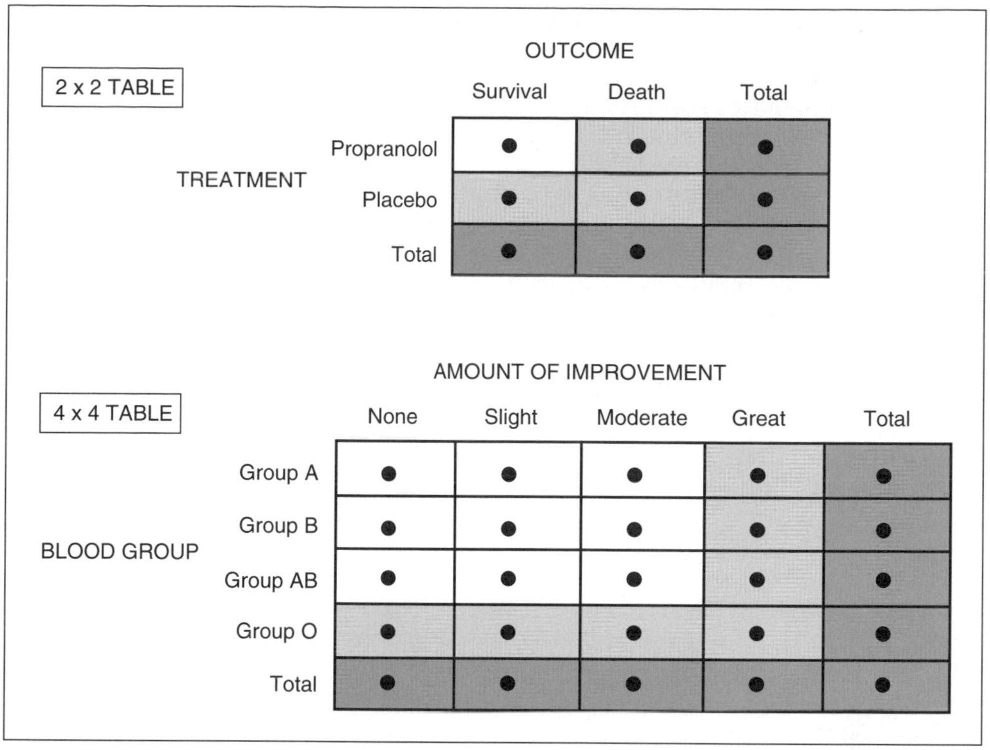

FIGURE 11–3 Conceptualization of the calculation of the degrees of freedom *(df)* in a 2 × 2 contingency table (top) and in a 4 × 4 contingency table (bottom). A white cell is free to vary; a light orange cell is not free to vary; and a dark orange cell is a row or column total. The formula is $df = (R - 1)(C - 1)$, where R denotes the number of rows and C denotes the number of columns. For the 2 × 2 table, $df = 1$. For the 4 × 4 table, $df = 9$.

provide the exact p value when calculating a chi-square; for the data in Box 11–2, the p value was 0.0205. Because the observed p was less than alpha (alpha = 0.05), the results were considered statistically significant.

If the chi-square value for the data in Box 11–2 had been calculated using the Yates correction, the result would have been 4.32, instead of 5.38, and the corresponding p value would have been somewhat larger (0.0376). Nevertheless, the results still would be statistically significant at the alpha = 0.05 level.

For the study of 91 patients reported in Box 11–2, the null hypothesis was that the outcome (survival versus death) was not related to the method of treatment (propranolol versus placebo). Because 24 of the total of 91 patients (26%) died, if the treatment had had no effect, the investigator would expect about 26% of the propranolol-treated patients and 26% of the placebo-treated patients to have died. Because the proportion who survived in each treatment group differed significantly from this expectation, the null hypothesis of independence between the variables can be rejected, and the alternative hypothesis that treatment had an effect on the survival rate can be accepted.

Note that the alternative hypothesis tested does not state whether the effect of the treatment would be to increase or decrease survival. This is because the null hypothesis was only that there would be no difference. In other words, the null hypothesis as stated required a two-tailed test of statistical significance (see Chapter 10). The investigator could have tested the null hypothesis that the propranolol-treated group would show a higher sur-

vival rate than the placebo-treated group, but this would have required interpreting the chi-square value as a one-tailed test of statistical significance. The choice of a one-tailed versus a two-tailed test does not affect the performance of a statistical test but does affect how the critical ratio thus obtained is converted to a p value in a statistical table. The direction of difference is obvious by inspection.

The Chi-Square Test for Paired Data (McNemar Test)

The chi-square test above was useful for comparing the distribution of a categorical variable in two or more different groups, but a new test is needed to compare before and after findings in the same individual or to compare findings in a matched analysis. The McNemar chi-square test does this for dichotomous variables.

The McNemar Test of Before and After Comparisons

In the discussion of t-tests in Chapter 10, it was noted that a study subject in a before and after study serves as his or her own control. For this reason, it was appropriate to use the paired t-test, instead of the Student's t-test. In the case of chi-square analysis, it would be appropriate to use the McNemar test, which is a modified chi-square test of data with 1 degree of freedom (Dawson-Saunders and Trapp 1994).

Suppose, for example, that an investigator wanted to compare the attitudes of the faculty of a certain medical school toward the second-year medical students before and after the "Second-Year Show," an event in which students traditionally perform skits about medical school life, often portraying favorite faculty with gentle humor and less-liked faculty with negative humor. Next, suppose that 200 faculty were asked to fill out questionnaires about their feelings toward the second-year medical students before and after attending the performance and that their responses were recorded as either positive or negative (i.e., dichotomous responses). The data could be set up in a 2×2 table with the preshow opinion on the left axis and the postshow opinion at the top, as shown in Box 11–3, and with each of the four cells representing one of the following four possible combinations: cell a = positive opinion before and after (no change); cell b = change from positive to negative opinion; cell c = change from negative to positive opinion; and cell d = negative opinion

before and after (no change). According to the hypothetical data from 200 faculty who participated in the study, the overall percentage reporting a favorable opinion of second-year students dropped from 86% (172/200) before the show to 79% (158/200) after the show, presumably reflecting a change in those faculty who were not treated kindly in the show. The null hypothesis to be tested is that the show produced no true change in faculty opinion about students, and the following formula would be used:

$$\text{McNemar } \chi^2 = \frac{(|b-c|-1)^2}{b+c}$$

Note that the formula uses only cells b and c in the 2×2 table. This is because cells a and d do not

---

BOX 11–3 McNemar Chi-Square Analysis of the Relationship Between Data Before and Data After an Event (Two Dichotomous Variables, Paired) in a Study of 200 Subjects (Fictitious Data)

Part 1 Standard 2 × 2 table format on which equations are based

		FINDINGS AFTER EVENT		Total
		Positive	Negative	
FINDINGS BEFORE EVENT	Positive	a	b	$a+b$
	Negative	c	d	$c+d$
	Total	$a+c$	$b+d$	$a+b+c+d$

Part 2 Data for a study of the opinions of medical school faculty toward second-year medical students before and after seeing a show presented by the students

		POSTSHOW OPINION		Total
		Positive	Negative	
PRESHOW OPINION	Positive	150	22	172
	Negative	8	20	28
	Total	158	42	200

Part 3 Calculation of the McNemar chi-square (χ^2) value

$$\text{McNemar } \chi^2 = \frac{(|b-c|-1)^2}{b+c}$$

$$= \frac{(|22-8|-1)^2}{22+8} = \frac{(13)^2}{30} = \frac{169}{30} = 5.63$$

Part 4 Calculation of the degrees of freedom (df) for a contingency table, based on the number of rows (R) and columns (C)

$$df = (R-1)(C-1) = (2-1)(2-1) = 1$$

Part 5 Determination of the p value

Value from the chi-square table for 5.63 on 1 df: $p < 0.025$ (statistically significant)

Interpretation: A statistically significant difference was noted between the faculty preshow opinion and postshow opinion. Specifically, if faculty changed their attitude toward second-year medical students after the show, most of these changes were from a positive attitude to a negative attitude, rather than vice versa.

change and therefore do not contribute to the standard error. Note also that the formula tests data with 1 degree of freedom, using a correction for continuity.

The McNemar chi-square value for the data shown in Box 11–3 is 5.63. This result is statistically significant ($p < 0.025$), so that the null hypothesis is rejected. Care must be taken in interpreting these data, however, because the test of significance only says the following: Among those faculty who *changed* their opinion, significantly more changed from positive to negative than vice versa.

The McNemar Test of Matched Data

In medical research, the McNemar chi-square test is often used in case-control studies, where the cases and controls are matched on the basis of some characteristics such as age, sex, and residence and then are compared for the presence or absence of a specific risk factor. Under these circumstances, the data can be set up in a 2×2 table similar to that shown in the first part of Box 11–4.

For purposes of illustrating the use of the McNemar test in matched data, the observations made by Cohen (1977) in a case-control study are discussed here and reported in the second part of Box 11–4. In this study, the investigator wanted to examine the association between mycosis fungoides (a type of lymphoma that begins in the skin and eventually spreads to internal organs) and a history of employment in an industrial environment with exposure to cutting oils. After matching 54 subjects who had the disease (the cases) with 54 subjects who did not have the disease (the controls), Cohen recorded whether or not the study subjects had a history of this type of industrial employment.

When the McNemar chi-square formula was used to test the null hypothesis that prior occupation was not associated with the development of mycosis fungoides (see Box 11–4), the chi-square value was 5.06. Because the result was statistically significant ($p = 0.021$), the null hypothesis could be rejected, and the alternative hypothesis that industrial exposure was associated with mycosis fungoides could be accepted.

Note that for Cohen's data, a **matched odds ratio** can also be calculated (see Chapter 6). When the data are set up as in Box 11–4, the ratio is calculated as b/c. Here, the ratio is 13/3, or 4.33, indicating that the odds of acquiring mycosis fungoides was over 4 times as great in those with a history of industrial exposure as in those without such a history.

The Fisher Exact Probability Test

When one or more of the expected counts in a 2×2 table is small (i.e., less than two), the chi-square test cannot be used. However, it is possible to calculate the exact probability of finding the observed numbers by using the Fisher exact probability test. The formula is as follows:

$$\text{Fisher } p = \frac{(a+b)\,!\,(c+d)\,!\,(a+c)\,!\,(b+d)\,!}{N\,!\,a\,!\,b\,!\,c\,!\,d\,!}$$

where p is probability; a, b, c, and d denote values in the top left, top right, bottom left, and bottom right cells, respectively, in a 2×2 table; N is the total number of observations; and ! is the symbol for factorial. (The factorial of $4 = 4! = 4 \times 3 \times 2 \times 1$.)

The Fisher exact probability is extremely tedious to calculate unless the investigator has a calculator with a function key that determines factorials. Moreover, unless one of the four cells contains a 0, the sum of more than one calculation is needed. For this reason, it is strongly recommended that the calculation be done using a computer statistical package. Most commercially available statistical packages now calculate the Fisher probability automatically when an appropriate situation arises in a 2×2 table.

Standard Errors for Data in 2×2 Tables

Standard errors for proportions, risk ratios, and odds ratios are sometimes calculated for data in 2×2 tables, although they are not used for data in larger $R \times C$ tables.

Standard Error for a Proportion

In a 2×2 table, the proportion of success (defined, for example, as survival) can be determined for each of the two levels (categories) of the independent variable, and the standard error can be calculated for each of these proportions. This is of value when the primary study objective was to estimate the true proportions of success in each of the two groups, rather than to compare the rates of success.

For example, in Box 11–2, the proportion of 28-day survivors in the propranolol-treated group was 0.84 (shown as 84% in the percentage column), and the proportion of 28-day survivors in the placebo-treated group was 0.63. Knowing this information allows the investigator to calculate both the standard error and the 95% confidence interval for each survival percentage by the methods described earlier (see Use of z-Tests, under Tests of Statistical Significance in Chapter 10). When the calculations are performed for the proportions surviving in Box 11–2, the 95% confidence interval for the propranolol-treated group is expressed as (0.73, 0.95), meaning that the true proportion probably is between 0.73 and 0.95, while the confidence interval for the placebo-treated group is expressed as (0.49, 0.77).

Standard Error for a Risk Ratio

If a 2×2 table is used to compare the proportion of disease in two different exposure groups or is used to compare the proportion of success in two different treatment groups, the relative risk or relative success

BOX 11–4 McNemar Chi-Square Analysis of the Relationship Between Data from Cases and Data from Controls (Two Dichotomous Variables, Paired) in a Case-Control Study of 54 Subjects

Part 1 Standard 2 × 2 table format on which equations are based

		CONTROLS		
		Risk Factor Present	Risk Factor Absent	Total
CASES	Risk Factor Present	a	b	$a + b$
	Risk Factor Absent	c	d	$c + d$
	Total	$a + c$	$b + d$	$a + b + c + d$

Part 2 Data for a case-control study of the relationship between mycosis fungoides (the disease) and a history of exposure to an industrial environment containing cutting oils (the risk factor)

		CONTROLS		
		History of Industrial Exposure	No History of Industrial Exposure	Total
CASES	History of Industrial Exposure	16	13	29
	No History of Industrial Exposure	3	22	25
	Total	19	35	54

Part 3 Calculation of the McNemar chi-square (χ^2) value

$$\text{McNemar } \chi^2 = \frac{(\mid b - c \mid - 1)^2}{b + c}$$

$$= \frac{(\mid 13 - 3 \mid - 1)^2}{13 + 3} = \frac{(9)^2}{16} = \frac{81}{16} = \mathbf{5.06}$$

Part 4 Calculation of the degrees of freedom (df) for a contingency table, based on the number of rows (R) and columns (C)

$$df = (R - 1)(C - 1) = (2 - 1)(2 - 1) = \mathbf{1}$$

Part 5 Determination of the p value

Value from the chi-square table for 5.06 on 1 df: $p = 0.021$ (statistically significant)

Interpretation: The data presented in this 2 × 2 table are statistically significant. The cases (subjects with mycosis fungoides) were more likely than expected by chance alone to have been exposed to an industrial environment with cutting oils than were the controls (subjects without mycosis fungoides).

Part 6 Calculation of the odds ratio (OR)

$$\text{OR} = b/c = 13/3 = \mathbf{4.33}$$

Interpretation: When a case and a matched control differed in their history of exposure to cutting oils, the odds that the case was exposed was 4.33 times as great as the odds that the control was exposed.

Source of data: Cohen, S. R. Mycosis fungoides: clinicopathologic relationships, survival, and therapy in 54 patients, with observation on occupation as a new prognostic factor. Master's thesis, Yale University School of Medicine, New Haven, Conn., 1977.

can be expressed as a risk ratio. Standard errors can be set around the risk ratio, and if the 95% confidence limits exclude the value of 1.0, there is a statistically significant difference between the risks, at an alpha level of 5%.

For example, in Box 11–2, because the proportion of 28-day survivors in the propranolol-treated group was 0.84 and the proportion of 28-day survivors in the placebo-treated group was 0.63, the risk ratio was 0.84/0.63, or 1.34. This ratio indicates that for the myocardial infarction patients studied, the 28-day survival probability with propranolol was 34% better than that with placebo.

There are several approaches to computing the standard error of a risk ratio. All of the methods are complicated, and they produce somewhat different estimates, so the methods will not be shown here. One or another of these methods is provided in every major statistical computer package. When the risk ratio in Box 11–2 is analyzed by the Taylor series approach used in the EPIINFO 5.01 computer package (Dean et al. 1991), for example, the 95% confidence interval around the risk ratio of 1.34 is reported as (1.04, 1.73). This means that the risk ratio has a 95% probability of being between 1.04 and 1.73. This finding confirms the chi-square test finding of statistical significance, because the 95% confidence interval does not include a risk ratio of 1.0 (which means no difference between the groups).

Standard Error for an Odds Ratio

If a 2×2 table provides data from a case-control study, the odds ratio can be calculated. Even though Box 11–2 is best analyzed by a risk ratio, because the study method is a cohort study (randomized control trial) rather than a case-control study, the odds ratio can also be examined. Here the odds of surviving in the propranolol-treated group are 38/7, or 5.43, and the odds of surviving in the placebo-treated group are 29/17, or 1.71. The odds ratio is therefore 5.43/1.71, or 3.18, which is much larger than the risk ratio. As was emphasized in Chapter 6, the odds ratio is a good estimate of the risk ratio only if the risk being studied by a case-control study is rare. Since the risk event (mortality) in Box 11–2 is not rare, the odds ratio is not a good estimate of the risk ratio.

Calculating the standard error for an odds ratio is also a complicated process and will not be discussed here. When the odds ratio in Box 11–2 is analyzed by the Cornfield approach used in the EPIINFO 5.01 computer package (Dean et al. 1991), the 95% confidence interval around the odds ratio of 3.18 is reported as (1.06, 9.85). The lower limit estimate of 1.06 with the odds ratio is close to the lower limit estimate of 1.04 with the risk ratio, so this approach also confirms statistical significance. However, the upper limit estimate for the odds ratio is much larger than that for the risk ratio, because the odds ratio itself is much larger than the risk ratio.

Strength of Association and Clinical Utility of Data in 2 × 2 Tables

Earlier in this chapter, the strength of association between two continuous variables was measured as r^2. For the data shown in 2×2 tables, an alternative method is used to estimate the strength of association. A fictitious scenario and set of data will be used here to illustrate how to determine strength of association and why it is important to examine associations for strength as well as statistical significance.

Assume that an eager male student was pursuing a master's degree and based his thesis on a study to determine if there was a true difference between the results of a certain blood test in males and the results in females. After obtaining the data shown in the first part of Box 11–5, he calculated the chi-square value and found that the difference between findings in males and findings in females was not statistically significant ($p = 0.572$). His advisor pointed out that even if the difference had been statistically significant, the data would not have been clinically useful because of the small gender difference in the proportion of subjects with positive findings in the blood test (52% of males versus 48% of females).

This eager student, however, decided to obtain a Ph.D. and to base his dissertation on a continued study of the same topic. Believing that small numbers were the problem with the master's thesis, he decided to obtain blood test findings this time in a sample of 20,000 subjects, half from each gender. As shown in the second part of Box 11–5, the difference in proportions was the same as before (52% of males versus 48% of females), so the results were still clinically unimportant (i.e., trivial). However, now the student had obtained (perhaps felt "rewarded" with) a statistical association that was highly significant ($p < 0.0001$).

Findings can have statistical significance and at the same time be of no clinical value, especially if the study involves a large number of subjects. This example shows an interesting point: because the sample size in the Ph.D. study was 100 times as large as that in the master's study, the chi-square value for the data in the Ph.D. study was also 100 times as large. It would be helpful to measure the strength of the association in Box 11–5, in order to show that the magnitude of the association was not important, even though it was statistically significant.

In 2×2 tables, the strength of association is measured using the **phi coefficient,** which basically adjusts the chi-square value for the sample size and can be considered the correlation coefficient (r) for the data in a 2×2 table. The formula is as follows:

$$\text{phi} = \sqrt{\frac{\chi^2}{N}}$$

The phi value in the first part of Box 11–5 is the same as that in the second part (i.e., 0.04) because the strength of the association is the same (i.e., very small). If phi is squared (like r^2), the proportion of variation in chi-square that is explained by gender in this example is less than 0.2%, which is extremely small. Note that although phi is not accurate in larger $(R \times C)$ tables, a similar test, called **Cramer's V,** can be used in these tables (see Blalock 1972).

Every association should be examined for strength of association and clinical utility as well as statistical significance. Strength of association can be shown by a risk ratio, a risk difference, an odds ratio, an r^2 value, a phi value, or a Cramer's V value. A **statistically significant association** implies that the association is real (i.e., is not due to chance alone) but not

BOX 11–5 Analysis of the Strength of Association (phi) Between Blood Test Results and Gender (Two Nonparametric Variables, Unpaired) in an Initial Study of 200 Subjects and a Subsequent Study of 20,000 Subjects (Fictitious Data)

Part 1 Data and calculation of the phi coefficient for the initial study (the master's thesis)

		GENDER				Total	
		Male		Female			
		Number	(Percentage)	Number	(Percentage)	Number	(Percentage)
BLOOD TEST RESULT	Positive	52	(52)	48	(48)	100	(50)
	Negative	48	(48)	52	(52)	100	(50)
	Total	100	(100)	100	(100)	200	(100)

chi-square (χ^2) value: 0.32
degrees of freedom *(df)*: 1
p value: **0.572** (not statistically significant)

$$\text{phi} = \sqrt{\frac{\chi^2}{N}} = \sqrt{\frac{0.32}{200}} = \sqrt{0.0016} = \mathbf{0.04}$$

Interpretation: The association between gender and the blood test result was neither statistically significant nor clinically important.

Part 2 Data and calculation of the phi coefficient for the subsequent study (the Ph.D. dissertation)

		GENDER				Total	
		Male		Female			
		Number	(Percentage)	Number	(Percentage)	Number	(Percentage)
BLOOD TEST RESULT	Positive	5,200	(52)	4,800	(48)	10,000	(50)
	Negative	4,800	(48)	5,200	(52)	10,000	(50)
	Total	10,000	(100)	10,000	(100)	20,000	(100)

chi-square (χ^2) value: 32.0
degrees of freedom *(df)*: 1
p value: **<0.0001** (highly statistically significant)

$$\text{phi} = \sqrt{\frac{\chi^2}{N}} = \sqrt{\frac{32}{20,000}} = \sqrt{0.0016} = \mathbf{0.04}$$

Interpretation: The association between gender and the blood test result was statistically significant. However, it was clinically unimportant (i.e., it was trivial), because the phi value was 0.04, and the proportion of chi-square that was explained by the blood test result was only $(0.04)^2$, or 0.0016, an amount that was much less than 1%.

necessarily that it is important. A **strong association** is likely to be important if it is real. Therefore, looking for both statistical significance and strength of association is as important as having both the right and left wings on an airplane.

There is, however, a danger of automatically rejecting as unimportant a statistically significant association that showed only limited strength of association. As discussed in Chapter 6, both the risk ratio (or odds ratio if from a case-control study) and the prevalence of the risk factor determine the population attributable risk. Thus, for a prevalent disease such as myocardial infarction, a common risk factor that showed a risk ratio of only 1.3 could be responsible for a large number of preventable infarctions.

Survival Analysis

In clinical studies of medical or surgical interventions for cancer, for example, success usually is measured in terms of the length of time that some desirable outcome (such as survival or remission of disease) is maintained. An analysis of the time-related patterns of survival commonly involves using life tables and techniques that were first developed in the insurance field, and survival analysis requires that the dependent (outcome) variable be dichotomous (e.g., survival/death, success/failure, or presence/absence of improvement).

The mere reporting of the proportion of patients who are alive at the termination of a study's observation period is obviously inadequate, because it does not account for how long the individual patients were observed, nor does it consider when they died or how many were lost to follow-up. Among the techniques that statisticians use to control for these problems are person-time methods and life table analysis using the actuarial method or the Kaplan-Meier method.

Person-Time Methods

In a survival study, some subjects are lost to follow-up and others die during the observation period. To control for the fact that the length of observation varies from subject to subject, the person-time methods introduced in an earlier discussion of **incidence density** (see Chapter 2) can be used in calculating risks and rates of death. Briefly, if one person is observed for 3 years and another for 1 year, the **duration of observation** would be equal to 4 **person-years.** Calculations can be made on the basis of years, months, weeks, or any other unit of time. The results can then be reported as the number of events (e.g., deaths or remissions) per person-time of observation.

Person-time methods are useful if the risk of death or some other outcome does not change greatly over the period of follow-up. If the risk of death does depend strongly on the amount of time since baseline (e.g., amount of time since diagnosis of a disease or since entry in a study), as is true with certain cancers that tend to kill quickly if they are going to be fatal, the overall risk using person-time methods will depend on the relative proportion of study subjects in the early versus late follow-up period, and the incidence density will not be useful. As mentioned in Chapter 2, person-time methods are especially useful for studies of phenomena that can occur repeatedly over time, such as otitis media and other acute infections.

Life Table Analysis

In follow-up studies of a single dichotomous outcome such as death, a major problem is that some subjects may be lost to follow-up (unavailable for examination) and some may be censored (when the time of observation of a patient is terminated early because the patient entered late and the study is ending). The most popular solution to this problem is to use life table analysis. The two main methods of life table analysis—the actuarial method and the Kaplan-Meier method—handle losses to follow-up and censorship in slightly different ways, but both methods make it possible to base the analysis on the findings in all of the subjects for whom there are data.

Both methods require the following information for each patient: (1) the date of entry into the study;

(2) the reason for withdrawal (death, loss to follow-up, or censorship); and (3) the date of withdrawal (date of death for those who died, the last time seen alive for those who were lost to follow-up, and the date withdrawn alive for those who were censored).

The Actuarial Method. The actuarial method, which was developed to calculate risks and premium rates for life insurance companies and retirement plans, was one of the earlier methods used in life table analysis. In medical studies, the actuarial method is used to calculate the survival rates of patients during *fixed* intervals, such as years. First, it determines the number of people surviving to the beginning of each interval. Next, it assumes that those who were censored or lost to follow-up during the interval were observed for only half of that interval. Then the method calculates the mortality rate for that interval (m_x in life tables) by dividing the number of deaths in the interval by the total person-years for all those who began the interval.

The survival rate for an interval (p_x) is 1.0 minus the mortality rate. The rate of survival of the study group to the end of, say, three of the fixed intervals (P_3) is the product of the survival of each of the three component intervals. For example, assume the following: the intervals were years; the survival rate to the end of the first interval (p_1) was 0.75 (i.e., 75%); for those who began the second year, the survival rate to the end of the second interval (p_2) was 0.80; and for those who began the third year, the survival rate to the end of the third interval (p_3) was 0.85. These three numbers would be multiplied together to arrive at a 3-year survival rate of 0.51, or 51%.

An important example of a study in which the actuarial method was used is the Veterans Administration study of the long-term effects of coronary artery bypass grafts (CABG) versus medical treatment of patients with stable angina (see Veterans Administration Coronary Artery Bypass Surgery Cooperative Study Group 1984). Fig. 11–4 shows the 11-year cumulative survival for surgically and medically treated patients who did not have left main coronary artery disease but were nevertheless at high risk according to angiographic analysis in the study.

The actuarial method can also be used in studies of outcomes other than death or survival. Currie, Jekel, and Klerman (1972), for example, used the method in a study of subsequent pregnancies among two groups of teenage mothers. The teenage mothers in one group were enrolled in special programs to help them complete their education and delay subsequent pregnancies, while those in the other group had access to the services that are usually available. The actuarial method was used to analyze data concerning the number and timing of subsequent pregnancies in each group, and when tests of significance were performed, the observed differences between the groups were found to be statistically significant.

The actuarial method continues to be used in the medical literature if there are large numbers of study subjects, but another method called the

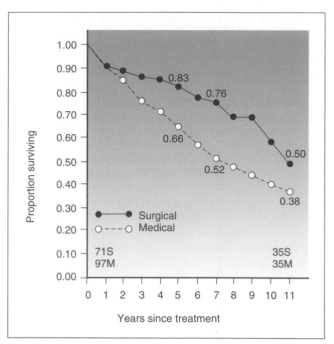

FIGURE 11–4 **Graph showing results of survival analysis using the actuarial method in a study of the long-term effects of coronary artery bypass grafts (CABG) versus medical treatment of patients with stable angina.** Depicted here is the 11-year cumulative survival for surgically and medically treated patients who did not have left main coronary artery disease but were nevertheless at high risk according to angiographic analysis in the study. Numbers of patients at risk at the beginning and end of the study are given at the bottom of the figure, where S denotes surgical and M denotes medical. (From Veterans Administration Coronary Artery Bypass Surgery Cooperative Study Group. Eleven-year survival in the Veterans Administration randomized trial of coronary bypass surgery for stable angina. New England Journal of Medicine 311: 1333–1339, 1984. Copyright © 1984, Massachusetts Medical Society. All rights reserved. Adapted with permission in 1996 and 1999.)

Kaplan-Meier method has many advantages, particularly if the sample size is small.

The Kaplan-Meier Method. The Kaplan-Meier method (Kaplan and Meier 1958) has become the most commonly used approach to survival analysis in medicine. In the medical literature, it is usually referred to as the **Kaplan-Meier life table method.** It is also sometimes referred to as the **product-limit method,** because it takes advantage of the fact that the N year survival rate (P_N) is equal to the product of all of the survival rates of the individual intervals (p_1, p_2, and so forth) leading up to year N.

The Kaplan-Meier method is different from the actuarial method in that it calculates a new line of the life table every time a new death occurs. Because deaths occur unevenly over time, the intervals are *uneven* and there are many of them. For this reason, the graph of a Kaplan-Meier life table analysis often looks like uneven stair steps.

In a Kaplan-Meier analysis, the deaths are not conceived of as occurring during an interval. Rather, they are seen as instantaneously terminating one interval and beginning a new interval at a lower survival rate. The periods of time between when deaths occur are death-free periods, and therefore the proportion sur-

viving between deaths does not change, and the curve of the proportion surviving is flat rather than sloping downward. A death produces an instantaneous drop in the proportion surviving, and then another death-free period begins.

To illustrate the method, the following example was taken from Kaplan and Meier's original (1958) article and is analyzed in Box 11–6. The study began with eight fictitious patients, four of whom died and the remaining four of whom were losses (i.e., either lost to follow-up or censored). The four deaths occurred at 0.8, 3.1, 5.4, and 9.2 months. The four losses occurred at 1.0, 2.7, 7.0, and 12.1 months. Because losses to follow-up and censored patients are removed from the study group during the between-death interval in which they occur, they do not appear in the denominator when the next death occurs.

In Box 11–6, p_x is the proportion surviving interval x (i.e., from the time of the previous death to just before the next death), and P_x is the proportion surviving from the beginning of the study to the end of that interval. (P_x is obtained by multiplying together the p_x values of all of the intervals up to and including the row of interest.) The p_x of the first interval is always 1.0, because the first death ends the first study interval and all of the patients not lost to follow-up survive until the first death.

To illustrate the use of Kaplan-Meier analysis in practice, Fig. 11–5 shows a Kaplan-Meier life table of the probability of remaining relapse-free over time for two groups of patients who had cancer of the bladder (Esrig et al. 1994). All of the patients had organ-confined transitional-cell cancer of the bladder with deep invasion into the muscularis propria (i.e., stage 3a disease) but without regional lymph node metastases. One group consisted of 14 patients with negative results in a test for p53 protein in the nuclei of tumor cells, and the other group consisted of 12 patients with positive results in the same test (Esrig et al. 1994). Despite small numbers, the difference in the survival curves for the p53-positive group and the p53-negative group was found to be statistically significant ($p = 0.030$).

Life table methods do not eliminate the bias that occurs if the losses to follow-up happen more frequently in one group than in another, particularly if the characteristics of the patients lost from one group differ greatly from those of the patients lost from the other group. (For example, in a clinical trial comparing the effects of an experimental antihypertensive drug with those of an established antihypertensive drug, the occurrence of side effects in the group treated with the experimental drug might cause many in this group to drop out of the study and no longer maintain contact with the investigators.) However, the life table method is a powerful tool if the losses are few, if the losses represent a similar percentage of the starting numbers in the groups to be compared, and if the characteristics of those lost to follow-up are similar. The life table method is usually considered the

BOX 11–6   Survival Analysis by the Kaplan-Meier Method in a Study of 8 Subjects

Part 1   Beginning data

Timing of deaths in 4 subjects: 0.8, 3.1, 5.4, and 9.2 months
Timing of loss to follow-up or censorship in 4 subjects: 1.0, 2.7, 7.0, and 12.1 months

Part 2   Tabular representation of the data

Number of Months at Time of Subject's Death	Number Living Just Before Subject's Death	Number Living Just After Subject's Death	Number Lost to Follow-Up Between This and Next Subject's Death	Fraction Surviving This Death	p_x	Survival Interval (for p_x)	P_x Surviving to End of Interval
—	—	—	—	—	1.000	$0 < 0.8$	1.000
0.8	8	7	2	7/8	0.875	$0.8 < 3.1$	0.875
3.1	5	4	0	4/5	0.800	$3.1 < 5.4$	0.700
5.4	4	3	1	3/4	0.750	$5.4 < 9.2$	0.525
9.2	2	1	0	1/2	0.500	$9.2 < 12.1$	0.263
No deaths	1	1	1	1/1	1.000	> 12.1	0.263

Note: p_x is the proportion surviving interval x (i.e., from the time of the previous death to just before the next death), and P_x is the proportion surviving from the beginning of the study to the end of that interval.

Part 3   Graphic representation of the data

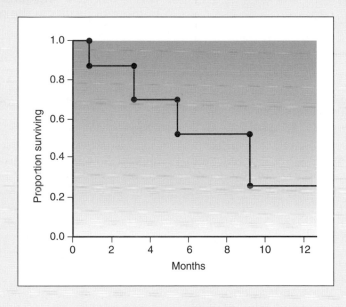

Source of data: Kaplan, E. L., and P. Meier. Nonparametric estimation from incomplete observations. Journal of the American Statistical Association 53:457–481, 1958.

method of choice for describing dichotomous outcomes in longitudinal studies, such as randomized clinical trials.

In statistics, it is always crucial to look at the raw data, and nowhere is this more important than in survival analysis, where examining the pattern of survival differences may be more important for making a clinical decision than examining whether the difference is statistically significant. For example, a new surgical cancer therapy may result in a greater initial mortality but a higher 5-year survival (i.e., the therapy is a "kill or cure" method), whereas a more traditional medical therapy results in a lower initial mortality but also a lower 5-year survival. It might be important for patients to know this difference in choosing between these therapies. For example, patients who preferred to be free of cancer quickly and at all costs might choose the surgical treatment. In contrast, patients who wanted to live for at least a few months in order to finish writing a book or to see the

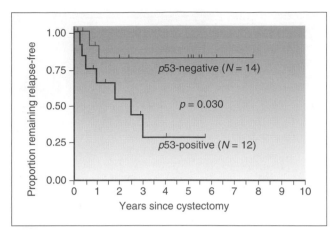

FIGURE 11–5   Graph showing a life table analysis using the Kaplan-Meier method in a study of the probability of remaining relapse-free over time for two groups of patients who had organ-confined transitional-cell cancer of the bladder with deep invasion into the muscularis propria (i.e., stage 3a disease) but without regional lymph node metastases. One group consisted of 14 patients with negative results in a test for p53 protein in the nuclei of tumor cells, and the other group consisted of 12 patients with positive results in the same test. (From Esrig, D., et al. Accumulation of nuclear p53 and tumor progression in bladder cancer. New England Journal of Medicine 331:1259–1264, 1994. Copyright © 1994, Massachusetts Medical Society. All rights reserved. Adapted with permission in 1996 and 1999.)

birth of a first grandchild might choose the medical treatment.

Tests of Significance for Differences in Survival

Two or more life table curves can be tested to see if they are significantly different. Statistical computer packages do this using some rather complicated tests, such as the Breslow test and the Cox test. However, reasonably good tests of significance between actuarial curves (such as the z-test for proportions) and between Kaplan-Meier curves (such as the logrank test) can be done by hand.

Significance Tests for Proportions. See Chapter 10 for a discussion of t-tests and z-tests. The t-test for a difference between actuarial method curves depends on the Greenwood formula for the standard error of a proportion. For details, see Cutler and Ederer (1958) or Dawson-Saunders and Trapp (1994).

The Logrank Test. Despite its name, the logrank test does not deal with logarithms or with ranked data. The test is often used to compare data in studies involving treatment and control groups and to test the null hypothesis that each group has the same force of mortality.

In the logrank test, each time a death occurs, the investigator calculates the probability that the observed death would have occurred in the treatment group and the probability that it would have occurred in the control group. These probabilities are proportional to the number of survivors to that point in time in each group. For example, suppose the study started with 100 patients in each group, but at a certain point there were 60 left in the treatment group and 40 in the control group. Under the null hypo-

thesis, the probability that the next death would occur in the treatment group is 0.6, and the probability that the next death would occur in the control group is 0.4.

Within each study group, the expected probabilities for each death are summed to form the total expected number of deaths *(E)* for that group. The actual deaths in each group are also summed to form the observed number of deaths *(O)*. Then the observed deaths are compared with the expected deaths in the following chi-square test on 1 degree of freedom:

$$\text{logrank } \chi^2 = \frac{(O_T - E_T)^2}{E_T} + \frac{(O_C - E_C)^2}{E_C}$$

where O_T and E_T are the observed and expected deaths in the treatment group and where O_C and E_C are the observed and expected deaths in the control group. Note that only two terms are needed, because the expected counts are not determined from row and column totals in a 2×2 table but instead are obtained by an independent method. There is only 1 degree of freedom here, because the total number of deaths is already known and because when the number of deaths in one of the two groups is known, the number of deaths in the other group is fixed and no longer free to vary.

Proportional Hazards Models (Cox Models). The Kaplan-Meier approach has been made even more powerful by the development of statistical models that enable dichotomous outcomes to be used as dependent variables in multiple logistic regression analyses, despite losses to follow-up and censorship of patients. Although a detailed discussion of these models is beyond the scope of this book, students should be aware that they are called proportional hazards models or Cox models and that their application is becoming increasingly common in medical studies. For more information, see Dawson-Saunders and Trapp (1994).

■ SUMMARY

Bivariate analysis is the analysis of the relationship between one independent variable and one dependent variable. The statistical significance tests frequently used for this purpose are listed in Table 11–1.

The relationships between two variables that are both continuous should first be examined graphically. Then the data can be analyzed statistically to determine whether there is a real relationship between the variables, whether the relationship is linear or nonlinear, whether the correlation *(r)* is positive or negative, and whether the association is sufficiently strong that it is not likely to have occurred by chance alone. The strength of an association between two continuous variables can be determined by calculating the value of r^2, and the impact that variable x has on variable y can be determined by calculating the slope of the regression.

Both correlation and regression analyses indicate whether there is an association between two continuous variables, such as weight *(y)* and height *(x)*. Correlation tells what proportion of the variation in y is explained by the variation in x. Linear regression estimates the value of y when the value of x is 0, and it also predicts the degree of expected change in y when x changes by one unit of measure.

There are numerous tests to determine the relationships between an ordinal variable and a noncontinuous variable. For example, the relationship between an ordinal variable and dichotomous variable can be determined by the Mann-Whitney U test (which is used for unpaired studies and is similar to the Student's t-test) and the Wilcoxon matched-pairs signed-ranks test (which is similar to the paired t-test). The relationship between an ordinal variable and a nominal variable can be determined by the Kruskal-Wallis test (which is similar to the F-test). Of the tests that measure the correlation between two ordinal variables, the most important are the Spearman and the Kendall correlation coefficients, which are rho and tau, respectively. There are no linear regression tests for ordinal variables.

The bivariate analysis of dichotomous or nominal data may begin by placing the data for the two variables in a 2×2 contingency table. Then the null hypothesis of independence between the two variables is usually tested by using the chi-square test for unpaired data or the McNemar chi-square test for paired data. Less frequently, the Fisher exact probability test is used in the analysis of dichotomous unpaired data. For data in 2×2 tables, the phi coefficient can be used to test the strength of association, and methods are available to calculate standard errors and confidence intervals for proportions, risk ratios, or odds ratios.

Survival analysis employs various methods to study dichotomous outcome variables (e.g., death/survival) over time. Although the actuarial method of analysis is still used, the Kaplan-Meier (product-limit) method has become the most frequently used approach. Life table curves are constructed from the data, and two or more curves can be tested to see if they are significantly different. For actuarial curves, significance tests for proportions can be used. For Kaplan-Meier curves, the logrank test and proportional hazards (Cox) models are among the statistical tests available.

■ QUESTIONS

Directions (Items 1–10). Each of the numbered items or incomplete statements in this section is followed by answers or by completions of the statement. Select the ONE lettered answer or completion that is BEST in each case. Correct answers and explanations are given at the end of the chapter.

1. To employ parametric methods of statistical analysis, the population distribution of the dependent variable must be

   (A)   age-matched
   (B)   dichotomous
   (C)   linear
   (D)   nominal
   (E)   normally distributed

2. A joint distribution graph can be used to display

   (A)   causality
   (B)   correlation
   (C)   kurtosis
   (D)   power
   (E)   specificity

3. A correlation is noted between putting on boxing gloves and acts of aggression. The correlation coefficient in this case

   (A)   cannot be determined, because the data are dichotomous
   (B)   may be close to 1
   (C)   may be greater than 1
   (D)   must be less than 0.05
   (E)   must be statistically significant

4. In the formula for linear regression, the term used to represent the slope is

   (A) a
   (B) b
   (C) m
   (D) x
   (E) y

5. A distinction between the one-tailed and two-tailed tests of significance is that a one-tailed test

   (A)   does not affect statistical significance but does affect power
   (B)   does not affect the performance of the statistical test but does affect the conversion to a p value
   (C)   is based on the number of independent variables
   (D)   requires that the sample size be doubled
   (E)   should be performed during data analysis

6. A study is conducted to determine the efficacy of influenza vaccine. Subjects agree to participate for 2 years. During the first year, subjects are randomly assigned to be injected with either an inert substance (a placebo) or the active vaccine. During the second year, each subject who previously received the placebo is given the active vaccine, and each subject who previously received the active vaccine is given the placebo. Thus, each subject serves as his or her own control. All incident cases of influenza are recorded, and the occurrence of influenza when vaccinated is compared with the occurrence when unvaccinated. The appropriate test of significance for this study is the

   (A)   Kaplan-Meier method
   (B)   Kruskal-Wallis test
   (C)   Mann-Whitney U test
   (D)   McNemar test
   (E)   Pearson correlation coefficient

7. The phi coefficient is defined as follows:

$$phi = \sqrt{\frac{\chi^2}{N}}$$

This is used to measure

(A) effect modification in a 2×2 table
(B) the p value of a 2×2 table
(C) the standard error of a 2×2 table
(D) the statistical power of a 2×2 table
(E) the strength of association in a 2×2 table

Items 8–10

Two groups of subjects are assembled on the basis of whether or not they can correctly identify a newt in a pond-life ensemble. The groups are asked to rate the probability that industrial emissions cause global warming. They are to use a scale with five choices, ranging from "improbable" to "highly probable."

8. The data in this study are

(A) continuous
(B) dichotomous
(C) nominal
(D) ordinal
(E) parametric

9. To analyze the responses of the two groups statistically, the data are compared on the basis of

(A) means
(B) ranking
(C) standard deviation
(D) standard error
(E) variance

10. The appropriate statistical method for this analysis is

(A) chi-square analysis
(B) linear regression analysis
(C) nonparametric analysis
(D) the Fisher exact probability test
(E) the Student's t-test

■ ANSWERS AND EXPLANATIONS

1. **The answer is E: normally distributed.** Data are parametric if their distribution is fully described by the mean and the standard deviation, which are the parameters. To meet this requirement, the data must be continuous and derived from an underlying set of data that is normally distributed (i.e., derived from the means of repeated samples drawn from the same population). Appropriate use of parametric methods further requires that the study population be a random sample of the larger population that it is intended to represent. Data need not be age-matched or linear for parametric methods to pertain. Dichotomous and nominal data require nonparametric analysis.

2. **The answer is B: correlation.** A joint distribution graph is a plot of the relationship between two continuous variables. The more closely the data points cluster about a line, the greater is the correlation between the two variables. If two variables are related in a nonlinear manner, the correlation may not be displayed as a line but, rather, as a curvilinear distribution of data points. Methods for calculating the correlation coefficient in such a setting are available, but their description is beyond the scope of this text. Correlation alone does not establish causality. For example, someone who owns a car is also likely to own a television set, but ownership of one item does not cause ownership of the other item.

3. **The answer is B: may be close to 1.** The Pearson product-moment correlation coefficient, also referred to as the r value, is a measure of the linear relationship between two variables. Its value range is the same as that for the slope of a line, from –1, through 0, to 1. Therefore, it cannot be greater than 1. A strong correlation, such as the one in the question, will produce a correlation coefficient close to 1. Statistical significance is certainly more likely when the correlation is strong but is also dependent on the sample size, about which we are told nothing in this case.

4. **The answer is B: b.** The formula for linear regression is $y = a + bx$, where a is the y-intercept and b is the slope. This formula is derived from the formula for a straight line, which is $y = mx + b$, where m is the slope and b is the y-intercept. Linear regression analysis is used to quantify the linear relationship between an independent variable (x) and a dependent variable (y).

5. **The answer is B: does not affect the performance of the statistical test but does affect the conversion to a p value.** The choice of a one-tailed or two-tailed test of significance should be made before a study is conducted, based on the hypothesis to be tested. If the outcome can differ from the null hypothesis in only one direction (e.g., if you are comparing a placebo with an antihypertensive drug that you are thoroughly convinced will not cause the blood pressure to increase), then a one-tailed test of significance is appropriate. If the outcome may differ from the null hypothesis in either direction (e.g., if you are comparing a placebo with a type of drug that may cause the blood pressure to increase or decrease), a two-tailed test of significance is warranted. The stipulation of a one-tailed test or two-tailed test affects the associated p value. When a one-tailed test is chosen, statistical significance (i.e., a p value less than alpha) is more readily achieved because the extreme 5% of the distribution that differs sufficiently from the null hypothesis to warrant rejection of the null hypothesis (when alpha is set at 0.05) is all to one side. When a two-tailed test of significance is

chosen, the rejection region is divided into two areas, with half (or 0.025 of the distribution when alpha is set at 0.05) at either extreme of the curve. The implications of choosing a one-tailed test or a two-tailed test are discussed in Chapter 10 and Box 10–6.

6. **The answer is D: McNemar test.** In the study described, the outcome for each subject is binary: the disease (influenza) occurs or does not occur. The proportion of subjects who acquire the disease in the year they were vaccinated will be compared with the proportion of subjects who acquire it in the year they were not vaccinated. Chi-square analysis is appropriate for this sort of comparison, and because each subject in the study serves as his or her own control, the McNemar test (chi-square test for paired data) is used. The contingency table for such a test contains paired data and would be set up as follows:

		YEAR VACCINATED	
		Diseased	Nondiseased
YEAR NOT VACCINATED	Diseased	a	b
	Nondiseased	c	d

The numbers placed in the various cells would represent the following: in cell a, subjects who acquired influenza both when vaccinated and not vaccinated; in cell b, subjects who acquired influenza only when not vaccinated; in cell c, subjects who acquired influenza only when vaccinated; and in cell d, subjects who remained free of influenza whether vaccinated or not.

7. **The answer is E: the strength of association in a 2 × 2 table.** A very large sample size is likely to result in statistical significance, even if the association under investigation is weak and trivial. The strength of the association between the two variables under study does not change with the sample size, however. The phi coefficient adjusts the chi-square value for the size of the sample. The phi coefficient squared is the proportion of variation in the dependent variable accounted for by the independent variable.

8. **The answer is D: ordinal.** Ordinal data are data that can be ranked from lowest to highest but not measured on an exact scale. In the study described, the scale clearly has directionality (with choices ranging from "improbable" to "highly probable"); therefore, the data are ordinal rather than nominal. There are more than two choices, so the data are not bivariate. The choices are discrete, so the data are neither continuous nor parametric.

9. **The answer is B: ranking.** Nonparametric methods of statistical analysis are used for ordinal data and are based on ranking of the data. Ordinal data do not have a mean or a definable variance and therefore cannot be characterized by a standard deviation or standard error. To analyze these data, which are the ordinal responses provided by the two groups of subjects, the Mann-Whitney U test is appropriate, as indicated in Table 11–1.

10. **The answer is C: nonparametric analysis.** Nonparametric methods of statistical analysis are used for ordinal data and are based on the ranking of the data. To analyze these data, which are the ordinal responses provided by the two groups of subjects, the Mann-Whitney U test is appropriate, as indicated in Table 11–1.

References Cited

Blalock, H. M., Jr. Social Statistics, 2nd ed. New York, McGraw-Hill Book Company, 1972.

Cohen, S. R. Mycosis fungoides: clinicopathologic relationships, survival, and therapy in 54 patients, with observation on occupation as a new prognostic factor. Master's thesis, Yale University School of Medicine, New Haven, Conn., 1977.

Currie, J., J. F. Jekel, and L. V. Klerman. Subsequent pregnancies among teenage mothers enrolled in a special program. American Journal of Public Health 62:1606–1611, 1972.

Cutler, S. J., and F. Ederer. Maximum utilization of the life table method in analyzing survival. Journal of Chronic Disease 8:699–713, 1958.

Dawson-Saunders, B., and R. G. Trapp. Basic and Clinical Biostatistics, 2nd ed. Norwalk, Conn., Appleton and Lange, 1994.

Dean, J., et al. EPIINFO, Version 5.01. Atlanta, Centers for Disease Control, Epidemiology Program Office, 1991.

Emerson, J. D., and G. A. Colditz. Use of statistical analysis. New England Journal of Medicine 309:709–713, 1983.

Esrig, D., et al. Accumulation of nuclear p53 and tumor progression in bladder cancer. New England Journal of Medicine 331:1259–1264, 1994.

Kaplan, E. L., and P. Meier. Nonparametric estimation from incomplete observations. Journal of the American Statistical Association 53:457–481, 1958.

Kleinbaum, D. G., and L. L. Kupper. Applied Regression Analysis and Other Multivariable Methods. North Scituate, Mass., Duxbury Press, 1978.

Phillips, D. S. Basic Statistics for Health Science Students. San Francisco, W. H. Freeman and Company, 1978.

Siegel, S. Nonparametric Statistics. New York, McGraw-Hill Book Company, 1956.

Snow, P. J. Effect of propranolol in myocardial infarction. Lancet 2:551–553, 1965.

Veterans Administration Coronary Artery Bypass Surgery Cooperative Study Group. Eleven-year survival in the Veterans Administration randomized trial of coronary bypass surgery for stable angina. New England Journal of Medicine 311:1333–1339, 1984.

Selected Readings

Dawson-Saunders, B., and R. G. Trapp. Basic and Clinical Biostatistics, 2nd ed. Norwalk, Conn., Appleton and Lange, 1994.

Inglefinger, J. A., et al. Biostatistics in Clinical Medicine, 2nd ed. New York, Macmillan Publishing Company, 1987.

Kleinbaum, D. G., and L. L. Kupper. Applied Regression Analysis and Other Multivariable Methods. North Scituate, Mass., Duxbury Press, 1978.

Lee, E. T. Statistical Methods for Survival Data Analysis. Belmont, Calif., Lifetime Learning Publications, 1980.

12 Sample Size, Randomization, and Probability Theory

■ SAMPLE SIZE

The determination of sample size is critical in planning clinical research, because sample size is usually the most important factor determining the time and funding necessary to perform the research. Members of committees responsible for funding clinical studies look closely at the assumptions used to estimate the number of study subjects needed and at the way in which calculations of sample size were performed. Part of their task in reviewing the sample size is to determine whether the proposed research is realistic—e.g., whether there are enough available subjects to comprise the group at risk in a cohort study or to comprise the group of cases in a case-control study. In research that is already reported, inadequate sample size may explain why apparently useful clinical results may not be statistically significant.

Statisticians are probably consulted more often because an investigator wants to know the sample size needed for a study than for any other reason.

Sample size calculations can be confusing even for many people who can do ordinary statistical analyses without trouble. As a test of intuition regarding sample size, try to answer the following three questions:

(1) What size sample—large or small—would be needed if there was a very large variance?

(2) What size sample would be needed if the investigator wanted the answer to be very close to the true value (i.e., have very narrow confidence limits or a very small p value)?

(3) What size sample would be needed if the difference that the investigator wanted to be able to detect was extremely small?

If intuition suggested that all of the above requirements would create the need for a large sample size, that is correct. If intuition did not suggest the correct answers, review these questions again after reading the following information about how the basic formula for sample size is derived.

Among other factors affecting the number of subjects required for a study are whether the research design involves paired data (e.g., observations before treatment and after treatment in the same group of subjects) or unpaired data (e.g., observations in an experimental group and a control group); whether the investigator wishes to consider beta (type II or false-negative) errors in addition to alpha (type I or false-positive) errors; whether the investigator anticipates a large or small variance in the data sets; whether the investigator chooses the usual alpha level (p value of 0.05 in the two-tailed test and a confidence interval of 95%) or a smaller level; and whether the investigator wants to be able to detect a fairly small or extremely small difference between the means or proportions of the outcome variable.

Derivation of the Basic Sample Size Formula

To derive the basic formula for calculating the sample size, it is easiest to start with the formula for the paired t-test:

$$t_\alpha = \frac{\bar{d}}{\dfrac{s_d}{\sqrt{N}}}$$

where $\bar{d}$ is the mean difference that was observed, s_d

is the standard deviation of that mean difference, and N is the sample size.

To solve for N, several rearrangements and substitutions of terms in the equation must be made. First, everything can be squared and the equation rearranged so that N is in the numerator and s^2 is the variance of the distribution of d:

$$t_\alpha^2 = \frac{(\overline{d})^2}{(s_d/\sqrt{N})^2} = \frac{(\overline{d})^2 \cdot N}{(s)^2}$$

Next, the terms can be rearranged so that the equation for N in a paired (before and after) study becomes:

$$N = \frac{t_\alpha^2 \cdot (s)^2}{(\overline{d})^2}$$

Now the t in the formula must be replaced with z. This provides a solution to a circular problem: In order to know the value of t, the degrees of freedom (df) must be known. However, the df is dependent on N, which is what the investigator is trying to calculate in the first place. Because the value of z is not dependent on df and because z is equal to t when the sample size is large, z can be used instead of t. The formula therefore becomes:

$$N = \frac{z_\alpha^2 \cdot (s)^2}{(\overline{d})^2}$$

In theory, using z instead of t might produce a slight underestimate of the sample size needed. In practice, however, using z seems to work well, and its use is customary.

Note that the above formula is for a study using the paired t-test, in which each subject serves as his or her own control. For a study using the Student's t-test, such as a randomized controlled trial with an experimental group and a control group, it would be necessary to calculate N for each group. Note also that the above formula considers only the problem of alpha error; to minimize the possibility of beta error, a z term for beta error must be introduced as well. Before these topics are discussed, however, the answers to the three questions posed earlier should be explored more fully in light of the information provided by the basic formula for N.

(1) The larger the variance (s^2) is, the larger the sample size must be, because the variance is in the numerator of the above formula for N. This makes sense intuitively, because with a large variance (and therefore a large standard error), a bigger N is needed to compensate for the greater uncertainty of the estimate.

(2) To have considerable confidence that a mean difference shown in a study is real, the analysis must produce a small p value for the observed mean difference, which in turn implies that the value for t_α or z_α was large. Because z_α is in the numerator of the sample size formula, the larger z_α is, the larger the N (the sample size needed) will be. For example, for a two-tailed test, a p value of 0.05 (the alpha level chosen) would require a z_α of 1.96, which, when squared as in the formula, would equal 3.84. To be even more confident, the investigator might set alpha at 0.01. This would require a z_α of 2.58, which equals 6.66 when squared, 73% greater than when alpha is set at 0.05. To decrease the probability of being wrong from 5% to 1% would thus require the sample size to be almost doubled.

(3) If the investigator wanted to detect with confidence a very small difference between the mean values of two study groups (i.e., a small $\overline{d}$), a very large N would be needed, because the difference (squared) is in the denominator. The smaller the denominator is, the larger the ratio is and, hence, the larger the N must be. A precise estimate and therefore a large sample size are needed to detect a small difference. Whether a small difference is considered clinically important often depends on factors such as the area of research. For example, studies showing that a new treatment for hypertension reduces the systolic blood pressure by 2–3 mm Hg would be considered clinically trivial. However, studies showing that a new treatment for pancreatic cancer improves the survival rate by 10% (0.1) would be considered a major advance. Clinical judgment is involved in determining the minimum difference that should be considered clinically important.

The Problem of Beta Error

If a mean difference is examined with a t-test and it is statistically significant at the prestated level of alpha (e.g., 0.05), there is no need to worry about beta error (type II or false-negative error). If, however, an investigator observes a mean difference in the data that appears to be clinically important but the null hypothesis cannot be rejected at the desired level of confidence (e.g., alpha = 0.05), beta error may have occurred because the sample size was small. In planning a study, investigators want to avoid the likelihood of beta (false-negative) error as well as the likelihood of alpha (false-positive) error.

The need to be concerned about beta error was illustrated in a seminal article by Freiman et al. (1978). They found that in most of 71 "negative" randomized controlled trials of new therapies, the sample sizes were too small "to provide reasonable assurance that a clinically meaningful 'difference' (i.e., therapeutic effect) would not be missed." In their study, "reasonable assurance" was 90%. In fact, in 94% of these negative studies, the sample size was too small to detect a 25% improvement in outcome with reasonable (90%) assurance. In 75% of the studies, the sample size was too small to detect a 50% improvement in outcome with the same level of assurance.

A study with a large beta error has a low sensitivity for detecting a mean difference because, as discussed in Chapter 7:

Sensitivity + False-negative (beta) error = 1.00

When investigators speak of a study as opposed to a clinical test, however, they usually use the term "statistical power" instead of "sensitivity." With this substitution in terms,

$$\text{Statistical power} + \text{Beta error} = 1.00$$

which means that statistical power is equal to (1 − beta error). Therefore, in calculating a sample size, if the investigators accept a 20% possibility of missing a true finding (beta error = 0.2), the study should have a statistical power of 0.8, or 80%. That means the investigators are 80% confident that they will be able to detect a true mean difference of the size they specify with the sample size they determine.

The best way to incorporate beta error into a study is to include it beforehand in the determination of sample size. Incorporating beta in the sample size calculation is easy, but it is likely to increase the sample size considerably.

Steps in the Calculation of Sample Size

The first step in calculating sample size is to choose the appropriate formula to be used, based on the type of study and the type of error to be considered. Four common formulas for calculating sample size are discussed in this chapter and listed in Table 12–1. In the second step in calculating sample size, the investigators must specify the following values: the variance expected (s^2); the z_α value for the alpha desired; the smallest clinically important difference ($\bar{d}$); and, usually, beta (actually, z_β). All but the variance must come from clinical and research judgment. The estimated variance, however, should be based on knowl-

edge of data. If the outcome variable being studied is continuous, such as blood pressure, the estimate of variance can be obtained from the literature or from a small pilot study.

If the outcome is the proportion surviving for 5 years, for example, the variance is easier to estimate. The investigators need to estimate only the proportion that would survive 5 years with the new experimental treatment (which is p_1 and is, say, 60%) and the proportion expected to survive with the control group's treatment (which is p_2 and is, say, 40%). Assuming the two study groups are of approximately equal size, the investigators must determine the mean survival in the entire group (which would be $\bar{p} = 50\%$ in this example). The formula for the variance of a proportion is simply the following:

$$\text{Variance (proportion)} = \bar{p}\,(1 - \bar{p})$$

Once the investigators are armed with all of the above information, it is straightforward to compute the needed sample size, as shown in Boxes 12–1 through 12–4 and discussed below. Note that the N determined using the formulas in Boxes 12–2, 12–3, and 12–4 is only for the experimental group. This N must be doubled to include both the experimental and the control group. For some studies, investigators may find it easier to obtain control subjects than cases (or vice versa). When cases are scarce or costly, it is possible to increase the sample size by matching two or three controls with each case in a case-control study or by obtaining two or three control group subjects for each experimental subject in a clinical trial. However, the incremental benefits in statistical power decline as the number of cases per control increases, so it is seldom cost-effective to have more than three controls for each case. If the number of controls exceeds the number of cases, the sample size formulas discussed in this chapter will need to be modified. For details, see Kelsey et al. 1996.

Sample Size for Studies Using t-Tests

Box 12–1 shows the formula and the calculations for a before and after study of an antihypertensive drug—that is, a study for which a **paired t-test** will be used. Given the variance, alpha, and difference chosen by the investigator, only 9 subjects would be needed altogether. Clearly, this kind of study is efficient in terms of the sample size required. However, even most paired studies require far more than 9 subjects.

Box 12–2 shows the formula and the calculations for a randomized controlled trial of an antihypertensive drug—that is, a study for which the **Student's t-test** will be used. This formula differs from the Box 12–1 formula only in that the variance estimate must be multiplied by 2. Given the same assumptions as in Box 12–1 concerning variance, alpha, and difference, it would be necessary to have a total of 36 study subjects for this randomized controlled trial, which is four times the number of subjects required for the before and after study described in Box 12–1. The larger sample size is needed for studies using the Stu-

TABLE 12–1 Formulas for the Calculation of Sample Size for Studies Commonly Pursued in Medical Research

Type of Study and Type of Errors to Be Considered	Appropriate Formula to Be Used*
Studies using the paired t-test (e.g., before and after studies) and considering alpha (type I) error only	$N = \dfrac{(z_\alpha)^2 \cdot (s)^2}{(\bar{d})^2}$
Studies using the Student's t-test (e.g., randomized controlled trials with one experimental group and one control group) and considering alpha error only	$N = \dfrac{(z_\alpha)^2 \cdot 2 \cdot (s)^2}{(\bar{d})^2}$
Studies using the Student's t-test and considering alpha (type I) and beta (type II) errors	$N = \dfrac{(z_\alpha + z_\beta)^2 \cdot 2 \cdot (s)^2}{(\bar{d})^2}$
Studies using a test of differences in proportions and considering alpha and beta errors	$N = \dfrac{(z_\alpha + z_\beta)^2 \cdot 2 \cdot \bar{p}(1 - \bar{p})}{(\bar{d})^2}$

*The appropriate formula is based on the study design and the type of outcome data. In these formulas, N = sample size; z_α = z value for alpha error; z_β = z value for beta error; s^2 = variance; $\bar{p}$ = mean proportion of success; and $\bar{d}$ = difference to be detected. See Boxes 12–1, 12–2, and 12–4 for examples of calculations using these formulas.

BOX 12–1   Calculation of Sample Size for a Study Using the Paired *t*-Test and Considering Alpha Error Only

Part 1   Data on which the calculation will be based

Study Characteristic	Assumptions Made by Investigator
Type of study	Before and after study of an antihypertensive drug
Data sets	Pretreatment and post-treatment observations in the same subjects
Variable	Systolic blood pressure
Losses to follow-up	None
Standard deviation *(s)*	15 mm Hg
Variance *(s²)*	225 mm Hg
Data for alpha *(z_α)*	$p = 0.05$; therefore, 95% confidence desired (two-tailed test); $z_\alpha = 1.96$
Difference to be detected $(\overline{d})$	10 mm Hg or larger difference between pretreatment and posttreatment blood pressure values

Part 2   Calculation of sample size *(N)*

$$N = \frac{(z_\alpha)^2 \cdot (s)^2}{(\overline{d})^2} = \frac{(1.96)^2 \cdot (15)^2}{(10)^2}$$

$$= \frac{(3.84)(225)}{100} = \frac{864}{100} = 8.64 - 9 \text{ subjects total}$$

Interpretation: Only 9 subjects would be needed for this study, because each paired subject serves as his or her own control in a before and after study. Note that when the estimated *N* is a fraction, the *N* used should be rounded up to be safe.

---

calculations show that 72 study subjects are needed for the randomized controlled trial. In contrast, 36 subjects were needed if only alpha was considered, as shown in Box 12–2.

The issue of adequate versus excessive sample sizes continues to be debated. Some believe that the

---

BOX 12–2   Calculation of Sample Size for a Study Using the Student's *t*-Test and Considering Alpha Error Only

Part 1   Data on which the calculation will be based

Study Characteristic	Assumptions Made by Investigator
Type of study	Randomized controlled trial of an antihypertensive drug
Data sets	Observations in one experimental group and one control group of the same size
Variable	Systolic blood pressure
Losses to follow-up	None
Standard deviation *(s)*	15 mm Hg
Variance *(s²)*	225 mm Hg
Data for alpha *(z_α)*	$p = 0.05$; therefore, 95% confidence desired (two-tailed test); $z_\alpha = 1.96$
Difference to be detected $(\overline{d})$	10 mm Hg or larger difference between mean blood pressure values of the experimental group and control group

Part 2   Calculation of sample size *(N)*

$$N = \frac{(z_\alpha)^2 \cdot 2 \cdot (s)^2}{(\overline{d})^2} = \frac{(1.96)^2 \cdot 2 \cdot (15)^2}{(10)^2}$$

$$= \frac{(3.84)(2)(225)}{100} = \frac{1728}{100} = 17.28$$

$$= 18 \text{ subjects per group} \times 2 \text{ groups}$$

$$= \textbf{36 subjects total}$$

Interpretation: For the type of study depicted in this box, 18 subjects will be needed in the experimental group and 18 in the control group, for a total *N* of 36 study subjects. Note that the *N* needed is rounded up. Note also that the total *N* needed in this box is four times as large as the total *N* needed in Box 12–1, even though the values for z_α, *s*, and $\overline{d}$ are the same in both boxes. The need for two groups is one reason that the total *N* is larger in a randomized controlled trial. The other is the fact that there are two variances to consider, so the estimated variance must be multiplied by 2.

---

dent's *t*-test because there are two sources of variance instead of one (hence the number 2 in the numerator) and because a second person serves as the control for each experimental subject (so that the total sample size for equal numbers of cases and controls would be 2*N*).

The only difference between the formula shown in Box 12–2 and the one shown in Box 12–3 is that the latter considers **beta error** in addition to alpha error. Although there is no complete agreement on the level of beta error acceptable for most studies, usually a beta error of 20% (one-tailed test) is used; this corresponds to a *z* value of 0.84. When these beta estimates are used in Box 12–3, with the same z_α, variance, and mean difference as in Box 12–2, the

BOX 12–3　Calculation of Sample Size for a Study Using the Student's *t*-Test and Considering Alpha and Beta Errors

Part 1　Data on which the calculation will be based

Study Characteristic	Assumptions Made by Investigator
Type of study	Randomized controlled trial of an antihypertensive drug
Data sets	Observations in one experimental group and one control group of the same size
Variable	Systolic blood pressure
Losses to follow-up	None
Standard deviation *(s)*	15 mm Hg
Variance *(s²)*	225 mm Hg
Data for alpha (z_α)	$p = 0.05$; therefore, 95% confidence desired (two-tailed test); $z_\alpha = 1.96$
Data for beta (z_β)	20% beta error; therefore, 80% power desired (one-tailed test); $z_\beta = 0.84$
Difference to be detected $(\overline{d})$	10 mm Hg or larger difference between mean blood pressure values of the experimental group and control group

Part 2　Calculation of sample size *(N)*

$$N = \frac{(z_\alpha + z_\beta)^2 \cdot 2 \cdot (s)^2}{(\overline{d})^2}$$

$$= \frac{(1.96 + 0.84)^2 \cdot 2 \cdot (15)^2}{(10)^2}$$

$$= \frac{(7.84)(2)(225)}{100} = \frac{3528}{100} = 35.28$$

$$= 36 \text{ subjects per group} \times 2 \text{ groups} = \textbf{72 subjects total}$$

Interpretation: The total number of subjects needed is 72. Including z_β (for beta error) in the calculation approximately doubled the sample size in this box, compared with the sample size in Box 12–2. If the investigators had insisted on an even smaller beta error, the sample size would have increased even more.

ance (i.e., the estimate was too small), the sample size would be too small, and the study might miss showing statistical significance for a difference that was clinically important. Therefore, for safety, the actual sample size that investigators use when planning a study probably should be somewhat larger than that calculated from the formula in Box 12–2.

On the other hand, when z_α and z_β are added together before squaring (as shown in the formula in Box 12–3), the sample size may be excessive. Depending on the value of z_β used, this could as much as quadruple the *N* estimated, which would increase the cost of a study astronomically. The large sample sizes required are one of the reasons for the limited number of major studies that can now be funded nationally. Moreover, a needlessly large sample size introduces other problems for the investigators, who previously set the minimum difference they thought was worthwhile to detect. If the sample size is larger than necessary, when the analysis is done, differences smaller than those the investigators considered clinically important are now likely to become statistically significant, creating problems for the interpretation and possibly forcing the investigators to confront statistically significant differences that they did not consider clinically important. In the research described in Boxes 12–2 and 12–3, for example, investigators were trying to detect a difference of 10 mm Hg or more in systolic blood pressure, presumably because they felt that a smaller difference would not be clinically important. With a total sample size of 36 (see Box 12–2), a difference smaller than 10 mm Hg would not be significantly significant. However, with a total sample size of 72 (see Box 12–3), a difference of only 8 mm Hg would be statistically significant ($t = 2.26$; *p* is approximately 0.03 on 70 degrees of freedom). In cases such as this, it is important to focus on the original hypotheses of the research.

Sample Size for a Test of Differences in Proportions

Often a dependent variable is measured as success/failure and is described as the proportion of outcomes that represent some form of success, such as improvement in health, remission of disease, or reduction in mortality. In this case, the formula for sample size must be expressed in terms of proportions, as shown in the formula in Box 12–4.

Box 12–4 provides an example of how to calculate the sample size for a randomized controlled trial of a drug to reduce the 5-year mortality in patients with a particular form of cancer. Before the calculations can be made, the investigators must decide which values they will use for z_α, z_β, variance, and the smallest difference to be detected. For alpha and beta, they decide to use a level of 95% confidence (two-tailed test, $p = 0.05$) and 80% power (one-tailed test), so that z_α equals 1.96 and z_β equals 0.84.

Initially, as shown in the first part of Box 12–4, the investigators decide they want to detect a 10% improvement in survival (i.e., a difference of 0.1 between the 5-year mortality of the experimental group and that of the control group). They also assume that

medical world may have overreacted to the beta error study by Freiman et al. (1978), with the result that investigators began using samples that were larger than necessary.

On the one hand, if the estimated variance used in the calculations was smaller than the observed vari-

BOX 12–4   Initial and Subsequent Calculation of Sample Size for a Study Using a Test of Differences in Proportions and Considering Alpha and Beta Errors

Part 1A   Data on which the initial calculation is based

Study Characteristic	Assumptions Made by Investigator
Type of study	Randomized controlled trial of a drug to reduce the 5-year mortality in patients with a particular form of cancer
Data sets	Observations in one experimental group *(E)* and one control group *(C)* of the same size
Variable	Success = 5-year survival after treatment (0.6 in the experimental group and 0.5 in the control group); failure = death within 5 years of treatment
Losses to follow-up	None
Variance, expressed as $\overline{p}(1-\overline{p})$	$\overline{p} = 0.55$; therefore, $(1-\overline{p}) = 0.45$
Data for alpha (z_α)	$p = 0.05$; therefore, 95% confidence desired (two-tailed test); $z_\alpha = 1.96$
Data for beta (z_β)	20% beta error; therefore, 80% power desired (one-tailed test); $z_\beta = 0.84$
Difference to be detected $(\overline{d})$	0.1 or larger difference between the success (survival) of the experimental group and that of the control group (i.e., 10% difference—because $p_E = 0.6$, and $p_C = 0.5$)

Part 1B   Initial calculation of sample size *(N)*

$$N = \frac{(z_\alpha + z_\beta)^2 \cdot 2 \cdot \overline{p}(1-\overline{p})}{(\overline{d})^2} = \frac{(1.96 + 0.84)^2 \cdot 2 \cdot (0.55)(0.45)}{(0.1)^2}$$

$$= \frac{(7.84)(2)(0.2475)}{0.01} = \frac{3.88}{0.01} = 388$$

$$= 388 \text{ subjects per group} \times 2 \text{ groups} = \textbf{776 subjects total}$$

Interpretation: A total of 776 subjects would be needed, 388 in each group.

Part 2A   Changes in data on which the initial calculation was based

Study Characteristic	Assumptions Made by Investigator
Difference to be detected $(\overline{d})$	0.2 or larger difference between the success (survival) of the experimental group and that of the control group (i.e., 20% difference—because $p_E = 0.7$, and $p_C = 0.5$)
Variance, expressed as $\overline{p}(1-\overline{p})$	$\overline{p} = 0.60$; therefore, $(1-\overline{p}) = 0.40$

Part 2B   Subsequent (revised) calculation of sample size *(N)*

$$N = \frac{(z_\alpha + z_\beta)^2 \cdot 2 \cdot \overline{p}(1-\overline{p})}{(\overline{d})^2} = \frac{(1.96 + 0.84)^2 \cdot 2 \cdot (0.60)(0.40)}{(0.2)^2}$$

$$= \frac{(7.84)(2)(0.2400)}{0.04} = \frac{3.76}{0.04} = 94$$

$$= 94 \text{ subjects per group} \times 2 \text{ groups} = \textbf{188 subjects total}$$

Interpretation: Now a total of 188 subjects would be needed, 94 in each group. As a result of changes in the data on which the initial calculation was based, the number of subjects needed would be reduced from 776 to 188.

the survival rate will be 60% (0.6) in the experimental group and 50% (0.5) in the control group. Therefore, the mean proportion of success $(\overline{p})$ for all subjects enrolled in the study will be 0.55. Based on these assumptions, the calculations show that they would need 388 subjects in the experimental group and 388 in the control group, for a total of 776 subjects. In all probability, it would be difficult to find that many subjects or fund a study this large. What can be done? Theoretically, any of the estimated values in the formula might be altered. However, the alpha and beta values that they chose are the ones customarily used, and the best estimate of variance should always be used. Therefore, the only place to rethink the sample size calculation is the requirement for the minimum difference to be detected. Perhaps a 10% improvement is not large enough to be very meaningful. What if it were changed to 20% (a difference of 0.2, based on a survival rate of 70% in the experimental group and 50% in the control group)? As shown in the second part of Box 12–4, changing the improvement requirement to 20% changes the variance estimate, so that $\overline{p}$ is equal to 0.6. Based on these revised assumptions, the calculations show that the investigators would need 94 subjects in the experimental group and 94 in the control group, for a total of 188 subjects. A study with this smaller sample size appears much more reasonable and more likely to be funded, but changing the difference the investigators want to detect after a sample size calculation is made may be trying to adjust truth to what is convenient. If the investigators really believe the small difference is clinically important, they should try to obtain funding for the large sample required.

In choosing the 10% difference initially, the investigators may have intuitively assumed (incorrectly) that it is easier to detect a small difference than a large one. Or they may just have had an interest in detecting a small difference, even though it would not be clinically important. In either case, the penalty in sample size may alert the investigators to the statistical realities of the situation and force them to think seriously about the smallest difference that would be clinically important. Once they have agreed on the minimal clinically important difference, they should retain it in their research, despite any sample size difficulties.

■ ENLISTING STUDY SUBJECTS

Most funding organizations award clinical research grants only to institutions that have a committee specifically charged with the responsibility of reviewing all proposed research and ensuring that it is ethical. In federal legislation, this type of committee is called an **institutional review board** (IRB). IRBs have their foundation in the World Medical Association's Declaration of Helsinki, which was originally drafted in June 1964 and was subsequently amended in 1975, 1983, 1989, and 1996. The primary goals of IRBs are to ensure the following: that all research involving human subjects is of high quality (so that any risks involved are justified); that the potential benefits to the study subjects or to society in general are greater than the potential harm from the research; that researchers will obtain documented **informed consent** from study subjects or their guardians; that researchers will protect the confidentiality of their research data; and that study subjects will be allowed to withdraw from the research at any time, without this action's adversely affecting their care. Most universities and hospitals now require that all **human research protocols** be approved by an IRB, whether or not the research is externally funded.

■ RANDOMIZING STUDY SUBJECTS

There is a distinction between **randomization,** which entails allocating the available subjects to one or another study group, and **random sampling,** which entails selecting a small group for study from a much larger group of potential study subjects. Randomization is usually used in clinical studies.

Goals of Randomization

An experimental design, of which the randomized clinical trial is the standard in clinical research, depends on an **unbiased allocation of study subjects** to the experimental and control groups. For most purposes, the only evidence of an unbiased allocation that will be accepted is randomization. Contrary to popular opinion, randomization does not guarantee that the two (or more) groups created by random allocation are identical in either size or subject characteristics. What randomization does guarantee, if properly done, is that the different groups will be free of selection bias and problems resulting from regression toward the mean.

Selection bias can occur if subjects are allowed to choose whether they will be in an intervention group or a control group, as occurred in the 1954 polio vaccine trials (see Chapter 4). Selection bias can also occur if investigators influence the assignment of subjects to one group or another. There may be considerable pressure from a patient and from his or her family members or other care givers to alter the randomization process and let the patient into the intervention group, especially in studies involving a community intervention (Lam, Hartwell, and Jekel 1994), but this pressure must be resisted.

Regression toward the mean, which is also known as the **statistical regression effect,** affects patients who were chosen to participate in a study precisely because they had an extreme measurement on some variable (e.g., a high number of throat infections during the past year). They are likely to have a measurement that is closer to average at a later time (e.g., during the subsequent year) for reasons unrelated to the type or efficacy of the treatment they are given. In a study comparing treatment methods in two groups of patients, both of which had extreme measurements at the beginning of the study, randomization cannot eliminate the tendency to regress toward the mean. However, randomization can equalize the tendency between the study groups, thereby preventing bias in the comparison. When Paradise et al. (1984), for example, undertook a randomized clinical trial of surgical treatment (tonsillectomy and adenoidectomy) versus medical treatment (antibiotics) of children with recurrent throat infections, they found that the children in both groups had fewer episodes of throat infection in the year following treatment than in the year before (an effect attributed to regression toward the mean) but that the surgically treated patients showed more improvement than the medically treated patients (an effect attributed to the intervention).

Methods of Randomization

Before and after studies sometimes randomize the study subjects into two groups, so that one group is given the experimental intervention first and the other group is given the placebo first. Then, after a **washout period** (a period in which no intervention is given and physiologic values are expected to return to baseline), the group that was previously given the experimental intervention now receives the placebo and vice versa. By careful analysis, it is possible to see whether being randomized to receive the experimental intervention first or second made any difference.

When a study involving an experimental group and a control group is planned, the investigators must decide what method of randomization will be used to ensure that each subject has an equal probability of being assigned to the experimental group. As described below, some methods incorporate the use of a random number table such as that shown in the Appendix. Regardless of the method chosen, the best way to keep human preferences from creeping into the randomization process is to hide the results of randomization until they are needed for the analysis. If possible, the study subjects should not know which group they are in. This often can be accomplished by "blinding" the study subjects (e.g., giving the control group a placebo that looks, tastes, and smells the same as the treatment for the experimental group) and blinding the persons who record the findings from the study subjects. If both of these are done, it is a **double-blind study.**

The methods described below all assume that an equal number of subjects is desired in the experimental and control groups. However, the methods can easily be modified to provide two or more control subjects for each experimental subject.

Simple Random Allocation

In this method, the investigators begin with a random number table (see the Appendix) and a stack of sequentially numbered envelopes (e.g., numbered from 1 to 100 in a study with 100 participants). They blindly put a pencil on a number in the random number table and proceed from that number in a predetermined direction (e.g., up the columns of the table). If the first number is even, they write "experimental group" on a slip of paper and put it in the first envelope. If the next number is odd, they write "control group" on a slip of paper and insert it in the second envelope. They continue until all of the envelopes contain a random group assignment.

The first patient enrolled in the study is assigned to whatever group is indicated in the first envelope. As each new eligible patient is enrolled, the investigators open the next sequentially numbered envelope to find out the patient's group assignment.

Randomization into Groups of Two

Patients can be randomized two at a time. Envelopes are numbered sequentially (e.g., from 1 to 100) and separated into groups of two. As in the above method, the investigators begin by blindly putting down a pencil on a number in the random number table and proceeding in a predetermined direction. If the first number is even, they write "experimental group" on a slip of paper and put it in the first envelope. For the paired envelope, they automatically write the alternative group—in this case, "control group." They use the random number table to determine the assignment of the first envelope in the second pair and continue in this manner for each pair of envelopes. Thus, any time an even number of patients have been admitted into the study, half will be in the experimental group and half in the control group.

Systematic Allocation

Systematic allocation in research studies is equivalent to the old military "Sound off!" The first patient is randomly assigned to a group, and the next patient is automatically assigned to the alternative group. Subsequent patients are given group assignments on an alternating basis. This will ensure that the experimental and control groups are of equal size if there is an even number of patients entered in the study.

There are advantages to this method beyond simplicity. Usually, the variance of the data from a systematic allocation is smaller than that from a simple random allocation, so the statistical power is improved. However, if there is any kind of "periodicity" in the way patients enter, there may be a bias. For example, suppose systematic sampling is used to allocate patients into two groups, and only two patients are admitted each day to the study (e.g., the first two new patients who enter the clinic each morning). If each intake day started so that the first patient was assigned to the experimental group and the second was assigned to the control group, all of the experimental group subjects would be the first patients to arrive at the clinic, perhaps very early in the morning. They might be systematically different (e.g., employed, eager, early risers) compared to those who come later in the day, in which case bias might be introduced into the study. This danger is easy to avoid, however, if the investigator reverses the sequence frequently, sometimes taking the first person each day into the control group. The convenience and statistical advantages of systematic sampling make it desirable to use whenever possible.

The systematic allocation method can also be used for allocating study subjects to three, four, or even more groups.

Stratified Allocation

In clinical research, stratified allocation is often called **prognostic stratification.** It is used when the investigators want to assign patients to different risk groups depending on such baseline variables as the severity of disease (e.g., stage of cancer) and age. When such risk groups have been created, each stratum can then be allocated randomly to the experimental group or the control group. This is usually done to ensure homogeneity of the study groups by severity of disease. If the experimental and control groups have been made prognostically similar, the analysis can be done both for the entire group and within the prognostic groups.

Special Issues Concerning Randomization

Randomization does not guarantee that two or more groups will be identical. Suppose an investigator, when checking how similar the experimental and control groups were after randomization, found that the two groups were of somewhat different size and that 1 out of 20 characteristics being compared showed a statistically significant difference between the groups. The fact that there are occasional differences which are statistically significant does not mean that the randomization was biased; some differences are expected by chance alone. However, there may be a legitimate concern that some of the observed differences between the randomized groups could confound the analysis. In that case, the variables of concern can be controlled for in the analysis.

Even though randomization is the fundamental technique of clinical trials, many other precautions must still be taken in clinical trials, including ensuring the accuracy of all of the data by blinding patients and observers, standardizing data collection instruments, and so forth.

One of the biggest problems of randomization has to do with the generalizability of findings of the study. Obviously, patients have the right to refuse to participate in a study. This means that a particular study is limited to patients who are willing to participate. Are these patients typical of patients who refused to participate, or are they an unusual subset of the entire population with the problem being studied? The results of a clinical trial can only be generalized to similar patients.

What happens if, following randomization, a patient is not doing well and the patient or physician wishes to switch from the experimental treatment to another medication? Ethically, the patient cannot be forced to continue a particular treatment. Once the switch occurs, it will be necessary to choose an alternative way of analyzing the data. There are several possible strategies, and the choice between them represents a philosophical position. Currently, the popular approach is to analyze the data as if the patient had remained in his or her original group, so that any negative outcomes are assigned to their original treatment. This strategy, called the **"intention to treat" approach,** is based on the belief that if the patient was doing so poorly as to want to switch, a negative outcome should be ascribed to that treatment. Other investigators prefer to analyze the data as if the patient had never participated in the study, but this could lead to a small, and probably biased, sample. Still others prefer to reassign the patient to a third group and analyze the data separately from the original groups. The problem with this approach is that the original groups are changed and it is not clear whom the remaining groups represent.

Another problem in randomized trials of treatment is deciding what to consider as the starting point for measuring the outcome. For example, if surgical treatment and medical treatment are being compared, should surgical mortality be included as part of the debit side for surgical treatment, or is the question "Given survival from initial surgical or medical therapy, does the other treatment do better?" (Sackett and Gent 1979). Most investigators recommend counting from the point of randomization.

■ DANGERS OF DATA DREDGING

In studies with large amounts of data, there is a temptation to use modern computer techniques to see which variables are associated with which other variables and to grind out hundreds of associations. This process is sometimes referred to as data dredging.

The search for associations can be appropriate as long as the investigator keeps two points in mind. First, the scientific process requires that hypothesis development and hypothesis testing be based on different data sets. One data set is used to develop the hypothesis or model, which is used to make predictions, which are then tested on a new data set. Second, a correlational study (e.g., the Pearson correlation coefficient or the chi-square test) is useful only for developing hypotheses, not for testing them. Stated in slightly different terms, a correlational study is only a kind of screening method. Investigators who keep these points clearly in mind are unlikely to make the mistake of thinking every association found in a data set represents a true association.

One of the most celebrated examples of the problem of data dredging was seen in the report of an association between coffee consumption and pancreatic cancer (MacMahon et al. 1981), obtained by looking at many associations in a large data set, without repeating the analysis on another data set to see if it was consistent. This approach was severely criticized at the time (Feinstein et al. 1981), and several subsequent studies have failed to find a true association between coffee consumption and pancreatic cancer.

How does this problem arise? Suppose there were 10 variables in a descriptive study and the investigator wanted to try to associate each one with every other one. There would be 10×10 possible cells

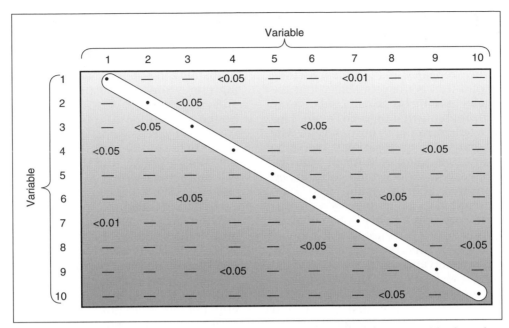

FIGURE 12–1   Matrix of possible statistical associations between 10 different variables from the same research study. Perfect correlations of one variable with itself are shown by dots; nonstatistically significant relationships are shown by dashes; and statistically significant associations are shown by the *p* values. (Redrawn from Jekel, J. F. Should we stop using the *p*-value in descriptive studies? Pediatrics 60:124–126, 1977. Reproduced by permission of Pediatrics, vol. 60, page 125, copyright 1977.)

represented (Fig. 12–1). However, 10 of these would be each variable times itself, which is always a perfect correlation. That leaves 90 possible associations, but half of these would be "*x* times *y*" and the other half "*y* times *x*." Because the *p* values for bivariate tests are the same regardless of which is considered the independent variable and which is considered the dependent one, there are only half as many truly independent associations, or 45. If the *p* = 0.05 cutoff point is used for alpha, then out of 45 independent associations, slightly more than 2 "statistically significant" associations would be expected to occur by chance alone (see Jekel 1977).

The problem with multiple hypotheses is similar to the problem with multiple associations: the greater the number of hypotheses that are tested, the more likely it is that at least one of them will be found "statistically significant" by chance alone. One possible way to handle this is to lower the *p* value required before rejecting the null hypothesis (e.g., make it less than 0.05). This was done in a study testing the same medical educational hypothesis at 5 different hospitals (Jekel et al. 1983). If the alpha level in the study had been set at 0.05, there would have been almost a 25% probability of finding a statistically significant difference by chance alone in at least 1 of the 5 hospitals, because each hospital had a 5% (alpha = 0.05) probability of showing a difference owing to chance alone. To keep the risk of a false-positive finding in the entire study to no more than 0.05, the alpha level chosen for rejecting the null hypothesis was made more stringent by dividing alpha by 5 (the number of hospitals) to make it 0.01. This method of adjusting for multiple hypotheses is called the **Bonferroni ad-**

justment to alpha. There are other possible adjustments that are less stringent, but they are more complicated and are used in different situations. Examples include the Tukey procedure, the Scheffe procedure, and the Newman-Keuls procedure (see Dawson-Saunders and Trapp 1994).

■ ELEMENTARY PROBABILITY THEORY

A newsletter from a local insurance agent recently made the following argument:

> Statistics indicate that if you are fortunate enough to reach age 65, the odds are . . . 50/50 you will spend time in a nursing home. . . . Ergo (our logic): If there are two of you, it would seem the odds are 100% that one of you will need . . . [nursing home] care.

Is this writer's logic correct when he states that if two married people reach the age of 65, there is essentially a 100% chance that at least one member of the couple will require nursing home care? Common sense would indicate that this is not true, because at least some couples are certain to escape. However, it is better to know where the fallacy in the writer's reasoning lies.

There are three basic rules of probability that should be kept in mind when considering arguments such as that used in the example: the independence rule, the product rule, and the addition rule.

The Independence Rule

If the insurance agent's statement that the husband and wife each have a 50% chance of requiring care in a nursing home is true and if the probabilities are independent of each other, the correct probability that one of them will require nursing home care can be obtained by many trials of flipping an unbiased coin, twice in a row, repeated many times. Assume that the first flip of a trial is the probability that the husband would need nursing home care and that the second flip is the probability that the wife would. Two successive heads would mean both husband and wife would need such care (not necessarily at the same time); one head and one tail would mean that one partner would need care and one would not; and two tails would mean that neither would need care. Heads could be recorded as a plus sign (+), meaning that nursing home care is necessary; tails could be recorded as a minus sign (–), meaning that nursing home care is unnecessary; and the symbols H and W could be used for husband and wife.

Repeated trials of two flips would show the following: a 25% chance of getting two heads in a row (H+ and W+); a 25% chance of getting first a head and then a tail (H+ and W–); a 25% chance of getting first a tail and then a head (H– and W+); and a 25% chance of getting two tails (H– and W–). Therefore, if each member of a couple has a 50% probability of requiring nursing home care at some time and if these probabilities are independent, the chances that at least one member of the couple would require nursing home care at some time would be 75%, not 100%.

In this example, independence means that the overall probability of the husband's being confined to a nursing home is the same whether the wife is confined or not (and vice versa). In statistical terms, this statement can be expressed as follows: $p\{H+ \mid W+\} = p\{H+ \mid W–\}$. Here, p denotes probability, H+ denotes confinement of the husband, the vertical line means "given that" or "conditional upon" what immediately follows, W+ denotes confinement of the wife, and W– denotes no confinement of the wife.

The independence rule does not mean that the husband and wife must have an equal probability of being confined to a nursing home; it requires only that the probability of one partner (whatever that probability is) is not influenced by what happens to the other.

The Product Rule

The product rule is used to determine the probability of two things being true. The manner of calculation depends on whether the two things are independent.

In the example of the husband and wife, if independence is assumed, this simplifies the calculation. The probability that *both* the husband and wife will be confined to a nursing home is simply the product of their independent probabilities. Thus, $p\{H+ \text{ and } W+\} = p\{H+\} \times p\{W+\} = 0.5 \times 0.5 = 0.25$. The probability that *neither* will be confined to a nursing home is the product of the probabilities of not being in a nursing home. Thus, $p\{H– \text{ and } W–\} = p\{H–\} \times p\{W–\} = (1 – p\{H+\}) \times (1 – p\{W+\}) = (1 – 0.5) \times (1 –$ 0.5) $= 0.25$. These answers are the same answers that were derived from flipping coins.

If independence cannot be assumed, a more general product rule must be used. In calculating the probability that *neither* would be confined to a nursing home, the general product rule says that $p\{H– \text{ and } W–\} = p\{H– \mid W–\} \times p\{W–\}$. The answer would be the same if the rule was expressed as $p\{H– \text{ and } W–\} = p\{W– \mid H–\} \times p\{H–\}$. In this example, the probability of the husband not being confined if the wife is not confined is 0.5, and the probability that the wife will not be confined is 0.5. Therefore, the $p\{H– \text{ and } W–\} = 0.5 \times 0.5 = 0.25$, again the same answer as derived from flipping coins.

Although the insurance agent assumed that the probabilities for the husband and wife were each 50%, a detailed study by Kemper and Murtaugh (1991) estimated that the probability of confinement in a nursing home after age 65 is 33% for the husband and 52% for the wife. If independence between these probabilities is assumed, the probability that they both will be confined to a nursing home would be calculated as the product of the separate probabilities: $0.33 \times 0.52 = 0.17 = 17\%$.

The Addition Rule

One of the insurance agent's errors was adding the probabilities when he should have multiplied them. A quick way to know that adding the probabilities was incorrect would have been to say, "Suppose each partner had a 90% chance of being confined." If adding were the correct approach, the total probability would be 180%, which is impossible. According to the addition rule, all of the possible different probabilities in a situation must add up to 1.0 (100%), no more and no less.

The addition rule is used to determine the probability of one thing being true under all possible conditions. For example, it may be used to determine the lifetime probability that the husband will be confined to a nursing home, taking into consideration that the wife may or may not be confined. In this case, the equation would be as follows: $p\{H+\} = p\{H+ \mid W+\} \times p\{W+\} + p\{H+ \mid W–\} \times p\{W–\}$. Box 12–5 shows the calculations for this formula, based on probabilities estimated from Kemper and Murtaugh (1991). Husbands have a lower probability of being in a nursing home than do wives, partly because wives are often younger and may take care of the husband at home, thus removing his need for a nursing home, and partly because women live longer and are more likely to reach the age at which many people require nursing home care.

Note that the numerator and the denominator of Bayes' theorem (see Chapter 8) are based on the general product rule and the addition rule, respectively.

■ SUMMARY

The most common reason biostatisticians are consulted is for help in calculating sample sizes needed

---

BOX 12–5   Calculation of All Possible Probabilities of Husband and Wife Requiring or Not Requiring Care in a Nursing Home

Part 1   Definitions

H+ = probability that the husband will require care in a nursing home at some time

H– = probability that the husband will not require care in a nursing home at some time

W+ = probability that the wife will require care in a nursing home at some time

W– = probability that the wife will not require care in a nursing home at some time

Part 2   Assumptions on which calculations are based

(1) The following holds true if the wife does not require care in a nursing home: H+ = 0.3 and H– = 0.7

(2) The following holds true if the wife does require care in a nursing home: H+ = 0.4 and H– = 0.6

(3) The following holds true whether or not the husband requires care in a nursing home: W+ = 0.52 and W– = 0.48

Part 3   Calculations

(1) Probability that neither the husband nor the wife will require care in a nursing home:

$$p\{H- \text{ and } W-\} = p\{H- \mid W-\} \times p\{W-\} = 0.7 \times 0.48 = \mathbf{0.336}$$

(2) Probability that both the husband and the wife will require care in a nursing home:

$$p\{H+ \text{ and } W+\} = p\{H+ \mid W+\} \times p\{W+\} = 0.4 \times 0.52 = \mathbf{0.208}$$

(3) Probability that the husband will require care and the wife will not require care in a nursing home:

$$p\{H+ \text{ and } W-\} = p\{H+ \mid W-\} \times p\{W-\} = 0.3 \times 0.48 = \mathbf{0.144}$$

(4) Probability that the husband will not require care and the wife will require care in a nursing home:

$$p\{H- \text{ and } W+\} = p\{H- \mid W+\} \times p\{W+\} = 0.6 \times 0.52 = \mathbf{0.312}$$

(5) Sum of the above probabilities (must always equal 1.00):

$$0.336 + 0.208 + 0.144 + 0.312 = \mathbf{1.00}$$

Note that, as it should, the sum of (1) and (3) equals the probability that the wife will not require care in a nursing home (0.336 + 0.144 = 0.48). Likewise, the sum of (1) and (4) equals the probability that the husband will not require care in a nursing home (0.336 + 0.312 = 0.648), on average.

Source of data on which probability estimates are based: Kemper, P., and C. M. Murtaugh. Lifetime use of nursing home care. New England Journal of Medicine 324:595–560, 1991.

---

for studies. Such help can be given only, however, if the investigator already has determined the basic numbers that will be used in the calculations: the level of alpha and beta to be used, the clinically important difference in outcome variables to be detected, and the variance expected. Determining the needed sample size is usually straightforward if these values are known. The equations commonly used are shown in Table 12–1.

Another process that is essential to much clinical research is random allocation. This is ordinarily not difficult to accomplish effectively if certain steps are followed carefully. It is especially important to keep the selection process secret until it is announced, and sealed envelopes are often a good way to achieve this. The basic methods of random allocation include simple random allocation, randomization into groups of two, systematic allocation, and stratified allocation.

In the analysis of data, investigators should be alert to the problem of multiple associations, which occurs when multiple hypotheses are tested. Without some statistical adjustment, testing multiple hypotheses increases the probability of false-positive statistical associations (alpha errors).

In the calculation of probabilities, three basic rules should be kept in mind: the independence rule, the product rule, and the addition rule. If the independence of two events can be assumed, then the probability of both events occurring jointly is the product of their separate probabilities. This is true whether the probability is that something will happen or that something will not happen.

■ QUESTIONS

Directions (Items 1–10). Each of the numbered items or incomplete statements in this section is followed by answers or by completions of the statement. Select the ONE lettered answer or completion that is BEST in each case. Correct answers and explanations are given at the end of the chapter.

1. The formula for a paired *t*-test is as follows:

$$t_\alpha = \frac{\overline{d}}{\dfrac{s_d}{\sqrt{N}}}$$

To calculate for sample size, this formula is often used and rearranged algebraically to solve for *N*. In the process, *z* must be substituted for *t* because

(A) *t* is dependent on degrees of freedom and *z* is not
(B) *t* provides too large a sample
(C) *t* provides too small a sample
(D) *z* is dependent on degrees of freedom and *t* is not
(E) *z* takes beta error into account

2. It is important to consider beta error when
(A) the difference under consideration is not clinically meaningful
(B) the difference under investigation is statistically significant
(C) the null hypothesis is not rejected
(D) the null hypothesis is rejected
(E) the sample size is excessively large

3. Which one of the following characteristics of a diagnostic test is analogous to the statistical power of a study?
(A) Positive predictive value
(B) Negative predictive value
(C) Sensitivity
(D) Specificity
(E) Utility

4. An investigator studying the health effects of rutabaga in subjects with arthritis tends to assign enthusiastic participants to rutabaga and skeptics to the placebo. The best way to avoid this form of bias is
(A) "intention to treat" analysis
(B) random sampling
(C) randomization
(D) self-selection
(E) statistical regression

5. Statistical methods of adjusting for the testing of multiple hypotheses from a single large data set, such as the Bonferroni adjustment to alpha, are designed to prevent
(A) bias
(B) confounding
(C) effect modification
(D) false-negative results
(E) false-positive results

6. Assume that the risk of myocardial infarction during the next year in a 60-year-old man is 20%

but is reduced by half if the man exercises regularly. Assume as well that the risk of the same event in the man's 58-year-old wife is 14% but is reduced by half if she uses hormone replacement therapy. What is the probability that neither husband nor wife will experience a myocardial infarction during the next year if the husband exercises but the wife is unwilling to take supplemental hormones?

(A) 17%
(B) 20%
(C) 37%
(D) 77%
(E) 93%

Items 7–10

A study is designed to test the effects of sleep deprivation on academic performance among medical students. Each subject serves as his or her own control. A 10-point difference (10% difference) in test scores is considered meaningful. The standard deviation of test scores in a similar study was 8. Alpha is set at 0.05 (two-tailed test), and beta is set at 0.2.

7. The appropriate sample size is
(A) 6
(B) 16
(C) 34
(D) 60
(E) 100

8. The study is conducted by another group that does not specify beta. The required sample size for this study is
(A) 3
(B) 6
(C) 8
(D) 30
(E) 60

9. The study in question 7 is conducted by yet another group. All the specified parameters remain the same, but the investigators use separate intervention and control groups. The required sample size for this study is
(A) 6
(B) 11
(C) 18
(D) 22
(E) 60

10. The study in question 7 is revised to detect a difference of only 2 points (2%) in test scores. All other parameters of the original study remain unchanged. The required sample size is
(A) 6
(B) 12
(C) 42
(D) 60
(E) 126

ANSWERS AND EXPLANATIONS

1. **The answer is A: *t* is dependent on degrees of freedom and *z* is not.** Both *z* and *t* are used to provide unit-free measures of dispersion about a mean value. When the sample size is small, the *t* distribution must be used (instead of the *z* distribution), and the *t* distribution varies with the size of the sample. Degrees of freedom derive from the sample size, which is the unknown in a sample size calculation. This means that *t* cannot be used to calculate sample size, because the sample size must be known to calculate *t*. Use of *z* circumvents this problem and is customary. The substitution confers a slight risk of underestimating the sample size required.

2. **The answer is C: the null hypothesis is not rejected.** Beta error (which is also called type II error and false-negative error) is the failure to detect a true difference when one exists. Only a negative result (i.e., failure to reject the null hypothesis) is at risk for being a false-negative result. If the null hypothesis is rejected (choice D) or if the difference under investigation is statistically significant (choice B), a difference is being detected, so neither of these choices can be correct. Beta error is the result of inadequate power to detect the difference under investigation and therefore occurs when the sample size is small, not large. Either enlarging the sample or pooling data to increase statistical power would be an appropriate means to correct beta error, provided that the difference is clinically meaningful.

3. **The answer is C: sensitivity.** The sensitivity of a diagnostic test, or $a/(a + c)$, is the ability of the test to detect a condition when it is present. Similarly, statistical power is the ability of a study to detect a difference when it exists. Beta error is (1 – sensitivity) or (1 – statistical power).

4. **The answer is C: randomization.** The bias described is selection bias. This type of bias can occur whenever an investigator believes in a particular intervention and has the ability to assign to that intervention those subjects most likely to respond well. Selection bias can also occur when subjects choose a particular study or a particular intervention. Randomization in the assignment of interventions is the best way to avoid selection bias. Randomization should not be confused with random sampling. Random sampling is a method of drawing a representative study sample from a larger population but does not pertain to assigning treatment interventions. In "intention to treat" analysis, study data are interpreted on the basis of a subject's assignment to a particular group, regardless of whether the subject actually complied with that assignment. Statistical regression is not a technique but, rather, a tendency against which one needs to be on guard. Extreme values tend to "regress" toward the mean when they are reassessed over time, simply because they had already become maximally extreme and the only direction they could go is back toward the population "norm." When randomization is used in the assignment of interventions, extreme values that are susceptible to the statistical regression effect will be distributed evenly between intervention groups. While randomization cannot ensure that groups will be comparable in all ways except for the intervention assigned, it is an unbiased means of allocating subjects to treatment assignments. Randomization has the potential to eliminate both known and unknown confounders.

5. **The answer is E: false-positive results.** When investigators set alpha at 0.05, this means that they are accepting a 5% risk of rejecting the null hypothesis on the basis of a random outcome. This risk is small when a single hypothesis is tested. However, if that same 5% risk pertains to each of many hypotheses being tested, the aggregate risk of rejecting one of the null hypotheses on the basis of chance becomes large. If 20 hypotheses are tested, a single false-positive result can be expected with some confidence. Various techniques, including the Bonferroni adjustment to alpha, can be used to maintain the aggregate risk of a false-positive result close to the 0.05 level. Such techniques place more stringent requirements on associations before the associations are deemed significant and the null hypothesis is rejected.

6. **The answer is D: 77%.** The probability that the husband will experience a myocardial infarction is 20% if he does not exercise and 10% if he does. We are told that he is exercising. Therefore, the probability that the husband will not experience a myocardial infarction during the next year is 90%. The wife's risk of myocardial infarction is 14%. Her risk is not reduced, because she is disinclined to use hormone replacement therapy. Her probability of not experiencing a myocardial infarction is therefore 86%. The risks for myocardial infarction are independent in the two individuals. Therefore, the probability that neither spouse will experience a myocardial infarction is the product of their separate probabilities of not experiencing a myocardial infarction, or (0.90)(0.86) = 0.774. This is approximately 77%.

7. **The answer is A: 6.** This is a study for which a paired *t*-test is appropriate. The corresponding sample size formula, as detailed in Box 12–1, is

$$N = \frac{(z_\alpha)^2 \cdot (s)^2}{(\overline{d})^2}$$

In this example, however, the value for beta is also specified, so that the formula becomes

$$N = \frac{(z_\alpha + z_\beta)^2 \cdot (s)^2}{(\overline{d})^2}$$

The value of z_α when alpha is 0.05 and the test is two-tailed is 1.96. The value of z_β when beta is 20%, or 0.2, is 0.84; z_β is one-tailed by convention. The standard deviation (s) is derived from a prior study and is 8. The difference sought is 10 points. The equation becomes the following:

$$N = \frac{(1.96 + 0.84)^2 \cdot (8)^2}{(10)^2}$$

$$= \frac{(7.84)(64)}{100}$$

$$= 501.76/100$$

$$= 5.02$$

By convention, all sample size calculations are rounded up to the nearest whole number. The correct answer is therefore 6. The small sample size required for this study is the result of the large difference sought (a 10% change in test scores is substantial), the small standard deviation, and the use of each subject as his or her own control. The sample required would be even smaller if beta were not specified (see the explanation for question 8, below).

8. **The answer is A: 3.** The sample size calculation here is the same as for question 7, but this time there is no beta term. Therefore, the equation is as follows:

$$N = \frac{(1.96)^2 \cdot (8)^2}{(10)^2}$$

$$= \frac{(3.8416)(64)}{100}$$

$$= 245.86/100$$

$$= 2.46 \text{ rounded to } 3$$

This is obviously a very small sample. A sample this small may make intuitive sense if you consider how many subjects you would need to demonstrate that test scores are higher if the test taker gets 8 hours of sleep the night before the test, rather than staying up all night.

9. **The answer is D: 22.** The formula for this calculation is shown in Box 12–2. The basic sample size formula for a trial using separate control and intervention groups is as follows:

$$N = \frac{(z_\alpha + z_\beta)^2 \cdot 2 \cdot (s)^2}{(\overline{d})^2}$$

Note that the term for z_β has been added to the numerator. The difference between this equation and the equation for the before and after study in question 7 is the 2 in the numerator, doubling the sample. When the numbers from question 7 are inserted, the equation becomes the following:

$$N = \frac{(1.96 + 0.84)^2 \cdot 2 \cdot (8)^2}{(10)^2}$$

$$= \frac{(7.84)(2)(64)}{100}$$

$$= 1003.52/100$$

$$= 10.04 \text{ rounded to } 11$$

N represents the number of subjects needed per group. As there are now separate control and intervention groups, the total sample is $2N$. The total number of subjects needed is therefore 22.

10. **The answer is E: 126.** The calculation is as shown in the answer to question 7, with one difference: the denominator is now $(2)^2$ instead of $(10)^2$. The numerator is again 501.76. When this is divided by $(10)^2$, or 100, it yields a sample size of 5.02, or 6. When divided by $(2)^2$, or 4, it yields a sample size of 125.44, or 126. As this example demonstrates, the size of the difference in outcome that the investigator is hoping to detect can have a profound effect on sample size requirements.

References Cited

Dawson-Saunders, B., and R. G. Trapp. Basic and Clinical Biostatistics, 2nd ed. Norwalk, Conn., Appleton and Lange, 1994.

Feinstein, A. R., et al. Coffee and pancreatic cancer: the problems of etiologic science and epidemiologic case-control research. Journal of the American Medical Association 246:957–961, 1981.

Freiman, J. A., et al. The importance of beta, the type II error, and sample size in the design and interpretation of the randomized control trial: a survey of 71 "negative" trials. New England Journal of Medicine 299:690–695, 1978.

Jekel, J. F. Should we stop using the p-value in descriptive studies? Pediatrics 60:124–126, 1977.

Jekel, J. F., et al. The regional educational impact of a renal stone center. Yale Journal of Biology and Medicine 56:97–108, 1983.

Kelsey, J. L., et al. Methods in Observational Epidemiology, 2nd ed. New York, Oxford University Press, 1996.

Kemper, P., and C. M. Murtaugh. Lifetime use of nursing home care. New England Journal of Medicine 324:595–600, 1991.

Lam, J. A., S. W. Hartwell, and J. F. Jekel. "I prayed real hard, so I know I'll get in": living with randomization. New Directions for Program Evaluation 63:55–66, 1994.

MacMahon, B., et al. Coffee and cancer of the pancreas. New England Journal of Medicine 304:630–633, 1981.

Paradise, J. L., et al. Efficacy of tonsillectomy for recurrent throat infection in severely affected children. New England Journal of Medicine 310:674–683, 1984.

Sackett, D. L., and M. Gent. Controversy in counting and attributing events in clinical trials. New England Journal of Medicine 301:1410–1412, 1979.

Selected Readings

Dawson-Saunders, B., and R. G. Trapp. Basic and Clinical Biostatistics, 2nd ed. Norwalk, Conn., Appleton and Lange, 1994.

Feinstein, A. R. The other side of "statistical significance": alpha, beta, delta, and the calculation of sample size. Clinical Pharmacology and Therapeutics 18:491–505, 1975.

Kelsey, J. L. et al. Methods in Observational Epidemiology, 2nd ed. New York, Oxford University Press, 1996.

13

Multivariable Analysis

■ AN OVERVIEW OF MULTIVARIABLE STATISTICS

However imperfect they may be, mathematical and statistical equations are attempts to model reality (Kac 1969). Statistical models often seek to represent only one dimension of reality, such as the effect of a change in one variable (e.g., a nutrient) on another variable (e.g., the growth rate of a rat). For such models to be meaningful, all factors other than the one being studied must be equalized to the extent possible in the research architecture—for example, by using genetically identical animals or by using randomization techniques to allocate human subjects to study groups. Often, however, either the other influences cannot be adequately controlled by design or the investigator may actually wish to study the relative size of simultaneous influences of several independent (possibly causal) variables on a dependent (outcome) variable.

Statistical models that have one outcome variable but include more than one independent variable are generally called **multivariable models.** (These are not the same as *multivariate* models, which have more than one outcome variable in addition to having more than one independent variable.) Multivariable models are intuitively attractive to investigators because they seem more true to life than the single-variable models. Multivariable analysis does not enable an investigator to ignore the basic principles of good research design and analysis, because

multivariable analysis also has many limitations. The methodology and interpretation of findings in this type of analysis are difficult for most physicians, despite the fact that the methods and results of multivariable analysis are reported frequently in the medical literature and their use is increasing (Concato, Feinstein, and Holford 1993). Their conceptual attractiveness and the availability of high-speed computers contribute to making these methods popular. In order to be intelligent consumers of the medical literature, health care professionals should understand how to interpret the findings of multivariable analysis as they are presented in the literature.

A Conceptual Understanding of Equations

One of the reasons people "turn off" statistics is that the equations appear to be a jumble of meaningless symbols. That is especially true of multivariable techniques, but it is possible to understand conceptually, rather than mathematically, what is generally going on in multivariable analysis. For example, suppose that there is a study of the prognosis of patients at the time of diagnosis for a certain cancer for which there is not, as yet, an effective treatment. The physician might surmise that the length of survival for a patient would depend on at least four things: the patient's age, the anatomic stage of the disease at the time of diagnosis, the presence or absence of other diseases (comorbidity), and the degree of systemic symptoms such as weight loss. That relationship could be explained conceptually as follows:

$$\text{Cancer prognosis varies with Age and}$$
$$\text{Stage and Comorbidity and Symptoms} \quad (13\text{--}1)$$

This statement could be made to look more mathematical simply by making a few slight changes:

$$\text{Cancer prognosis} \approx \text{Age} + \text{Stage}$$
$$+ \text{Comorbidity} + \text{Symptoms} \quad (13\text{--}2)$$

The four independent variables on the right side of the equation are not necessarily of equal importance. Expression 13–2 can be improved by giving each independent variable a **coefficient,** which is a **weighting factor** based on its relative importance in predicting prognosis. Thus, the equation becomes:

209

$$\text{Cancer prognosis} \approx (\text{Weight}_1)\,\text{Age} + (\text{Weight}_2)\,\text{Stage}$$
$$+ (\text{Weight}_3)\,\text{Comorbidity}$$
$$+ (\text{Weight}_4)\,\text{Symptoms} \qquad (13\text{--}3)$$

Before equation 13–3 can become useful, two more things are needed. First, some sort of **anchor point** for the equation is needed. This anchor point must be something comparable to the a of the formula for simple regression ($y = a + bx$). Second, an **error term** is needed to make the equation true if the prediction is not perfect. By inserting the anchor point and the error term, the $\approx$ symbol (meaning "varies with") can be replaced by an equals sign. Abbreviating the weights with a W, the equation now becomes:

$$\text{Cancer prognosis} = \text{Anchor point} + W_1\text{Age}$$
$$+ W_2\text{Stage} + W_3\text{Comorbidity}$$
$$+ W_4\text{Symptoms} + \text{Error term}$$
$$(13\text{--}4)$$

In common statistical symbols, y is the dependent (outcome) variable (e.g., cancer prognosis) and is customarily placed on the left; $x_1 + x_2 + x_3 + x_4$ are the independent variables 1 (age) through 4 (symptoms), and they are lined up on the right; b_i is the statistical symbol for the weight of the ith independent variable; a is the estimated y-intercept (the anchor point); and e is the error term. Now, purely in statistical symbols, the equation can be expressed as follows:

$$y = a + b_1x_1 + b_2x_2 + b_3x_3 + b_4x_4 + e \qquad (13\text{--}5)$$

Although equation 13–5 looks complex, it means exactly the same thing as equations 13–1 through 13–4.

Best Estimates

Equation 13–5 cannot be used to do any calculations, because the value for the error term *(e)* is not known until after the equation has been solved for a and all of the b's. Therefore, in multivariable statistics a further modification is made in the equation. Instead of y, the estimated value of y—namely, $\hat{y}$ is used, and there is no error term. (Because the estimate of y has a circumflex, or "hat," over it, it is usually called y-hat.) If the values of all of the observed y's and all of the x's are inserted, the following equation can be solved:

$$\hat{y} = a + b_1x_1 + b_2x_2 + b_3x_3 + b_4x_4 \qquad (13\text{--}6)$$

When equation 13–6 is subtracted from equation 13–5, the following equation for the error term emerges:

$$(y - \hat{y}) = e \qquad (13\text{--}7)$$

The error term is the observed value of the outcome variable y for a given patient minus the predicted value of y for the same patient.

What happens to indicate when the best estimates of the values of a and b_i have been obtained? The best estimate has been achieved in this equation when the sum of the squared error term has been minimized. That sum is expressed as:

$$\sum(y_i - \hat{y})^2 = \sum(y_O - y_E)^2 = \sum e^2 \qquad (13\text{--}8)$$

This idea is not new, because as was noted in previous chapters, variation in statistics is measured as the sum of the squares of the observed value *(O)* minus the expected value *(E)*. In multivariable analysis, the error term e is often called a **residual.**

In straightforward language, the best estimates for the values of a and b_1 through b_4 are found when the total quantity of error (measured as the sum of squares of the error term, or, most simply, e^2) has been minimized. Those values of a and of the several b_i's that, taken together, give the smallest value for the squared error term are the best estimates that can be obtained from that set of data. Appropriately enough, this approach is called the **least-squares solution,** because the process is stopped when the sum of squares of the error term is the least.

The General Linear Model

The multivariable equation, with one dependent variable and one or more independent variables, as shown in equation 13–6, is usually called the general linear model. The model is "general" because there are many variations regarding the types of variables for y and x_i as well as the number of x variables that can be used. The model is "linear" because it is a linear combination of the x_i terms. For the x_i variables, a variety of transformations (e.g., square of x, cube of x, square root of x, or logarithm of x) could be used and the combination of terms would still be linear, so that the model would remain linear. What cannot happen if the model is to remain linear is for any of the coefficients (the b_i terms) to be a square, a square root, a logarithm, or another transformation.

Numerous procedures for multivariable analysis are based on the general linear model. These include methods with such imposing terms as analysis of variance (ANOVA), analysis of covariance (ANCOVA), multiple linear regression analysis, multiple logistic regression, the log-linear model, and discriminant function analysis. As discussed below and outlined in Table 13–1, the choice of which procedure to use depends primarily on whether the dependent and independent variables are continuous, dichotomous, nominal, or ordinal. Knowing that the procedures are all variations of the same theme (the general linear model) helps to make them less confusing.

Uses of Multivariable Statistics

In some research, important findings can be presented more clearly in a contingency table (see Chapter 11) than by multivariable analysis. Sometimes, however, subtle findings and interactions cannot be discovered without multivariable analysis. One of the

TABLE 13–1   Choice of an Appropriate Procedure to Be Used in Multivariable Analysis (Analysis of One Dependent Variable and More Than One Independent Variable)

Characterization of Variables to Be Analyzed		Appropriate Procedure or Procedures
Dependent Variable	**Independent Variables***	
Continuous	All are categorical.	Analysis of variance (ANOVA).
Continuous	Some are categorical and some are continuous.	Analysis of covariance (ANCOVA).
Continuous	All are continuous.	Multiple linear regression.
Ordinal	—	There is no formal multivariable procedure for ordinal dependent variables. Either treat the variables as if they were continuous (see above procedures) or perform log-linear analysis.
Dichotomous	All are categorical.	Logistic regression; log-linear analysis.
Dichotomous	Some are categorical and some are continuous.	Logistic regression.†
Dichotomous	All are continuous.	Logistic regression; discriminant function analysis.
Nominal	All are categorical.	Log-linear analysis.
Nominal	Some are categorical and some are continuous.	Group the continuous variables and perform log-linear analysis.
Nominal	All are continuous.	Discriminant function analysis; group the continuous variables and perform log-linear analysis.

*Categorical variables include ordinal, dichotomous, and nominal variables.

†If the outcome is a time-related dichotomous variable (such as live/die), then proportional hazards (Cox) models are best.

disadvantages of contingency tables compared to multivariable analysis is that unless the sample size is very large, the numbers in the cells of the final contingency tables might become small. This is because controlling for other variables in contingency tables requires subdividing the total sample size into many smaller tables containing subgroups. Multivariable analysis uses all of the observations in the analysis and therefore is often more efficient and robust than is contingency table analysis.

A frequent purpose of multivariable analysis is to understand how important, both individually and when acting together, the independent variables are

for explaining the variation in the dependent variable y. Often, there is considerable overlap in the ability of independent variables to explain the dependent variable. For example, both height and age predict body weight, but age and height are usually correlated, particularly for the first two decades of life. During the growth years, height and weight both increase with age, so that age can be considered the underlying explanatory variable and height can be viewed as an intervening variable influencing weight. Children, however, grow at different rates, so that height would add explanatory power that age could not: those children who were tall for their age would, on the average, also be heavier than children of the same age who were short for their age. Thus, each independent variable explains some of the variation in y beyond what any other variable explains.

Multivariable techniques also make it possible to determine whether there is an **interaction between variables.** Interaction is present when the value of one independent variable influences the way another independent variable explains y. In a large blood pressure survey in Connecticut, for example, Freeman et al. (1983) found that in African-American people under about 50 years of age, hypertension was more likely to occur in men than in women. After age 50, however, that trend was reversed, and hypertension was more likely to occur in women than in men. Thus, there was an interaction between age and gender in explaining the prevalence of hypertension.

In a clinical setting, such as an emergency room, it would be helpful to have some kind of scale or index that predicts whether or not a patient with chest pain is likely to have a myocardial infarction. One of several multivariable techniques can be used to develop such a **prediction model,** complete with coefficients for use in prediction. For example, in a classic study, Goldman et al. (1982) used a multivariable technique to develop a protocol to assist in the diagnosis of myocardial infarction in patients presenting to an emergency room with chest pain. Using various combinations of symptoms, signs, laboratory values, and electrocardiographic findings, the authors developed estimates for the probability of myocardial infarction. More recently, multiple logistic regression has become the most common technique used to develop clinical prediction models (see Other Procedures for Multivariable Analysis, below).

Multivariable analysis was also used by investigators in the Framingham Study to develop prediction equations for the 8-year risk of developing cardiovascular disease in people with various combinations of the following factors: smoking, elevated cholesterol levels, hypertension, glucose intolerance, and left ventricular hypertrophy (see Table 5–2 and the references listed in the table). These prediction equations or updated versions of them are being used in various health risk assessment programs.

Another increasingly important role for multivariable analysis in clinical research is to adjust for intergroup differences that remain after randomization, matching, or other design attempts to equalize comparison groups. For example, van den Hoogen et al. (2000) studied the relation between blood pressure and mortality from coronary heart disease in men from different parts of the world, after using multivariable statistical methods to adjust for age, total cholesterol level, and cigarette smoking.

If all goes well, the net effect of the complex calculations of multivariable analysis is that the investigators can determine which of the independent variables are the strongest predictors of y and which of the independent variables overlap with one another or interact in their ability to predict y.

■ PROCEDURES FOR MULTIVARIABLE ANALYSIS

As shown in Table 13–1, the choice of an appropriate statistical method for multivariable analysis depends on whether the dependent and independent variables are continuous, ordinal, dichotomous, or nominal. In cases in which more than one method could be used, the final choice will depend on the investigator's experience, personal preference, and comfort with the methods that are appropriate. Because there are many potential pitfalls in the use of multivariable techniques in medical research (see Concato, Feinstein, and Holford 1993), these techniques should not be used without experience or expert advice.

Analysis of Variance (ANOVA)

If the dependent variable is continuous and all of the independent variables are categorical (i.e., nominal, dichotomous, or ordinal), the correct multivariable technique is analysis of variance (ANOVA). One-way ANOVA and N-way ANOVA are discussed briefly below. Both techniques are based on the general linear model and can be used to analyze the results of an experimental study. If the design includes only one independent variable (e.g., treatment), the technique is called one-way analysis, regardless of how many different treatment groups are present. If it includes more than one independent variable (e.g., treatment, age group, and gender), the technique is called N-way ANOVA.

One-Way ANOVA (The F-Test)

Suppose a team of investigators wanted to study the effects of drugs A and B on blood pressure. They might randomly allocate hypertensive patients into four treatment groups: those taking drug A alone, those taking drug B alone, those taking drugs A and B in combination, and those taking a placebo. The investigators would measure systolic blood pressure before and after treatment in each patient and calculate a difference score (posttreatment systolic pressure minus pretreatment systolic pressure) for each study subject. This difference score would become the outcome variable. They would then calculate a mean difference score for each of the four treatment groups (i.e., the three drug groups and the one placebo group) so that these mean scores could be compared in a test of statistical significance.

The investigators would want to determine whether the difference in blood pressure found in one or more of the drug groups was large enough to be clinically important, assuming it was a drop. For example, a drop in mean systolic blood pressure from 150 mm Hg to 148 mm Hg would be too small to be clinically useful. If the results were not clinically useful, there would be little point in looking for an appropriate test of significance. If, however, one or more of the groups showed a clinically important drop in blood pressure, the investigators would want to determine whether the difference was likely to have occurred by chance alone. To do this, an appropriate statistical test of significance is needed.

The Student's t-test could be used to compare each pair of groups, but this would require six different t-tests: each of the three drug groups (A, B, and AB) versus the placebo group; drug A group versus drug B group; drug A group versus drug combination AB group; and drug B group versus drug combination AB group. This raises the problem of multiple hypotheses and multiple associations (see the discussion of alpha and p values under Dangers of Data Dredging in Chapter 12). Even if the investigators decided that the primary comparison should be each drug or drug combination with the placebo, this would still leave three hypotheses to test instead of just one. Moreover, if two or three groups did significantly better than the placebo group, it would be necessary to determine if one effective drug was significantly better than the others.

There are numerous complex ways of handling the problem of multiple associations (see Dawson-Saunders and Trapp 1994), but the best approach in cases such as this is to begin by performing an F-test, which is the first step of ANOVA. The F-test is a kind of "super t-test" that allows the investigators to compare more than two means simultaneously. The null hypothesis for the F-test in the previous example is that the mean change in blood pressure $(\overline{d})$ will be the same for all four groups $(\overline{d}_A = \overline{d}_B = \overline{d}_{AB} = \overline{d}_P)$, indicating that all samples were from the same population and that any differences between the means are due to chance variation.

In creating the F-test (F is for Fisher), Sir Ronald Fisher reasoned that if two different methods could be found to estimate the variance and if all of the samples came from the same population, these two different estimates of variance should be similar. He therefore developed two measures of the variance of the observations. One is called **between-groups variance** and is based on the variation between (or among) the means. The other is called **within-groups variance** and is based on the variation within each group—i.e., variation around a single group mean. In ANOVA, these two measures of variance are also called the **between-groups mean square** and the **within-groups mean square.** (Mean square is simply another name for variance, which is defined as a sum of squares, or SS, divided by the appropriate number of degrees of freedom, or df.) The ratio of the two measures of variance can therefore be expressed as follows:

$$F\text{ ratio} = \frac{\text{Between-groups variance}}{\text{Within-groups variance}} = \frac{\text{Between-groups mean square}}{\text{Within-groups mean square}}$$

If the F ratio is fairly close to 1.0, the two estimates of variance are similar, and the null hypothesis that all of the means came from the same underlying population is not rejected. If the ratio is much larger than 1.0, there must have been some force, attributable to group differences, pushing the means apart, and the null hypothesis of no difference is rejected.

The assumptions for the F-test are similar to those for the t-test. First, the dependent variable (in this case, blood pressure difference scores) should be normally distributed, although with large samples this assumption can be relaxed because of the central limit theorem. Second, the several samples of the dependent variable should be independent random samples from populations with approximately equal variances. This concern is more acute in the F-test than it is in the t-test, where an adjustment is available to correct for a large difference between the two variances. As with the t-test, the F-test requires that

an alpha level be specified in advance. After the F statistic has been calculated, its p value can be looked up in a table of the F distribution to determine whether the results are statistically significant. This task, however, is more complicated with the F-test than with the t-test, because ANOVA has two different degrees of freedom to deal with, one for the numerator (the model mean square) and one for the denominator (the error mean square), as explained in Box 13–1. Therefore, the table of F distributions is more complicated than the table of t distributions. (For additional details, including an F table, see Dawson-Saunders and Trapp 1994).

If the results of the F-test are not statistically significant, either the null hypothesis must be accepted or the study must be repeated using a larger sample. However, if the results are statistically significant, the investigators must take additional steps to determine which of the differences in means are the "true" differences. In the case of the example introduced earlier, involving four treatment groups (drug A alone, drug B alone, drugs A and B combined, and placebo), statistical significance could be found if any of the following were true: (1) the mean difference of one

---

BOX 13–1   The Analysis of Variance (ANOVA) Table

The goal of ANOVA, stated in the simplest terms, is to explain (i.e., to model) the total variation found in a study. Because the total variation is equal to the sum of squares (SS), the process of explaining total variation is a process that entails partitioning the SS into component parts. The logic behind this process was introduced in Chapter 10 (see Variation Between Groups Versus Variation Within Groups), and the discussion there focused on the example of explaining the difference between the heights (fictitious data) of men and women. In the example, the heights of 100 female and 100 male university students were measured, the total variation was found to be 10,000 cm^2, and 4,000 cm^2 of the variation was attributed to gender. Because that example is uncomplicated and involves round numbers, it is used here to illustrate the format for an ANOVA table.

Source of Variation	Sum of Squares (SS)	Degrees of Freedom (df)	Mean Square (MS)	F Ratio
TOTAL	10,000	199		
Model (gender)	4,000	1	4,000.0	132.0
Error	6,000	198	30.3	

The model in this example has only one independent variable—namely, gender, a dichotomous variable.

In the column showing the sum of the squares (SS), the figure of 4,000 represents the amount of variation resulting from gender (i.e., the between-groups variation noted in the ANOVA), while 6,000 represents the amount of variation resulting from error (i.e., the within-groups variation).

In the column showing the degrees of freedom (df), the total df is listed as 199, reflecting the fact that there were 200 subjects and 1 df was lost in calculating the grand mean for all observations. The df for the model is calculated as the number of categories (groups) minus 1. Gender has only two categories (men and women), so 1 df is assigned to it. The df for error is calculated as the total df minus the number of df assigned to the model: $199 - 1 = 198$.

The mean square (MS) is simply another name for variance and is equal to the SS divided by the appropriate df: $4,000/1 = 4,000.0$, and $6,000/198 = 30.3$.

The F ratio is calculated by dividing the model mean square by the error mean square: $4,000/30.3 = 132.0$. To look up the p value that corresponds to this F ratio in the table of F distributions, it is necessary to know the df for the denominator and the df for the numerator. In this case, as described above, the df for the numerator would be 1 and the df for the denominator would be 198. Because the F ratio is so large (i.e., 132.0), the p value would be extremely small ($p < 0.00001$), and the null hypothesis that there is no true difference between the mean heights of men and women would be rejected.

Note that if there was more than one independent variable in the model being analyzed, there would be more entries under the column showing the source of variation: TOTAL, model, interaction, and error. Interaction would refer to the portion of the variation that is due to interactions between the independent variables in the model. Error would then be defined as the variation not explained by any of the independent variables or their interactions.

group differed greatly from that of the other three groups; (2) the means of two groups differed greatly from those of the remaining two groups; or (3) the means of the four groups were strung along a line representing values of the mean systolic blood pressure differences—for example, with drugs A and B combined showing the best results, drug A showing the second best, drug B showing the third best, and the placebo showing the worst.

Most advanced statistical computer packages include a program for ANOVA, allowing investigators to determine which of the differences are the "true" differences in cases such as this. While a detailed discussion of the various methods is beyond the scope of this book, it is important for readers to understand the logic behind this form of analysis and to recognize the circumstances under which one-way ANOVA is appropriate. As an example, Pearlman et al. (1992) performed a clinical trial in which asthma patients were randomized into three treatment groups: one that received 42 µg of salmeterol two times daily, one that received 180 µg of albuterol four times daily, and one that received a placebo. At the beginning and end of the study, the investigators measured the asthma patients' forced expiratory volume in 1 second (FEV_1), and they then used F-tests to compare the changes in FEV_1 values seen in the three different treatment groups. Based on the results of one-way ANOVA, they concluded that salmeterol was more effective than albuterol or placebo in increasing the morning peak expiratory flow rate.

N-Way ANOVA

The goal of ANOVA, stated in the simplest terms, is to explain (to "model") the total variation found in a study.

If only *one* independent variable is tested in a model and that variable happens to be gender, as shown in Box 13–1, the total amount of variation must be explained in terms of how much variation is due to gender and how much is not. Any variation (SS) that is not due to the model (gender) is considered to be error (residual) variation.

If *two* independent variables are tested in a model and those variables happen to be treatment and gender, the total amount of variation must be explained in terms of how much variation is due to each of the following: the independent effect of treatment, the independent effect of gender, the interaction between (joint effect of) treatment and gender, and error. If *more than two* independent variables are tested, the analysis becomes increasingly complicated, but the underlying logic remains the same. As long as the research design is balanced—that is, there are equal numbers of observations in all of the study groups—ANOVA can be used to analyze the individual and joint effects of the independent variables and to partition the total variation into the various component parts. Numerous computer programs are available to test significance using the F-test and to perform subsequent calculations of formulas based

on the general linear model described earlier in this chapter.

An example in which *N*-way ANOVA procedures were used is the study performed by Finkelstein et al. (1994) to determine whether supplementing gonadotropin-releasing hormone (GnRH) with parathyroid hormone (PTH) would reduce the osteoporosis-causing effect of GnRH. In this study, the investigators used ANOVA to examine the effects of treatment and other independent variables on the bone loss induced by estrogen deficiency.

Analysis of Covariance (ANCOVA)

As shown in Table 13–1, analysis of variance (ANOVA) and analysis of covariance (ANCOVA) are methods for evaluating studies in which the dependent variable is continuous. If the independent variables are all of the categorical type (nominal or dichotomous), then ANOVA is used. However, if some of the independent variables are categorical and some are continuous, then ANCOVA is appropriate. ANCOVA would be used, for example, in a study in which the goal was to test the effects of antihypertensive drugs on systolic blood pressure (a continuous variable that is the dependent variable here) and the independent variables were age (a continuous variable) and treatment (a categorical variable with four levels—i.e., those treated with drug A, those treated with drug B, those treated with both A and B, and those treated with a placebo).

The ANCOVA procedure adjusts the dependent variable on the basis of the continuous independent variable or variables, and it then does an *N*-way ANOVA on the **adjusted dependent variable.** In the above example, the ANCOVA procedure would remove the effect of age from the analysis of the effect of the drugs on systolic blood pressure. Controlling for age means that (artificially) all of the study subjects are made the same age. Suppose that the mean systolic blood pressure in the study group is 150 mm Hg at an average age of 50 years. The first step (and this is all done by the computer packages that have ANCOVA) is to do a simple regression between age and blood pressure, which shows that the blood pressure increases, say, an average of 1 mm Hg for each year of age over 50 years and decreases an average of 1 mm Hg for each year of age under 50. Thus, if a subject's age is 59, then 9 mm Hg would be subtracted from that subject's current blood pressure to arrive at the adjusted blood pressure. If another subject's age is 35, then 15 mm Hg would be added to that subject's current blood pressure to arrive at the adjusted value. If a subject's age is 50, no adjustment is necessary, because that subject is already at the population mean age. ANCOVA can adjust the dependent variable for several continuous independent variables (called covariates) at the same time.

Stacpoole et al. (1992) used ANCOVA to evaluate the results of a controlled clinical trial of dichloroacetate for treatment of lactic acidosis in adults.

ANCOVA adjusted the dependent variable for the pretreatment concentrations of arterial blood lactate in the study subjects, before the treatments were compared.

Multiple Linear Regression

If the dependent variable and all of the independent variables are continuous, the correct type of multivariable analysis is multiple linear regression. The formula looks like the general linear model formula as shown above in equation 13–6. Here, the intercept is really the mean of y, and each of the independent variables improves the prediction somewhat (depending on its strength of association).

There are several computerized methods of analyzing the data in a multiple linear regression. Probably the most common method is called stepwise linear regression. The investigator either chooses which variable to begin with (i.e., to enter first in the analysis) or else instructs the computer to start by entering the one variable that has the strongest association with the dependent variable. In either case, when only the first variable has entered, the result is a simple regression analysis. Next, the second variable is entered according to the investigator's instructions. The explanatory strength of the variable entered—that is, the r^2 (see Chapter 11)—changes as each new variable is entered. The "stepping" continues until none of the remaining independent variables meets the predetermined criterion for being entered (e.g., p is ≤ 0.1 or the increase in r^2 is ≥ 0.01) or until all of the variables have been entered. When the stepping stops, the analysis is complete.

In addition to watching for the statistical significance of the overall equation and of each variable entered, the investigator keeps a close watch on the overall r^2 for each step, which is the proportion of variation the model has explained so far. In multiple regression equations that are statistically significant, the increase in the total r^2 after each step, compared with the total r^2 after the previous step, indicates how much additional variation is explained by the variable just entered.

Multiple linear regression is not used very frequently in clinical medicine, because clinical variables are often nominal, dichotomous, or ordinal. However, it is used frequently in health services research. For example, the dependent variable in such research may be the amount of profit (or loss) in dollars for a hospital over a time period such as a year. The independent variables are often such factors as the average length of stay, the bed occupancy rate, and the proportion of patients who require surgical care.

Other Procedures for Multivariable Analysis

Other major multivariable procedures include **logistic regression, log-linear analysis,** and **discriminant function analysis.** Like the procedures discussed above, these too are forms of the general linear model and function in an analogous manner. Their uses are outlined in Table 13–1.

Multiple logistic regression is a procedure that is appropriate to use when the outcome variable in a clinical prediction model is a dichotomous variable (such as correct/incorrect). The procedure was used, for example, to test a model that was developed by Aronin, Peduzzi, and Quagliarello (1998) to predict on admission to the hospital whether patients with bacterial meningitis would experience a good outcome (complete recovery) or a poor outcome (residual neurologic sequelae or death).

Today, logistic regression is the most powerful procedure available to analyze the results of studies in which the outcome variable is dichotomous. In medicine, the most commonly used form of logistic regression is the proportional hazards (Cox) model. The Cox model enables logistic regression to be done on a time-related, dichotomous, dependent variable such as survival/death, even when there are losses to follow-up and censored cases. It is used to test for differences between Kaplan-Meier survival curves while controlling for other variables. It is also used to determine which variables are associated with better survival. Logistic regression was used, for example, by O'Connell et al. (1994) to compare the relapse-free survival of two groups of patients with rectal cancer: those treated with radiation plus a protracted infusion of fluorouracil and those given a bolus injection of fluorouracil. The patients treated with the combination of radiation and fluorouracil had a statistically lower rate of tumor recurrence, and the Cox analysis showed that increased age, greater lymph node involvement, and a higher tumor grade were associated with a shorter relapse-free time.

■ SUMMARY

Multivariable analysis is a statistical method of determining how well several independent (possibly causal) variables, both separately and together, explain the variation in a single dependent (outcome) variable.

In medical research, there are three common uses of multivariable analysis. The first is to improve the test of a hypothesis in a clinical trial by controlling for the independent and joint effects of independent variables on the dependent variable. The second is to shed light on the etiology of a disease by estimating the relative impact that several independent variables have on the disease. The third is to develop weights for the different variables used in a diagnostic or prognostic scoring system.

As shown in Table 13–1, the choice of an appropriate procedure to be used in multivariable analysis depends on whether the dependent and independent variables are continuous, dichotomous, nominal, ordinal, or a combination of these. Because there are many potential problems and pitfalls in the use of multivariable techniques in clinical research, these procedures should be used with care.

■ QUESTIONS

Directions (Items 1–7). Each of the numbered items or incomplete statements in this section is followed by answers or by completions of the statement. Select the ONE lettered answer or completion that is BEST in each case. Correct answers and explanations are given at the end of the chapter.

1. A multivariable analysis is appropriate when
   (A) bivariate analysis fails to reveal statistical significance
   (B) more than one independent variable is under investigation
   (C) multiple hypotheses are being tested
   (D) multiple outcome variables are under investigation
   (E) multiple repetitions of an experiment are planned

2. A multivariable model is best exemplified by which of the following statements?
   (A) Height and weight vary together
   (B) Height and weight vary with age and gender
   (C) Height varies with age and weight and gender
   (D) Height varies with gender
   (E) Height varies with gender, and weight varies with age

3. The basic equation for a multivariable model generally includes an outcome variable (y); an anchor point or y-intercept (a); weights (b terms); and a residual or error term (e). The least-squares solution to a multivariable equation is determined when
   (A) the model is statistically significant
   (B) the residual is maximized
   (C) the value of a is minimized
   (D) the value of e^2 is minimized
   (E) the y-intercept is 0

4. A particular advantage of multivariable analysis over contingency table analysis is that
   (A) multivariable methods exclude overlapping variables
   (B) multivariable methods exclude weak associations
   (C) multivariable methods permit examination of the interaction between independent variables
   (D) statistical significance is more easily achieved with multivariable methods
   (E) type I error is minimized with multivariable methods

5. In a survival study of patients with pancreatic cancer, one group was treated with a chemotherapeutic agent and another group was treated with a placebo. Which of the following procedures would be the best one for comparing the survival experience of the two groups over time

while adjusting for other variables, such as age, gender, and cancer stage?
   (A) Analysis of covariance (ANCOVA)
   (B) Linear regression analysis
   (C) Logrank test
   (D) McNemar chi-square test
   (E) Proportional hazards (Cox) model

Items 6–7

You are interested in comparing the effects of various agents on the management of pain caused by osteoarthritis. You design a study in which equal numbers of patients are assigned to three groups defined by treatment (acetaminophen treatment, ibuprofen treatment, or placebo treatment). Other independent variables are gender; age (dichotomous: <50 years or ≥50 years); and severity of arthritis (categorical: mild, moderate, or severe).

6. Which of the following would be the most appropriate statistical method for analyzing your data?
   (A) Analysis of covariance (ANCOVA)
   (B) Logistic regression analysis
   (C) N-way analysis of variance (N-way ANOVA)
   (D) One-way analysis of variance (one-way ANOVA)
   (E) Wilcoxon matched-pairs signed-ranks test

7. To analyze the data using the F ratio, you must first establish
   (A) the between-groups mean square and the degrees of freedom
   (B) the between-groups variance and within-groups variance
   (C) the degrees of freedom and the value of p
   (D) the least squares and the residual
   (E) the standard error and the mean for each group

■ ANSWERS AND EXPLANATIONS

1. **The answer is B: more than one independent variable is under investigation.** As defined in this chapter, multivariable models include multiple independent variables but only one dependent variable. In contrast, multivariate models include multiple independent variables and more than one dependent variable. The testing of multiple hypotheses does not per se indicate which analytic technique will be appropriate. The appropriate statistical methods depend on the nature of the hypotheses. Similarly, multiple repetitions of an experiment do not dictate the statistical method required. That is always determined by the number and nature of the variables involved and the types of hypotheses being tested. When bivariate analysis fails to reveal statistical significance, use of an alternative analytic technique is generally not indicated (and may be inappropriate). The appropriate responses in-

clude increasing the sample size or accepting the null hypothesis.

2. **The answer is C: height varies with age and weight and gender.** As described in this chapter, multivariable models may be expressed both conceptually and mathematically. A conceptual understanding of multivariable analysis is facilitated by a verbal description of the relationships under study. To conform to the requirements for multivariable analysis, the model must postulate the influence of more than one independent variable on one, and only one, dependent (outcome) variable. In general, such a model, expressed in words, would take the following form: dependent variable y varies with independent variables x_1, x_2, and so on. The only choice provided that fits this pattern is C.

3. **The answer is D: the value of e^2 is minimized.** The basic equation for a multivariable model is as follows:

$$y = a + b_1x_1 + b_2x_2 + b_3x_3 + b_4x_4 + e$$

The outcome variable is y; the y-intercept or anchor point is a; the b terms represent weights; and e is the residual or error term. The goal of the least-squares approach to multivariable analysis is to find the model that produces the smallest sum of squares of the error term, e. The values of a and the b_i's that lead to the smallest error term produce the best "fit," or model. The least-squares model may or may not be statistically significant, depending on the strength of association between the independent variables and the dependent variable under investigation.

4. **The answer is C: multivariable methods permit examination of the interaction between independent variables.** A contingency table may be used to show that more than one independent variable contributes independently to an outcome. While the use of a contingency table and tabular analysis may suggest an interaction between variables, it is generally not robust for this application. To demonstrate the interaction between or among independent variables reliably, multivariable methods are preferred. For example, the independent contributions of tobacco and alcohol to the risk of head and neck cancer can be shown with contingency table analysis, but the synergistic interaction between the two generally cannot. To demonstrate interaction such as synergy, multivariable methods are required. The achievement of statistical significance is no easier with multivariable methods. Weak associations may be studied by either method. Overlapping or interacting variables are purposefully studied in multivariable methods. With either method, type I error is minimized by setting an appropriately stringent alpha level.

5. **The answer is E: proportional hazards (Cox) model.** In a survival study, the outcome variable is dichotomous (live/die). Consequently, a standard chi-square can be used to test the hypothesis of independence (see Chapter 11); the McNemar chi-square is used for paired data. However, a survival study can provide much more information about the subjects in each group than simply the proportion of subjects who were alive at the end of the study. In a study that may span years, the timing of death is equally important. Thus, intergroup comparison should address the distribution as well as the number of deaths. The logrank test is designed for making such a comparison, but it cannot adjust for other independent variables. The multivariable method appropriate for survival analysis is the proportional hazards (Cox) model, a method now employed commonly in the analysis of clinical trial data. (For a description of the mechanics of the model, see Lee 1980 and Cantor 1997). Analysis of covariance (ANCOVA) is a multivariable method used with a continuous outcome variable when the independent variables are a mix of continuous and categorical. Linear regression is either a bivariate method or, in the case of multiple linear regression, a multivariable method; it is used to analyze a continuous outcome variable and exclusively continuous independent variables.

6. **The answer is C: N-way analysis of variance (N-way ANOVA).** As shown in Table 13–1, ANOVA is appropriate when the outcome variable is continuous and multiple independent variables are categorical. The study described meets these criteria. The method is N-way ANOVA, rather than one-way ANOVA, because the model includes several different independent variables.

7. **The answer is B: the between-groups variance and within-groups variance.** The F ratio is the ratio of between-groups variance to within-groups variance. Therefore, only these two parameters must be established to calculate the F ratio. Subsequently, a p value for a given F ratio is determined from a table of the F distribution. (In ANOVA, note that variance is often called the mean square.)

References Cited

Aronin, S. I., P. Peduzzi, and V. J. Quagliarello. Community-acquired bacterial meningitis: risk stratification for adverse clinical outcome and effect of antibiotic timing. Annals of Internal Medicine 129:862–870, 1998.

Breslow, L. Risk factor intervention for health maintenance. Science 200:908–912, 1978.

Cantor, A. B. Extending SAS Survival Analysis Techniques for Medical Research. Cary, N.C., SAS Institute, Inc., 1997.

Concato, J., A. R. Feinstein, and T. Holford. The risk of determining risk with multivariable models. Annals of Internal Medicine 118: 201–210, 1993.

Dawson-Saunders, B., and R. G. Trapp. Basic and Clinical Biostatistics, 2nd ed. Norwalk, Conn., Appleton and Lange, 1994.

Finkelstein, J. S., et al. Parathyroid hormone for the prevention of bone loss induced by estrogen deficiency. New England Journal of Medicine 331:1618–1623, 1994.

Freeman, D. H., Jr., et al. The prevalence distribution of hypertension: Connecticut adults, 1978–1979. Journal of Chronic Disease 36:171–181, 1983.

Goldman, L., et al. A computer-driven protocol to aid in the diagnosis of emergency room patients with acute chest pain. New England Journal of Medicine 307:588–596, 1982.

Kac, M. Some mathematical models in science. Science 166:695–699, 1969.

Lee, E. T. Statistical Methods for Survival Data Analysis. Belmont, Calif., Lifetime Learning Publications, 1980.

O'Connell, M. J., et al. Improving adjuvant therapy for rectal cancer by combining protracted-infusion fluorouracil with radiation therapy after curative surgery. New England Journal of Medicine 331:502–507, 1994.

Pearlman, D. S., et al. A comparison of salmeterol with albuterol in the treatment of mild-to-moderate asthma. New England Journal of Medicine 327:1420–1425, 1992.

Stacpoole, P. W., et al. A controlled clinical trial of dichloroacetate for treatment of lactic acidosis in adults. New England Journal of Medicine 327:1564–1569, 1992.

van den Hoogen, P. C. W., et al. The relation between blood pressure and mortality due to coronary heart disease among men in different parts of the world. New England Journal of Medicine 342:1–8, 2000.

Selected Readings

Dawson-Saunders, B., and R. G. Trapp. Basic and Clinical Biostatistics, 2nd ed. Norwalk, Conn., Appleton and Lange, 1994. [Tests for multiple comparisons.]

Freeman, D. L., Jr. Applied Categorical Data Analysis. New York, Marcel Dekker, 1987. [Advanced text.]

Kleinbaum, D. G., and L. L. Kupper. Applied Regression Analysis and Other Multivariable Methods. North Scituate, Mass., Duxbury Press, 1978. [Moderately advanced text.]

PREVENTIVE MEDICINE AND PUBLIC HEALTH

14 Introduction to Preventive Medicine

◼ BASIC CONCEPTS

The fields of preventive medicine and public health share the goals of promoting general health, preventing specific diseases, and applying the concepts and techniques of epidemiology toward these goals. While preventive medicine seeks to enhance the lives of individuals by helping them improve their own health, public health attempts to promote health in populations through the application of organized community efforts. Although preventive medicine and public health are discussed somewhat separately here, there should be a seamless continuum between the following: the practice of preventive medicine by physicians and other health professionals (clinical preventive services); the attempts of individuals and families to promote their own and their neighbors' health; and the efforts of governments and voluntary agencies to achieve the same health goals for populations.

By traditionally focusing on the diagnosis and treatment of disease, Western medical education and medical practice have tended to obscure the importance, scientific basis, and clinical process of promoting the overall health of individuals. Diagnosis and treatment of disease will always be important aspects of health care, but increasing emphasis is also being placed on the preservation and enhancement of health. There are specialists who undertake research, teaching, and clinical practice in the field of preventive medicine, but prevention is no more the exclusive province of preventive medicine specialists than, for example, the care of older people is limited to geriatricians. On the contrary, prevention should be incorporated into the practice of all physicians and other health care professionals.

Health

Health is more difficult to define than is disease. Perhaps the best-known definition of health comes from the preamble to the constitution of the World Health Organization: "Health is a state of complete physical, mental, and social well-being and not merely the absence of disease or infirmity." This definition has the strengths of recognizing that any meaningful concept of health must include all the dimensions of human life and that such a definition must be positive (i.e., "not merely the absence of disease or infirmity"). Nevertheless, the definition has been criticized for two weaknesses. It is too idealistic in its expectations for complete well-being, and it is too static in viewing health as a state rather than as a dynamic process that requires constant effort and activity to maintain.

Successful Adaptation

Decades ago, Dubos pointed out that "the states of health or disease are the expressions of the success or failure experienced by the organism in its efforts to respond adaptively to environmental challenges" (Dubos 1965:xvii). Those who developed the concept of **stress** used today correctly understood that different stressors could induce helpful and harmful forms of stress ("eustress" and "dystress"). That is, good health requires the presence of eustress. It may also require some dystress, but this must be limited to a level to which the organism can adapt (Selye 1973). Even though the body may adapt successfully to environmental stressors in the short term, if continual major adaptation is required, it may exact a serious toll on the body, particularly the neural, neuro-endocrine, and immune systems. The ongoing level of demand for adaptation in an individual is called the **allostatic load** on that person, and it may be an important contributor to many chronic diseases (McEwen and Stellar 1993).

Satisfactory Functioning

Often what matters most to people is how they function in their own environment. The inability to function will bring many people to a doctor more quickly than the presence of discomfort per se: "Clearly, health and disease cannot be defined merely in terms of anatomical, physiological, or mental attributes. Their real measure is the ability of the individual to function in a manner acceptable to himself and to the group of which he is a part" (Dubos 1961:214).

However health is defined, it derives principally from forces other than medical care. Appropriate nutrition, adequate shelter, a nonthreatening environment, and a prudent life-style contribute far more to health and well-being than does the medical care system. Nevertheless, medicine contributes to health both directly through patient care and indirectly through the development and dissemination of knowledge about disease prevention and treatment.

■ MEASURES OF HEALTH STATUS

Historically, measures of health status have been based primarily on **mortality data** (see Chapter 2). Researchers assumed that a low age-adjusted death rate and a high life expectancy reflected good health in a population. Currently, a higher proportion of the population lives to old age than ever before, and this group accumulates various chronic and disabling illnesses. Consequently, health care investigators and practitioners have increasingly expressed dissatisfaction with using mortality data as the sole index for the overall level of health in a population and have also shown an increased concern with improving the **health-related quality of life.** Unfortunately, much more research needs to be done before quality of life can be adequately measured (Gill and Feinstein 1994). An appropriate societal goal is for people to age in a healthy manner, with minimal disability until shortly before death (Fries and Crapo 1981).

Considerable research effort now goes into the development of **health status indexes.** Most indexes require that each subject complete some form of questionnaire, and most do not incorporate mortality data (see McDowell and Newell 1996). Many health status indexes seek to adjust life expectancy on the basis of morbidity, the perceived quality of life, or both. Such indexes can also be used to help guide clinical practice and research. For example, they can show that a nation's emphasis on reducing mortality may not be producing parallel results in improving the function or self-perceived health of the nation's population. When physicians consider which treatments to recommend to patients with a chronic dis-ease, such as prostate cancer, it is important to consider the side effects of treatment, such as incontinence and impotence, as well as the impact on mortality (Bogardus, Holmboe, and Jekel 1999). Describing survival estimates in terms of quality-adjusted life years (see below) can help to communicate a fuller picture to patients than using survival rates alone.

Life expectancy is traditionally defined as the average number of years of life remaining at a given age. **Quality-adjusted life years** (QALY) incorporates both life expectancy and the perceived impact of illness and disability on the quality of life (Last 1988). People who have had a stroke and now suffer from hemiparesis, for example, may be asked to estimate how many years of life with their disability would have a value to them equal to 1 year of life with good health (healthy years). If the answer was that 2 limited years is equivalent to 1 healthy year, a year of life following a stroke might be given a weight of 0.5. If 3 limited years were equivalent to 1 healthy year, each limited year would contribute 0.33 years to the QALY. Some people might consider being confined to a nursing home and unable to speak (as occurs with some strokes) to be as bad as or worse than no life at all, and, if so, the weighting factor would be 0.0 for such years.

Healthy life expectancy is a somewhat less subjective measure that attempts to combine both mortality and morbidity into one index (see Barendregt et al. 1994). The index reflects the number of years of life remaining that are expected to be free of serious disease. The onset of a serious disease with permanent sequelae—for example, a stroke with serious permanent residual effects—reduces the index as much as if the person who has the sequelae had died from the disease.

Other indexes combine several measures of health status. For example, the **General Well-Being Adjustment Scale** is an index that measures "anxiety, depression, general health, positive well-being, self-control, and vitality" (Revicki et al. 1994). Another index is called the **Life Expectancy Free of Disability,** which is just what the name suggests. The US Centers for Disease Control and Prevention (CDC) developed an index called the **Health Related Quality of Life** (HR-QOL) based on data from the Behavioral Risk Factor Surveillance System (BRFSS) (see Centers for Disease Control and Prevention 1994). Using the BRFSS data, CDC investigators found that 87% of adults in the USA considered their health to be good to excellent. They also found that the mean number of good health days—i.e., the number of days free of both physical and mental health problems during the 30-day period preceding the interview—was 25 days in the adults surveyed (see Centers for Disease Control and Prevention 1995).

■ THE NATURAL HISTORY OF DISEASE

Before a disease process begins in an individual—that is, during the **predisease stage**—the individual can be thought of as possessing various factors that promote or resist disease. These factors include genetic makeup, demographic characteristics (especially age), environmental exposures, nutritional history, social environment, immunologic capability, and behavioral patterns.

Over time, the sum total of these and other factors may cause a disease process to begin, either slowly (as is usually the case with noninfectious diseases) or quickly (as is commonly the case with infectious diseases). If the disease-producing process is under way but no symptoms of disease have become apparent, the disease is said to be in the **latent (hidden) stage.** If the underlying disease is detectable by a reasonably safe and cost-effective means during this stage, then screening may be feasible. In this sense, the latent stage may represent a **window of opportunity,** during which detection followed by treatment provides a better chance of cure or at least of effective treatment. For some diseases, there is no window of opportunity, because safe and effective screening technology is not available. For other diseases, such as rapidly progressive conditions, the window of opportunity may be too short to be useful for screening programs.

When the disease is advanced enough to produce clinical manifestations, it is said to be in the **symptomatic (manifest) stage.** Even in this stage, the earlier the condition is diagnosed and treated, the more likely the treatment is to delay death or serious complications or at least to provide the opportunity for effective rehabilitation.

The natural history of a disease is its normal course in the absence of intervention. The central question for studies of prevention (field trials) and studies of treatment (clinical trials) is whether the institution of a particular preventive or treatment measure will change the natural history of disease in a favorable direction, by delaying or preventing clinical manifestations, complications, or deaths. Many interventions do not prevent the progression of disease but instead slow the progression so that the disease either does not occur in the patient's lifetime or occurs later in life than it would have occurred if there had been no intervention.

In the case of myocardial infarction, for example, risk factors include male gender, a family history of myocardial infarction or other illnesses (e.g., diabetes mellitus and hypertension), elevated serum lipid levels, a high-fat diet, cigarette smoking, sedentary life-style, and advancing age. Genotype is only one of many factors influencing the composition of serum lipids and the development of atherosclerosis. The speed with which coronary atherosclerosis develops in an individual will be modified not only by the diet but also by the pattern of physical activity over the course of a lifetime. Hypertension may accelerate the development of atherosclerosis, and it also may lead to increased myocardial oxygen demand, thus precipitating infarction earlier than it otherwise might have occurred and also making recovery more difficult.

After a myocardial infarction occurs, some patients die, some recover completely, and others recover but suffer serious sequelae that limit their function. Treatment may improve the outcome so that death or serious sequelae are avoided. Intensive changes in diet, exercise, and behavior (such as cessation of smoking) may actually stop the progression of atheromas or even reverse them.

■ LEVELS OF PREVENTION

A useful concept of prevention that was developed or at least popularized in the classic account by Hugh Leavell (see Leavell and Clark 1965) has come to be known as **Leavell's levels.** Based on this concept, all of the activities of physicians and other health professionals have the goal of prevention. There are three levels of prevention, as shown in Table 14–1 and described below. What is to be prevented depends on the stage of health or disease in the individual receiving preventive care. **Primary prevention** keeps the disease process from becoming established by elimi-

TABLE 14–1   **Modified Version of Leavell's Levels of Prevention***

Stage of Disease	Level of Prevention	Appropriate Response
Predisease		
No known risk factors	Primary prevention	Health promotion (e.g., encourage healthy changes in life-style, nutrition, and environment).
Disease susceptibility	Primary prevention	Specific protection (e.g., recommend nutritional supplements, immunizations, and occupational and automobile safety measures).
Latent Disease	Secondary prevention	Screening (for populations) or case finding (for individuals in medical care) and treatment if disease is found.
Symptomatic Disease		
Initial care	Tertiary prevention	Disability limitation (i.e., institute medical or surgical treatment to limit damage from the disease and also institute primary prevention measures).
Subsequent care	Tertiary prevention	Rehabilitation (i.e., identify and teach methods to reduce social disability).

*Modified from Leavell, H. R., and E. G. Clark. Preventive Medicine for the Doctor in His Community, 3rd ed. New York, McGraw-Hill Book Company, 1965. Although Leavell originally categorized disability limitation under secondary prevention, both in Europe and in the USA it has become customary to classify it as tertiary prevention because it involves the management of symptomatic disease.

nating causes of disease or increasing resistance to disease (see Chapters 15 and 16). **Secondary prevention** interrupts the disease process before it becomes symptomatic (see Chapter 17). **Tertiary prevention** limits the physical and social consequences of symptomatic disease (see Chapter 18).

Primary Prevention and Predisease

Most noninfectious diseases can be seen as having an early stage, during which the causal factors will start to produce physiologic abnormalities. In atherosclerosis, for example, there may be high levels of low-density lipoprotein (LDL) cholesterol and very low density lipoprotein (VLDL) cholesterol and there may be low levels of high-density lipoprotein (HDL, or "scavenger" lipoprotein) cholesterol in the blood but no signs of atheroma during the predisease stage. The goal of a health intervention at this time is to modify risk factors in a favorable direction. Life-modifying activities, such as changing to a low-fat diet, pursuing a consistent program of aerobic exercise, and ceasing to smoke cigarettes, are considered to be methods of primary prevention because they are aimed at keeping the pathologic process and disease from occurring.

Health Promotion

Health-promoting activities usually contribute to the prevention of a variety of diseases as well as enhancing a positive feeling of health and vigor. They consist of nonmedical changes, such as changes in life-style, nutrition, and the environment. Such activities may require structural improvements in society to enable the majority of people to take part in them. Structural improvements require societal changes that make healthy choices easier. For example, dietary modification may be difficult unless a variety of low-fat, low-salt, low-sugar, yet tasty and nutrient-rich foods are available in stores at a reasonable cost. Exercise will be more difficult if bicycling or jogging is a risky activity because of automobile traffic or social violence. Even more basic to health promotion is the assurance of the basic necessities of life, including freedom from poverty, environmental pollution, and violence.

Health promotion applies both to noninfectious diseases and to infectious diseases. Infectious diseases are reduced in frequency and seriousness where the water is pure, liquid and solid wastes are disposed of in a sanitary manner, and arthropod and animal vectors of disease are controlled. Crowding promotes the spread of infectious diseases, whereas adequate housing and working environments tend to minimize the spread of disease. In the barracks of soldiers, for example, even a technique as simple as requiring some soldiers to sleep with their pillows at the head of the bed and others to sleep with their pillows at the foot of the bed, in an alternating pattern, can reduce the spread of respiratory diseases because it doubles the distance between upper respiratory tracts during sleeping time.

Specific Protection

If health-promoting changes in environment, nutrition, and behavior are not fully effective, it may be necessary to employ specific protection (see Table 14–1). This form of primary prevention is targeted at a specific disease or type of injury. Examples include immunization against poliomyelitis; pharmacologic treatment of hypertension to prevent subsequent end-organ damage; use of ear-protecting devices in loud working environments, such as around jet airplanes; and use of seat belts, air bags, and helmets to prevent bodily injuries in automobile and motorcycle crashes. Some measures provide specific protection while also contributing to the more general goal of health promotion. Fluoridation of water supplies, for example, not only prevents dental caries but is a nutritional intervention that promotes stronger bones and teeth.

Secondary Prevention and Latent Disease

Sooner or later, depending on the individual, a disease process such as coronary artery atherosclerosis will progress far enough to become detectable by medical tests, even though the individual is still asymptomatic. This may be thought of as the latent (hidden) stage of disease.

For many infectious and noninfectious diseases, the development of screening tests has made it possible to detect latent disease in individuals considered to be at high risk. Presymptomatic diagnosis and treatment through screening programs is referred to as secondary prevention because it is the secondary line of defense against disease. Although it does not prevent the cause from initiating the disease process, it may prevent progression to the symptomatic stage.

Tertiary Prevention and Symptomatic Disease

When disease has become symptomatic and medical assistance is sought, the goal of the clinician is to provide tertiary prevention in the form of disability limitation for patients with early symptomatic disease or in the form of rehabilitation for patients with late symptomatic disease (see Table 14–1).

Disability Limitation

Disability limitation describes medical and surgical measures aimed at correcting the anatomic and physiologic components of disease in symptomatic patients. The majority of care provided by physicians meets this description. It can be considered prevention because its goal is to halt the disease process and thereby prevent or limit the impairment (disability) caused by it. An example is the surgical removal of a tumor, which may prevent the spread of disease locally or by metastasis to other sites.

Discussions about a patient's disease may provide an opportunity to convince the patient to begin health promotion techniques designed to delay disease progression (e.g., to begin exercising and improving the diet and to stop smoking after a myocardial infarction).

Rehabilitation

Although many are surprised to see rehabilitation designated a form of prevention, this designation is appropriate because rehabilitation may mitigate the effects of disease and thereby prevent it from resulting in total social and functional disability. For example, a person who has been injured or who has suffered a stroke may be taught how to care for himself or herself in the **activities of daily living** (feeding, bathing, and so forth). This may enable him or her to avoid the adverse sequelae associated with prolonged inactivity (e.g., increasing muscle weakness).

Rehabilitation of a stroke patient begins with early and frequent mobilization of all joints during the period of maximum paralysis. This permits recovery of limb use, rather than the development of stiff joints and flexion contractures. Next, physical therapy helps the stroke patient to strengthen remaining muscle function and to use this remaining function to maximum effect in performing the activities of daily living. Occupational and speech therapy may enable the patient to gain skills and perform some type of gainful employment, thereby preventing complete economic dependence on others. It is legitimate, therefore, to view rehabilitation as a form of prevention.

■ THE ECONOMICS OF PREVENTION

In an era of cost consciousness, there are increasing demands that health promotion and disease prevention be proven economically worthwhile either by means of **cost-benefit analysis** or by means of **cost-effectiveness analysis** (see Box 14–1 and Petitti 1994). The results of these forms of analysis are commonly expressed in terms of mortality, disease, and costs or in terms of their inverse (longevity, disease-free time, and savings). When other measures of desirable outcome are used (usually, scales of quality of life), the method is generally referred to as **cost-utility analysis.** In other respects, the techniques of cost-utility analysis are similar to those of cost-effectiveness analysis.

Although most people believe it makes sense to invest resources to maintain health and prevent disease, there are numerous factors that make it difficult to demonstrate that special programs devoted to these goals produce benefits that are greater than or equal to the associated costs (Russell 1986).

Demonstration of Benefits

Scientific proof of benefits may be difficult because it is often unpractical or unethical to undertake randomized trials using people as subjects. For example, it is not possible to randomly assign people to smoking and nonsmoking groups. Therefore, apart from some research done on animal models, investigators are limited to observational studies, which usually

are not as convincing as experiments. Moreover, life is filled with risks for one disease or another, and many of these operate together to produce the levels of health observed in a population. These risks may be changing in frequency in different subpopulations, making it impossible to infer what proportion of the improvement observed over time is due to a particular preventive measure. For example, if there is a reduction in the incidence of lung cancer, it is difficult to infer what proportion is due to smoking reduction programs and what proportion is due to the elimination of smoking in workplaces and public areas, the increase in public awareness of (and action against) the presence of radon in homes, and other factors as yet poorly understood.

Delay of Benefits

With most preventive programs, there is a long delay between the time that the preventive measures are instituted and the time that positive health changes become discernible. For example, because the latent period (incubation period) for lung cancer caused by cigarette smoking is 20 years or more, investments made now in smoking reduction programs may not be clearly identified until many years have passed. There are similar delays between the time of smoking cessation and the demonstration of effect for other smoking-related cancers and for chronic obstructive pulmonary disease.

Accrual of Benefits

Even if a given program could be shown to produce meaningful economic benefit, it is critical to know where the benefits would accrue. For example, a financially stressed health insurance plan or health maintenance organization might cover a preventive measure if the financial benefit were fairly certain to be as great as or greater than the cost of the program and if most or all of this financial benefit would accrue to the insurance plan. If most of the financial benefit would go to the enrollees rather than to the insurance plan, the prevention program would be seen as only a financial cost by the insurance plan.

The same principle is true for even more financially strapped government budgets, such as local, state, and federal budgets. If the savings from prevention efforts would go directly to individuals, rather than to a government budget, the elected representatives might not support the prevention effort, even if the benefits clearly outweighed the costs. Elected representatives seek to show results before the next election campaign. Disease prevention often shows results only over an extended time period and therefore does not often lend itself to political popularity.

Discounting

If a preventive effort is made now by a government body, the costs are present-day costs, but the savings may not be evident until many years from now. Even if the savings are expected to accrue to the same bud-

---

BOX 14–1   Cost-Benefit and Cost-Effectiveness Analysis

Cost-benefit analysis measures the costs and the benefits of a proposed course of action in terms of the same units, usually monetary units such as dollars. For example, a cost-benefit analysis of a poliomyelitis immunization program would determine the number of dollars to be spent toward vaccines, equipment, personnel, and so forth, to immunize a particular population. It then would determine the number of dollars that would be saved by not having to pay for the hospitalizations, medical visits, and lost productivity that would occur if poliomyelitis were not prevented in that population.

Incorporating ideas such as the dollar value of life, suffering, and the quality of life into such an analysis is difficult. However, cost-benefit analysis is useful if a particular budgetary entity (such as a government or business) is trying to determine whether the investment of resources in health would save money in the long run. It is also useful if a particular entity with a fixed budget is trying to make informed judgments concerning allocations in various sectors (health, transportation, education, and so forth) and to determine the sector in which an investment would produce the greatest economic benefit.

Cost-effectiveness analysis provides a way of comparing different proposed solutions in terms of the most appropriate measurement units. For example, by measuring hepatitis B cases prevented, deaths prevented, and life-years saved per 10,000 population, Bloom et al. (1993) were able to compare the effectiveness of four different strategies of dealing with the hepatitis B virus: (1) no vaccination; (2) universal vaccination; (3) screening followed by vaccination of unprotected individuals; and (4) a combination of the screening of pregnant women at delivery, the vaccination of the newborns of women found to be antibody-positive during screening, and the routine vaccination of all 10-year-old children.

After Bloom et al. estimated the numbers of persons involved in each step of each method, they determined the costs of screening, of purchasing and administering the vaccine, and of medical care for various forms and complications of hepatitis. They calculated that the fourth strategy

would have an undiscounted cost of about $367 (or a discounted cost of $1205) per case of hepatitis B prevented, and they concluded that this was clearly the strategy with the lowest cost.

The rather chaotic situation in the USA regarding costs and charges under different health insurance plans and in different hospitals makes it difficult to estimate medical care costs. The situation can be partly dealt with by performing a "sensitivity analysis" with spreadsheets in which different costs per item are substituted to see how they affect the total cost.

In addition, the concept of **discounting,** which is important in business and finance, must be used in medical cost-benefit and cost-effectiveness analysis when the costs are incurred in the present but the benefits will occur some time in the future. Discounting is a reduction in the present value of delayed benefits (or an increase in their present costs) to account for the time value of money. If the administrators of a prevention program spend $1000 now to save $1000 of expenses in the future, they will take a net loss. This is because they will lose the use of $1000 in the interim and also because of the effects of inflation (the $1000 eventually saved will not be worth as much as the $1000 initially spent). Discounting attempts to adjust for these forces.

To discount a cost-benefit or cost-effectiveness analysis, the easiest way is to increase the present costs by a yearly factor, which can be thought of as the interest that would have to be paid in order to borrow the prevention money until the benefits occurred. For example, if it costs $1000 today to prevent a disease that would have occurred 20 years in the future, the present cost can be multiplied by $(1 + r)^n$, where r is the yearly interest rate for borrowing and n is the number of years until the benefit is realized. If the average yearly interest rate is 5% over 20 years, the formula becomes: $(1 + 0.05)^{20} = (1.05)^{20} = 2.653$. When this is multiplied by the present cost of $1000, the result is $2653. Thus, the expected savings 20 years in the future from a $1000 investment today would have to be greater than $2653 in order for the initial investment to be a net (true) financial gain.

---

getary unit that provided the money for the preventive program, the delay in economic return means that the benefits are worth less to that unit now. In the jargon of economists, the present value of the benefits must be discounted (see Box 14–1), making it more difficult to demonstrate cost-effectiveness or a positive benefit-cost ratio.

Priorities

As the saying goes, the squeaky wheel is the one that gets greased. Current, obvious problems usually attract far more attention and concern than future, subtle problems. Emergency care for victims of motor vehicle crashes is easy to justify, regardless of costs. Even though prevention may be far more cost-effective, it is difficult to justify money for medi-

cal crises that have not yet appeared. The same dilemma applies to essentially every phase of life. It is difficult to get money for programs to prevent the loss of topsoil, to prevent illiteracy, and to prevent the decay of roads and bridges. Even on an individual level, many patients will not want to make changes in fundamental aspects of their lives, such as eating a healthier diet, exercising, and stopping smoking, because the risk of future problems does not speak to them urgently in the present.

■ SUMMARY

Preventive medicine seeks to enhance the lives of patients by helping them promote their own health and prevent specific diseases. Preventive medicine also tries to apply the concepts and techniques of health promotion and disease prevention to the organization and practice of medicine (clinical preventive services). Health is an elusive concept, but there is general agreement that it means much more than the absence of disease; it is a positive concept that includes the ability to adapt to stress and the ability to function in society.

The three levels of prevention define the various strategies that are available to practitioners to promote health and prevent disease, impairment, and disability at various stages of the natural history of disease. Primary prevention keeps a disease from becoming established by eliminating the causes of disease or increasing resistance to disease. Secondary prevention interrupts the disease process by detecting and treating it in the presymptomatic stage. Tertiary prevention limits the physical impairment and social consequences from symptomatic disease.

It is not easy for prevention programs to compete for funds in a tight fiscal climate because of the frequently long delays before the benefits of such investments are noted. One of the purposes of specialty training in preventive medicine is to prepare investigators who can demonstrate the cost-effectiveness and cost benefits of prevention.

■ QUESTIONS

Directions (Items 1–8). Each of the numbered items or incomplete statements in this section is followed by answers or by completions of the statement. Select the ONE lettered answer or completion that is BEST in each case. Correct answers and explanations are given at the end of the chapter.

1. Measures of health status have traditionally been based on mortality data. The principal reason this is no longer satisfactory is that
   - (A) changes in diagnostic technology permit earlier detection of disease
   - (B) the infant mortality rate has declined so much that it no longer serves as a useful index
   - (C) the population is older and more subject to chronic illness than in the past
   - (D) there is less risk of fatal infection than in the past
   - (E) traditional sources of mortality data have failed to include women

2. Following the onset of blindness resulting from diabetic retinopathy, a 54-year-old man seems depressed. When you question him regarding the quality of life, he dejectedly tells you that 10 years "like this" is not worth 1 year of good health. The patient's statement indicates that
   - (A) blindness is associated with depression
   - (B) each year of life contributes less than 0.1 quality-adjusted life years
   - (C) each year of life contributes 10 quality-adjusted life years

   - (D) the healthy life expectancy is 2 years
   - (E) the life expectancy is less than 10 years

3. In which of the following ways is health promotion distinguished from disease prevention?
   - (A) Only health promotion can begin before a disease becomes symptomatic
   - (B) Only health promotion involves materials and methods that are generally nonmedical
   - (C) Only health promotion is applied once a disease has developed
   - (D) Only health promotion is targeted at populations rather than individuals
   - (E) Only health promotion is targeted at specific diseases

4. Which of the following is an example of secondary prevention?
   - (A) Cholesterol reduction in a patient with asymptomatic coronary artery disease
   - (B) Hormone replacement therapy for menopause
   - (C) Physical therapy following lumbar disk herniation
   - (D) Pneumococcal vaccine in a patient who has undergone splenectomy
   - (E) Thrombolysis for acute myocardial infarction

Items 5–8

You are interested in helping a 45-year-old perimenopausal woman to avoid osteoporosis. The patient is motivated but has a fixed income and is concerned about the expense. Assume that the cost of hormone replacement therapy is fixed at $660 per year, that this therapy will prevent the development of a hip fracture in the patient at age 68 years, that the current cost of surgical fixation of the hip fracture is $12,000, and that the yearly rate of inflation is 4%.

5. If the patient had no insurance to offset prescription expenses, how much money would she spend to prevent a hip fracture at age 68 years if she started hormone replacement therapy now?
   - (A) $4,260
   - (B) $12,000
   - (C) $15,180
   - (D) $18,000
   - (E) The amount cannot be determined from the information provided

6. When inflation is taken into account, what is the cost of surgery to repair a hip fracture in the patient at age 68 years?
   - (A) $11,620
   - (B) $17,580
   - (C) $29,580
   - (D) $42,814
   - (E) The amount cannot be determined from the information provided

7. Based on your answers to questions 5 and 6, above, you decide that hormone replacement therapy
    (A) has a favorable cost-benefit ratio
    (B) has an unfavorable cost-benefit ratio
    (C) is appropriate for your patient
    (D) is cost-effective
    (E) is not cost-effective

8. If the cost of preventing a hip fracture is greater than the cost of surgical repair, then which of the following is true?
    (A) A preventive strategy may still be indicated
    (B) If a hip fracture occurs, it should be managed nonsurgically
    (C) No attempt should be made to prevent hip fracture until a more cost-effective strategy is devised
    (D) The least costly preventive strategy should be chosen
    (E) The most effective preventive strategy should be chosen

Directions (Items 9–12). The set of matching questions in this section consists of a list of lettered options followed by several numbered items. For each numbered item, select the ONE lettered option that is most closely associated with it. To avoid spending too much time on matching sets with large numbers of options, it is generally advisable to begin each set by reading the list of options. Then, for each item in the set, try to generate the correct answer and locate it in the option list, rather than evaluating each option individually. Each lettered option may be selected once, more than once, or not at all.

Items 9–12

(A) Health promotion
(B) Secondary prevention
(C) Specific protection
(D) Tertiary prevention

Match the procedure to the corresponding category (level) of prevention.

9. Vaccinating a health care worker against hepatitis B
10. Giving isoniazid for 1 year to a 28-year-old medical student whose result in the tuberculin skin test using purified protein derivative (PPD) recently converted from negative to positive
11. Performing carotid endarterectomy in a patient with transient ischemic attacks
12. Recommending regular physical activity to a patient with no known medical problems

■ **ANSWERS AND EXPLANATIONS**

1. **The answer is C: the population is older and more subject to chronic illness than in the past.** When many deaths occur among young people in a population, prolongation of life expectancy is a strong indicator that public health is improving. Until the 20th century, relatively few individuals in most societies lived long enough to die of processes principally related to senescence, or aging. With the advances in medical technology and hygiene of the past decades, life expectancy has increased to the point where most deaths in adults are related to chronic diseases, many of which compromise the quality of life over a number of years before causing death. Thus far, the state of medical care is better suited to stave off death than to prevent disease. Consequently, the measurement of quality of life has assumed greater importance as the burden of chronic disease on an aging population has increased.

2. **The answer is B: each year of life contributes less than 0.1 quality-adjusted life years.** Quality-adjusted life years (QALY) is a measure of the quality as well as the length of life. Each year of life with a disability represents some portion of the quality of that year of life without disability. In this case, if 1 year of good health is worth more to the patient than 10 years with blindness, then the disability results in less than 10% of the quality of life with intact health, and each year of life with disability contributes less than 0.1 QALY. While this scale is useful in comparing the relative impact of various disabilities on quality of life, the absolute measure may not be meaningful. In some instances, the more years spent with a disability, the more miserable a person becomes. In this case, 10 years of life with the disability may not truly add up to the value, or quality, of 1 year of good health.

3. **The answer is B: only health promotion involves materials and methods that are generally nonmedical.** Both health promotion and disease prevention share the goal of keeping people well. Disease prevention is generally directed specifically at a disease or a related group of diseases; the tools of disease prevention, such as vaccines, are generally medical. Health promotion is not disease-oriented but, rather, is an effort to enhance overall health. The materials and methods of health promotion, such as regular physical activity, proper nutrition, safe sexual practices, and the provision of adequate housing and transportation, are generally related to life-style and are therefore nonmedical entities. While health promotion and disease prevention are closely linked in efforts to enhance the public health, they are somewhat disparate in both philosophy and application.

4. **The answer is A: cholesterol reduction in a patient with asymptomatic coronary artery disease.** As defined in this chapter and discussed in greater detail in Chapter 17, secondary prevention interrupts the disease process before it becomes symptomatic. The implication of this definition is that there must be a disease process

in order for secondary prevention to take place. The reduction of an elevated cholesterol level in a patient without coronary artery disease is an example of primary prevention; once the disease process has begun, however, the modification of causal factors to prevent the development of symptoms is secondary prevention. In this case, angina pectoris and myocardial infarction are the symptomatic states at which preventive efforts are directed.

5. **The answer is C: $15,180.** The scenario stipulated that the yearly cost of hormone replacement therapy was fixed at $660. Therefore, to prevent a hip fracture at age 68 years, a 45-year-old patient would need to spend $660 each year for 23 years, or a total of $15,180. In reality, the cost of any prescription medication is likely to change over time to keep pace with inflation. In addition, the cost of treatment should be inflated to include lost investment revenue, since money not spent on medication might be invested to generate more money. Many insurance plans include at least partial coverage of prescription drugs, so the cost of these drugs is generally not fully borne by an insured patient. The inadequacy or lack of prescription drug benefits in the Medicare program is currently a topic of intense public and political interest.

6. **The answer is C: $29,580.** The means for answering this question are provided in Box 14–1. The rate of inflation is analogous to the annual interest rate on money borrowed now to prevent a future event. The current cost of surgical fixation of the hip is provided as $12,000. However, the patient will require this surgery 23 years in the future unless a fracture is avoided. To obtain the cost of the operation for the patient at age 68 years, the current cost is multiplied by (1 + inflation) raised to the number of years, which is $(\$12,000)(1 + 0.04)^{23} = (\$12,000)(2.465) = \$29,580$.

7. **The answer is A: has a favorable cost-benefit ratio.** Cost-benefit analysis is the process of determining and then comparing the cost and financial benefit of an intervention. In the scenario, the financial benefit of prevention is greater than the cost, so the cost-benefit ratio is favorable. However, the cost-effectiveness of hormone replacement therapy has not been assessed. Cost-effectiveness analysis requires that alternative means of achieving the same goal be compared on the basis of cost; the least costly is the most cost-effective. Hormone replacement therapy would not be cost-effective if an alternative strategy, such as calcium and vitamin D supplementation, were as effective at preventing osteoporotic hip fracture at a lower cost. Finally, the scenario does not provide enough information to determine whether hormone replacement therapy is indicated for the patient. Such a determination is contingent not only on the pa-

tient's risk of osteoporosis and hip fracture but also on estimates of the risk of cardiovascular disease and breast cancer, as well as on the patient's preferences after alternative preventive strategies are discussed.

8. **The answer is A: a preventive strategy may still be indicated.** The scenario provided for questions 5 through 8 is a simplistic one. The cost of preventing a hip fracture is compared with the cost of repairing one. However, a great deal of pertinent information is not addressed by this cost-benefit analysis. One of the principal deficiencies of cost-benefit analysis is the expression of human morbidity or mortality in financial terms. The pain and disability associated with a hip fracture are not discussed. The effort required to recover from a fracture is not considered. Even the financial losses that might result from transient or permanent disability, as well as the financial burden associated with rehabilitation, are ignored. A realistic cost-benefit analysis must be far more comprehensive.

9. **The answer is C: specific protection.** Vaccinating a health care worker against hepatitis B is specific protection, because it prevents the initial establishment of the disease process in the host. In contrast to health promotion, which is generally nonmedical, specific protection is often medical, as in this case.

10. **The answer is B: secondary prevention.** The goal of secondary prevention is the avoidance of symptoms once a disease process has begun. Conversion of the tuberculin skin test result from negative to positive implies that exposure to and latent infection with tuberculosis has occurred. Postexposure treatment with isoniazid for a period of up to 1 year is recommended to reduce the risk of developing active (symptomatic) tuberculosis in the future (Barnes and Barrows 1993).

11. **The answer is D: tertiary prevention.** The goal of tertiary prevention is the limitation of physical consequences of symptomatic disease. Although carotid endarterectomy is generally *not* recommended in asymptomatic patients with low-grade stenosis and carotid bruits (secondary prevention), it is recommended to reduce the risk of cerebrovascular accidents in patients who have carotid disease with symptoms such as transient ischemic attacks (tertiary prevention) (see Riggs and DeWeese 1998).

12. **The answer is A: health promotion.** Recommending regular physical activity to a patient with no known medical problems is a health-promoting strategy. Health promotion is an attempt to preserve good health, rather than an effort to avoid or prevent a particular disease. Regular physical activity is associated with better

health and greater life expectancy (Lee, Hsieh, and Paffenberger 1995) and with a reduced risk of several specific diseases (Abbott et al. 1994; Lakka et al. 1994).

References Cited

Abbott, R. D., et al. Physical activity in older middle-aged men and reduced risk of stroke: the Honolulu Heart Program. American Journal of Epidemiology 139:881–893, 1994.

Barendregt, J. J., et al. Health expectancy: an indicator for change? Journal of Epidemiology and Community Health 48:482–487, 1994.

Barnes, P. F., and S. A. Barrows. Tuberculosis in the 1990s. Annals of Internal Medicine 119:400–410, 1993.

Bloom, B. S., et al. A reappraisal of hepatitis B virus vaccination strategies using cost-effectiveness analysis. Annals of Internal Medicine 118:298–306, 1993.

Bogardus, S. T., E. Holmboe, and J. F. Jekel. Perils, pitfalls, and possibilities in talking about medical risk. Journal of the American Medical Association 281:1037–1041, 1999.

Centers for Disease Control and Prevention. Health-related quality of life measures: United States, 1993. Morbidity and Mortality Weekly Report 44:195–200, 1995.

Centers for Disease Control and Prevention. Quality of life as a new public health measure: Behavioral Risk Factor Surveillance System. Morbidity and Mortality Weekly Report 43:375–380, 1994.

Dubos, Rene. Man Adapting. New Haven, Conn., Yale University Press, 1965.

Dubos, Rene. Mirage of Health. New York, Doubleday and Company, 1961.

Fries, J. F., and L. M. Crapo. Vitality and Aging. San Francisco, W. H. Freeman and Company, 1981.

Gill, T. M., and A. R. Feinstein. A critical appraisal of the quality of quality-of-life measurements. Journal of the American Medical Association 272:619–626, 1994.

Lakka, T. A., et al. Relation of leisure-time physical activity and cardiorespiratory fitness to the risk of acute myocardial infarction in men. New England Journal of Medicine 330:1549–1554, 1994.

Last, J. M. A Dictionary of Epidemiology, 2nd ed. New York, Oxford University Press, 1988.

Leavell, H. R., and E. G. Clark. Preventive Medicine for the Doctor in His Community, 3rd ed. New York, McGraw-Hill Book Company, 1965.

Lee, I. M., C. Hsieh, and R. S. Paffenberger. Exercise intensity and longevity in men. Journal of the American Medical Association 273:1179–1184, 1995.

McDowell, I., and C. Newell. Measuring Health: A Guide to Rating Scales and Questionnaires, 2nd ed. New York, Oxford University Press, 1996.

McEwen, B. S., and E. Stellar. Stress and the individual. Archives of Internal Medicine 153:2093–2101, 1993.

Petitti, D. B. Meta-analysis, Decision Analysis, and Cost-Effectiveness Analysis: Methods for Quantitative Synthesis in Medicine. New York, Oxford University Press, 1994.

Revicki, D. A., et al. Responsiveness and calibration of the General Well Being Adjustment Scale in patients with hypertension. Journal of Clinical Epidemiology 47:1333–1342, 1994.

Riggs, P. N., and J. A. DeWeese. Carotid endarterectomy. Surgical Clinics of North America 78:881–900, 1998.

Russell, L. B. Is Prevention Better than Cure? Washington, D. C., Brookings Institution, 1986.

Selye, H. The evolution of the stress concept. American Scientist 61:692–699, 1973.

Selected Readings

Dubos, Rene. Mirage of Health. New York, Doubleday and Company, 1961. [The concept of prevention.]

Evans, R. G. Manufacturing consensus, marketing truth: guidelines for economic evaluation. Annals of Internal Medicine 123:59–60, 1995. [Cost-effectiveness and cost-benefit analysis.]

Fries, J. F., and L. M. Crapo. Vitality and Aging. San Francisco, W. H. Freeman and Company, 1981. [The concept of prevention.]

Goldbloom, R. B., and R. S. Lawrence. Preventing Disease. New York, Springer-Verlag, 1990. [Techniques of prevention.]

Leavell, H. R., and E. G. Clark. Preventive Medicine for the Doctor in His Community, 3rd ed. New York, McGraw-Hill Book Company, 1965. [The concept of prevention.]

Petitti, D. B. Meta-analysis, Decision Analysis, and Cost-Effectiveness Analysis: Methods for Quantitative Synthesis in Medicine. New York, Oxford University Press, 1994. [Various methods of analysis.]

Russell, L. B. Is Prevention Better than Cure? Washington, D. C., Brookings Institution, 1986. [The concept of prevention.]

Task Force on Principles for Economic Analysis of Health Care Technology. Economic analysis of health care technology: a report on principles. Annals of Internal Medicine 123:61–70, 1995. [Cost-effectiveness and cost-benefit analysis.]

Udvarhelyi, S., et al. Cost-effectiveness and cost-benefit analyses in the medical literature: are the methods being used correctly? Annals of Internal Medicine 116:238–244, 1992. [Cost-effectiveness and cost-benefit analysis.]

US Preventive Services Task Force. Guide to Clinical Preventive Services. Baltimore, Williams and Wilkins, 1989. [Techniques of prevention.]

15 Methods of Primary Prevention: Health Promotion

Chapters 15 through 18 follow the outline of Leavell's levels of prevention. Primary prevention consists of health promotion (the focus of Chapter 15) and specific protection (the focus of Chapter 16). Secondary prevention and tertiary prevention are discussed in Chapters 17 and 18, respectively.

■ SOCIETY'S CONTRIBUTION TO HEALTH

In the absence of serious genetic disease, the most fundamental sources of health are adequate nutrition, a safe environment, and prudent behavior. Society provides the basic structure for these three sources of health, through the socioeconomic conditions, opportunities for safe employment, environmental systems (such as water supply and sewage disposal), and the regulation of the environment, commerce, and public safety. Society also helps to sustain social support systems such as families, neighborhoods, and churches, which are fundamental to health (Pratt 1976).

Because socioeconomic and other conditions vary greatly from country to country and from time to time, health problems and the success of health promotion efforts vary as well. For example, recent conditions in areas such as East Timor, Ethiopia, and Sudan precluded adequate nutrition, and even international relief efforts were hindered. Immediately following the chemical disaster in Bhopal, India, or the radiation disaster in Chernobyl, Ukraine, it was impossible for people in the immediate area to find a safe environment. And during wars, ordinary standards of safe, civil behavior may be abandoned.

Even in the presence of a reasonably ordered society, income must be sufficient to allow for adequate nutrition and a safe environment for individuals and families. Education is needed both to enhance employment opportunities and to provide sufficient understanding of the forces that promote good health.

In the United Kingdom, the relationship between socioeconomic status and health has been studied more than in most other nations. This is because for decades people in the UK have been assigned to one of the following five "social classes," based on their occupations and "general standing" in the community (Morris 1967): class I, professionals (e.g., company directors and physicians); class II, teachers, shopkeepers, and farm owners; class III, skilled workers (e.g., clerks and miners); class IV, partly skilled workers (including most agricultural and assembly line workers); and class V, laborers. Although this social classification system is controversial, studies using it have consistently shown that according to almost every measure, the best health is found in class I, with health measures declining steadily as one proceeds to class V. This trend applies not only to direct measures of health or lack of it (e.g., perinatal death rates) but also to nutrition, health behaviors, and fertility (Morris 1967).

The best known socioeconomic scale in the USA was developed by Hollingshead in the 1950s and is based on education, occupation, and residence. Using this scale to study the relationship between social class and mental illness, Hollingshead and Redlich (1958) showed a strong social class trend, with fewer cases of mental illness found in the upper classes than in the lower classes. It is difficult, however, to know whether the level of mental illness was the result of or the cause of the social class observed. In the 1990s, using educational background as a measure of socioeconomic status, investigators showed that disparities between socioeconomic groups in the USA persist in health care delivery and health care access, as shown by differences in infant mortality rates, age-adjusted death rates, use of mammography, and immunization levels (see Pappas 1993 and US Department of Health and Human Services 1999).

In the USA, as in the UK and elsewhere, there has been and continues to be much debate about what factors should be taken into account in defining socioeconomic groups. Some authors have suggested that other social classifications are more adequate for African-Americans in the USA (for example, see Billingsley 1968). In developing nations, social classifications also tend to show that the amount and types of illnesses are quite different among the middle and upper classes as opposed to those living in the rural areas and in poor urban areas. Even in poor nations, the wealthier persons tend to die of "Western" diseases, especially cardiovascular diseases and cancer, whereas the poor tend to die of infections and the sequelae of malnutrition.

■ NUTRITIONAL FACTORS IN HEALTH PROMOTION

Nutrition has a profound and largely incalculable impact on human health. Only a few other factors, including breathable air, drinkable water, and a habitable environment, are as fundamental to health as is nutrition.

Deficiencies of particular nutrients and deficiencies of total nutrient energy have been the principal nutritional threats to human beings throughout nearly all of evolutionary history. These threats continue to plague, at least episodically, a large proportion of the world's population in developing countries and a disenfranchised minority in the USA and other industrialized countries. However, for the majority of people in the so-called developed countries, the threat has shifted to nutritional excess. In the USA, for example, the combination of overnutrition and a sedentary life-style has been cited as the second leading cause of preventable, premature death, accounting for about 300,000 deaths per year (McGinnis and Foege 1993).

Undernutrition

Starvation, Marasmus, and Kwashiorkor

Most of the frank starvation in recent decades has occurred as a result of war or civil unrest. Events in places such as Ethiopia, Sudan, Kosovo, and Bosnia serve as reminders that adequate nutrition depends on a fragile chain of production, transportation, storage, processing, and marketing. Wars interfere with all of these steps.

In infants, severe malnutrition results in a wasting syndrome called marasmus. Marasmus causes almost total growth retardation and is the result of

deficiencies in all nutrients, as occurs when the mother's milk fails and no substitute is available. Breast-feeding is absolutely essential for infant survival in most developing nations, because formula milk is often unavailable and because breast milk is nutritionally well-balanced, contains antibodies that help infants fight off infection, and is usually sterile (although in infected mothers it may contain the human immunodeficiency virus and other pathogens).

In slightly older children, nutritional deficiencies tend to develop during the weaning process, when the greatest deficiency is usually in vitamins and essential amino acids, while caloric intake may be closer to normal. In developing nations, gruel and other foods used to wean children tend to be starchy, are apt to be deficient in one or more essential amino acids, and are often prepared with polluted water. Under these circumstances, a condition called kwashiorkor (visceral protein malnutrition) can develop and lead to serious morbidity and mortality. The resulting infections and kwashiorkor produce liver damage and a reduction in serum proteins, both of which lead to ascites (fluid in the abdominal cavity). Because the abdominal ascites causes the stomach to swell, observers may think that affected children are fat, when actually they are severely undernourished.

The extent to which marasmus and kwashiorkor occur varies with many factors, including the type of staple food crops. In areas where the diet consists primarily of cassava, plantain, bananas, or a combination of these crops, the protein intake may be especially low (Hegsted 1978). But even in areas where the staple crops are relatively rich in amino acids, if the economy is based largely on a single staple crop, a deficiency of one or more amino acids may occur (King 1969). Corn, for example, is low in tryptophan, and beans are low in methionine. However, by mixing starchy crops that are deficient in different amino acids, it is possible to obtain a diet that is adequate in all of the essential amino acids. Successful programs based on this principle have been developed, making it possible to reduce the incidence of weaning malnutrition and child mortality resulting from amino acid deficits (King 1969).

Vitamins, in particular, may be deficient where nutrition is poor, and supplying vitamins alone may markedly reduce mortality from infectious disease. For example, Rahmathullah et al. (1990) showed that the mortality of preschool children in southern India could be reduced by more than half merely by giving the children vitamin A supplements.

Synergism of Malnutrition and Infection

In developing nations, there is a significant risk of both malnutrition and infection among children who are between their first and fifth birthday, particularly those in the process of being weaned from breast milk. Not only are malnutrition and infection frequently present together, but each makes the other worse (Scrimshaw, Taylor, and Gordon 1968; Hansen et al. 1968). This synergism between malnutrition and infection, which is discussed in Chapter 1 (see the section entitled Synergism of Factors Predisposing to Disease), is the underlying cause of a large proportion of deaths of young children in poor countries and is therefore the target of many programs designed to promote health.

Because the prevention of infection will improve the ratio of caloric intake to caloric need, programs that provide measles vaccinations and programs that make uncontaminated water supplies more accessible to the population will have a positive effect on the nutritional status of children in that population. Similarly, programs that provide improved nutrition, especially for young children, will help the children avoid death or permanent organ damage caused by infections during the highest risk period of life. An important lesson of research on synergism, however, is that the approach to nutritional and infectious disease problems in regions of scarcity should be broad-based, attempting to improve all dimensions of life simultaneously.

Overnutrition

Factors Contributing to Nutritional Excesses and Imbalances

In the USA and other industrialized countries, a confluence of economic and sociocultural trends has served to render overnutrition a threat to the health of the general public for the first time in history. These trends include the following: the proliferation of mechanized devices and systems that obviate the need for physical work; the implementation of agricultural methods that allow for production of food in excess of the amount needed for industrialized populations; the accumulation of sufficient capital to use grains to feed animals and then to purchase and consume animal products, rather than directly consuming the grains; the popularization of sedentary activities, such as television and computer use; an increase in the influence of food advertising on dietary behavior; and an increase in the availability of affordable and easy-to-prepare foods that are energy-dense and nutrient-dilute. As industrialization and affluence spread globally, so, too, do the "Western" diet and the associated risks of nutritional imbalances and obesity (see Axelson 1986; Nestle et al. 1998; Glanz et al. 1998; Hill and Melanson 1999; James and Ralph 1999; and Katz 2000).

While it is clear that a balance between energy ingestion and energy consumption is the principal determinant of weight maintenance in an individual, the factors responsible for the wide variations in the set-point for that equilibrium are uncertain. Genetic factors influence the propensity for weight gain or loss, apparently playing both a direct role (e.g., by determining levels of leptin) and an indirect role (e.g., by affecting levels of thyroid hormone, the degree of postprandial thermogenesis, and the mass of brown fat). Environmental influences, such as the prevailing food supply and the accessibility of opportunities for physical activity, are comparably important. The rising prevalence of obesity in industrialized countries makes it clear that, rather than being a problem of impaired self-restraint in individuals, obesity can be seen as a public health threat mediated by a "toxic" nutritional environment.

The imbalance between energy intake and energy expenditure that is fundamental to obesity is largely the product of an interaction between physiologic traits and sociocultural factors. Human metabolism is the product of millions of years of natural selection, the overwhelming majority of which occurred in an environment demanding vigorous physical activity and providing access to a largely nutrient-dense but energy-dilute diet (Eaton, Eaton, and Konner 1997). In such an environment, characterized by cyclical feast and famine, metabolic efficiency would be favored, as would a capacity to store nutrient energy in the body. Such an environment would likely shape behavioral responses as well. For example, in hunter-gatherer societies, the tendency to binge eat, the preference for naturally sweet foods (such as fruit and honey, which provide readily metabolizable energy and are rarely toxic), and the affinity for dietary fat (which represents a source of concentrated energy and essential nutrients) all represent adaptive behavioral responses. However, in highly industrialized societies in which food is abundantly and constantly available, these same tendencies and preferences are conducive to excess energy consumption.

Excess Weight and Obesity

The **body mass index,** or BMI, of an individual is calculated as the weight in kilograms (kg) divided by the square of the height in meters (m^2). **Overweight** is defined as a BMI of 25–29.9. **Stages of obesity** are defined as follows: stage I, a BMI of 30–34.9; stage II, a BMI of 35–39.9; and stage III, a BMI of 40 or more.

In the USA, excess weight and obesity may be the most common conditions seen in primary care. In addition to affecting more than 50% of the adult population, these conditions are being found in increasing proportions of the adolescent and pediatric populations. Obesity represents a major public health problem because it is associated with an increased risk of a wide range of chronic and degenerative diseases, including cardiovascular disease, diabetes, cancer, and arthritis. Obesity is also associated with an increased risk of premature death and is now considered to be directly or indirectly responsible for approximately 300,000 deaths per year (McGinnis and Foege 1993; Allison et al. 1999). Based on findings in an observational cohort of more than 1 million subjects who were followed for 14 years, Calle and colleagues (1999) reported a linear relationship between the BMI and the mortality risk.

Recent studies based on computer modeling have highlighted the health and economic consequences of obesity and demonstrated that greater efforts at prevention and treatment would likely be both beneficial and cost-effective. For example, when Oster et al. (1999) and Thompson et al. (1999) used computer modeling to estimate the health and economic benefits of a sustained modest (10%) weight loss in persons with varying degrees of obesity, they concluded that in addition to meaningful improvements in health, there would be health care cost reductions ranging from $2200 to $5300 per person.

Although obesity may be the single most common condition encountered in primary care, it is often not addressed by primary care providers (Nawaz, Adams, and Katz 1999). This is unfortunate, because counseling by physicians and other health care professionals can be an important factor in helping patients select safe and appropriate methods to lose weight. Recommendations should take into account the degree and duration of obesity, its refractoriness to life-style interventions (such as increased exercise and improved nutrition), and its physical and psychologic sequelae. The risk-benefit ratio of specific treatment methods should also be considered.

Weight loss is promoted by a diet that is consistent with general recommendations for health promotion. As discussed in Box 15–1, these recommendations include exercising regularly, eating appropriately sized portions of food, limiting the intake of fat (to reduce the energy density of the diet), and eating an abundant amount of whole grains, vegetables, and fruits. There is some evidence that within the context of a fat- and energy-restricted diet, the intake of relatively more protein (in the form of beans, legumes, fish, poultry, and egg whites) and relatively less carbohydrate may result in lower fasting insulin levels. However, weight loss consistently lowers insulin levels as well. Moreover, because studies that have varied carbohydrate and protein content have generally stayed within close proximity to the recommended levels of carbohydrate and protein intake, there is no meaningful evidence that extreme alterations of the basic health-promoting diet are indicated to achieve or maintain weight loss. To date, there is also no evidence that commercially available programs for weight loss are successful in the long term. Programs promoting diets that are alternatives to the basic health-promoting diet, whether or not they facilitate short-term weight loss, are inconsistent with the long-term dietary pattern advised for health maintenance and the prevention of disease.

The majority of patients who have a weight control problem and are seen in the primary care setting either are considered overweight or have stage I obesity (as defined above). Evidence that pharmacotherapy is beneficial in these patients is currently lacking. Therefore, the use of pharmacotherapy for patients who have minimal weight problems without sequelae is generally not indicated. However, as an adjunct to life-style changes in the management of patients with more severe weight problems, clinicians should be prepared to consider the long-term use of pharmacologic agents (as is commonly done with other diet-sensitive conditions, such as hypertension and hyperlipidemia). Although stage II and stage III obesity can sometimes be managed effectively in the short term with low-calorie liquid diets, these benefits are difficult to sustain. Surgery is beneficial in carefully selected patients with severe obesity, but intensive behavioral intervention is required to sustain the weight loss achieved.

Physical activity is among the best predictors of long-term weight maintenance. Given the many impediments to lifelong compliance with health-promoting dietary guidelines, the ultimate control of epidemic obesity in industrialized countries will almost certainly require environmental changes that facilitate consistent physical activity and consumption of a nutrient-dense but relatively energy-dilute diet.

Nutritional Counseling

Routine counseling to promote healthy eating is encouraged by the US Preventive Services Task Force (1996). As discussed earlier, dietary and life-style patterns are predicated on many considerations other than health. Given the multiple biologic, economic, and sociocultural influences on dietary selection, professional guidance is clearly required to encourage individuals to follow a health-promoting diet. Expertise in clinical nutrition has traditionally been the purview of dietitians, to whom only a minority of patients are ever referred. The institution of routine nutritional counseling by physicians has been hampered by the lack of nutrition education in most medical schools, as well as by time pressures, competing demands, and lack of conviction that the effort would be productive. Effective dietary counseling leans heavily on the power of persuasion, and it may seem a potentially thankless task. However, the aggregate toll of diet-related health problems is enormous. Even when not discernibly contributing to the development or prevention of a particular disease, nutrition plays a role in lifelong health, influencing appearance, functional status, self-esteem, socialization, energy level, athletic performance, susceptibility to infection, and longevity.

When patients visit their physicians, the information elicited during the history and physical examination should routinely include information about dietary habits and exercise. All patients, with or without chronic diseases or risk factors for particular diseases, should be encouraged to comply with the health-promoting diet outlined in Box 15–1. Patients with one or more predominant risk factors or diseases may benefit from modest adjustments to the diet that are disease- or factor-specific. While the advice may not change much with the development of disease, the conviction and frequency with which counseling is provided should increase.

Nutritional counseling should always be linked to advice about physical activity, because the health benefits of each support those of the other and because there is evidence that counseling provided by physicians effectively promotes physical activity (Calfas et al. 1996). Difficulties involved in making dietary and other life-style changes should be discussed briefly. If more involved dietary counseling is indicated as part of the disease management or

BOX 15–1 Health-Promoting Dietary Guidelines

In the past, various expert panels and organizations have recommended different types of diets for the prevention of particular diseases. These individual disease-preventing diets have largely been supplanted by one **health-promoting diet** that is based on the **food guide pyramid** depicted below and is designed to prevent multiple diseases by enhancing health. Consensus opinion regarding nutrition is reflected in the fact that dietary guidelines generated by the US Surgeon General, the American Heart Association, the American Cancer Society, the National Cancer Institute, and other organizations differ only in minor points, while all support the goal of maintaining and promoting health by exercising regularly, eating appropriately sized portions of food, limiting the intake of fat, and eating an abundant amount of whole grains, vegetables, and fruits.

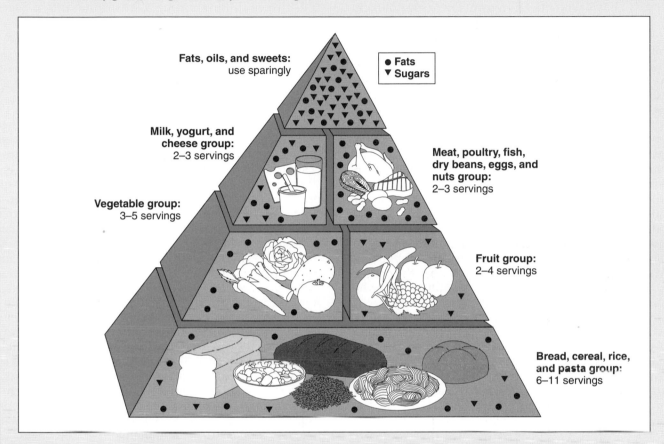

The recommended diet is schematically represented by the food pyramid. Cereal grains are the foundation of the health-promoting diet. Vegetables and fruits should be consumed in variety and abundance, with a total of five servings of these items a day representing the minimal recommendation. The consumption of fat-restricted (or, preferably, fat-free) dairy products is advisable to increase calcium intake; the intake of full-fat dairy products should be restricted. Items in the meat and fish group should generally be eaten as peripherals to vegetable-based meals. Poultry should be eaten without skin, with white meat consumed preferentially. The intake of red meat should generally be limited and lean cuts selected. The advantages of fish consumption should be emphasized. Fatty, dark-meat fish, such as salmon, is particularly rich in omega-3 fatty acids. Beans and legumes are a good source of protein and should be eaten regularly as an alternative to meat. A variety of seeds and nuts should be consumed, but they should be eaten in modest quantities because of their caloric density. Highly refined foods, sweets, and oils should be used sparingly.

With regard to macronutrient distribution, guidelines call for 30% or less of total calories from fat, 55–60% from carbohydrates, and 10–15% from proteins. With regard to fat, more specific recommendations are for an intake of monounsaturates at approximately 10–15% of total calories, polyunsaturates at approximately 10% of total calories, and saturated fats below 10% of total calories. Specific recommendations for the intake of *trans*-fatty acids are lacking, but the evidence suggests that *trans*-fatty acids and saturated fat should be combined and collectively restricted to below 10% of total caloric intake. Total calorie consumption should be limited to the amount required to maintain a healthful body weight. At least 30 g of dietary fiber should be consumed daily, achieved by complying with the recommendations for abundant intake of grains, beans, fruits, and vegetables. Sodium intake should be restricted to not more than 3 g/d, a figure supported by recommendations to eat processed foods sparingly. Alcohol consumption should be modest, with ethanol levels not exceeding 15 g/d for women or 30 g/d for men (one drink for women or two drinks for men).

Source of figure: http://www.nal.usda.gov:8001/py/pmap.htm. US Department of Agriculture and US Department of Health and Human Services. Nutrition and Your Health: Dietary Guidelines for Americans, 4th ed., 1995.

weight loss plan for a particular patient, the responsibilities for counseling should generally be shared with a dietitian. Under these circumstances, the physician's role is to reinforce the detailed counseling provided by the dietitian, to incorporate the dietary recommendations within the overall clinical plan, and to encourage the patient's efforts by applying realistic behavior modification principles (see Rollnick, Mason, and Butler 1999; Katz 2001).

Some patients will need to be motivated before they are willing to consider changes; others will need help developing strategies to maintain changes that are currently under way; and still others will need help overcoming the sequelae of prior failed attempts. This latter group, perhaps predominant, may be harmed by counseling efforts that focus only on motivation. Much effort at dietary modification fails because of the diverse and challenging obstacles to a healthy diet in the modern "toxic" nutritional environment (Katz 2000). Physicians committed to promoting the nutritional health of patients must commit to devising strategies that are tailored to individual patients and that work around such obstacles by distinguishing between responsibility and blame and by offering both rationales and methods for dietary change.

While the evidence that dietary counseling in the context of clinical care can change behavior or outcomes is limited, such evidence does exist. The application of methods specifically tailored to the setting of clinical practice should lead to better outcomes than have been described to date. A concerted effort by physicians to incorporate nonjudgmental dietary guidance into routine clinical care is clearly indicated by the importance of good nutrition and its universal relevance to health.

◼ ENVIRONMENTAL AND OCCUPATIONAL FACTORS IN HEALTH PROMOTION

Environmental conditions affecting health may be harmful (producing "dystress") or helpful (producing "eustress"). The environment should be understood in a broad sense to include not only microbiologic and chemical agents but also physical, social, and psychologic sources of dystress or eustress.

Public concern about the environment today tends to focus on hazards such as chemical toxins (e.g., dioxin), radiation (including electromagnetic, ionizing, and solar ultraviolet radiation), radon, "sick" buildings, and other relatively new and "high-tech" environmental and occupational hazards. In contrast, hazards related to crowding or loud noise from music or industrial exposure elicit little public concern or interest, because in general people tend to be more fearful about risks over which they believe they have no control than about those with which they are familiar. People have control over some aspects of their environment (such as whether or not to smoke) but little control over other aspects of their environment (such as the quality of the air where they live).

Among the tasks of physicians in environmental health are the following: (1) helping patients interpret the dangers of environmental risks about which they are concerned, (2) exploring the possibility of environmental and occupational causes of acute and chronic disease in patients by performing histories and physical examinations that are environmentally sensitive, and (3) reporting diseases that might have an environmental source to public health agencies (see Chapter 19).

Routes and Effects of Exposure to Environmental Hazards

Chemical and biologic hazards ordinarily enter the body through one of its protective surfaces: the skin for external hazards, the gastrointestinal tract for ingested hazards, and the lung for inhaled hazards. Therefore, it is not surprising that all three of these organ systems are heavily affected by the environment. The environment also can damage the vision and hearing, which often happens in an occupational or recreational setting.

Knowledge of the probable **route of entry** of an environmental hazard is essential in devising adequate protection. The **skin** is damaged by microbial hazards, by chemicals (both direct damage and allergic reaction), and by heat and other energy sources, including ultraviolet radiation and kinetic energy that causes cuts or contusions. The **gastrointestinal tract** is particularly subject to microbial hazards, but it is also a portal of entry for ingested chemical toxins, including lead. The gastrointestinal tract also is sensitive to large doses of ionizing radiation. The **lung** is especially sensitive to airborne microbes, chemical aerosols, fumes, dusts, and allergens in the environment (including pollens, dust mites, animal danders, and molds).

Exposure to an environmental hazard can be classified as acute or chronic. The negative effects of **acute exposure** may result from short-term, high-level exposure to an infectious organism; to certain toxic substances, such as potassium cyanide or carbon monoxide; or to a source of high energy, such as heat (resulting in burns), noise (resulting in acute deafness), or a heavy blow (resulting in crushing or penetrating wounds). The negative effects of **chronic exposure** may result from cumulative contact with or irritation of human tissues, as occurs, for example, with long-term exposure to asbestos, lead, mercury, and certain types of dust; with repetitive motion injuries (e.g., carpal tunnel syndrome); or with repeated exposure to loud noise of the type faced by airport ground crew and baggage handlers and by members or aficionados of rock bands.

Chronic exposures often show a **dose-response relationship** (see Chapter 4), such as that between the quantity of cigarette smoking and the risk of lung cancer. For cigarette smoking, a dose-response relationship has been found, whether the "dose" is estimated by duration of smoking, depth of inhalation, or pack-years (see US Department of Health and Human Services 1980). In research concerning a potential carcinogen, the dose-response relationship is measured beyond the usual **latent period** for the carcinogen (i.e., the period between the onset of exposure and the development of cancer). The latent period for lung cancer caused by cigarette smoking is approximately 20 years, while the latent period for mesothelioma caused by asbestos exposure is about 15–20 years.

Environmental and occupational exposures may or may not have a **threshold level** below which the human body can adapt successfully and no harm will come. For example, exposure to noise has a threshold level, whereas exposure to ionizing radiation does not.

Moderate decibel levels of noise, such as those associated with normal speech, do not injure the ear; however, high decibel levels, such as those associated with explosions or jet engines, can produce permanent nerve damage to the inner ear. For this reason, **threshold limit values** (TLVs), reflecting the maximum allowed concentration of a particular risk factor, are set for many exposures, including noise. The hope is that if the exposure levels do not exceed the TLVs, no harm will come to workers.

Unlike noise, some occupational and environmental exposures are **nonthreshold exposures.** These cause increases in the risk of damage and in the level of damage in proportion to the intensity and duration of the exposure, even down to extremely low levels. A small amount of ionizing radiation, for instance, will produce a small risk (but not a zero risk) of cancer. Nonthreshold exposures are usually monitored to limit the monthly, yearly, or lifetime exposure. In the case of exposure to ionizing radiation, each worker is usually required to carry a badge that shows the total amount of radiation received during the time the badge is worn. Maximum exposure limits are set for defined time periods.

Another way to monitor nonthreshold exposures, particularly for chemical toxins, is to monitor levels of the toxin or its metabolites in each worker's blood. For many chemicals, **biologic exposure indexes** (BEIs) are set, and if a worker shows a level above the BEI, he or she will be moved to another job.

The **Ames test** is used as a quick and inexpensive test to estimate the mutagenic potential of a chemical substance. In the Ames test, *Salmonella typhimurium* bacteria are exposed to the suspected toxin in the presence of mammalian enzymes and then observed for the mutation of a specific gene. Although the Ames test looks for mutagenesis, rather than carcinogenesis, a high proportion of the chemicals that cause mutations in this test are also found to be carcinogenic in other, more complicated assays.

Assessment of Environmental Risks

Table 15–1 lists five suggested steps in the assessment of an environmental risk. These steps have parallels in the investigation of a disease outbreak (see Chapter 3) and in the determination of causation (see Chapter 4). Risk can be assessed in terms of the prob-

TABLE 15–1   Suggested Steps in the Assessment of an Environmental Risk

(1) Identify the environmental substance presumed to be a hazard.

(2) Establish diagnostic criteria for the outcome of concern (e.g., injury or disease).

(3) Characterize the contact with the presumed hazard in terms of the number of exposures, the duration and intensity of each exposure, and the timing of exposures (to establish that the cause came before the effect).

(4) Determine whether there is a statistical association between the exposure to the presumed hazard and the outcome of concern. Use methods that control for possible alternative explanations. Look for dose-response relationships.

(5) On the basis of the first four steps, determine the risks for an exposed individual. From known population exposure levels, determine the probable impact on the population.

ability (risk) that some untoward outcome will result (e.g., lead toxicity) and in terms of the seriousness of that outcome (e.g., toxicity with or without neurologic damage).

First, the presumed environmental hazard must be identified. This step is qualitative. In the case of lead exposure, it would consist of identifying the form or forms of lead that are thought to represent a hazard. Similarly, in the case of a disease outbreak, it consists of identifying the organism or organisms thought to be responsible. Careful surveillance is the foundation for effective control.

Second, the damage thought to result from the presumed hazard must be identified, and criteria for the diagnosis must be established. This step is similar to establishing a case definition. In the example of lead exposure, the investigator might describe toxicity characterized by central nervous system damage in growing children or characterized by abdominal symptoms or motor neuropathy in adults.

Third, the quantitative and qualitative aspects of the exposure to the presumed hazard must be determined, including the number of exposures, the duration and intensity of each exposure, and the timing of exposures (to determine whether the exposures came before the neurologic damage or other symptoms).

Fourth, the presumed hazard and the outcome of concern should be studied to look for statistical associations. It may be difficult to determine whether an environmental exposure is actually associated with a disease or injury, because it would be unethical to test human subjects by exposing them to a substance that is a presumed hazard. It may be possible to demonstrate that mutagenesis occurs in bacteria after they are exposed to the substance in the Ames test (see above), and it may also be possible to demonstrate that animals exposed to the substance developed a disease similar to that seen in humans exposed to the same substance. However, this would not prove that the environmental exposure caused the disease in humans. The search for true associations requires that the disease be diagnosed accurately, that exposure be quantified carefully, and that possible alternative explanations be controlled for, either in the research design or in the statistical analysis. It is important to look for dose-response relationships, because these enable investigators to predict the risk to individuals.

Fifth, the risks for an exposed individual and for the population must be assessed (see Chapter 6). This step is particularly difficult for many types of environmental hazards, because much of what is known about them is based on data concerning fairly high levels of exposure and the resulting risk of acute toxic effects. It is not clear to what extent such data can be extrapolated to low levels of exposure for a long period of time. Nevertheless, an estimate of risk for low levels of exposure is often obtained by plotting observed levels of exposure against associated known risks of death, disease, or damage and then calculating the regression line for this relationship and examining the risks predicted for lower exposures.

Methods of Environmental Modification

The basic approach to environmental control is first to identify specific biologic, chemical, social, and physical factors that represent hazards to health or well-being and then to modify the environment in a manner that protects people from harmful exposures.

There are two basic methods for modifying the environment. The first method consists of eliminating or reducing the offending agent—for example, eradicating microorganisms such as the smallpox virus, discontinuing most production of chemicals such as the insecticide DDT in the USA, switching to lead-free gasoline, or controlling the level of heat in buildings. The second method consists of preventing contact between people and the environmental hazard. In some cases, this is accomplished by public measures, such as water sanitation, sewage disposal, restaurant sanitation, and control of disease vectors (e.g., mosquitoes and ticks). In other cases, it is accomplished by individual measures that are strongly encouraged (e.g., good hygiene, proper food handling practices in the home, and wearing of protective clothing and repellents in areas of ticks or mosquitoes) or legislatively mandated (e.g., requirements that motorcyclists wear helmets, that airport ground crew members wear devices for ear protection, and that septic tanks and private wells pass inspection).

Major Sources of Environmental Hazard

Air pollution, water pollution, solid wastes, radiation, contaminated food, and disease vectors represent major sources of environmental hazard.

Air Pollution

The air contains a variety of substances that not only affect the health, longevity, and quality of life for people and plants but also have positive and negative effects on nonliving aspects of the environment. In addition to playing a vital role in human respiration and metabolism, air is the source of entry for a variety of environmental hazards other than those normally considered under the term "air pollution." For example, because sound results from rapid variation in the air pressure on the eardrums, "noise pollution" is airborne. Moreover, many illnesses are caused by airborne microorganisms, with the rate of spread of the organisms influenced by the distance between people and their behavior (e.g., sneezing), by the degree of ventilation of indoor air spaces, and by the humidity of the ambient air.

Types of Air Pollutants. The lung is the most frequent site of serious contact with environmental hazards, not only because the lung tissue is extremely sensitive and absorptive but also because the volume of air inhaled and exhaled each day is so great—i.e., about 50 pounds per day (Moeller 1997). The lung is easily damaged by a variety of airborne pollutants, including particulate matter, metal fumes, gases, dusts, and allergens.

Particulate matter, whether from cigarette smoking or from fuel combustion, often contains carcinogenic substances, such as benzpyrene and other hydrocarbons and arsenic. The normal respiratory defense mechanisms are usually adequate against these unless they have been damaged by cigarette smoking or are overwhelmed during an episode of acute air pollution.

Metal fumes are gaseous metal oxides that come primarily from activities in occupational settings, such as welding without adequate ventilation. An acute syndrome called metal fume fever may occur a few hours following exposure and characteristically consists of flu-like symptoms, including fever, weakness, muscle aches, and headache, which subside within a day if exposure is stopped or within a few days if exposure is continued. Frequently, the syndrome is due to zinc oxide, copper oxide, or a combination of both, and these metals can be detected in the urine. Other metals responsible for air pollution include arsenic, beryllium, cadmium, lead, and mercury. Lead in the air has been markedly reduced in most areas since the use of lead in gasoline has been restricted.

Gases of various types have negative effects on the lung. **Ozone,** a component of smog, is created by the action of sunlight on the reaction of nitrogen oxides and hydrocarbons. Inhalation of ozone produces acute and chronic changes in the respiratory tract, and these changes can predispose to respiratory infections. **Nitrogen dioxide** is produced from fuel combustion and automobile exhausts. Acute exposure may exacerbate bronchoconstriction, and chronic exposure may predispose to respiratory infections. **Sulfur dioxide** forms complexes with particulates. These complexes are toxic to the respiratory tract and can exacerbate respiratory infections and asthma. **Hydrocarbons** are emitted into the atmosphere in huge amounts (almost 30 million metric tons per year) from burning fossil fuels and from solvents and other chemicals. **Carbon monoxide** is an asphyxiant that is produced by sources of incomplete combustion, especially automobiles, poorly ventilated space heating devices, and cigarette smoking.

Dusts are an important cause of chronic lung disease. Inhalation of **coal dust** over a long period of time causes chronic bronchitis and fibrosis ("black lung" disease), which may result in death. Inhalation of **silica dust** is an occupational hazard for miners, stone masons, quarry workers, and foundry workers. The silica dust appears to stimulate varying degrees of pulmonary fibrosis and sometimes causes considerable interference with respiration. Occupational asthma (discussed in greater detail in Chapter 19) affects workers in a number of occupations and may be due to dusts from grain, wood, cotton, hemp, or flax, as well as to certain chemicals, especially isocyanates.

Outdoor Versus Indoor Air Pollution. The importance of the distinction between outdoor and indoor air pollution has become clear only since World War II. The indoor environment protects people and objects from some types of air pollution (e.g., pollens) but concentrates other types (e.g., cigarette smoke). Among the factors that influence the relative concentration outdoors and indoors include where the pollutant is produced or released, the nature of the pollutant, the size of the air space available for dilution, and the rate of air exchange indoors.

Pollutants produced or released outdoors tend to be most concentrated outdoors. Examples include pollen, ozone, sulfur and nitrogen oxides, gasoline, and solvents. Fuel combustion is the greatest single source of particulate matter in the air. Most carbon monoxide comes from automobiles, whereas most sulfur and nitrogen oxides come from fuel combustion for power production and space heating.

Outdoor air is naturally mixed when there are lateral winds and when cooler air, which is usually above, sinks and the warmer air below rises. These diluting and cleansing mechanisms are usually fairly effective. Occasionally, however, **air inversions** occur, when the cooler air is found close to the earth and the warmer air is above, so that natural vertical mixing does not occur. This allows a much greater than normal buildup of air pollutants in the outdoor environment. At such times, a large geographic area can become like a huge indoor environment, capable of concentrating all pollutants released in the area. In valleys protected from lateral winds, air inversions can be disastrous, as was the case with a fatal smog episode in Donora, Pennsylvania, in 1948, which killed 20 people (Roueché 1953) and with periodic smog episodes that have occurred in Mexico City.

Control of outdoor air pollution must come from a reduction in the release of pollutants, achieved either by altering the production process or by using filters, precipitators, or scrubbers before the pollutants are released into the ambient air.

Pollutants produced or released indoors almost always show higher concentrations indoors. Examples include microorganisms, allergens (such as those from pets and dust mites), allergenic molds, aerosols from products used indoors, cooking products, radon, tobacco smoke, and chemicals or fumes released by building or consumer products (such as urethane or formaldehyde from plywoods and carpets).

There have been cases in which significant numbers of people in a building complain of headaches, difficulty in concentrating or staying awake, wheezing or difficulty in breathing, watery eyes, and other such complaints whenever they work long hours or even enter a certain building. This is sometimes referred to as the **sick building syndrome.** Usually, it occurs in buildings that are tightly sealed for energy conservation, but increasing the ventilatory rate does not always ameliorate the symptoms (Menzies et al. 1993). Often, the sick building syndrome appears to be due to the joint action of many factors. Recently, for example, an older building was discovered to have elevated levels of carbon monoxide, and it appeared that a combination of heavy traffic outside and poor ventilation inside was responsible for the carbon monoxide buildup (Goldberg 1995).

Probably the most common and most serious indoor air pollutant is environmental tobacco smoke. According to the US Environmental Protection Agency (1992), environmental tobacco smoke causes lung cancer in nonsmoking adults; increases the risk of developing asthma and acute lower respiratory tract irritation and infections in children; and is associated with a higher risk of sudden infant death syndrome. The Council on Scientific Affairs of the American Medical Association concurred with these conclusions and recommended a number of steps that physicians should take, including (1) educating their patients about the risks associated with exposure to environmental tobacco smoke at home and at work; (2) encouraging parents to insist on smoke-free environments for children at day-care and preschool facilities; (3) supporting efforts to ban smoking from public places and workplaces; and (4) informing elected representatives about the dangers of environmental tobacco smoke (see American Medical Association 1994).

Control of other indoor pollutants also focuses on methods to reduce the production or release of the pollutants. Examples include improving stoves for better burning and changing behaviors that contribute to pollution (e.g., encouraging people to avoid the use of aerosols and poorly designed stoves). The next line of defense involves increasing the rate of air exchange (ventilation) at the source of the pollutant (e.g., by installing a hood over a cooking stove). The least effective approach is cleaning the air in a room or building by such methods as air filters or electrostatic precipitators.

Water Pollution

Water constitutes about two-thirds of the body weight in humans. Water contributes directly to health when ingested in liquids and as a constituent of food. It also contributes indirectly to health and well-being through its uses in agriculture, industry, power generation, waste disposal, recreation, and transportation.

Pollution of oceans, rivers, and lakes may cause human disease when toxins move through the food chain and enter into fish, which are subsequently caught and consumed by people. Perhaps the most striking example of this occurred in 1958 among the people who lived along Minamata Bay in Japan. Over 100 cases of central nervous system damage and some deaths occurred when the people ate fish contaminated by methylmercury from the dumping of toxic wastes by a vinyl chloride plant on the bay (Kurland et al. 1960). Pollution of sources of drinking water can also cause serious illnesses and deaths.

Sources of Potable Water. Potable water is water that does not contain harmful types or levels of microorganisms, chemical toxins, dissolved metals, or radioactivity and is therefore safe for human consumption. The provision of potable water has been one of the major methods of lowering the rates of death and disease throughout the world, and the decade from 1990 to 2000 was proclaimed the "Water Decade" by the World Health Organization. Surface water and ground water are the major sources of water for drinking.

Surface water includes protected surface reservoirs, lakes, and rivers. **Protected surface reservoirs** are usually the safest water sources. **Lakes** may be an excellent primary water source for a city if little or no pollution drains into the lakes from rivers or from cities and industries on the lake shores. However, many lakes are highly polluted. For example, the Great Lakes in the USA became seriously polluted after World War II, but environmental control efforts have helped them to recover considerably. The water from **rivers** may be polluted by a variety of sources and may therefore require considerable treatment to meet acceptable standards of potability. First, rivers are frequently used for the dumping of sewage by cities, often with only primary sewage treatment (i.e., letting the solids settle out first) or sometimes with no sewage treatment. Second, river water may contain industrial pollutants, such as chemical, biologic, or radioactive wastes. Third, rivers often are contaminated by runoff from farms, including biologic pollutants (animal waste) and chemical pollutants (fertilizers, pesticides, and fungicides).

Ground water exists in underground domes of water called **aquifers.** The rate of turnover of water in aquifers varies considerably, and when an aquifer becomes contaminated by chemical pollutants, such as gasoline from a leaking underground tank at a service station, it may be years or decades before the aquifer can cleanse itself to the point at which it is considered potable again. Therefore, protecting underground water sources is as important as protecting surface water sources.

Water Treatment. Although some surface and ground water supplies are safe for drinking without treatment, most states have laws requiring the treatment of any water supply going to more than one dwelling.

The treatment of water involves removing some substances and adding others.

Filtration is the fundamental method for removing unwanted substances, including the cysts of *Giardia lamblia,* which are spread by beavers and other wild animals. Even if the water seems pure, as in the case of water from a mountain stream, there is a danger of giardiasis and other infectious diseases if the water has not been properly filtered.

The most common filtration methods are slow sand filtration and rapid sand filtration. **Slow sand filtration** requires the use of a large bed of packed sand, on which an organic layer forms and assists in the filtration process. The organic layer is called a *Schmutzdecke,* the German term for "dirt layer." When the *Schmutzdecke* becomes too thick, filtration is slowed and the layer must be shoveled off so water can get through and a new *Schmutzdecke* can form. In **rapid sand filtration,** a flocculent (usually aluminum sulfate, called alum) is added to the water before filtration. The flocculent coagulates and traps suspended materials, preventing them from passing through the sand with the filtered water. The flocculent is removed periodically by back flushing, and new flocculent is added to the next batch of water.

If the water contains chemicals that are hazardous or give the water a bad taste, they can be removed by **chemical filtration processes,** such as passing the water through activated carbon, but such techniques are expensive.

Additions are often made to drinking water. For example, chlorine is added to kill vegetative forms of microorganisms. Filtration of chlorinated water is necessary, however, because chlorination fails to kill many types of cysts and because even vegetative bacteria and viruses may be protected from the chlorine by the organic matter in unfiltered water. In many water systems, fluoride is added to help prevent dental caries. Despite considerable concern among some community groups that fluoride might be dangerous, no good evidence of danger from fluoridation (in the range of one part per million in tap water) has been found. There is now good evidence that a considerable drop in the rate of decayed, missing, and filled teeth (called the DMF rate in dental epidemiology) has occurred in communities with fluoridated water.

Sewage Treatment. Human sewage poses a threat to more than just other human beings. Biologic wastes, rather than chemical toxins, are responsible for many, if not most, of the episodes of mass death occurring in fresh water fish. All living creatures in rivers and lakes, including fish at the top of the food chain, use dissolved oxygen in the water to sustain life. If the level of dissolved oxygen is too low, they will die. Sewage from humans and domestic animals contains aerobic bacteria (bacteria whose metabolism requires oxygen), and these bacteria lower the oxygen level in water. The quantity of oxygen that aerobic bacteria in a given amount of sewage will deplete from the water is called their **biochemical oxygen demand.** A related measure, which reflects the effect of industrial wastes, is the **chemical oxygen demand.** Two goals of sewage treatment are to remove as much of the organic material as possible from the water (primary treatment) and then to reoxygenate the water (secondary treatment).

In the process of **primary sewage treatment,** water is held in a large basin until most of the solids have settled to the bottom. If the basin is long enough and the rate of water flow into the basin is slow enough, the water flowing out the top of the basin at the far end can be considered to have had primary treatment. Periodically, the basin is emptied and the sludge in the bottom is removed to dry either in sunlight or in a digester. If the sludge does not contain harmful metals or other toxins, it can sometimes be used as a fertilizer. Otherwise, the treated sludge is buried or dumped at sea (this is not the same as dumping raw garbage at sea, a practice that is gradually being discontinued).

In the process of **secondary sewage treatment,** the water is aerated, usually by means of an activated sludge process or a trickling filter process. If the treated sewage water (called the effluent) must be essentially as clean as drinking water, it may be subjected to sand filtration and may even be chlorinated at the end of this process. Although secondary treatment usually destroys harmful bacteria, it does not always destroy viruses.

Solid Wastes

Each year, the average person in the USA generates between 1000 and 1500 pounds of garbage and related solid wastes that must be disposed of by city governments and other governing bodies. The volume of solid waste produced by the industrial sector is even greater than that generated by the private sector. Both citizens and industry discard toxic waste, some of which is radioactive. Most of this waste goes to sanitary landfills, but it is becoming increasingly difficult to find locations for new landfills, and the existing landfills frequently leach toxic chemicals into the ground water. Recognizing that hazardous wastes are becoming an increasing problem, the US Congress passed the Superfund Act (Public Law 96-150) in 1980, the Superfund Amendments and Reauthorization Act (Public Law 99-499) in 1986, and subsequent acts to strengthen these. It is clear more than a decade after the Superfund Act that the problem of toxic wastes is still enormous and probably getting worse.

Physicians may see patients who believe that their symptoms (or even frank diseases, such as cancer) are due to their living in proximity to a facility that produces, releases, or disposes of toxic substances. Although such proximity has seldom been clearly established to cause disease in nearby residents (it is more likely to cause symptoms or disease in those working in the facility), such complaints by patients must be dealt with. Often, this will require communication with the local or state department of health or with the state pollution control agency if it is not in the department of health.

Additional information concerning toxic agents and other potential health hazards is presented in Chapter 19.

Electromagnetic Radiation

Electromagnetic radiation produces injurious effects roughly proportional to the energy level (in electron volts). Radiation rays in the higher energy ranges (e.g., cosmic, gamma, x, and some ultraviolet rays) have enough energy to cause damage to cells by ionizing atoms. This type of radiation, called **ionizing radiation,** may damage DNA and produce free radicals, which speed up the cellular aging process. Radiation rays in lower energy ranges (e.g., infrared radiation, radar, microwaves, radio waves, magnetic fields, and some ultraviolet rays) are called **nonionizing radiation.** Scientists continue to debate about the amount of tissue damage that the forms of nonionizing radiation can cause, apart from actual heat production.

Terminology. The terms used to describe radiation effects in biology can be confusing. The easiest approach is to consider terminology historically. The first unit was the **roentgen,** which is no longer used. Then came the **rad** (an acronym for radiation absorbed dose), which is a unit of the amount of energy absorbed by tissues (about 100 ergs per gram of tissue). The rad proved to be an inadequate unit of measure because different forms of radiation, although equal in rads, may not cause the same amount of tissue damage. Therefore, the **rem** (an acronym for roentgen equivalent man) was developed. One rad of absorbed dose from beta, gamma, or x radiation is equal to 1 rem. However, 1 rad of absorbed dose from alpha radiation equals 20 rems, although alpha radiation penetrates only a few millimeters of tissue. The danger from radon (a gaseous radioactive element) comes mostly from alpha radiation, which when inhaled can penetrate most of the lung parenchyma. Both rads and rems have units to use for large doses: 1 **gray** (Gy) equals 100 rads, and 1 **sievert** (Sv) equals 100 rems.

Biologic Effects. The biologic effects of radiation depend on how much of the body is irradiated, which parts of the body are irradiated, and how much radiation is given (dose per time period). For comparison purposes, usually "whole body" radiation doses are used, although some tissues (e.g., bone marrow and testes) are especially sensitive to ionizing radiation.

Acute effects are seen when a large dose (e.g., 100 rems or more) of whole body radiation is given over a short time. The lethal dose for 50% of adults given whole body radiation (the LD_{50}) is about 600 rems. A dose of 1000 rems or more given over a short time is fatal to 100% of persons, initially causing gastrointestinal symptoms and soon destroying bone marrow.

Chronic effects of radiation are harder to measure, but in those affected by the Chernobyl nuclear disaster in the Ukraine, the effects included cellular mutations, with an increased incidence of cancers, abnormal genetic material in ova and sperm, abnormalities in offspring of women exposed to radiation during pregnancy, and damage to specific sites receiving high doses, such as the thyroid gland.

Control. Several forms of ionizing radiation, including x-rays, are used in medicine and industry for research, diagnosis, treatment, and quality control. The general methods for controlling exposure to ionizing radiation include reducing the intensity and duration of the source, focusing the source, and shielding people from the radiation.

It is difficult or impossible to limit most natural background radiation. The primary method for reducing contact with radiation from sunlight is to avoid exposure, although shielding by use of clothing and sunblock is also important. Keeping at a distance from the source is the primary protection against microwaves, radio waves, and electric or magnetic fields, especially those emitted from appliances inside the home. Some geographic areas have higher levels of background radiation from uranium, owing to the seepage of radon and radon daughters from the ground. To some extent, radon exposure can be controlled by home construction methods. The biggest concern is to avoid future nuclear power plant disasters or nuclear war. A related issue, the disposal of nuclear wastes, is becoming more difficult throughout the world.

Contaminated Food

Worldwide, foods contaminated with enteric bacteria, viruses, or parasites are a major source of reported morbidity. In the developing countries, they are also a source of mortality in infants who are not being breast-fed. In the USA, despite the fact that many outbreaks of food-borne illness are reported, it is believed that most individual cases go unreported. In addition to contamination by microbes, food may be contaminated by microbial toxins (e.g., botulinum toxin, staphylococcal toxin, and toxins found in algae, fish, or shellfish) and by residual amounts of insecticides, fungicides, or weed killers.

To avoid contamination of food, a chain of safety procedures must be followed during production, transportation, storage, processing, marketing, and preparation. Contamination is possible at each stage. Examples of the ways in which hazards can be eliminated are adequate pasteurization of milk, ice cream, eggnog, and other milk products; proper sanitation in facilities handling food; and adequate refrigeration and cooking of foods.

Environmental Vectors

Until Lyme disease became a problem in the USA and was discovered to be a tick-borne illness, North Americans did not think much about the hazards of environmental vectors. Two serious types of mosquito-borne disease, malaria and dengue, were no longer spread indigenously, and various types of mosquito-borne encephalitis were rare. Tick-borne diseases, such as Rocky Mountain spotted fever, were not feared. However, the development of Lyme disease and, more recently, the development of West Nile virus infection in the northeastern USA have called the public's attention to potential insect- and arthropod-borne disease hazards. West Nile virus will probably spread to most of the North American continent and become endemic. Dengue may reemerge as a threat in the southern part of the USA, and malaria and tick-borne diseases continue to be leading killers in other parts of the world.

Prevention of vector-borne diseases usually consists of a variety of health promotion and specific protection methods, such as identifying and controlling mosquito-breeding swamps and encouraging travelers to take personal precautions (e.g., wear appropriate clothing, sleep under mosquito netting, use mosquito repellent, and take prophylactic antimicrobial agents) when visiting areas where the risk of malaria is high.

■ BEHAVIORAL FACTORS IN HEALTH PROMOTION

Human behavior is difficult to separate from nutrition and the environment, because human choices and behaviors have a profound influence on both. This is true, for example, of decisions regarding the types, quantities, and methods of preparation of the foodstuffs that are available to an individual or family.

Similarly, people make choices from the range of possible environments in which they live, work, and play. For example, the choice of a rural or semirural home environment means that the water supply and sewage disposal are likely to be individual responsibilities; the control of vectors (such as the ticks that carry Lyme disease) is a greater problem than in urban residential areas; there is a reduced threat of gang-related violence but probably more time is spent traveling in automobiles; and loneliness and isolation may cause social or psychologic problems. Choices regarding substances that are released into the indoor air space, such as cigarette smoking and aerosols, will influence the indoor ambient environment.

Because the level of education influences the types of jobs available to an individual, it also influences the environment in which he or she will work (office, factory, mine, farm, and so forth) and thereby determines the types of occupational risks that will be faced. Like occupational pursuits, recreational pursuits have an effect on the level of risk faced by individuals. Although mountain climbing, hang gliding, sky diving, and scuba diving are known to involve high risks, some risk is involved in almost any sport, including jogging, even though jogging is touted to have a net benefit of extending life.

Physicians may not be aware of individual behavioral choices made by their patients and may not feel comfortable in trying to influence them. Rather, physicians are more likely to counsel a patient in a special situation or concerning a special topic, such as family planning, nutrition and behavior during pregnancy, and care of a newborn infant. Physicians may also decide to counsel a patient when they discover definite risk factors for disease, such as obesity, hypertension, elevated cholesterol levels, or unprotected sexual activity. Another window of opportunity for counseling occurs following the development of symptomatic disease, such as coronary artery disease, when a patient's motivation to modify the diet, begin exercising regularly, and quit smoking may be at its peak.

Boxes 15–1 and 15–2 provide specific recommendations for promoting a healthy diet and for smoking cessation. The second report of the US Preventive Services Task Force (1996) offers recommendations for physician counseling concerning a variety of additional topics, including the prevention of motor vehicle injuries, household injuries, recreational injuries, youth violence, sexually transmitted diseases, unintended pregnancies, gynecologic cancers, low back pain, and dental and periodontal disease.

Counseling of Women Before and During Pregnancy

Family planning and the counseling of pregnant women are generally discussed in textbooks of obstetrics and gynecology. However, recent research has emphasized the importance of certain items that will be discussed here.

A woman who might become pregnant should seriously consider taking supplements of folic acid to reduce the risk of neural tube defects in the fetus. For folic acid supplementation to be of benefit, the woman must begin taking it before conception and during the first weeks following conception. Even early prenatal visits are too late to provide the benefit of folic acid supplements. In the USA, enriched cereal grain products have been required since January 1998 to be fortified with 140 µg of folic acid per 100 g of grain (see Centers for Disease Control and Prevention 1999), so women who eat these products will receive some folic acid via this source. In addition to cereal grains, leafy green vegetables are an excellent natural source of folic acid.

Currently, cigarette smoking is one of the most frequent factors contributing to premature delivery and the delivery of infants with low birth weight or intrauterine growth retardation. Maternal alcohol consumption, even in small quantities, can have serious negative effects on the developing fetus, and consumption in large quantities can cause fetal alcohol syndrome in the newborn. The intake of illegal drugs, particularly opiates and cocaine, can have negative effects on the infant. The exact nature and magnitude of these effects are difficult to predict, however, and the impact of illegal drugs is difficult to separate from the impact of medical, psychosocial, and economic problems that often accompany illegal drug use.

Because the ingestion of alcohol and illegal drugs and cigarette smoking are personal choices that involve habituation or addiction, solutions are not easy for the patient or physician. Nevertheless, identification of problems, counseling, and appropriate referrals are necessary steps, even if they are not always successful.

Counseling of Parents

Topics to be discussed with parents of infants and toddlers include nutrition (e.g., breast-feeding); safety (e.g., use of car seats, placement of barriers at the tops of stairs to prevent falls, and proper storage of harmful substances that might be ingested); immunizations (see Chapter 16); and the scheduling of routine medical examinations. The counseling of parents becomes more difficult and specialized when their offspring reach adolescence, a time during which behavioral problems may develop or become more pronounced. Most pediatric and adolescent medicine books offer guidelines concerning the types of health and safety topics that become pertinent as children reach specific ages.

Counseling of Patients with Risk Factors

Patients in whom a physician discovers risk factors often need and want counseling. If there are medications that could be prescribed, it is tempting for the physician to give them as the first line of attack for obesity, smoking, hypertension, and elevated cholesterol levels. Nevertheless, unless the problem is severe when the patient is first seen, generally the best approach is to try first to modify diet, exercise, or other aspects of life-style, such as eliminating smoking. If these approaches to reducing risk factors are refused or are not successful within a reasonable time, medications should be introduced.

Even if a physician is not comfortable with risk factor counseling, because of either perceived lack of counseling skills or shortage of time, he or she does have the responsibility to identify the problem, state firmly that it affects the patient's health and therefore requires attention, and offer recommendations to the patient concerning how to proceed (e.g., refer the patient to a specialist, such as a dietitian or nutritionist, or to a smoking-cessation program).

Perhaps the single most important behavior change for improving health is smoking cessation. Each year about 3.3 million smokers quit smoking, because they want to and because they are concerned about their health (see National Heart, Lung, and Blood Institute 1992). Signs of tobacco dependence include the continuous use of tobacco for at least 1 month plus at least one of the following: a history of unsuccessful attempts to stop smoking on a permanent basis, withdrawal symptoms after an attempt to stop smoking, or continuing use of tobacco despite a serious physical disorder the patient knows is made worse by tobacco use, such as lung or heart disease. Box 15–2 summarizes the approach that the National Heart, Lung, and Blood Institute and the American Lung Association recommend for use by physicians in counseling their patients.

Regardless of the extent of the physician's activity in behavior change, the physician has the responsibility for monitoring the progress of the patient on a regular basis and for changing the approach if sufficient progress is not being made. If necessary, the physician can assist the process of risk factor modification by recommending appropriate medications, such as nicotine patches or nicotine inhalers for cessation of smoking or such as acetyl-CoA reductase inhibitors for reduction of cholesterol levels (see US Preventive Services Task Force 1996). Patients using these medications require close monitoring for potential side effects.

In patients with hypertension (see Chapter 18), antihypertensive medications are indicated immediately if at the time of diagnosis the patient has a severely elevated blood pressure or evidence of end-organ damage. If the patient has a moderately elevated blood pressure with no evidence of end-organ damage, dietary change and exercise should be tried first. Only if these measures do not reduce blood pressure to satisfactory levels in an ac-

ceptable period of time should medication be started.

■ SUMMARY

Primary prevention begins with health promotion, which is working to improve the nutritional, environmental, social, and behavioral conditions in which people are conceived, born, and raised and live out their lives.

Proper nutrition is fundamental to good health and requires the intake of adequate amounts of proteins, carbohydrates, fats, vitamins, and minerals. In the developing nations, undernutrition is frequently a problem and usually takes the form of starvation, marasmus, or kwashiorkor. In industrialized nations, nutritional excesses and imbalances can lead to malnutrition and obesity.

The physical, biologic, and social environment has an impact on health and safety, with environmental threats taking the form of air pollution, water pollution, improper disposal of solid wastes, exposure to electromagnetic radiation, ingestion of contaminated food, contact with environmental disease vectors, and problems associated with crowded living conditions.

Many behavioral factors contribute to good or poor health. Negative factors include dangerous personal habits (such as smoking, use of illegal drugs,

---

BOX 15–2 The Approach to Smoking Cessation that the National Heart, Lung, and Blood Institute and the American Lung Association Recommend for Use by Physicians in Counseling Their Patients

Step 1. Act as a role model by not smoking. Measures include adopting a no-smoking policy in the physician's office, posting no-smoking signs, and making pamphlets about smoking cessation available in the office.

Step 2. Provide the patient with information on the risks associated with smoking and the reduction of risks if smoking is stopped. In addition to outlining the patient's risks for specific diseases, the information should outline the risks faced by members of the patient's household, particularly children.

Step 3. Encourage abstinence by direct advice and suggestions. The patient is more likely to stop smoking if the physician recommends it clearly and forcefully. The approach should be brief, direct, unambiguous, and informative. Instead of using a "scare tactic," which is likely to arouse defense mechanisms, the physician should emphasize the benefits that will result from cessation of smoking. The reasons for smoking should be taken into account, and the advice should be tailored to individual needs. For example, an emphasis on the health benefits that will result may be most effective for an individual who has symptoms of heart or lung disease, whereas an emphasis on sports performance or how one

smells to others may be more effective for an adolescent. If the patient is willing to try smoking cessation, it is important to set a quit-smoking date. If the patient is unwilling to do this, it may be possible to persuade him or her to take some other positive action, such as contacting a smoking-cessation program, by a defined time. Most successful quitters have tried and failed several times before they finally succeed, and knowing this may help the patient.

Step 4. Refer the patient to a smoking-cessation program. Local hospitals or offices of the American Lung Association or American Cancer Society are good sources to find smoking-cessation programs.

Step 5. Follow up on the use of specific cessation and maintenance strategies. The patient must know that the physician is not abandoning him or her by referral but only enlisting specialized assistance. The physician should schedule specific follow-up visits for physical checkups and for emotional support both during and after the smoking-cessation process. Continual emotional support may be helpful in preventing the patient from smoking again or in encouraging the patient to cease smoking if relapse does occur.

Source of data: National Heart, Lung, and Blood Institute. Clinical Opportunities for Smoking Intervention: A Guide for Busy Physicians. NIH Publication No. 92-2178. Washington, D. C., Government Printing Office, June 1992.

excessive intake of alcohol, and excessive intake of saturated fats), risk taking (such as risky driving or recreational activities), and failure to use available preventive measures (such as failure to be immunized). The physician's role in counseling patients regarding personal habits is underutilized. In particular, many physicians do not counsel patients until after a health problem is detected or an adverse event occurs.

■ QUESTIONS

Directions (Items 1–9). Each of the numbered items or incomplete statements in this section is followed by answers or by completions of the statement. Select the ONE lettered answer or completion that is BEST in each case. Correct answers and explanations are given at the end of the chapter.

1. In the 1950s, Hollingshead and Redlich demonstrated an association between social class and mental illness, with more cases of mental illness found in the lower social classes. This finding
   (A) indicates that although mental illness and social class may be correlated, the direction of causality is uncertain
   (B) indicates that poverty is causally related to mental illness but the relationship may be indirect
   (C) indicates that poverty produces mental illness directly
   (D) indicates that the treatment of mental illness should include social welfare
   (E) is spurious because it is not biologically plausible

2. Visceral protein malnutrition that tends to occur in developing nations during the weaning of children from breast milk is known as
   (A) anabolism
   (B) anasarca
   (C) cachexia
   (D) kwashiorkor
   (E) marasmus

3. The current recommendation for the dietary fat intake in adults is to reduce the intake to
   (A) 10% of total daily calories
   (B) 20% of total daily calories
   (C) 30% of total daily calories
   (D) 65 g/d
   (E) 75 g/d

4. The best explanation for the prevalence of obesity in the USA is
   (A) a deficiency of dietary fiber and an excess of protein
   (B) a genetic defect resulting in low basal metabolism
   (C) a high-fat diet and a sedentary life-style

   (D) an aversion to broccoli at the highest levels of American society
   (E) an innate preference for sweet food, compounded by insulin resistance

5. Of the following environmental hazards, the only one categorized as a nonthreshold hazard is
   (A) carbon monoxide
   (B) heat
   (C) ionizing radiation
   (D) lead
   (E) noise

6. The Ames test is used to
   (A) determine antibiotic susceptibility
   (B) establish environmental standards for heavy metals
   (C) estimate the adequacy of ventilation in a building
   (D) estimate the mutagenic potential of a chemical
   (E) quantify radiation exposure

7. The most frequent site of serious contact with environmental hazards is the
   (A) eye
   (B) gastrointestinal tract
   (C) hand
   (D) lung
   (E) skin

8. The indoor air pollutant of greatest public health importance is
   (A) carbon monoxide
   (B) dioxin
   (C) dust
   (D) radon
   (E) tobacco smoke

9. Public reaction to environmental health risks
   (A) is always commensurate with the magnitude of risk
   (B) is often greater when control over the exposure is high
   (C) is often greater when control over the exposure is low
   (D) tends to be greater than the magnitude of risk
   (E) tends to be less than the magnitude of risk

■ ANSWERS AND EXPLANATIONS

1. **The answer is A: indicates that although mental illness and social class may be correlated, the direction of causality is uncertain.** An association or correlation between two variables may suggest causality but cannot definitively establish causality. While there is evidence that lower social class and mental illness are correlated, causality is plausible in either direction. The stresses of poverty may lead to malnutrition, physical abuse, fractured social supports, and,

consequently, poor mental health. Alternatively, poor mental health may lead to unemployability and eventually to poverty. Moreover, some factors, such as racially motivated discrimination, are plausible causes of both low social class and poor mental health. For these reasons, an association should serve as a basis for further research or testing but not as sufficient evidence for causality.

2. **The answer is D: kwashiorkor.** Kwashiorkor is characterized by severe protein deficiency that occurs in the context of adequate or nearly adequate intake of calories. In developing countries, kwashiorkor tends to develop at the time when young children are weaned from breast milk to subsist on gruel or porridge.

3. **The answer is C: 30% of total daily calories.** As defined in *Healthy People 2000* (see US Department of Health and Human Services 1990), one of the US goals for the year 2000 was to reduce the intake of dietary fat to no more than 30% of total daily calories. The goal of 30% represents a compromise, since most nutrition experts concur that an even lower fat intake would be preferable but is unrealistic at least for the near future. The associations among dietary fat intake, elevated serum lipid levels, and heart disease risk are now well established. Increasingly, though, evidence suggests that the risk of heart disease is influenced as strongly by the type of dietary fat as by the quantity of it. Saturated and *trans*-fatty acids are associated with an increased heart disease risk. Monounsaturated and omega-3 polyunsaturated fatty acids are associated with a reduced heart disease risk. Beneficial effects on the rates of coronary atherosclerosis and adverse cardiac events have been shown both with fat restriction to 10% of calories and with a "Mediterranean" dietary pattern that provides nearly 40% of calories as predominantly monounsaturated fat (see Katz 2000).

4. **The answer is C: a high-fat diet and a sedentary life-style.** Obesity is a complex and multifactorial condition, about which a vast and at times controversial literature continues to proliferate. Fundamentally, though, obesity is known to represent an imbalance between the body's fuel intake and fuel consumption. A high intake of fat is tantamount to a high intake of calories, because fat is calorie-dense (there are approximately 9 kcal per gram of fat). Low-fat diets may or may not be low-calorie diets, as excessive intake of either carbohydrate or protein can lead to caloric excess. Fuel consumption is largely due to basal metabolism, but it can be substantially modified by the level of physical activity. Having evolved over 4 million years under the pressures of strenuous activity and dietary deficiency, humans are ill-prepared to defend themselves against a con-

veniently available abundance of calorie-dense foods and a host of energy-saving devices. An extremely high prevalence of obesity is the apparent consequence. Obesity and insulin resistance are associated, but at this time it is unclear which condition precedes the other.

5. **The answer is C: ionizing radiation.** Exposures to most hazards must exceed some threshold to produce a harmful effect. This is true of physical and chemical toxins, as well as microbial pathogens. However, current theory holds that no measurable level of ionizing radiation is entirely innocuous. This is because radiation-induced injury to even a single gene might be sufficient to ultimately produce cancer, although the risk is known to be greater with a more substantial exposure. Until or unless measurement technology improves and demonstrates otherwise, ionizing radiation is considered a hazard at any level above zero.

6. **The answer is D: estimate the mutagenic potential of a chemical.** In the Ames test, strains of *Salmonella typhimurium* are exposed to a suspected toxin in the presence of certain enzymes. The bacteria are then observed for the mutation of a specific gene. A high proportion of the chemicals that cause mutation in this assay can be shown by more complex methods to be carcinogenic.

7. **The answer is D: lung.** The lungs are extremely vulnerable to environmental hazards. This is because it is difficult to control the dispersion of substances in air and because the volume of air exchanged in the lungs is tremendous. An adult inhales and exhales about 50 pounds of air per day.

8. **The answer is E: tobacco smoke.** Individuals who smoke cigarettes have been shown to be at increased risk for a variety of health problems, and there is now a substantial body of evidence that passive exposure to tobacco smoke increases the risk of reactive airway disease (such as asthma), respiratory tract infections, and lung cancer. Significant exposure to carbon monoxide is potentially lethal but is rare compared with significant exposure to tobacco smoke. Both the intensity and the frequency of exposure to radon are small compared with those of exposure to tobacco smoke. Dust may lead to allergic reactions but is relatively innocuous under most circumstances. Dioxin is a chemical carcinogen that is introduced into the environment by industries.

9. **The answer is C: is often greater when control over the exposure is low.** The magnitude of environmental health risks and the reactions that they elicit from the public often diverge, based

on the level of actual or perceived control over the hazard. For example, while the public health impact of dioxin exposure is apparently small, concern about the elimination of dioxin from the environment has tended to be great. This is related, at least in part, to the fact that individuals cannot control their own exposure to environmental dioxin. On the other hand, although individuals can substantially reduce their risk of injuries by using automobile seat belts and motorcycle helmets, legislation has been required to induce them to do so. The discrepancies between actual and perceived risk are an important consideration when providing health behavior counseling.

References Cited

Allison, D. B., et al. Annual deaths attributable to obesity in the United States. Journal of the American Medical Association 282: 1530–1538, 1999.

American Medical Association, Council on Scientific Affairs. Environmental tobacco smoke: health effects and prevention policies. Archives of Family Medicine 3:865–871, 1994.

Axelson, M. L. The impact of culture on food-related behavior. Annual Review of Nutrition 6:345–363, 1986.

Billingsley, A. Black Families in White America. Englewood Cliffs, N. J., Prentice-Hall, 1968.

Calfas, K. J., et al. A controlled trial of physician counseling to promote the adoption of physical activity. Preventive Medicine 25: 225–233, 1996.

Calle, E. E., et al. Body mass index and mortality in a prospective cohort of US adults. New England Journal of Medicine 341: 1097–1105, 1999.

Centers for Disease Control and Prevention. Folic acid campaign and evaluation, southwestern Virginia, 1997–1999. Morbidity and Mortality Weekly Report 48:914–917, 1999.

Eaton, S. B., S. B. Eaton III, and M. J. Konner. Paleolithic nutrition revisited: a twelve-year retrospective on its nature and implications. European Journal of Clinical Nutrition 51:207–216, 1997.

Glanz, K., et al. Why Americans eat what they do: taste, nutrition, cost, convenience, and weight control concerns as influences on food consumption. Journal of the American Dietetic Association 98:1118–1126, 1998.

Goldberg, C. When office air is hazardous. The New York Times, June 14, 1995.

Hansen, J. D., et al. Evaluating the synergism of infection and nutrition in the field. In Scrimshaw, N. S., and J. E. Gordon, eds. Malnutrition, Learning, and Behavior. Cambridge, Mass., MIT Press, 1968.

Hegsted, D. M. Protein-caloric malnutrition. American Scientist 66:61–65, 1978.

Hill, J. O., and E. L. Melanson. Overview of the determinants of overweight and obesity: current evidence and research issues. Medicine and Science in Sports and Exercise 31(supplement 11):S515–S521, 1999.

Hollingshead, A. B., and F. C. Redlich. Social Class and Mental Illness: Appendix 2. New York, John Wiley and Sons, 1958.

James, W. P., and A. Ralph. New understanding in obesity research. Proceedings of the Nutrition Society 58:385–393, 1999.

Katz, D. L. Behavior modification in primary care: the pressure system model. Preventive Medicine 32:66–77, 2001.

Katz, D. L. Nutrition in Clinical Practice. Philadelphia, Lippincott Williams & Wilkins, 2000.

King, K. W. The world food crisis: a partial answer. Research/ Development, September, pp. 22–25, 1969.

Kurland, L. T., et al. Minamata disease. World Neurology 1:370, 1960.

McGinnis, J. M., and W. H. Foege. Actual causes of death in the United States. Journal of the American Medical Association 270: 2207–2212, 1993.

Menzies, R., et al. The effect of varying levels of outdoor air supply on the symptoms of sick building syndrome. New England Journal of Medicine 328:821–827, 1993.

Moeller, D. W. Environmental Health, revised ed. Cambridge, Mass., Harvard University Press, 1997.

Morris, J. N. The Uses of Epidemiology, 2nd ed. Edinburgh, E. and S. Livingstone, Ltd., 1967.

National Heart, Lung, and Blood Institute. Clinical Opportunities for Smoking Intervention: A Guide for Busy Physicians. NIH Publication No. 92-2178. Washington, D. C., Government Printing Office, June 1992.

Nawaz, H., M. L. Adams, and D. L. Katz. Weight loss counseling by health care providers. American Journal of Public Health 89: 764–767, 1999.

Nestle, M., et al. Behavioral and social influences on food choice. Nutrition Reviews 56(supplement 2):S50–S74, 1998.

Oster, G., et al. Lifetime health and economic benefits of weight loss among obese persons. American Journal of Public Health 89:1536–1542, 1999.

Pappas, G., et al. The increasing disparity in mortality between socioeconomic groups in the United States, 1960 and 1986. New England Journal of Medicine 329:103–109, 1993.

Pratt, L. Changes in health care ideology in relation to self-care by families. Paper presented at the annual meeting of the American Public Health Association, Miami Beach, Fla., 1976.

Rahmathullah, L., et al. Reduced mortality among children in southern India receiving a small weekly dose of vitamin A. New England Journal of Medicine 323:929–935, 1990.

Rollnick, S., P. Mason, and C. Butler. Health Behavior Change: A Guide for Practitioners. Edinburgh, Churchill Livingstone, 1999.

Roueché, B. Eleven Blue Men. New York, Berkeley Publishing Corporation, 1953.

Scrimshaw, N. S., C. E. Taylor, and J. E. Gordon. Interactions of Nutrition and Infection. Geneva, World Health Organization, 1968.

Thompson, D., et al. Lifetime health and economic consequences of obesity. Archives of Internal Medicine 159:2177–2183, 1999.

US Department of Health and Human Services. Healthy People 2000: National Health Promotion and Disease Prevention Objectives. DHHS Publication No. (PHS)91-50212. Washington, D. C., Government Printing Office, 1990.

US Department of Health and Human Services. The Surgeon General's Report on the Health Consequences of Smoking for Women. Washington, D. C., Government Printing Office, 1980.

US Department of Health and Human Services, Centers for Disease Control and Prevention, and National Center for Health Statistics. Health, United States, 1999. DHHS Publication No. (PHS)99-1232. Washington, D. C., Government Printing Office, 1999.

US Environmental Protection Agency, Indoor Air Division, Office of Air and Radiation. Respiratory Health Effects of Passive Smoking: Lung Cancer and Other Disorders. Washington, D. C., Government Printing Office, 1992.

US Preventive Services Task Force. Guide to Clinical Preventive Services, 2nd ed. Baltimore, Williams and Wilkins, 1996.

Selected Readings

Burkitt, D. P., and N. J. Temple, eds. Western Diseases: Their Dietary Prevention and Reversibility. Totowa, N. J., Humana Press, 1994.

Cassens, B. J., ed. Preventive Medicine and Public Health, 2nd ed. Malvern, Pa., Harwal Publishing Company, 1992.

Institute of Medicine. Environmental Health: Integrating a Missing Element into Medical Education. Washington, D. C., National Academy Press, 1995.

Katz, D. L. Nutrition in Clinical Practice. Philadelphia, Lippincott Williams & Wilkins, 2000.

Last, J. M., and R. B. Wallace. Public Health and Preventive Medicine, 13th ed. Norwalk, Conn., Appleton and Lange, 1992.

Moeller, D. W. Environmental Health, revised ed. Cambridge, Mass., Harvard University Press, 1997.

16

Methods of Primary Prevention: Specific Protection

Three major goals of primary prevention by specific protection are (1) prevention of **specific diseases** (e.g., by using vaccines and antimicrobial prophylaxis); (2) prevention of **specific deficiency states** (e.g., by using iodized salt to prevent iodine deficiency goiter and by using fluoride to prevent dental caries); and (3) prevention of **specific injuries and toxic exposures** (e.g., by using helmets to prevent head injuries in construction workers, goggles to prevent eye injuries in machine tool operators, and filters and ventilation systems to control dusts). Vaccines will be discussed as the prototype of a scientifically developed specific method of protection.

■ PREVENTION OF DISEASES BY USE OF VACCINES

An intact immune system in a well-nourished and otherwise healthy person provides basic protection against infectious diseases. **Intact immunity** implies that the immune system has not suffered damage from a disease such as infection with human immunodeficiency virus (HIV) or damage from medications such as certain anticancer drugs or long-term steroid use. Besides infections and medications, there is some evidence that depression and loneliness can suppress normal functioning of the immune system (Roitt 1991). There are also reports that experimental animals are more resistant to infections when in the presence of (but not crowded by) other animals of the same species (Cassel 1974).

Types of Immunity

Passive immunity is protection against an infectious disease provided by circulating antibodies made in another organism. Newborn infants are protected, for example, by **maternal antibodies** transferred through the placenta before birth and through breast milk after birth. If a person has recently been exposed to hepatitis B virus and has not been immunized with hepatitis B vaccine, he or she can be given **human immune globulin,** which confers passive immunity and protects against infection with this virus. In an emergency, a specific type of **antitoxin,** if available, can be used to confer passive immunity. For example, diphtheria antitoxin is used in the presence of clinical diphtheria, and trivalent botulinum antitoxin is used in the presence of botulism. Passive immunity provides incomplete protection and usually is of short duration.

Vaccines confer **active immunity.** Some types of vaccines, such as the inactivated polio vaccine (see Chapter 1), do this by stimulating the production of **humoral (blood) antibody** to the antigen in the vaccine. Other types, such as the live attenuated polio vaccine, not only elicit this humoral antibody response but also stimulate the body to develop **cell-mediated immunity.** This tissue-based cellular response to foreign antigens involves mobilization of killer T cells. Active immunity is far superior to passive immunity, because active immunity lasts longer (a lifetime in some cases) and is rapidly stimulated to high levels by a reexposure to the same or closely related antigens.

All types of vaccines provide the immunized person with some level of **individual immunity** to a specific disease. Some vaccines also reduce or prevent the shedding (spread) of infectious organisms from an immunized person to others, and this contributes to **herd immunity,** a phenomenon discussed in Chapter 1 and illustrated in Fig. 1–2.

Types of Vaccines

As shown in Table 16–1, some vaccines are **inactivated** (killed), some are **live attenuated** (altered), and others are referred to as **toxoids** (inactivated or altered bacterial exotoxins).

The older pertussis and typhoid vaccines are examples of **inactivated bacterial vaccines,** while influenza vaccine and the inactivated polio vaccine are examples of **inactivated viral vaccines.** The bacillus Calmette-Guérin (BCG) vaccine against tuberculosis is an example of a **live attenuated bacterial vaccine,** and the measles and oral polio vaccines are examples of **live attenuated viral vaccines.** Live attenuated vaccines are created by altering the organisms so

TABLE 16–1 Prevention of Infectious Diseases by Vaccines Available in the USA

Disease	Vaccine
Anthrax	Anthrax vaccine contains inactivated bacteria and is administered subcutaneously.
Cholera	Cholera vaccine contains inactivated bacteria and is administered subcutaneously or intradermally.
Diphtheria	Several combination vaccines are available: DTP is a combined diphtheria, tetanus, and pertussis vaccine; DTaP is a combined diphtheria, tetanus, and acellular pertussis vaccine; DT is a combined diphtheria and tetanus vaccine; Td is like DT but with a reduced amount of diphtheria antigen; and Tetramune is the trade name for a tetravalent vaccine combining DTP and *Haemophilus* b conjugate vaccine. In all cases, the diphtheria component is a toxoid and the intramuscular route of administration is used.
Haemophilus influenzae infection	The *H. influenzae* type b conjugate vaccine (Hib) contains bacterial polysaccharide conjugated to protein. It is administered intramuscularly. A tetravalent vaccine against diphtheria, tetanus, pertussis, and *H. influenzae* type b is also available and is marketed under the trade name Tetramune.
Hepatitis A	Hepatitis A vaccine contains inactivated viral antigen and is injected into the deltoid muscle.
Hepatitis B	Hepatitis B conjugate vaccine (HBV) contains inactivated viral antigen and is administered intramuscularly.
Influenza	Influenza vaccine contains inactivated virus or viral components and is administered intramuscularly.
Japanese encephalitis	Encephalitis vaccine contains inactivated virus and is administered subcutaneously.
Lyme disease	Lyme disease vaccine contains recombinant *Borrelia burgdorferi* lipidated outer surface protein A (OspA) and is administered intramuscularly.
Measles	A vaccine against measles, mumps, and rubella (MMR) is available and contains live viruses. The vaccine is administered subcutaneously.
Meningococcal disease	Meningococcal vaccine contains bacterial polysaccharides of serotypes A, C, Y, and W-135 and is administered subcutaneously.
Mumps	A vaccine against measles, mumps, and rubella (MMR) is available and contains live viruses. A vaccine against mumps alone is also available. The vaccines are administered subcutaneously.
Pertussis	Three combination vaccines are available: DTP, DTaP, and Tetramune (see discussion under diphtheria, above). A vaccine against pertussis alone is also available. In all cases, the pertussis component consists of inactivated bacteria and the intramuscular route of administration is used.
Plague	Plague vaccine contains inactivated bacteria and is administered intramuscularly.
Pneumococcal disease	Pneumococcal vaccine for adults contains bacterial polysaccharides from 23 strains of *Streptococcus pneumoniae;* it is administered intramuscularly or subcutaneously. Pneumococcal vaccine for children contains 7 strains of pneumococcal antigen, it is given intramuscularly.
Poliomyelitis	Two vaccines are available. The oral polio vaccine (OPV) contains live polioviruses of all three types. The inactivated polio vaccine (IPV) contains inactivated polioviruses of all three types. The OPV, which is administered orally, is also referred to as the Sabin vaccine. The IPV, which is administered subcutaneously, is also referred to as the Salk vaccine.
Rabies	Human diploid cell vaccine (HDCV) contains inactivated virus and can be administered subcutaneously or intramuscularly. The subcutaneous dose is lower than the intramuscular dose and is used only for preexposure vaccination.
Rubella	A vaccine against measles, mumps, and rubella (MMR) is available and contains live viruses. A vaccine against rubella alone is also available and contains live attenuated virus. The vaccines are administered subcutaneously.
Tetanus	Several combination vaccines are available: DTP, DTaP, DT, Td, and Tetramune (see discussion under diphtheria, above). A vaccine against tetanus alone is also available. In all cases, the tetanus component is a toxoid and the intramuscular route of administration is used.
Tuberculosis	The bacillus Calmette-Guérin (BCG) vaccine contains live attenuated mycobacteria and is administered intradermally or subcutaneously.
Typhoid	The older typhoid vaccine contains inactivated bacteria and is administered subcutaneously. Two newer vaccines appear to be as antigenic as the older vaccine and to have fewer side effects. One is called the Ty21A oral vaccine and contains live attenuated bacteria. The other contains capsular polysaccharide and is administered intramuscularly.
Varicella	Varicella (chickenpox) vaccine contains live virus and is administered subcutaneously.
Yellow fever	Yellow fever vaccine contains live virus and is administered subcutaneously.

Sources of data: (1) Centers for Disease Control and Prevention (CDC). Advisory Committee on Immunization Practices (ACIP): general recommendations on immunization. Morbidity and Mortality Weekly Report 43(RR-1), 1994. (2) American Academy of Pediatrics (AAP). Report of the Committee on Infectious Diseases, 22nd ed. Elk Grove Village, Ill., AAP, 1991. (3) CDC. ACIP: recommendations for use of *Haemophilus* b conjugate vaccine and a combined diphtheria, tetanus, pertussis, and *Haemophilus* b vaccine. Morbidity and Mortality Weekly Report 42(RR-13), 1993. (4) CDC. ACIP: typhoid immunization. Morbidity and Mortality Weekly Report 43(RR-14), 1994. (5) CDC. ACIP: diphtheria, tetanus, and pertussis—recommendations for vaccine use and other preventive measures. Morbidity and Mortality Weekly Report 40(RR-10), 1991. (6) CDC. Varicella vaccination. Morbidity and Mortality Weekly Report 44:264, 1995. (7) CDC. Prevention of hepatitis A through active or passive immunization. Morbidity and Mortality Weekly Report 48(RR-12), 1999. (8) Chin, J. Control of Communicable Diseases Manual, 17th ed. Washington, D. C., American Public Health Association, 2000. (9) CDC. Recommended childhood immunization schedule: United States, 2001. Morbidity and Mortality Weekly Report 50:7–10, 2001.

that they are no longer pathogenic but still have antigenicity.

Diphtheria vaccine and tetanus vaccine are the primary examples of **toxoids.** *Corynebacterium diphtheriae,* the organism that causes diphtheria, produces a potent toxin when it is in the lysogenic state with corynebacteriophage. *Clostridium tetani,* an organism that is part of the normal flora of many animals and is frequently found in the soil, can cause tetanus in unimmunized people with infected wounds. This is because *C. tetani* produces a potent toxin when it grows under anaerobic conditions, such as those found in wounds with necrotic tissue. Tetanus is almost nonexistent in populations with high immunization levels.

Immunization Recommendations and Schedules

Active Immunization of Children

The Advisory Committee on Immunization Practices (ACIP) of the Centers for Disease Control and Prevention (CDC) publishes immunization schedules and other information in the *Morbidity and Mortality Weekly Report.* The recommendations of the American Academy of Pediatrics (AAP) and the ACIP are similar, but because the latter are more frequently updated, they are discussed here and form the basis for Table 16–2.

Table 16–2 shows the recommended immunization schedule for healthy children without specific contraindications (such as immunodeficiency). The recommendations for immunizing children who did not start immunizations as infants have similar intervals between vaccine doses, and the most important difference is that the measles, mumps, and rubella (MMR) vaccine should be started immediately in older children.

Children with altered immunocompetence, whether due to HIV infection or another reason, should not be given live attenuated virus vaccines, including oral polio vaccine; measles, mumps, and rubella vaccine; varicella (chickenpox) vaccine; and yellow fever vaccine. Killed vaccines may be given according to clinical judgment.

Active Immunization of Adults

The need for adequate immunization levels in adults was shown by the dramatic epidemic of diphtheria

---

TABLE 16–2   Recommended Schedule for Active Immunization of Healthy Infants and Children

Recommended Age	Vaccine and Dose Number*	Comments
Birth	HBV #1	HBV #1 must be given to the infant at birth if the mother is HBsAg-positive, but HBV #1 can be given to the infant at birth or at 1 or 2 months if the mother is HBsAg-negative.
2 months	DTaP #1 IPV #1 Hib #1 HBV #1 or #2 PCV7 #1	DTaP #1 and Hib #1 can be given earlier in areas of high endemicity. HBV #2 is given at 2 months if HBV #1 was given earlier.
4 months	HBV #2 DTaP #2 IPV #2 Hib #2 PCV7 #2	HBV #2 is given at 4 months if it was not given sooner.
6 months	DTaP #3 IPV #3 Hib #3 PCV7 #3	DTaP #3 should be given at 6 months in areas of high endemicity; otherwise, it can be given at 6 months or any time up to18 months.
15 months	MMR #1 DTaP #4 Hib #4	
6–18 months	HBV #3	
12–18 months	Var PCV7 #4	
4–6 years	DTaP #5 IPV #4 MMR #2	DTaP #5 and MMR #2 are given at or before school entry.
14–16 years	Td	Td is given as a booster at 14–16 years of age and every 10 years thereafter. HBV, MMR, and Var may be given as boosters.

*Abbreviations are as follows: DTaP = diphtheria, tetanus, and acellular pertussis vaccine; HBsAg = hepatitis B surface antigen; HBV = hepatitis B conjugate vaccine; Hib = *Haemophilus influenzae* type b conjugate vaccine; IPV = inactivated polio vaccine; MMR = measles, mumps, and rubella vaccine; PCV7 = heptavalent pneumococcal conjugate vaccine; Td = tetanus and diphtheria vaccine with a reduced amount of diphtheria antigen; and Var = varicella vaccine.
Source of data: Centers for Disease Control and Prevention. Recommended childhood immunization schedule: United States, 2001. Morbidity and Mortality Weekly Report 50:7–10, 2001.

TABLE 16–3   Indications for Use of Immune Globulins and Antitoxins Available in the USA

Biologic Agent	Type	Indication
Botulinum antitoxin	Specific equine antibody	Treatment of botulism.
Cytomegalovirus immune globulin	Specific human antibody	Prophylaxis for bone marrow and renal transplant recipients.
Diphtheria antitoxin	Specific equine antibody	Treatment of respiratory diphtheria.
Hepatitis B immune globulin	Specific human antibody	Hepatitis B postexposure prophylaxis.
Immune globulin (intramuscular)	Pooled human antibody	Hepatitis A preexposure and postexposure prophylaxis.
Immune globulin (intravenous)	Pooled human antibody	Replacement therapy for antibody deficiency disorders.
Rabies immune globulin	Specific human antibody	Rabies postexposure management of persons not previously immunized with rabies vaccine.
Tetanus immune globulin	Specific human antibody	Treatment of tetanus; postexposure management of persons not previously immunized wth tetanus vaccine.
Vaccinia immune globulin	Specific human antibody	Postexposure prophylaxis for susceptible immunocompromised persons and for perinatally exposed newborns.

Source of data: Centers for Disease Control and Prevention (CDC). Advisory Committee on Immunization Practices (ACIP): general recommendations on immunization. Morbidity and Mortality Weekly Report 43(RR-1), 1994.

that occurred in the independent states of the former Soviet Union, where over 50,000 cases were reported between 1990 and 1994. In 70% of the cases, diphtheria occurred in persons 15 years or older. Almost 2000 deaths resulted (see Centers for Disease Control and Prevention 1995).

The immunization of adults builds on the foundation of vaccines given during childhood. If an adult is missing polio, diphtheria, and tetanus vaccines, these should be started immediately. Many adults need boosters because they were immunized as children and their immunity levels have declined since they were immunized. A booster is indicated for adults who have had a primary series of immunizations against poliomyelitis, regardless of whether the inactivated polio vaccine (IPV) or oral polio vaccine (OPV) was used in the primary series. The polio booster may consist of either IPV or OPV, and one dose appears to be adequate (see Centers for Disease Control and Prevention 1997b). For protection against tetanus, several combination preparations are available (see Table 16–1); however, adults are usually given the combined tetanus and diphtheria (Td) vaccine, which contains a reduced amount of diphtheria antigen to decrease the number of reactions. For adults who have a high risk of exposure to pertussis, some experts recommend that adults be immunized with the acellular pertussis (aP) vaccine because it may provide some herd immunity against pertussis to children.

The measles, mumps, and rubella (MMR) vaccine should be administered to adults who were born after 1956 and lack evidence of immunity to measles (a definite history of measles or measles immunization after age 12 months). The exceptions are pregnant women and immunocompromised patients.

Pneumococcal polysaccharide vaccine should be given at least once to persons 65 years and older; to persons with chronic diseases that increase their risk of mortality or serious morbidity from pneumococcal infection, such as chronic pulmonary or cardiac disease, cancer, renal or hepatic disease, asplenia, and immunosuppression; and to persons with a history of pneumococcal pneumonia. Experts recommend that influenza vaccine be given annually in the late autumn to the same risk groups, and some believe that the influenza vaccine should be given to the general population, although this is not a national recommendation.

Immunization against hepatitis A, a disease acquired by eating or drinking contaminated substances, is recommended for persons living in or traveling to areas of high or moderate risk. It is also recommended for persons who have significant occupational exposure, engage in homosexual activities, or use illegal drugs (see Centers for Disease Control and Prevention 1999b).

Immunization against hepatitis B, a disease acquired via contact with blood and other body fluids, is recommended for persons who are at high risk because of their professions (health care workers, persons with jobs in certain countries overseas, etc.); homosexual activities; intravenous drug use; or frequent exposure to blood or blood products.

International travelers should make sure that they are up to date on all of their basic immunizations, including those against poliomyelitis, tetanus, diphtheria, and measles. Before traveling to less developed countries, it may be necessary or desirable to receive immunizations against hepatitis A, hepatitis B, typhoid, cholera, yellow fever, or other diseases shown in Table 16–1. For recommendations and help in determining requirements, those planning to travel abroad should consult their local and state health departments or the CDC.

Passive Immunization

The medical indications for passive immunization are far more limited than those for active immunization. Table 16–3 provides information about the biologic agents available in the USA and the indications for their use in immunocompetent persons (those with normal immune systems) and immunocompromised persons (those with impaired immune systems).

For immunocompetent persons who are at high risk for exposure to hepatitis A, usually because of travel to a country where it is common, hepatitis A vaccine can be administered if there is time (see Medical Letter on Drugs and Therapeutics 1995), or immune globulin can be administered prior to the travel as a method of preexposure prophylaxis. For those who were recently exposed to hepatitis B or rabies, a specific immune globulin can be used as a method of **postexposure prophylaxis.** For those who lack active immunity to exotoxin-producing bacteria already causing symptoms (such as *Clostridium botulinum,* the organism responsible for botulism), the injection of a specific antitoxin is recommended after tests are performed to rule out hypersensitivity to the antitoxin (see Chin 2000).

For immunocompromised persons who have been exposed to a common but potentially life-threatening infection such as chickenpox, immune globulin can be lifesaving if given intravenously soon after exposure.

Vaccine Surveillance and Testing

As discussed in Chapter 3, the rates and patterns of reportable diseases are monitored, and any cases that are thought to be vaccine-associated are investigated. The goals are to monitor the effectiveness of vaccines and to detect vaccine failures or adverse effects.

Randomized Field Trials

The standard way to measure the effectiveness of a new vaccine is through a randomized field trial (the public health equivalent of a randomized controlled trial, although the level of "control" usually is somewhat less). In this type of trial, susceptible persons are randomized into two groups and are then given the vaccine or a placebo, usually at the beginning of the high-risk season of the year. The vaccinated subjects and unvaccinated controls are followed through the high-risk season to determine the **attack rate** (AR) in each group:

$$AR = \frac{\text{Number of persons ill}}{\text{Number of persons exposed to the disease}}$$

Next, the **vaccine effectiveness** (VE) is calculated:

$$VE = \frac{AR_{(unvaccinated)} - AR_{(vaccinated)}}{AR_{(unvaccinated)}} \times 100$$

In the VE equation, the numerator is the observed reduction in AR due to the vaccination, and the denominator represents the total amount of risk that could be reduced by the vaccine. The VE formula is a specific example of the general formula for the **relative risk reduction.**

Testing the efficacy of vaccines by randomized field trials is very costly, but it may be required the first time a new vaccine is introduced. Field trials were used to evaluate inactivated polio vaccine (see Chapter 1 and Francis et al. 1955), oral polio vaccine, and measles, influenza, and varicella vaccines.

Retrospective Cohort Studies

The antigenic variability of influenza virus (see Chapter 1) necessitates frequent (often yearly) changes in the constituents of influenza vaccines to keep them up to date with new strains of the virus. This in turn requires constant surveillance of the disease and of the protective efficacy of the vaccine. Because there are insufficient resources and time to perform a randomized controlled trial of each new influenza vaccine, retrospective cohort studies are sometimes done during the influenza season to evaluate the protective efficacy of the vaccines.

In these studies, because there is no randomization, investigators cannot be sure that there was no selection bias on the part of the physicians who recommended the vaccine or the individuals who agreed to be immunized. If selection bias were present, those who were immunized might be either sicker or more interested in their health than those who were not immunized. Studies of influenza vaccine effectiveness in nursing homes have indicated that rates vary from near 0% to about 40% (for example, see Cartter et al. 1990). The low protection rates may be due to inadequate antibody production by older people and to the delay from the time that vaccine is given until an outbreak appears.

Case-Control Studies

Because randomized field trials require large sample sizes (often over 100,000), they are almost impossible to perform for relatively uncommon diseases, such as *Haemophilus influenzae* infections or pneumococcal pneumonia. To overcome this problem, many investigators have recommended using case-control studies (see, for example, Clemens and Shapiro 1984; Shapiro et al. 1991). Their recommendation is based on the fact that when the risk of disease in the population is low, the vaccine effectiveness (VE) formula above may be rewritten as follows:

$$VE = 1 - \left[\frac{AR_{(vaccinated)}}{AR_{(unvaccinated)}} \right] = (1 - RR) \cong (1 - OR)$$

The risk ratio (RR) is closely approximated by the odds ratio (OR) when the disease is uncommon, as in the cases of *H. influenzae* infections in children and pneumococcal infections in adults.

When Shapiro et al. (1991) performed a case-control study of pneumococcal vaccine, which is a polyvalent vaccine containing capsular polysaccharide antigens of 23 strains of *Streptococcus pneumoniae,* they found that the vaccine showed fairly good efficacy against the strains contained in the vaccine and no efficacy against other *S. pneumoniae* strains. The fact that the risks from strains not in the vaccine were comparable in the case and control groups suggests that the differences in protective efficacy for strains that were in the vaccine were not due to selection bias.

Incidence Density Measures

Among the questions that vaccine research and surveillance are designed to answer are the following: When should a new vaccine be given? What is the duration of the immunity produced?

In the case of measles vaccine, surveillance studies suggested that when the vaccine was given to infants before 12 months of age, often it was not effective, presumably because the vaccine antigen was neutralized by residual maternal antibody. To determine the answers to both of the questions above, Marks, Halpin, and Orenstein (1978) performed a study in which they monitored the incidence density of measles cases in Ohio over an extended period of time. In order to adjust for the duration of exposure to measles, which varied between individuals, they used incidence density (see Chapter 2) as their measure of measles incidence. The formula for incidence density (ID) is as follows:

$$ID = \frac{\text{Number of new cases of a disease}}{\text{Person-time of exposure}}$$

The denominator (person-time) can be expressed in terms of the number of person-days, person-weeks, person-months, or even person-years of exposure to the risk.

Marks, Halpin, and Orenstein obtained the results shown in Box 16–1, which, along with other studies, suggested that measles vaccine should be postponed until children reach approximately 15 months of age. One concern in delaying the vaccine is the fact that measles is more severe in newborns than in older infants. Partly to reduce the likelihood that new schoolchildren will be exposed to measles and will bring the disease home to younger siblings, experts recommend that all children be revaccinated with measles vaccine before they enter school, at age 5 or 6 years. Another concern has been the duration of immunity. As shown in the second part of Box 16–1, the measles vaccine lost its protective ability slowly during the first 6 years, but the relative risk of acquiring measles had almost tripled by 10–12 years after immunization. This is another line of evidence that led to the recommendation that children be revaccinated at the age of 5 or 6 years.

Immunization Goals

The strategy of developing disease control programs through the use of vaccines depends upon the objectives of the vaccine campaign. The goal may be **eradication of disease** (as has been achieved for smallpox), **regional elimination of disease** (as has been achieved for poliomyelitis in the western hemisphere), or **control of disease** to reduce morbidity and mortality. Global efforts to eradicate poliomyeli-

---

BOX 16–1   Data Showing Why Measles Vaccine Is Now Postponed Until Children Reach the Age of 15 Months

Part 1   Correlation of age at vaccination with data on measles incidence (rate of disease per 1000 person-weeks) and data on measles risk (relative risk of those vaccinated at the age shown in comparison with those vaccinated at 15 months of age)

Age at Vaccination	Measles Incidence per 1000 Person-Weeks	Relative Risk Compared to Risk in Children Vaccinated at 15 Months
Never	155.3	33.0
< 11 months	39.6	8.5
11 months	15.0	3.2
12 months	7.1	1.5
13 months	5.2	1.1
14 months	4.7	1.0

Part 2   Correlation of time since vaccination with data on measles incidence (rate of disease per 1000 person-weeks) and data on measles risk (relative risk)

Time Since Vaccination	Measles Incidence per 1000 Person-Weeks	Relative Risk
0–3 years	4.0	1.0
4–6 years	4.2	1.1
7–9 years	5.4	1.4
10–12 years	11.7	2.9

Source of data: Marks, J., T. J. Halpin, and W. A. Orenstein. Measles vaccine efficacy in children previously vaccinated at 12 months of age. Pediatrics 62:955–960, 1978.

tis are under way (see, for example, Centers for Disease Control and Prevention 2000b).

Disease eradication by immunization is feasible only for diseases in which human beings are the sole reservoir of the infectious organism. Although vaccines are available to prevent some diseases with reservoirs in other animals (e.g., rabies, plague, and encephalitis) and some diseases with reservoirs in the environment (e.g., typhoid fever), they are not candidates for eradication programs. The surveillance systems to achieve eradication or regional elimination must be excellent, and any eradication or elimination program would require considerably more resources and time, as well as general political and popular support, than would a disease control program. For these reasons, immunization strategies are frequently the subject of much scrutiny and debate.

For years, for example, immunization experts in the USA debated about whether to recommend routine immunization of children against varicella (chickenpox). In 1996, the CDC's Advisory Committee on Immunization Practices (ACIP) concluded that the varicella vaccine was efficacious and that the benefits of instituting a routine immunization program against chickenpox outweighed a number of concerns, including those about whether the protection would last for an adequate period of time, whether unimmunized adults would develop serious symptoms of disease if exposed, and whether a new form of herpes zoster might result (see Centers for Disease Control and Prevention 1996). The CDC now recommends that the varicella live attenuated vaccine be given to children during any visit on or after the first birthday (see Centers for Disease Control and Prevention 2001).

The Expanded Program on Immunization

In May of 1974, the World Health Assembly adopted a global Expanded Program on Immunization (EPI), with the goal of cooperation between the World Health Organization and the member governments in establishing or expanding existing national immunization programs. A particular emphasis of the EPI has been the surveillance of vaccine-preventable illnesses and the monitoring of immunization levels in the member countries (see Centers for Disease Control and Prevention 1994a and 1994c).

The Childhood Immunization Initiative

In the USA, because of requirements for complete immunization before children enter school at the age of approximately 5 years, the rate of vaccine-preventable diseases has generally been falling and levels of adequate immunization have been high in school-age children. In 2-year-old children, however, the immunization rates have remained disappointing. **Adequate immunization** is defined as receiving the recommended number of doses of vaccines by the ages shown in Table 16–2. In 1999, the National Immunization Survey found that the percentages of children who were between the ages of 19 and 35

months and had adequate vaccine levels were as follows: 96% for diphtheria, tetanus, and pertussis vaccine (4+ doses of DTP); 90% for polio vaccine (3 doses of IPV or OPV); 92% for measles-containing vaccine (usually 1 dose of MMR); 94% for *Haemophilus influenzae* type b vaccine (3 doses of Hib); 88% for hepatitis B vaccine (3 doses); 59% for varicella vaccine (1 dose); and 80% for DTP plus polio plus a measles-containing vaccine (see Centers for Disease Control and Prevention 2000c). These 1999 percentages are considerably higher than earlier percentages and reflect an increase that began after 1993, when the federal government started the Childhood Immunization Initiative (see Centers for Disease Control and Prevention 1994b).

For a while, a trivalent rotavirus vaccine (Rota-Shield, produced by Wyeth Laboratories) was recommended in the USA for vaccination of healthy infants. However, postvaccination surveillance revealed that infants who were immunized with the rotavirus vaccine had a much higher relative risk of intussusception than did infants who were unimmunized (see Centers for Disease Control and Prevention 1999a). Therefore, rotavirus vaccine was removed from the list of recommended vaccines.

Reasons for Low Immunization Levels

Despite major improvements in national childhood immunization levels in the 1990s, the reported levels still fall short of the goal. In an attempt to improve the knowledge of physicians in training, the Association of Teachers of Preventive Medicine (ATPM) has developed a series of aids for the teaching of immunization, called Teaching Immunization for Medical Education (TIME). Other obstacles that remain include personal beliefs about health, concerns about vaccine-related lawsuits, and missed opportunities for immunization.

Health Beliefs

Research concerning why people may not seek immunizations or other preventive measures for themselves or their children led to the development of what is often called the **health belief model** (see Rosenstock 1974). According to the model, before seeking preventive measures, people generally must believe (1) that the disease at issue is serious, if acquired; (2) that they or their children are personally at risk for the disease; (3) that the preventive measure is effective in warding off the disease; and (4) that there are no serious risks or barriers involved in obtaining the preventive measure. In addition, there need to be cues to action, consisting of information regarding how and when to obtain the preventive measure, as well as the encouragement from or support of other people.

The health belief model is useful in guiding the educational aspect of an immunization program. The "swine flu" (H1N1 viral influenza) vaccine campaign in 1976 had major difficulties, partly because the public was not convinced of any of the four items above. First, the public was not sure whether the disease would be a pandemic (as in 1918–1919) or just another outbreak which, while annoying and dangerous for a few, was not cause for alarm. Second, people were not sure if they were personally at risk. A few people had been found to harbor the H1N1 virus, but it was not clear that it would spread to large numbers of people. Third, experts were involved in debates about how effective the vaccine would be in preventing influenza if the H1N1 virus did establish a widespread infection. Fourth, there were conflicting stories about possible side effects from the vaccine.

In the case of pertussis vaccine, debates and continued concerns about the potential for serious side effects caused the British population largely to abandon its use of the vaccine and to suffer epidemics of pertussis as a consequence (Johnstone 1983). These concerns were also present in the USA but to a lesser extent than in Great Britain. Most of the US public's fears have been allayed by the development of the acellular pertussis (aP) vaccine, which is now incorporated into a triple vaccine against diphtheria, tetanus, and pertussis (the DTaP vaccine) and is associated with a much lower rate of adverse reactions (see Centers for Disease Control and Prevention 1997a). The media, however, have continued to raise concerns about the pertussis component of vaccines (see, for example, Goodwin 2000).

Vaccine-Related Lawsuits

In the USA, the number of lawsuits related to vaccine use increased from 1 lawsuit in 1978 to 219 lawsuits in 1985, and the damages claimed (but not necessarily awarded) increased from $10 million to over $3 billion (Herwaldt 1993). As a consequence of naming vaccine manufacturers in many of these lawsuits, there was a decrease in the number of companies making vaccines.

In response to the problem, the federal government instituted the National Vaccine Injury Compensation Program. This program covers diphtheria, tetanus, pertussis, measles, mumps, rubella, and both oral and inactivated polio vaccines. It is limited to claims for injuries or deaths that are attributable to vaccines given after October 1, 1988. Claims concerning injury must be filed within 3 years of the first symptoms (e.g., anaphylactic shock, paralytic poliomyelitis, seizure disorders, or encephalopathy). Claims concerning death must be filed within 4 years of the first symptoms and 2 years of death. The program essentially protects vaccine manufacturers from liability lawsuits, unless it can be shown that their vaccines differed from the federal requirements. It also simplifies the process and reduces the costs for those people making a claim, and almost all of the costs are borne by the federal government.

Missed Opportunities

In the USA, the immunization levels are consistently lower in the poorer population groups. It is not clear whether this is due to less education among these groups, inadequate medical care, or inability to put such things as immunization high on a struggling family's list of priorities. One of the problems is that both the medical care system and the physicians have largely failed to adapt immunization practices to accommodate the special needs of the poor and, hence, have missed many opportunities for immunizing poor children.

Studies have been undertaken to determine how many and what kind of missed opportunities for immunization occur in the context of medical care, especially during sick child visits (see Centers for Disease Control and Prevention 1994d). Often, physicians do not vaccinate children who have mild upper respiratory tract infections without complications, even though part of the reason for their office visit may have been to receive a vaccination. More recent guidelines have emphasized that children with these mild infections should receive the appropriate vaccines. Frequently, the siblings of a child who is being seen by the physician or nurse will be brought along by the parent, and these siblings should receive vaccinations if their immunization records are not up to date, although this is seldom done. These two scenarios are especially common in emergency departments, but opportunities are often missed here because providers lack records, time, and a relationship with the patients.

Hospitalized children and adults whose immunization records are not up to date should be given the appropriate vaccines unless there are clear contraindications. Unfortunately, clinicians are often ill-informed about contraindications. The following are *not* considered contraindications to immunizing children: a mild reaction to a previous DTP or DTaP dose, consisting of redness and swelling at the injection site, a temperature under 40.5° C (105° F), or both; the presence of nonspecific allergies; the presence of a mild illness or diarrhea with low-grade fever in an otherwise healthy child who is scheduled for vaccination; current therapy with an antimicrobial drug in a child who is convalescing well; breast-feeding of an infant scheduled for immunization; and pregnancy of someone else in the household. False contraindications account for part of the reason that US physicians have not adequately immunized children.

■ PREVENTION OF DISEASES BY USE OF ANTIMICROBIAL DRUGS

Another form of specific protection, which can be used for varying lengths of time, is **antimicrobial prophylaxis.**

For travelers to countries where malaria is endemic, antimicrobial protection against the causative organism, *Plasmodium,* is desirable. Oral chemoprophylaxis for adults may consist of the use of chloroquine phosphate before and during travel, followed by the use of primaquine for a few weeks after returning home. However, if chloroquine-resistant strains of *Plasmodium* have been reported in the area to be visited, proguanine should be added or an alternative drug, such as mefloquine, may be given instead (Chen 2000).

The chemoprophylaxis of tuberculosis is discussed in detail in Chapter 19. The usual prophylaxis is isoniazid (INH), given daily for 6 months, beginning from the time of the recognition of a recent exposure or the diagnosis of skin test conversion. This chemoprophylaxis reduces the probability of active tuberculosis, but it is associated with a risk of hepatitis. Because the risk of INH-induced hepatitis increases with age, only individuals who are under 35 years old should be routinely considered for prophylactic INH use.

In patients who have had rheumatic fever with valvular disease, a short-term course of bactericidal antibiotics is recommended before dental or other manipulative medical procedures are performed.

Individuals who have been exposed to a virulent meningococcal disease (either meningitis or meningococcal sepsis) should receive prophylactic treatment with an antibiotic such as rifampin, ciprofloxacin, or ceftriaxone. The tetravalent meningococcal vaccine is recommended to control outbreaks of serogroup C meningococcal disease and possibly also to control outbreaks of serogroup A, W-135, and Y disease (see Centers for Disease Control and Prevention 2000a).

A large dose of ceftriaxone is sometimes given to prevent syphilis or gonorrhea in people who are known to have had sexual contact with an infected person during the period in which the disease was communicable.

■ PREVENTION OF DEFICIENCY STATES

When specific vitamin and mineral deficiencies were identified in the past, it was possible to fortify food or water to ensure that most people would obtain sufficient amounts of nutrients of a specific type. The most well-known examples are iodine in salt, which has essentially eliminated goiter; vitamin D in milk, which has largely eliminated rickets; and fluoride ion in water, which has markedly reduced the incidence of dental caries in children who grow up in areas with fluoridated water. The most recent example is the enrichment of cereal grain products with folic acid; this practice was initiated in January 1998 to prevent neural tube defects.

The frequent use of vitamin and mineral supplements and the fortification of most breakfast cereals with a number of vitamins and minerals have largely eliminated vitamin B deficiencies in populations with reasonably normal nutrition. Nevertheless, vitamin B deficiencies are still found in some elderly persons.

■ PREVENTION OF INJURIES AND TOXIC EXPOSURES

In the USA today, there is intense activity, often mandated through government regulations or carried out by government agencies, to protect the population from specific injuries and exposure to harmful environmental agents. These activities are so broad in scope that just a few can be mentioned.

The activities of the Department of Agriculture are designed to protect the food sold in the USA. They include supervision of meat packing and milk production in the country, as well as inspection of imported food products. The regulations of the Food and Drug Administration are designed to ensure that prescription and over-the-counter drugs are safe and effective and that foods are safe and properly labeled. Food labels are now required to list the fat and salt content, and in the future they are expected to require more details about the content of different types of fat.

Continual efforts are made to protect the public through federal or state laws governing land, sea, and air transportation and equipment, ranging from regulations for those who construct highways and automobiles to regulations for those who use them (e.g., laws about seat belts, air bags, speed limits, maximum lengths of air time or driving time in a day or a week for pilots or truck drivers, and penalties for operating equipment under the influence of drugs or alcohol).

Local regulations regarding building codes are largely for home and workplace safety and include requirements for hard-wired smoke alarms in new houses and hotels, as well as for properly lighted safety exits and automatic sprinklers in public buildings. Workplace protection regulations are enforced by the Occupational Safety and Health Administration (OSHA). These consist of regulations in **chemical safety** (e.g., publication of all chemicals used in a manufacturing or research setting); **biologic safety** (e.g., protection for laboratory technicians working with hazardous microorganisms and proper immunizations for health care workers); and **physical safety** (e.g., protection against repetitive motion injuries and against harmful levels of exposure to noise, heat, and cold). Some common specific protection devices include helmets for construction workers, ear protection for those working around jet aircraft, and masks for those removing asbestos from old buildings or working in dusty areas.

■ PREVENTION OF IATROGENIC DISEASES AND INJURIES

Among the most preventable of health problems are those generated during the process of treatment— i.e., diseases and injuries that are iatrogenic (from the Greek *iatros,* which means physician, and *gennao,* which means to produce). Examples include infections, falls, medication errors, unnecessary surgery, and surgical and medical errors (see, for example, Bates et al. 1995; Inlander et al. 1988; and Leape et al. 1991). The Institute of Medicine recently released a report addressing the urgent need for improvement in health care quality (see Kohn, Corrigan, and Donaldson 1999).

Nosocomial infections (hospital-acquired infections) are more common than often supposed. Based on a review of the literature, Inlander et al. (1988)

concluded that there were at least 100,000 nosocomial infection–related deaths each year in the USA. Ensuring that all health care workers wash their hands before going from one patient to another is the single most important method of reducing the spread of infections in hospitals. Proper sterile techniques, appropriate isolation techniques, and proper disposal of needles and other sharp objects are also critical.

Medication errors include incorrect dosages, incorrect medications, and drug interactions. The incidence of these errors can be reduced by computer entry of medication orders, which eliminates the problem of physicians' handwriting, as well as by pharmacy information systems that automatically check dosages and determine potential drug interactions.

Unnecessary surgery is being reduced by increasing the requirements for second opinions concerning elective surgical procedures.

Surgical and medical errors will always occur, but their frequency can be limited by the proper training and evaluation of surgeons and physicians, by the surveillance of complications, and by medical care studies of morbidity and mortality in patients undergoing surgical or medical procedures. A classic example of a health problem produced by medical error was the epidemic of retrolental fibroplasia that occurred when 100% oxygen was delivered to preterm infants because it was thought to be beneficial. It actually caused vasoconstriction and destruction of small blood vessels, followed by an overgrowth of capillaries and fibrous tissue in the eye. Usually, keeping the oxygen tension in the infant's air at 40% or less, for as short a time as possible, will prevent retrolental fibroplasia.

SUMMARY

Many primary prevention strategies focus on the use of specific biologic, nutritional, or environmental interventions to protect individuals against certain diseases, deficiency states, injuries, or toxic exposures. The prototype of specific protection is the vaccine, which is directed against one disease and prevents the disease by increasing host resistance. Host resistance can be temporarily increased by passive immunization or sometimes by prophylactic antibiotic therapy.

Nutritional deficiencies can be eliminated by adding nutrients (such as iodine) to commonly used foods (such as salt) to prevent a particular disease (in this case, goiter). Among construction workers, the incidence of head injury and eye injury can be reduced by the use of helmets and goggles, two examples of specific protection against environmental hazards.

Both specific protection and health promotion may be used together. In the case of noise produced by jet aircraft, for example, the ear protection devices worn by aircraft mechanics and airport personnel who cannot avoid exposure to the noise would be considered specific protection against hearing loss. Engineering changes designed to reduce the general level of noise produced by jets could be considered health promotion.

QUESTIONS

Directions (Items 1–10). Each of the numbered items or incomplete statements in this section is followed by answers or by completions of the statement. Select the ONE lettered answer or completion that is BEST in each case. Correct answers and explanations are given at the end of the chapter.

1. The administration of human immune globulin after exposure to hepatitis B is an example of
   (A) cross-reactivity
   (B) health promotion
   (C) hypersensitivity
   (D) passive immunity
   (E) secondary prevention

2. Which of the following vaccines would most likely be dangerous to a person with immunodeficiency?
   (A) Diphtheria vaccine
   (B) Hepatitis B vaccine
   (C) Measles vaccine
   (D) Tetanus vaccine
   (E) Typhoid vaccine

3. The goal of a randomized field trial is to determine vaccine effectiveness (VE). Which of the following equations (in which AR is the attack rate) is a correct expression for VE?
   (A) $VE - AR \times 100$

   (B) $VE = \dfrac{AR_{(unvaccinated)} - AR_{(vaccinated)}}{AR_{(unvaccinated)}} \times 100$

   (C) $VE = \dfrac{AR_{(vaccinated)} - AR_{(unvaccinated)}}{AR_{(vaccinated)}} \times 100$

   (D) $VE = \dfrac{AR_{(vaccinated)} + AR_{(unvaccinated)}}{AR_{(vaccinated)}} \times 100$

   (E) $VE = \dfrac{AR_{(vaccinated)} + AR_{(unvaccinated)}}{AR_{(population)}} \times 100$

4. A modified influenza vaccine must be produced every year because of the antigenic drift of the influenza virus. Which of the following is appropriate for determining the efficacy of the vaccine for a particular year?
   (A) A randomized field trial
   (B) A retrospective cohort study
   (C) Administration of the vaccine by random assignment
   (D) Review of data from previous years
   (E) Routine surveillance

5. Measles vaccine used to be given to children under 1 year of age but is now delayed until children are 15 months of age. The principal reason for the change is that
   (A) herd immunity protects infants from exposure to measles
   (B) infants are immune to measles
   (C) maternal antibody inactivates the measles vaccine in infants
   (D) measles infection is less severe in infants
   (E) measles vaccine is a live vaccine that causes acute disease in infants

6. What characteristic must a disease have in order for its eradication to be feasible?
   (A) The disease must be epidemic rather than endemic
   (B) The disease must be geographically isolated
   (C) The disease must be spread by the fecal-oral route
   (D) The disease must lack an animal reservoir
   (E) The disease must lack an arthropod vector

7. The approval of the varicella vaccine and the decision to provide it routinely to children were most clearly supported by
   (A) evidence about the effects of the vaccine on herd immunity
   (B) evidence about the effects of the vaccine on the occurrence of herpes zoster
   (C) evidence of the efficacy of the vaccine
   (D) evidence regarding the duration of immunity
   (E) the relatively mild illness caused by the varicella-zoster virus

8. A relatively new acellular vaccine is available to prevent which of the following diseases?
   (A) Lyme disease
   (B) Measles
   (C) Pertussis
   (D) Rubella
   (E) Tuberculosis

9. Specific protection against malaria is provided by
   (A) antimicrobial prophylaxis
   (B) mosquito repellant
   (C) passive immunization
   (D) vaccination and active immunity
   (E) vitamin A supplementation

10. In the USA, nosocomial infections result in about how many deaths each year?
    (A) 10,000
    (B) 25,000
    (C) 50,000
    (D) 75,000
    (E) 100,000

■ ANSWERS AND EXPLANATIONS

1. **The answer is D: passive immunity.** Passive immunity is the protection of an individual from an infection by antibodies received passively, rather than by antibodies produced by the individual himself or herself. This occurs when newborn infants receive maternal antibodies in breast milk. It also occurs with various immunizations intended to provide postexposure prophylaxis (prevention of infection after exposure to the pathogen has occurred). The treatment of a wild animal bite often includes postexposure prophylaxis against rabies, with a regimen that involves both active and passive immunization. In this setting, the delivery of preformed antibodies confers protective immunity immediately, albeit temporarily, whereas active immunization requires the longer period of time needed for the exposed individual to produce antibodies to rabies virus. Human immune globulin contains preformed antibodies to hepatitis B virus, which protect individuals exposed to this virus. Generally, as with rabies, active immunization against hepatitis B is provided at the same time.

2. **The answer is C: measles vaccine.** Unlike the other vaccines that are listed (i.e., the diphtheria, hepatitis B, tetanus, and typhoid vaccines), the measles vaccine delivers a live attenuated pathogen. The process of attenuation reduces the pathogenicity of the measles virus so that infection, but not overt disease, will occur, and this produces lasting immunity. The advantage of this approach is the robustness and longevity of the immunity conferred. The danger of administering a live pathogen is that infection might actually lead to symptomatic disease, particularly in those who have marginal immunocompetence or are immunocompromised. Except in circumstances of compelling need, the use of live attenuated vaccines should be avoided in individuals known to be immunocompromised, because the risk exceeds the potential benefit for these individuals.

3. **The answer is B:**

$$VE = \frac{AR_{(unvaccinated)} - AR_{(vaccinated)}}{AR_{(unvaccinated)}} \times 100$$

Vaccine efficacy (VE) is an expression of how well a vaccine prevents disease. If the vaccine has no effect (no efficacy), the same attack rate (AR) would be expected in the vaccinated and unvaccinated groups, and the numerator in the formula above would approximate 0. If no infections occurred in the vaccinated group during the time that infections were occurring in the unvaccinated group, the vaccine efficacy would obviously be high (perfect, in fact). This is reflected in the formula. Subtracting 0 from the attack rate in the unvaccinated group, then dividing the sum by the attack rate in the unvaccinated group, and then multiplying the result by 100 provides a vaccine efficacy of 100%.

4. **The answer is B: a retrospective cohort study.** The influenza virus usually modifies its surface antigens every year (antigenic drift). Therefore, the efficacy of the previous year's influenza vaccine cannot be guaranteed. Determination of vaccine efficacy requires more than surveillance, because a defined population of vaccinated and unvaccinated subjects must be studied. A randomized field trial conducted prospectively is a hopelessly impractical approach for studying a vaccine that must be reconstituted annually. Administration of the vaccine by random assignment would be an essential component of such a field trial, but this is unethical in any condition other than a research setting. A retrospective cohort study allows for the rapid assembly of unvaccinated and vaccinated groups, which can be followed from the time of vaccination to the present and compared on the basis of disease outcome. As explained in the answer to question 3, above, this type of data permits the calculation of vaccine efficacy.

5. **The answer is C: maternal antibody inactivates the measles vaccine in infants.** The measles vaccine is a live vaccine. Because infants are protected by maternal antibodies to measles virus, the live vaccine does not cause acute disease in infants. The maternal antibodies attack the live vaccine so efficiently that the immune system of an infant does not have enough exposure to the virus for antibody production to occur. For this reason, administration of the vaccine is delayed until a child reaches 15 months of age, by which time the maternal antibodies have largely disappeared from the child's circulation (Marks, Halpin, and Orenstein 1978).

6. **The answer is D: the disease must lack an animal reservoir.** Poliomyelitis has been eradicated in the western hemisphere. Thus far, however, smallpox is the only infectious disease that has been eradicated throughout the world. In order to completely eradicate a disease, the disease must lack an animal reservoir. Otherwise, a residual source of the pathogen will remain, and susceptible individuals will eventually become infected. Means are not yet available to eliminate diseases in animal populations in the wild.

7. **The answer is C: evidence of the efficacy of the vaccine.** The one thing about the varicella vaccine that has been clearly established is that it effectively protects against chickenpox (Weibel et al. 1984). Controversy arose because of the unique natural history of the varicella-zoster vi-

rus and specifically its propensity to lie dormant in the dorsal root ganglia and regroup after years or decades to cause herpes zoster (shingles). To determine the effects of the vaccine on the occurrence of herpes zoster, decades of study would be required; for this reason, uncertainty persists about the duration of immunity with use of the vaccine and about the effects of the vaccine on herd immunity. Controversy also arose because chickenpox is usually a mild illness and some investigators argued that the risks of vaccination could not be offset by the benefits of preventing so mild a disease. Arguments in favor of the vaccine prevailed, however, and it is now recommended by the CDC for routine immunization of children.

8. **The answer is C: pertussis.** A relatively new acellular vaccine is available to prevent pertussis. The acellular vaccine exposes subjects to antigens derived from the pathogen, rather than to the whole pathogen.

9. **The answer is A: antimicrobial prophylaxis.** Specific protection, as the name implies, is the use of a targeted strategy to prevent a particular disease. Mosquito repellant may help protect against malaria but is not specific to malaria and may, in fact, fail to provide protection. Immunization, active or passive, is the archetype of specific protection, but there is, as yet, no effective vaccine against malaria. The consumption of supplemental vitamin A is a nonspecific and generally nonprotective measure. The use of antimalarial drugs in advance of exposure can provide specific protection against the disease.

10. **The answer is E: 100,000.** Nosocomial infections result in at least 100,000 deaths each year in the USA. The problem of nosocomial infections is certainly not new, and because it is unlikely to represent a marked divergence from precedent, it cannot be considered an epidemic. Quality-of-care review in hospitals provides data on iatrogenic complications, including nosocomial infections, but many of these infections are not specifically reported. To date, there is no comprehensive system for active surveillance of nosocomial infections.

References Cited

Bates, D. W., et al. Incidence of adverse drug events and potential adverse drug events. Journal of the American Medical Association 274:29–43, 1995.

Cartter, M. L., et al. Influenza outbreaks in nursing homes: how effective is influenza vaccine in the institutionalized elderly? Infection Control and Hospital Epidemiology 11:473–478, 1990.

Cassel, J. Psychological processes and stress: theoretical formulation. International Journal of Health Services 4:471–482, 1974.

Centers for Disease Control and Prevention. Advisory Committee on Immunization Practices: general recommendations on immunization. Morbidity and Mortality Weekly Report 43(RR-1), 1994a.

Centers for Disease Control and Prevention. Childhood Immunization Initiative. Morbidity and Mortality Weekly Report 43:57–60, 1994b.

Centers for Disease Control and Prevention. Diphtheria epidemic: new independent states of the former Soviet Union, 1990–1994. Morbidity and Mortality Weekly Report 44:177–181, 1995.

Centers for Disease Control and Prevention. Intussusception among recipients of rotavirus vaccine: United States, 1998–1999. Morbidity and Mortality Weekly Report 48:577–581, 1999a.

Centers for Disease Control and Prevention. National, state, and urban area vaccination coverage levels among children aged 19–35 months, United States, 1999. Morbidity and Mortality Weekly Report 49:585–589, 2000c.

Centers for Disease Control and Prevention. Pertussis vaccination: use of acellular pertussis vaccines among infants and young children. Morbidity and Mortality Weekly Report 46(RR-7), 1997a.

Centers for Disease Control and Prevention. Poliomyelitis prevention in the United States: introduction of a sequential vaccination schedule of inactivated poliovirus vaccine followed by oral poliovirus vaccine. Morbidity and Mortality Weekly Report 46(RR-3), 1997b.

Centers for Disease Control and Prevention. Prevention and control of meningococcal disease, and meningococcal disease and college students. Morbidity and Mortality Weekly Report 49(RR-7), 2000a.

Centers for Disease Control and Prevention. Prevention of hepatitis A through active or passive immunization. Morbidity and Mortality Weekly Report 48(RR-12), 1999b.

Centers for Disease Control and Prevention. Prevention of varicella. Morbidity and Mortality Weekly Report 45(RR-11), 1996.

Centers for Disease Control and Prevention. Progress toward global poliomyelitis eradication, 1999. Morbidity and Mortality Weekly Report 49:349–354, 2000b.

Centers for Disease Control and Prevention. Recommended childhood immunization schedule: United States, 2001. Morbidity and Mortality Weekly Report 50:7–10, 2001.

Centers for Disease Control and Prevention. Update: childhood vaccine—United States, 1994. Morbidity and Mortality Weekly Report 43:718—720, 1994c.

Centers for Disease Control and Prevention. Vaccines for Children Program, 1994. Morbidity and Mortality Weekly Report 43:705, 1994d.

Chin, J., ed. Control of Communicable Diseases Manual, 17th ed. Washington, D. C., American Public Health Association, 2000.

Clemens, J. D., and E. D. Shapiro. Resolving the pneumococcal vaccine controversy: are there alternatives to randomized clinical trials? Reviews of Infectious Diseases 6:589–600, 1984.

Francis, T., Jr., et al. An evaluation of the 1954 poliomyelitis vaccine trials. American Journal of Public Health, April supplement, 1955.

Goodwin, J. The trouble with DTP. McCall's Magazine, pp. 158–176, Sept. 2000.

Herwaldt, L. A. Pertussis and pertussis vaccines in adults. Journal of the American Medical Association 269:93–94, 1993.

Inlander, C. B., et al. Medicine on Trial. New Jersey, Prentice-Hall Press, 1988.

Johnstone, T. Whooping cough in the United States and Britain (letter). New England Journal of Medicine 309:108–109, 1983.

Kohn, L. T., J. M. Corrigan, and M. Donaldson, eds. To Err Is Human: Building a Safer Health System. Washington, D. C., Institute of Medicine, 1999.

Leape, L. L., et al. Adverse events and negligence in hospitalized patients. Iatrogenics 1:17–21, 1991.

Marks, J., T. J. Halpin, and W. A. Orenstein. Measles vaccine efficacy in children previously vaccinated at 12 months of age. Pediatrics 62:955–960, 1978.

Medical Letter on Drugs and Therapeutics. Hepatitis A vaccine. Medical Letter on Drugs and Therapeutics 37:51–52, 1995a.

Roitt, I. M. Essential Immunology, 7th ed. Oxford, Blackwell Scientific Publications, 1991.

Rosenstock, I. M. Historical origins of the health belief model. Health Education Monographs 2:328–335, 1974.

Shapiro, E. D., et al. The protective efficacy of polyvalent pneumococcal polysaccharide vaccine. New England Journal of Medicine 325:1453–1460, 1991.

Weibel, R. E., et al. Live attenuated varicella virus vaccine: efficacy trial in healthy children. New England Journal of Medicine 310:1409–1415, 1984.

Selected Readings

Centers for Disease Control and Prevention. Recommended childhood immunization schedule: United States, 2001. Morbidity and Mortality Weekly Report 50:7–10, 2001.

Chin, J., ed. Control of Communicable Diseases Manual, 17th ed. Washington, D. C., American Public Health Association, 2000.

17

Methods of Secondary Prevention

Secondary prevention is aimed at early detection of disease, through either screening or case finding, followed by treatment.

Screening is the process of identifying a subgroup of people in whom there is a high probability of finding asymptomatic disease or a risk factor for developing a disease or becoming injured. Unlike case finding, which is defined below, screening takes place in a **community setting** and is applied to a community population, such as students in a school or workers in an industry. A positive screening test result in an individual usually is not diagnostic of a disease. It must be followed by a diagnostic test (for example, a positive mammogram finding must be followed by a biopsy). As shown in Fig. 17–1, the process of screening is complex and involves a cascade of actions that should follow if each step along the way yields positive results. In this regard, initiating a screening program is like getting on a roller coaster, and those involved must continue until the end of the process is reached.

Screening is usually distinguished from **case finding,** which is the process of searching for asymptomatic diseases and risk factors among people in a **clinical setting** (i.e., among people who are under medical care). If a patient is being seen for the first time in a medical care setting, whether it is in a pri-

vate or group practice or a health maintenance organization (HMO), physicians and other health care workers will usually take a thorough medical history and perform a careful physical examination and any indicated laboratory tests. Establishing baseline values in this way may produce case finding (if problems are discovered) and is considered by many to be good medicine, but it is not screening.

A program to take annual blood pressures of the people employed in a business or industry would be considered "screening," whereas performing a chest x-ray or measuring the blood pressure of a patient who was just admitted to a hospital for elective surgery would be called "case finding." Unfortunately, the distinction between screening and case finding is frequently ignored in the literature and in practice. The distinction is important because many of the criteria for deciding to perform community screening do not need to be met during the process of case finding. Because the purposes and criteria for community screening differ considerably from those for case finding, the discussion of these will be separated below.

In Chapter 7, some of the quantitative issues involved in screening were considered, including sensitivity, specificity, and predictive value of tests. In this chapter, it is assumed that the reader is comfortable with these concepts. The purpose here is to discuss broader issues concerning screening and case finding.

■ COMMUNITY SCREENING

Objectives of Screening

Community screening programs seek to test large numbers of persons for one or more diseases or risk factors in a community setting (e.g., in an educational, employment, or recreational setting), on a voluntary basis, usually with little or no direct financial outlay by the persons being screened. Table 17–1 lists several possible objectives of community screening and provides examples.

Ethical and Practical Concerns About Community Screening

If a patient comes to see a physician because of a medical problem, the practitioner is ethically and le-

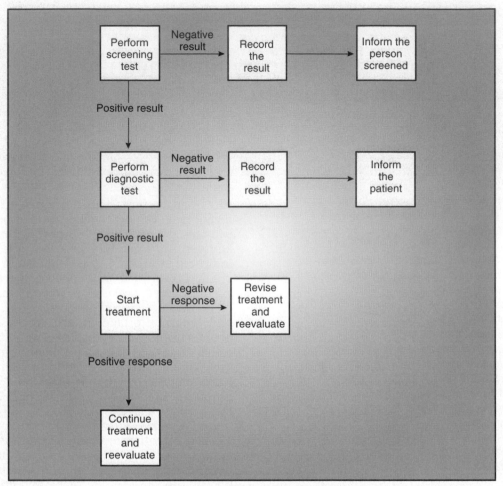

FIGURE 17–1 The process of screening.

gally obligated to provide the best of medical care but is not obligated to guarantee the success of an appropriate and standard treatment. However, when an apparently well population of individuals who have not sought medical care is screened, the professionals involved in the screening program have a greater obligation to show that the benefits of being screened outweigh the costs. The methods used in performing any public screening program, therefore, should be safe, with minimal side effects.

Test errors are a major concern in screening. **False-positive test results** lead to extra time and costs

and can also cause anxiety and discomfort to those whose results were in error. In the case of screening for breast cancer, Elmore et al. (1998) demonstrated that the more mammograms or clinical breast examinations a woman was given, the more likely the woman was to have one or more false-positive results. For example, an estimated 49% of women who had undergone ten mammograms had at least one false-positive reading. This was equal to a false-positive error rate of 6–7% on each mammogram. **False-negative test results** are, in some ways, even worse. One implied promise made to people is that if

TABLE 17–1 **Different Possible Objectives of Screening Programs**

Target	Objective	Example
Disease	Treatment to reduce mortality	Cancer
Disease	Treatment to prevent complications	Hypertension
Disease	Treatment to eradicate infection and prevent its spread	Gonorrhea, syphilis, or tuberculosis
Disease	Change in diet and life-style	Coronary artery disease or type II diabetes mellitus
Behavioral risk factor	Change in life-style	Cigarette smoking or unsafe sexual practices
Environmental risk factor	Change in occupation	Chronic obstructive pulmonary disease from work in a dusty trade
Metabolic risk factor	Treatment or change in diet and life-style	Elevated serum cholesterol levels

they are screened for a particular disease and found to have negative results, they do not have to worry about that disease. False-negative test results may lead people with early symptoms to be less concerned and therefore to delay medical visits that they might otherwise have made promptly. Thus, false-negative test results can be detrimental to the health of the people whose results were in error, and if the results delay the diagnosis in people who have an infectious disease, such as tuberculosis, they can be dangerous to the health of others as well.

It is not easy to establish the value of a community screening effort unless a randomized controlled trial is conducted. One of the scientific reasons that this type of trial is needed is that an association between having been screened and longer survival does not necessarily prove a cause-and-effect relationship, since problems such as selection bias, lead-time bias, and length bias could have occurred (Bailar 1976).

Lead-time bias occurs when screening detects disease earlier in its natural history than would otherwise have happened, so that the period of time from diagnosis to death is lengthened. Having additional lead time (the increased time during which the diagnosis is known) may not alter the natural history of the disease and, therefore, may not extend the length of life. This lead-time bias tends to operate in screening for cancers, no matter how aggressive the tumors are. **Length bias** occurs when the full spectrum of a particular tumor, such as prostate cancer, is composed of cancers that range from very aggressive to indolent. Persons discovered by screening programs are more likely to have a less aggressive tumor (because such persons survive longer to be detected) and therefore are likely to survive longer after detection, regardless of the treatment given. It should be noted that both lead-time bias and length bias apply to case finding as well as to community screening.

Given all of the potential problems in demonstrating the true effectiveness of screening, a great deal of care must be exercised to make sure a community screening program is worthwhile.

Minimum Requirements for Community Screening Programs

The minimum requirements for establishing a safe, ethical, and cost-effective screening program fall into three areas: disease requirements, screening test requirements, and health care system requirements. If any of the requirements is not at least partially met, population-wide screening may be inappropriate.

Disease Requirements

(1) The disease must be serious (i.e., produce significant morbidity or mortality), or there is no reason to screen in the first place.

(2) Even if a disease is serious, there must be an effective therapy for the disease if it is detected. Screening is of no value unless there is a good chance

that detecting the disease in the presymptomatic stage will result in effective therapy. At the present time, there is no value in screening for pancreatic cancer, because the chance of cure by standard medical and surgical methods is extremely small.

(3) The natural history of a disease must be understood clearly enough to know that there is a significant window of time during which the disease is detectable and during which detection would probably lead to a cure or at least to effective treatment. For example, early detection and surgical removal of a malignant tumor in the colon could prevent intestinal obstruction and considerable morbidity, and it might be curative if all of the tumor was removed.

(4) The disease or condition must not be too rare or too common. Screening for a rare disease usually means that many false-positive test results would be expected (see Chapter 7). This increases the cost and difficulties of discovering those who truly are ill or at high risk, and it also causes anxiety and inconvenience for those who must undergo retesting because of erroneous test results. Unless the benefits from discovering one case are very high (such as in the case of treating a newborn child who has phenylketonuria or congenital hypothyroidism), it will seldom be cost-effective to screen general populations for a rare disease. However, screening for some common conditions, such as elevated cholesterol levels, may provide opportunities for education and motivation, if it occurs in the context of medical care.

Screening Test Requirements

(1) The screening test must be reasonably quick, easy, and inexpensive, or the costs of large-scale screening in terms of time, effort, and money will be prohibitive.

(2) The screening test must be safe and acceptable both to the persons being screened and to their physicians. If the persons to be screened object to a procedure (as frequently occurs with colonoscopies), they are unlikely to participate.

(3) The sensitivity, specificity, positive predictive value, and other operating characteristics of a screening test must be known and be acceptable. As discussed above, both false-positive and false-negative test results are serious.

Health Care System Requirements

(1) Follow-up must be available for all persons who have positive results in the screening test. Because screening only sets apart a high-risk group, persons who have positive results must receive further diagnostic testing to rule in or rule out actual disease, even though the follow-up testing may be expensive, time-consuming, and painful and even entail some risk. With some screening programs, the majority of effort and costs are in the follow-up phase, not in the initial screening.

(2) Before a screening program for a particular disease is undertaken, treatment should already be

available for people known to have that disease. If there are limited resources, it does not make sense, either ethically or in terms of cost-effectiveness, to allow persons with symptoms of the disease to go untreated and yet look for the same disease in persons without symptoms.

(3) Those who are screened and diagnosed as having the disease in question must have access to treatment, or the process is ethically flawed. In addition to being unethical, it makes no medical sense to bring the persons screened to the point of informing them of a positive test result and then to abandon them. This is a major problem for community screening efforts, because many people who come for screening will have little or no medical care coverage, and the cost for their treatment will need to be borne by a local hospital or other institution.

(4) The treatment should be acceptable to those being screened. Otherwise, those who require treatment will not undertake it and the screening will have accomplished nothing. For example, some men will not want treatment for prostate cancer, because of possible incontinence and impotence.

(5) The population to be screened should be clearly defined, so that the resulting data will be epidemiologically useful. Although screening at "health fairs" and in shopping centers provides the opportunity to educate the public about health matters, the data obtained are seldom useful because the screening population is not well-defined and tends to be self-selected and highly biased in favor of those concerned about their health (Berwick 1985).

(6) It should be clear who is responsible for the screening, what the cutoff points are for calling a test result positive, and how the findings will become part of a participant's medical record at his or her usual place of care.

Application of the Criteria to Examples

Table 17–2 applies the above criteria to four conditions for which community screening has commonly been undertaken: (1) hypertension, tested by a sphygmomanometer reading of blood pressure; (2) elevated cholesterol levels, with total cholesterol measurement based on a rapid screening of blood; (3) breast cancer, tested by mammography; and (4) lung cancer, tested by chest x-ray.

Investigators have agreed that a screening program using chest x-rays to detect lung cancer fails at two critical points. First, the yield of detection is low. Second, as numerous studies have shown, only a small proportion of cancers that are detected by chest x-rays can be cured by the time they are visible (see, for example, Greenberg 1956; Brett 1968; Boucot and Weiss 1973). Because of these problems, community screening for lung cancer by chest x-rays is no longer recommended. However, the possible use of

TABLE 17–2   Requirements for Screening Programs and Ratings of Example Methods to Detect Hypertension, Elevated Cholesterol Levels, Breast Cancer, and Lung Cancer

Requirements	Screening Method and Rating*			
	Sphygmomanometer Reading (Hypertension)	Serum Cholesterol Test (Hypercholesterolemia)	Mammogram (Breast Cancer)	Chest X-Ray (Lung Cancer)
Disease Requirements				
(1) The disease is serious.	++	++	++	++
(2) Effective treatment exists.	++	+	+	+/–
(3) The natural history of the disease is understood.	++	+	+	+
(4) The disease occurs frequently.	++	++	++	++
(5) Other diseases or conditions may be detected.	–	–	–	+
Screening Test Requirements				
(1) The test is quick to perform.	++	+	+	++
(2) The test is easy to administer.	++	+	+	+
(3) The test is inexpensive.	++	+	+	+
(4) The test is safe.	++	++	+	+
(5) The test is acceptable to participants.	++	+	+	++
(6) The sensitivity, specificity, and other operating characteristics of the test are acceptable.	++	+	+	–
Health Care System Requirements				
(1) The method meets the requirements for screening in a community setting.	++	++	+	–
(2) The method meets the requirements for case finding in a medical care setting.	++	++	++	+

*Ratings are applied to four conditions for which community screening has commonly been undertaken: hypertension, tested by a sphygmomanometer reading of blood pressure; elevated cholesterol levels, with total cholesterol measurement based on a rapid screening of blood; breast cancer, tested by mammography; and lung cancer, tested by chest x-ray. Ratings are as follows: ++ means good, + means satisfactory, and – means unsatisfactory.

computed tomography (CT) scans for this purpose is being investigated.

Although the other screening methods indicated in Table 17–2 are now generally accepted, as is cervical cancer screening by Papanicolaou test, there is still considerable debate about general screening issues, such as what age to start the screening, how often to repeat it, and whether the methods yield accurate results (see Elmore et al. 1994 and 1998 regarding breast cancer).

Newer screening methods are being debated even more sharply. For example, investigators are questioning whether active treatment of prostate cancer detected by prostate-specific antigen (PSA) testing really changes the natural history of the disease. On the one hand, some studies indicate that mortality is reduced in areas with high rates of prostate cancer screening and radical treatment (surgical or radiation therapy). On the other hand, several studies suggest that aggressive treatment of prostate cancer detected through PSA screening may actually decrease the quality of life without adding compensatory benefits (see, for example, Krahn et al. 1994; Litwin et al. 1995; Potosky et al. 1995). In its 1996 report, the US Preventive Services Task Force recommends against routine screening with transrectal ultrasound, tests for serum tumor markers such as PSA, or digital rectal examination. The American College of Preventive Medicine generally concurs, but it states that men who are over 50 years old and have a life expectancy of more than 10 years should be given information about the benefits and harm of PSA screening and treatment, as well as information about the limits of current evidence, so they can make informed decisions (see Ferrini and Woolf 1998). There is now a strong interest in improving the efficiency of screening by such means as measuring the percentage of free PSA in serum samples, determining the rate of increase ("velocity") in an individual's PSA levels, and adjusting the PSA criteria according to age and prostate volume.

Repetition of Screening Programs

There are dangers in not giving careful thought to the details of repeat screening efforts. Strangely enough, this is particularly true if an initial major screening effort is considered a great success, in which case enthusiasm may lead the organizers to repeat the screening too soon (e.g., a year later). Almost inevitably, unless the population screened the second time is very different from the one screened the first time, a screening effort repeated after a short interval will be quite disappointing. This is because the initial screening will have detected prevalent cases (cases accumulated over many years), whereas the repeated screening will detect only incident cases (new cases since the last screening), making the number of cases detected in the second screening effort smaller (Christopherson, Parker, and Drye 1962).

TABLE 17–3 Correlation Between Number of Screening Tests Performed and Percentage of Persons with at Least One False-Positive Test Result

Number of Screening Tests Performed*	Percentage of Persons with at Least One False-Positive Test Result†
1	5.0
2	9.8
4	18.5
5	22.6
10	40.1
20	64.2
25	72.3

Source of data: Schoenberg, B. S. The "abnormal" laboratory result. Postgraduate Medicine 47:151–155, 1970.
*It is assumed that the tests measure different values (i.e., the tests are independent).
†Percentages are based on tests that each have a 5% false-positive error rate.

Multiphasic Screening

Multiphasic screening programs are those that involve screening for a variety of diseases in the same individual. Some investigators have argued that multiphasic screening makes community efforts more efficient. Once a sample of blood is drawn, for example, it is easy to perform a variety of tests, using modern, automated laboratory equipment. The yield of multiphasic screening, however, has come under serious question (Bates and Yellin 1972).

One problem is that multiphasic screening in an elderly population will often detect diseases or abnormal conditions that have been found earlier and are already being treated, in which case funds are being used for unnecessary testing. Another problem is that multiphasic screening results in a relatively high frequency of false-positive results, and this requires many participants to return for more expensive follow-up tests.

For each disease-free person screened with a battery of independent tests (i.e., tests that measure different values), the probability that at least one of the screening tests will yield a false-positive finding can be expressed as $[1 - (1 - \text{alpha})^n]$, where alpha is the false-positive error rate (see Chapter 7) and n is the number of screening tests done. If two screening tests are performed and alpha is 5% (making the test specificity 95%), the probability of a disease-free person's being recalled for further testing is $[1 - (0.95)^2] = [1 - (0.9025)] =$ almost 10%. If four tests are performed, the probability is $[1 - (0.95)^4] = [1 - (0.8145)] = 18.5\%$. As Table 17–3 shows, if 25 tests are performed, over 70% of disease-free individuals would be brought back for unnecessary but often costly follow-up testing.

Persons with one or more diseases or conditions that would be detected by multiphasic screening would have a slightly smaller probability of having one or more false-positive findings, only because the number of tests eligible to be falsely called positive would be reduced by the number of truly positive tests.

When Olsen, Kane, and Proctor (1976) undertook a controlled trial of multiphasic screening, they subjected one group of individuals to a battery of special screening tests that included hearing and vision tests, ocular pressure measurements, blood pressure measurements, spirometry, electrocardiography, mammography and breast examination, Papanicolaou smear, chest x-ray, urinalysis, complete blood count, and 12 blood chemistry tests. When they compared the findings in this group with the findings in a control group that was not subjected to the battery of special tests, they found that there were no major differences in the health knowledge or the mortality and morbidity rates of the two groups. However, the group that underwent multiphasic screening did spend more nights in the hospital.

■ INDIVIDUAL CASE FINDING
The Periodic Health Examination

Historically, the most common method of prevention in clinical medicine, especially in adults, has been the annual physical checkup, which has come to be known as the periodic health examination.

After World War II, the number of available treatments for chronic illnesses increased greatly, and more people began to have an annual checkup, usually consisting of a medical history, physical examination, complete blood count, urinalysis, chest x-ray, and electrocardiogram. Despite the popularity of these checkups, the number of people who received them was limited by the fact that many insurance plans would not cover their costs, although some corporations provided them as a benefit for high-level managers. In fact, most research on the periodic health examination prior to the 1960s concerned examinations that were sponsored by businesses or industries or were conducted by the few large health plans existing at the time.

An annotated bibliography of 152 early studies of periodic health examinations (Siegel 1963) showed that reports published prior to 1940 were mostly anecdotal and were enthusiastic about the examinations. Reports published between 1940 and 1962 were more likely to include quantitative data and, although still supportive, increasingly raised serious questions about "routine" use of examinations. With the subsequent increase in the number of health maintenance organizations (HMOs) came an increase in the use of periodic examinations, and even though most investigators agreed that examinations in children were beneficial, more and more studies began to cast doubts about the cost-effectiveness of examinations in adults (for example, see Schor et al. 1964; Roberts et al. 1969; Spitzer and Brown 1975; Spark 1976).

During the 1970s, investigators began moving toward the idea of modifying the periodic examination to focus only on those conditions and diseases that would be most likely to be found in a person of a given age, gender, and family history. This approach was given the term "lifetime health monitoring" by Breslow and Somers (1977). The biggest support for a new approach came in 1979, when the Canadian Task Force on the Periodic Physical Examination recommended that the traditional form of periodic checkup be replaced by the use of **health protection packages** that included sex-appropriate and age-appropriate immunizations, screening, and counseling of patients on a periodic basis. Specifically, the task force recommended that "with certain exceptions, the procedures be carried out as case finding rather than screening techniques; that is, they should be performed when the patient is attending for unrelated symptoms rather than for a specific preventive purpose." Among the "certain exceptions" noted by the task force were pregnant women, the very young, and the very old, for whom they recommended regular visits specifically for preventive purposes.

US Preventive Services Task Force

In an effort to clarify many of the issues concerning screening and case finding and to make well-studied recommendations, the US Department of Health and Human Services created the US Preventive Services Task Force (USPSTF). In its investigations, the USPSTF reviews data concerning the efficacy of a variety of interventions, including the following: (1) immunizations in children and adults; (2) postexposure prophylaxis of certain infectious diseases, such as *Haemophilus influenzae* type b diseases, meningococcal infections, hepatitis A and B, tuberculosis, and rabies; (3) aspirin use to prevent myocardial infarction; (4) counseling to prevent dental disease, tobacco use, motor vehicle injuries, household and environmental injuries, unintended pregnancy, and type 1 human immunodeficiency virus (HIV-1) infection and other sexually transmitted diseases; and (5) counseling to increase exercise and improve nutrition.

The first report of the USPSTF was issued in 1989. The updated report, published in 1996, offers recommendations concerning the interventions that physicians should include in the periodic health examination, based on assessments of the value of more than 100 interventions to prevent 60 illnesses and conditions. These recommendations, which are summarized in Box 17–1, take into account not only the efficacy of screening tests in detecting disease and adverse conditions but also the extent to which early detection actually improves health. In this regard, the US task force borrowed much of the methodology developed by the Canadian task force and applied it more broadly. For example, using the latter's idea of "health protection packages," the USPSTF listed the following for four major age groups and for pregnant women: (1) conditions to be the subject of screening efforts using the medical history, physical examination, and laboratory or other diagnostic procedures; (2) items for counseling regarding diet, exercise, substance use, sexual practices, injury prevention, dental

BOX 17–1 Summary of Major Recommendations from the US Preventive Services Task Force (USPSTF) Regarding the Screening of Asymptomatic Persons During Periodic Health Examinations Given by Primary Care Physicians

Disease, Condition, or Risk Factor	Recommendations*
Cancers	
Bladder cancer	Routine screening with urine dipstick, microscopic urinalysis, or urine cytology is not recommended.†
Breast cancer	For women aged 50–69 years, screening every 1–2 years with mammography alone or with mammography and a clinical breast examination (CBE) is recommended. For women aged 40–49 or aged 70 and older, there is insufficient evidence to recommend for or against routine mammography or CBE.
Cervical cancer	For women who are or have been sexually active and who have a cervix, screening with Papanicolaou testing is recommended. Pap smears should begin with the onset of sexual activity and should be repeated at least every 3 years.
Colorectal cancer	For men and women aged 50 years and older, screening with fecal occult blood testing (FOBT), sigmoidoscopy, or both is recommended. The FOBT should be given annually; the periodicity of sigmoidoscopy is unspecified. There is insufficient evidence to recommend for or against routine screening with digital rectal examination, barium enema, or colonoscopy. Persons with a family history of hereditary syndromes associated with a high risk of colon cancer should be referred for diagnosis and treatment.
Lung cancer	Routine screening with chest radiography or sputum cytology is not recommended.†
Oral cancer	There is insufficient evidence to recommend for or against routine screening, but clinicians should remain alert to signs and symptoms of oral cancer in persons who use tobacco or alcohol.†
Ovarian cancer	Routine screening with ultrasound, the measurement of serum tumor markers, or pelvic examination is not recommended.
Pancreatic cancer	Routine screening with ultrasound, the measurement of serum tumor markers, or abdominal palpation is not recommended.
Prostate cancer	Routine screening with transrectal ultrasound, measurement of serum tumor markers (e.g., prostate-specific antigen), or digital rectal examination is not recommended.
Skin cancer	There is insufficient evidence to recommend for or against either performing routine screening or counseling patients to perform periodic self-examination.†
Testicular cancer	There is insufficient evidence to recommend for or against either performing routine screening or counseling patients to perform periodic self-examination.
Thyroid cancer	Routine screening with ultrasound or neck palpation is not recommended.
Cardiovascular diseases	
Abdominal aortic aneurysm	There is insufficient evidence to recommend for or against routine screening with ultrasound or abdominal palpation.
Carotid artery stenosis	There is insufficient evidence to recommend for or against routine screening with carotid ultrasound or physical examination.†
Coronary artery disease	For children, adolescents, and young adults, routine screening is not recommended as part of the periodic health visit or preparticipation sports examination. For middle-aged and older men and women, there is insufficient evidence to recommend for or against screening with resting electrocardiography (ECG), ambulatory ECG, or exercise ECG.†
Hypercholesterolemia and other lipid abnormalities	For men aged 35–65 years and women aged 45–65 years, periodic screening for high blood cholesterol levels is recommended. There is insufficient evidence to recommend for or against routine screening for other lipid abnormalities.†
Hypertension	For all children and adults, screening is recommended.†
Peripheral artery disease	Routine screening is not recommended.
Hearing and visual disorders	
Glaucoma	There is insufficient evidence to recommend for or against routine screening.
Hearing impairment	For older adults, screening by periodically asking questions about hearing is recommended.
Visual impairment	For children, screening to detect amblyopia and strabismus is recommended. Screening should be performed once prior to the start of elementary school but preferably between the ages of 3 and 4 years. For older adults, screening with the Snellen visual acuity chart is recommended.

Box continued on following page

BOX 17–1   Summary of Major Recommendations from the US Preventive Services Task Force (USPSTF) Regarding the Screening of Asymptomatic Persons During Periodic Health Examinations Given by Primary Care Physicians *Continued*

Disease, Condition, or Risk Factor	Recommendations*
Infectious diseases	
Bacteriuria	For pregnant women, screening with a urine culture is recommended. For others, routine screening is not recommended.
Chlamydial infections	For all sexually active female adolescents and for other women at high risk of *Chlamydia trachomatis* infections (including pregnant women considered at high risk), screening with cultures or other tests is recommended. For others, routine screening is not recommended.†
Genital herpes infections	Routine screening with viral cultures or other tests is not recommended.†
Gonorrhea	For women at high risk of *Neisseria gonorrhoeae* infections (including pregnant women considered at high risk), screening with cultures is recommended.
Hepatitis B	For all pregnant women, screening with serologic tests for hepatitis B surface antigen (HBsAg) is recommended at the first prenatal visit. For others, routine screening is not recommended.
Human immunodeficiency virus (HIV) infections	For men and women at increased risk of HIV infections (including pregnant women considered at risk), screening with serologic tests is recommended. For infants born to high-risk mothers, screening is recommended if the mother's antibody status is not known.†
Rubella	For all women of childbearing age, screening for rubella susceptibility by asking about vaccination or by performing serologic tests is recommended at the first clinical encounter.†
Syphilis	For all pregnant women and for men and women at increased risk of *Treponema pallidum* infections, screening with serologic tests is recommended.
Tuberculosis	For children and adults at high risk of *Mycobacterium tuberculosis* infections (including pregnant women considered at high risk), screening with the tuberculin skin test is recommended.
Mental disorders and substance abuse	
Dementia	There is insufficient evidence to recommend for or against routine screening with standardized screening instruments.
Depression	There is insufficient evidence to recommend for or against routine screening with standardized questionnaires.
Drug abuse	There is insufficient evidence to recommend for or against routine screening with standardized questionnaires or biologic assays, but clinicians should be alert to the signs and symptoms of drug abuse in their patients.†
Family violence	There is insufficient evidence to recommend for or against routine screening with specific screening instruments, but clinicians should be alert to the various presentations of child abuse, spouse and partner abuse, and elder abuse.
Problem drinking	For all adolescents and adults, screening by taking a careful history of alcohol use or giving standardized screening questionnaires is recommended. Routine measurement of biochemical markers is not recommended.†
Suicidal intent	There is insufficient evidence to recommend for or against routine screening with specific screening instruments, but clinicians should routinely ask patients about their use of alcohol and other drugs and should be alert to signs of suicidal ideation in persons with established risk factors.
Metabolic, nutritional, and environmental disorders	
Diabetes mellitus	There is insufficient evidence to recommend for or against routine screening for any form of diabetes mellitus, including gestational diabetes.
Iron deficiency anemia	For all pregnant women and for infants at high risk of iron deficiency anemia, screening by measuring the hemoglobin or hematocrit is recommended.
Lead toxicity	For children at increased risk of exposure to lead in their homes or communities, screening by measuring blood lead levels is recommended at least once, preferably at the age of 12 months.
Obesity	For all persons, periodic height and weight measurements are recommended.
Thyroid disease	For newborn infants, screening for congenital hypothyroidism is recommended during the first week of life.

BOX 17–1   Summary of Major Recommendations from the US Preventive Services Task Force (USPSTF) Regarding the Screening of Asymptomatic Persons During Periodic Health Examinations Given by Primary Care Physicians *Continued*

Disease, Condition, or Risk Factor	Recommendations*
Musculoskeletal disorders	
Adolescent idiopathic scoliosis	There is insufficient evidence to recommend for or against routine screening in adolescents.
Postmenopausal osteoporosis	There is insufficient evidence to recommend for or against routine screening with bone densitometry in postmenopausal women.†
Perinatal disorders‡	
Chromosomal defects	In areas where adequate counseling and follow-up services are available, screening for chromosomal defects should be offered to pregnant women.† For those whose offspring are at low risk for these defects, a maternal serum multiple-marker screening should be offered to detect Down syndrome (characterized by a low level of alpha-fetoprotein, high level of human chorionic gonadotropin, or low level of unconjugated estriol) and to detect neural tube defects (characterized by a high level of alpha-fetoprotein). If there is a positive result in the maternal serum multiple-marker screen, then amniocentesis or chorionic villus sampling should be offered. For pregnant women whose offspring are at high risk for chromosomal defects, a choice of any of the above screening measures should be offered.
Metabolic defects	For newborn infants, screening for congenital hypothyroidism and phenylketonuria (PKU) should be performed during the first week of life. If the PKU test is performed during the first 24 hours of life and the results are negative, the test should be repeated within 2 weeks.

Sources of data: US Preventive Services Task Force (USPSTF). Guide to Clinical Preventive Services, 2nd ed. Baltimore, Williams & Wilkins, 1996. The recommendations are made by the USPSTF, Department of Health and Human Services, Office of Disease Prevention and Health Promotion, and are constantly being revised on the basis of the latest research. Updates can be found at the following Web site: www.ahcpr.gov/clinic/uspstfix.htm.

*Note: Recommendations are for screening only in asymptomatic individuals. Moreover, recommendations concern only the members of the specific groups mentioned (e.g., those with the specific age, gender, or other characteristics listed). For those in other groups, there is insufficient evidence to recommend for or against routine screening. Nevertheless, there may be valid reasons to perform screening tests in individuals, based on other grounds (e.g., family history or occupational exposure).

†For this condition, consult the sources of data listed above regarding related health promotion activities (counseling, vaccination, etc.).

‡The listings under perinatal disorders do not include screening tests that are accepted as a part of good prenatal care, such as tests for toxemia of pregnancy, syphilis, hemoglobinopathies, and D(Rh) incompatibility. The USPSTF does not support the routine use of electronic monitoring or ultrasonography. The USPSTF indicates that there is insufficient evidence to recommend for or against routine screening of pregnant women for lead toxicity and gestational diabetes.

health, and other matters; and (3) immunizations and chemoprophylaxis.

Health Risk Assessments

Health risk assessments (HRAs) use questionnaires or computer programs to elicit and evaluate information concerning individuals in a clinical or industrial medical practice. Each assessed person receives information concerning his or her life expectancy and the types of interventions that are likely to have a positive impact on health or longevity.

For more than 25 years, the idea of HRAs has been promoted by physicians who are enthusiastic about detecting disease and risk factors in individuals. Based on the original work of Robbins and Hall (1970), a professional organization called the Society for Prospective Medicine has been formed. Its members seek to improve the construction and use of HRAs and the practice of preventive ("prospective") medicine in the context of a clinical or industrial medical practice (see Society for Prospective Medicine 1995). Toward this end, they promote the use of

HRAs for (1) assessing the needs of individual patients as they enter a medical care system or of employees in an industrial setting, (2) developing health education information for those who complete the assessment, and (3) developing cost-containment strategies based on better acquisition of health risk information from individuals.

Most HRAs use questionnaires or interactive computer programs to gather data concerning each person being assessed. In addition to data such as height, weight, blood pressure, cholesterol level, and previous and present diseases, the information usually includes details concerning the person's life-style and his or her family history. A computer then calculates the person's "risk age" on the basis of the data and an algorithm. Most HRAs use an algorithm based on findings of the Framingham Study. The **risk age** is defined as the age at which the average individual would have the same risk of dying as the person being assessed. If the assessed person's risk age is older than his or her chronologic age, that means that he or she has a higher risk of dying than the average individual of the same chronologic age. Likewise, if the assessed person's risk age is younger than the chronologic age, the person has a lower risk of dying than the average individual of the same chronologic age.

The HRAs usually provide a printed report about the assessed person's relative risk of dying or risk age, combined with some sort of educational message regarding the types of interventions that would have the most positive effect on the person's life expectancy if they were instituted. The printed reports have become more sophisticated in recent years and are sometimes supplemented with video cassettes providing tailor-made educational messages.

HRAs have been extensively evaluated, with mixed results (see, for example, Foxman and Edington 1987; Kirscht 1989; Schoenbach 1987; Smith, McKinlay, and McKinlay 1989; Smith, McKinlay, and Thorington 1987). So far, criticisms have focused on errors or lack of information by the persons entering the data; difficulties in validating the predictions; uncertainties concerning the correct reference population for baseline risks; and limitations related to the fact that the instruments focus mainly or exclusively on mortality and not on morbidity or the quality of life. The greatest strength of HRAs may be their ability to clarify how nutritional and life-style factors affect an assessed person's risk of death and to motivate that person to make changes in a positive direction.

■ SUMMARY

The goal of secondary prevention is the detection of disease or risk factors in the presymptomatic stage, when medical, environmental, nutritional, and life-style interventions can be most effective. Screening is carried out in a community setting, whereas case finding is carried out in a clinical setting.

For community screening programs to be beneficial and cost-effective, they must fulfill various requirements concerning the health problem to be detected, the screening test to be used, and the system available to provide health care for those with positive screening results. Lead-time bias and length bias can cause health care personnel and analysts to overestimate the benefit produced by a screening program, particularly when the program is aimed at detection of cancer. Although multiphasic screening seeks to make the process more efficient by searching for many conditions at the same time, the high incidence of false-positive test results and other associated problems have made this technique less successful than was originally anticipated.

Historically, the periodic health examination has been the most common method of case finding. Because it has provided disappointing benefits when examined carefully, it is now being replaced by lifetime health monitoring. This approach focuses on monitoring individuals for the specific set of conditions and diseases most likely to be found in persons of a certain age and gender, and its use has been advocated by experts on preventive medicine in Canada and the USA. However, many practitioners who emphasize preventive medicine prefer to see their patients for checkups more often than may be recommended, such as every year or two, in order to maintain a relationship of trust and to repeat health promotion messages that are important for efforts to change behavior.

■ QUESTIONS

Directions (Items 1–9). Each of the numbered items or incomplete statements in this section is followed by answers or by completions of the statement. Select the ONE lettered answer or completion that is BEST in each case. Correct answers and explanations are given at the end of the chapter.

1. An example of secondary prevention is
   - (A) detection and treatment of hypertension
   - (B) early treatment of diabetic nephropathy
   - (C) hormone replacement therapy at menopause
   - (D) percutaneous transluminal coronary angioplasty
   - (E) vaccination against hepatitis B

2. A screening program is designed for the early detection of lung cancer. The survival time in individuals whose lung cancer was detected by screening is found to be 3 months longer than the survival time in individuals who did not undergo screening and presented with symptoms of lung cancer. This difference is most likely due to
   - (A) better treatment options for those found through screening
   - (B) effect modification
   - (C) lead-time bias
   - (D) length bias
   - (E) observer bias

3. A screening program designed to find candidates for liver transplantation would be ill-advised because
   - (A) false-negative results might occur
   - (B) the condition is common
   - (C) the necessary resources for treatment are in short supply
   - (D) the population at risk is unknown
   - (E) the treatment is invasive

4. Data that are obtained through screening at health fairs are of little epidemiologic value because
   - (A) comorbid conditions may go undetected
   - (B) false-positive results are common
   - (C) follow-up is not adequate
   - (D) most conditions are rare in random samples
   - (E) self-selection produces a biased sample

5. There is controversy regarding the use of prostate-specific antigen to screen for prostate cancer because
   - (A) prostate cancer cannot be detected until it is symptomatic

(B)   prostate cancer is a rare disease
(C)   prostate cancer is uniformly fatal
(D)   the appropriate management of asymptomatic prostate cancer is uncertain
(E)   there is no effective treatment for prostate cancer

6. Twenty-five tests are being performed together in a multiphasic screening program. If the tests measure different values (i.e., the tests are independent) and if each test has a 5% false-positive error rate, the approximate percentage of healthy subjects in whom at least one false-positive result would be found is

(A)   25%
(B)   33%
(C)   50%
(D)   70%
(E)   85%

7. The concept of "lifetime health monitoring" refers to

(A)   modification of the periodic physical examination to focus on likely conditions in a given individual
(B)   routine performance of a comprehensive physical examination
(C)   the aggregate use of diagnostic technology during an individual's lifetime
(D)   the compilation of a comprehensive list of risk factors for chronic disease
(E)   the completion of periodic health surveys compiled in a national data base

8. The US Preventive Services Task Force, which issued its first report in 1989, was created by the US Department of Health and Human Services to

(A)   control the spread of human immunodeficiency virus (HIV) infection
(B)   curtail population growth
(C)   devise a strategy for the prevention of antimicrobial resistance
(D)   eradicate poliomyelitis
(E)   recommend the appropriate role for screening and case finding in the periodic physical examination

9. Health risk assessments (HRAs) are used to determine an individual's "risk age." Which of the following is a correct interpretation of the risk age?

(A)   If the chronologic age exceeds the risk age, the risk of death is below average
(B)   If the risk age exceeds the chronologic age, the risk of death is below average
(C)   If the risk age is low, the risk of death is high
(D)   The risk age is defined by the onset of risk factors for chronic disease
(E)   The risk of death is greatest when the risk age equals the chronologic age

■ ANSWERS AND EXPLANATIONS

1. **The answer is A: detection and treatment of hypertension.** It is only fair to acknowledge that the distinctions between levels of prevention can at times be vague. The distinctions have both clinical and policy implications, however, so a physician must be familiar with them. Vaccination is an effort to prevent disease in an unaffected individual and is therefore an example of primary prevention. Hormone replacement therapy at menopause is usually a factor in the primary prevention of osteoporosis and ischemic heart disease. Hypertension is commonly asymptomatic and often detected through screening or case finding; the detection and treatment of an asymptomatic disease constitute secondary prevention. The early treatment of diabetic nephropathy is an attempt to limit the complications of an established disease and is therefore tertiary prevention. Percutaneous transluminal coronary angioplasty is a method to prevent the complications of established symptomatic coronary artery disease and is therefore tertiary prevention.

2. **The answer is C: lead-time bias.** Lead-time bias results when a disease is detected by screening at an earlier point in its natural history than it would be if a screening program were not in effect. The patient survives for a longer time after diagnosis only because the diagnosis is made at an earlier stage of the disease and not because detection changes the natural progression of the disease. Length bias results when cases of relatively indolent disease are preferentially detected by screening because cases of fulminant disease tend to produce early deaths and are therefore not in the population at the time of screening. If better treatment options are available for a disease found through screening (as is the case, for example, with early breast cancer detected by mammography, as compared with more advanced breast cancer), a longer survival time might be the result of alteration of the natural history of the disease, and this would represent a true effect and not a form of bias.

3. **The answer is C: the necessary resources for treatment are in short supply.** Organs for transplantation are generally in short supply, and waiting lists of desperately ill recipients are long. If a treatment for a disease is not available in adequate supply to meet and exceed the needs of symptomatic patients, then screening for the disease would be inappropriate because the asymptomatic or less symptomatic patients who were detected through screening would merely be added to the list of patients who could not be treated.

4. **The answer is E: self-selection produces a biased sample.** For a screening program to have

epidemiologic value, the relevant population must be identifiable. Community-based health fairs usually appeal only to health-conscious individuals. These individuals are perhaps less likely to have a particular condition (e.g., hypertension) than are those who are less interested in attending health fairs. Because of this self-selection bias, the utility of health fairs in screening a community for diseases is highly questionable. False-positive results may or may not be common in such screening efforts, depending on the specificity of the diagnostic test used and the prevalence of the condition. In any screening program, lack of adequate follow-up and inattention to comorbid conditions are potential deficiencies.

5. **The answer is D: the appropriate management of asymptomatic prostate cancer is uncertain.** The best way to detect and treat prostate cancer is the subject of ongoing debate in the medical literature (Ross et al. 2000; Small and Reese 2000). The disease is rapidly progressive and even fatal in some men but indolent in others, and there is no reliable way to distinguish between the two types early enough to affect the outcome. Those with rapidly progressive disease would clearly benefit from early detection and aggressive treatment. However, for the majority destined to have indolent disease, treatment may do more harm than good (e.g., surgical prostatectomy can result in erectile dysfunction as well as bladder and bowel incontinence). Prostate cancer can be detected while it is asymptomatic through digital rectal examination and perhaps also with the prostate-specific antigen assay. In 1998, the American College of Preventive Medicine advised against routine prostate cancer screening (see Ferrini and Woolf 1998), but this recommendation may be changed if the performance of screening tests is improved or if reliable methods to distinguish indolent cancer from aggressive cancer become available. There is effective treatment for prostate cancer, depending on the stage of disease. Prostate cancer is by no means rare, as it is the second leading cause of deaths from cancer among men in the USA (Catalona 1994).

6. **The answer is D: 70%.** For each disease-free person screened, the probability of at least one false-positive result is $[1 - (1 - \text{alpha})^n]$, where alpha is the false-positive error rate and n is the number of screening tests done. In this case, alpha is 0.05 and n is 25. Therefore, $[1 - (0.95)^{25}] = [1 - (0.277)] = 0.723 = 72.3\%$, or approximately 70%.

7. **The answer is A: modification of the periodic physical examination to focus on likely conditions in a given individual.** Lifetime health monitoring is an effort to detect and respond to

changes in the status of an individual's health over the course of his or her lifetime. To this end, age-specific and gender-specific examination and diagnostic screening have been recommended by the Canadian Task Force on the Periodic Physical Examination (1979) and by the US Preventive Services Task Force (1996). The routine performance of a comprehensive physical examination is essentially what lifetime health monitoring is intended to replace. Advocates of this type of monitoring emphasize that it is important to be cautious in the use of diagnostic techniques (since these techniques are costly and may expose patients to potential harm as well as potential benefit) and that it is necessary to consider the sensitivity and specificity of the tests employed, the disease prevalence, and the implications for the predictive value associated with diagnostic testing. Routine comprehensive physical examinations, which subject patients to what is arguably the most potent of diagnostic devices, the physician's brain, have not traditionally been grounded in such rational considerations. The concept of lifetime health monitoring treats the physical examination more like other modalities of screening and diagnosis, stipulating that it not be applied universally but that it instead be applied as indicated by the circumstances and attributes characterizing a particular patient.

8. **The answer is E: recommend the appropriate role for screening and case finding in the periodic physical examination.** The annual physical examination became popular in the USA in the 1940s, as advances in diagnostic and therapeutic technology raised expectations of medical care. The actual utility of an annual examination was first assessed in the 1970s. In 1979, the Canadian Task Force on the Periodic Examination advised that screening, counseling, and interventions be age-specific and gender-specific, rather than comprehensive. The US Preventive Services Task Force was later convened to review a variety of issues and to make recommendations regarding appropriate use of the periodic physical examination in the USA. The comprehensive examination became a fixture of the medical landscape before its value was established. With unmodified applications, it is a low-yield procedure.

9. **The answer is A: if the chronologic age exceeds the risk age, the risk of death is below average.** The risk age is the age of the average individual from a population whose risk of death equals that of the patient in question. If risk age and chronologic age are equivalent, the patient in question has the average risk of death for his or her age group. Because the risk of death rises with advancing age, if risk age is below chronologic age, the implication is that the patient has the same risk of death as an average younger per-

son. The lower the risk age, the lower the risk of death.

References Cited

Bailar, J. D., III. Mammography: a contrary view. Annals of Internal Medicine 84:77–84, 1976.

Bates, B., and J. A. Yellin. The yield of multiphasic screening. Journal of the American Medical Association 222:74–78, 1972.

Berwick, D. M. Screening in health fairs: a critical review of benefits, risks, and costs. Journal of the American Medical Association 254:1492–1498, 1985.

Boucot, K. R., and W. Weiss. Is curable lung cancer detected by semiannual screening? Journal of the American Medical Association 224:1361–1365, 1973.

Breslow, L., and A. R. Somers. The lifetime health monitoring program: a practical approach to preventive medicine. New England Journal of Medicine 296:601–608, 1977.

Brett, G. Z. The value of lung cancer detection by six-monthly chest radiographs. Thorax 23:414–420, 1968.

Canadian Task Force on the Periodic Physical Examination. The periodic health examination. Canadian Medical Association Journal 121:1193–1254, 1979.

Catalona, W. J. Management of cancer of the prostate. New England Journal of Medicine 331:996–1004, 1994.

Christopherson, W. M., J. E. Parker, and J. C. Drye. Control of cervical cancer: preliminary report on a community program. Journal of the American Medical Association 182:179–182, 1962.

Elmore, J. G., et al. Ten-year risk of false-positive screening mammograms and clinical breast examinations. New England Journal of Medicine 338:1089–1096, 1998.

Elmore, J. G., et al. Variability in radiologists' interpretations of mammograms. New England Journal of Medicine 331:1493–1499, 1994.

Ferrini, R., and S. H. Woolf. American College of Preventive Medicine practice policy: screening for prostate cancer in American men. American Journal of Preventive Medicine 15:81–84, 1998.

Foxman, B., and D. W. Edington. The accuracy of health risk appraisal in predicting mortality. American Journal of Public Health 77:971–974, 1987.

Greenberg, R. A. Mass survey detected lung cancer in Connecticut, 1949–1953. Connecticut State Medical Journal 20:857–863, 1956.

Kirscht, J. P. Process and measurement issues in health risk appraisal (editorial). American Journal of Public Health 79:1598–1599, 1989.

Krahn, M. D., et al. Screening for prostate cancer: a decision analytic view. Journal of the American Medical Association 272:773–780, 1994.

Litwin, L. S., et al. Quality of life outcomes in men tested for prostate cancer. Journal of the American Medical Association 273:129–135, 1995.

Olsen, D. M., R. L. Kane, and P. H. Proctor. A controlled trial of multiphasic screening. New England Journal of Medicine 294:925–930, 1976.

Potosky, A. L., et al. The role of increasing detection in the rising incidence of prostate cancer. Journal of the American Medical Association 273:548–552, 1995.

Robbins, L. C., and J. Hall. How to Practice Prospective Medicine. Indianapolis, Ind., Methodist Hospital of Indiana, 1970.

Roberts, N. J., et al. Mortality among males in periodic health examination programs. New England Journal of Medicine 281:20–24, 1969.

Ross, K. S., et al. Comparative efficiency of prostate-specific antigen screening strategies for prostate cancer detection. Journal of the American Medical Association 284:1399–1405, 2000.

Schoenbach, V. J. Appraising health risk appraisal (editorial). American Journal of Public Health 77:409–411, 1987.

Schor, S. S., et al. An evaluation of the periodic health examination. Annals of Internal Medicine 61:999–1005, 1964.

Siegel, G. S. Periodic Health Examinations: Abstracts from the Literature. Washington, D. C., US Department of Health, Education, and Welfare, 1963.

Small, E. J., and D. M. Reese. An update on prostate cancer research. Current Opinion in Oncology 12:265–272, 2000.

Smith, K. W., S. M. McKinlay, and J. B. McKinlay. The reliability of health risk appraisals: a field trial of four instruments. American Journal of Public Health 79:1603–1607, 1989.

Smith, K. W., S. M. McKinlay, and B. D. Thorington. The validity of health risk appraisal instruments for assessing coronary heart disease risk. American Journal of Public Health 77:419–424, 1987.

Society for Prospective Medicine: Managing Health Care, Measuring Lives: Expanding the Definition and Scope of Health Risk Appraisal. Thirty-First Annual Meeting of the Society for Prospective Medicine, New Orleans, April 2–3, 1995.

Spark, R. The case against regular physicals. New York Times Magazine, July 25, 1976.

Spitzer, W. O., and B. P. Brown. Unanswered questions about the periodic health examination. Annals of Internal Medicine 83:257–263, 1975.

US Preventive Services Task Force. Guide to Clinical Preventive Services, 2nd ed. Baltimore, Williams & Wilkins, 1996.

Selected Readings

Brownson, R. C., P. L. Remington, and J. R. Davis (editors). Chronic Disease Epidemiology and Control. Washington, D. C., American Public Health Association, 1993.

Canadian Task Force on the Periodic Physical Examination. The periodic health examination. Canadian Medical Association Journal 121:1193–1254, 1979.

US Preventive Services Task Force. Guide to Clinical Preventive Services, 2nd ed. Baltimore, Williams & Wilkins, 1996.

18 Methods of Tertiary Prevention

Methods of tertiary prevention are designed to limit the physical and social consequences of an injury or disease after it has occurred or become symptomatic. There are two basic categories of tertiary prevention. The first, called **disability limitation,** has the goal of halting the progress of the disease or limiting the damage caused by an injury. In fact, this category of tertiary prevention is probably better thought of as "the prevention of further impairment" (Leavell and Clark 1965). The second category, called **rehabilitation,** focuses on reducing the social disability produced by a given level of impairment, both by strengthening the patient's remaining functions and by helping the patient learn to function in alternative ways. Disability limitation and rehabilitation should ordinarily be initiated at the same time—i.e., when the disease is detected or the injury occurs—but the emphasis on one or the other depends on factors such as the type and stage of disease, the type of injury, and available methods of treatment.

■ OPPORTUNITIES FOR PREVENTION

The first sign of an illness is often an excellent opportunity to initiate methods of tertiary prevention. The sooner disability limitation (therapy) is begun, the greater the chance of preventing significant impairment. In fact, in the case of infectious diseases such as tuberculosis and sexually transmitted diseases, early treatment of a health problem in one person may prevent transmission of the disease to other persons and therefore constitute primary prevention of that health problem in others. Similarly, early treatment of alcoholism or drug addiction in one family member may prevent social and emotional problems, including codependency, from developing in other family members.

Symptomatic illness can guide physicians to those persons most in need of preventive efforts. In this sense, the symptoms function in a manner somewhat similar to screening by defining especially needy individuals. People may not be convinced by a preventive message when they feel well, but when they become symptomatic, they frequently are alerted for the first time to the importance of changing their diet, behavior, or environment. For example, a person who is at risk for coronary artery disease will usually be more open to changes in diet and exercise after experiencing angina pectoris or myocardial infarction. The onset of symptoms, therefore, may provide a window of opportunity for health promotion to prevent progression of the disease. Such opportunities are often called "teachable moments." Primary health care personnel are in the most strategic position to initiate preventive measures in symptomatic patients.

■ DISABILITY LIMITATION

Most medical or surgical treatment of symptomatic disease is directed at preventing or minimizing impairment over the short and long run. This is true, for example, of coronary angioplasty and coronary artery bypass grafting, which are aimed at both extending life and improving function. There is, however, a useful distinction between therapy and symptomatic stage prevention. Whereas **therapy** seeks to undo the threat or damage from an existing disease (e.g., coronary artery disease), **symptomatic stage prevention** attempts to halt or limit the future progression of disease. The strategies of symptomatic stage prevention are taken both from primary prevention (e.g., modification of diet, behavior, and environment) and from secondary prevention (e.g., frequent screening for incipient complications, followed by treatment when complications are discovered).

In this section of the chapter, coronary artery disease, hyperlipidemia, hypertension, and diabetes mellitus will be used to illustrate how methods of disability limitation can be applied to patients with chronic diseases. The emphasis will be on symptomatic stage prevention. Although a brief outline of therapy will be given, a detailed discussion of medical and surgical treatment is beyond the scope of this book.

Coronary Artery Disease

If coronary occlusion has already occurred, the goal is to prevent death and permanent damage. Whether or not coronary occlusion has occurred, the goal is also to slow, stop, or even reverse the progression of the disease process.

Risk Factors

Male Gender. Men are much more likely than women to show signs of atherosclerotic heart disease before the age of 60 years. In postmenopausal women, the rate of coronary artery disease rises as rapidly as that in men, but it never fully catches up on an age-specific basis. Nevertheless, in the USA, coronary artery disease is the leading cause of death in women as well as in men.

Family History of Myocardial Infarction. If an individual has a parent or sibling who had a myocardial infarction before the age of 60 years, the individual is at increased risk for coronary artery disease, unless the relatives had behavioral risk factors (such as cigarette smoking) that are not shared by the individual.

Cigarette Smoking. Smoking accelerates blood clotting, increases blood carbon monoxide levels, and causes a reduction in the delivery of oxygen. In addition, nicotine is vasoconstrictive. The age-related risk of myocardial infarction in smokers is approximately twice as high as that in nonsmokers. For those who stop smoking, the excess risk drops fairly quickly and appears to be minimal after a year of nonsmoking.

Diabetes Mellitus. The age-related risk of myocardial infarction in diabetics is about twice as high as that in nondiabetics. This risk may be attenuated by tight glycemic control, use of angiotensin-converting enzyme (ACE) inhibitors, and modification of other risk factors.

Hypertension. Severe hypertension (systolic blood pressure $\geq$ 195 mm Hg) approximately quadruples the risk of cardiovascular disease in middle-aged men (Breslow 1978). Lesser degrees of hypertension appear to increase the risk to a smaller degree.

Sedentary Life-Style. It appears that at least 20 minutes of vigorous exercise (fast walking or better) at least 3 times per week reduces the risk of cardiovascular disease. There is still debate regarding how large the negative impact of a sedentary life-style is on the risk of myocardial infarction. The uncertainty occurs because it is difficult to design observational

studies that completely avoid the potential bias of self-selection (i.e., people with incipient heart disease may have cues that tell them to avoid such exercise). Nevertheless, there is increasing emphasis on the large potential benefits of even modest physical activity.

Excess Weight. In people who are overweight, the risk for coronary artery disease depends on how the body fat is distributed. When fat is distributed in the hips and legs (giving the body the shape of a pear), there does not appear to be an increased risk of cardiovascular disease. In contrast, when fat is found primarily in the abdominal cavity (giving the body the shape of an apple, a shape more common in men than in women), the fat appears to be more metabolically active and the risk of cardiovascular disease is increased. This is not surprising, because fat mobilized from the omentum goes directly to the liver, which is the center of the body's lipid metabolism. Moreover, centrally located body fat is implicated in the insulin resistance syndrome and is associated with increased sympathetic tone and hypertension.

It is unclear what effect weight reduction per se has on the risk of heart disease. Some studies have suggested that alternating dieting and nondieting ("weight cycling") is a risk factor in itself (Lissner et al. 1991), but other studies have questioned this conclusion (Wing, Jeffery, and Hellerstedt 1995). Nevertheless, expert opinion supports a benefit from weight loss.

Hyperlipidemia. The risk of coronary artery disease is increased in patients with hyperlipidemia. As discussed below, the lipid profile is important and must be interpreted in light of the age, gender, and clinical history of the patient.

Interaction of Risk Factors

The best data on the risk factors for coronary heart disease are derived from the Framingham Study (see Dawber, Meadors, and Moore 1951; see also Breslow 1978). As discussed earlier and outlined in Table 5–2, data from the Framingham Study suggest that multiple risk factors interact in a synergistic manner. For example, the risk that a 45-year-old man would have cardiovascular disease (mostly coronary heart disease) within 8 years varied greatly, depending on whether none, one, or all of the following risk factors were present: (1) smoking, (2) glucose intolerance, (3) hypertrophy of the left ventricle, (4) severe hypertension (systolic blood pressure $\geq$ 195 mm Hg), and (5) high cholesterol level ($\geq$ 335 mg/dL).

As Table 5–2 shows, if none of these five risk factors was present, the 8-year risk was 2.2%, based on age and gender. In contrast, if all of the five risk factors were present, the risk was 77.8%—i.e., more than 35 times as high. Note that if one simply added the five individual risk percents, the expected 8-year risk would have been 3.8% + 3.9% + 6.0% + 8.4% + 8.5%, for a total of 30.6%. The observed 8-year risk, however, was 77.8%, which was more than 2.5 times as high as would be expected by simply adding the five individual risks. This suggests that the five factors (or unmeasured factors that vary with them) act synergistically to produce the final risk for heart disease.

Therapy

Obviously, the immediate and long-term care of patients with symptomatic coronary artery disease will depend on the extent to which the disease has progressed when the patient seeks or is placed under medical care. Even in the presence of severe disease, there may be little or no warning before myocardial infarction occurs. After acute medical and surgical care is provided, efforts at symptomatic stage prevention also begin.

Symptomatic Stage Prevention

The evaluation of risk factors and the development of a plan to reduce the risk of adverse cardiac events are necessary for every patient with symptomatic cardiac disease. If the patient has already had a myocardial infarction and undergone bypass surgery, the goals include preventing restenosis of the bypass grafts and slowing the progression of atherosclerosis elsewhere.

Behavior Modification. Patients should be questioned about cigarette smoking, exercise, and eating habits, all of which affect the risks of heart disease. Smokers should be encouraged to stop smoking (see Chapter 15 and Box 15–2), and all patients should receive counseling about the types and appropriate levels of exercise to pursue as well as about nutrition. Hospitalized patients should be placed on a low-fat, "heart healthy" diet and encouraged to continue this type of diet when they return home.

Other Measures. The assessment and appropriate management of other known risk factors, such as hyperlipidemia, hypertension, and diabetes mellitus, are essential for reducing the risk of adverse cardiac events in patients with symptomatic coronary artery disease. Each of these problems is the focus of a subsequent section of this chapter.

Hyperlipidemia

Hyperlipidemia is a general term used to describe an abnormal elevation in one or more of the lipids found in the blood. The **complete lipid profile** provides information on the following: total cholesterol (TC), high-density lipoprotein (HDL), low-density lipoprotein (LDL), very low density lipoprotein (VLDL), and triglycerides.

The **TC** level is equal to the sum of the HDL, LDL, and VLDL levels:

$$TC = HDL + LDL + VLDL$$
$$= (HDL) + (LDL) + (triglycerides/5)$$

HDL, the "good" cholesterol, acts as a scavenger of other types of cholesterol. **LDL** is one of the "bad" cholesterols, elevated levels of which are associated with increased cardiovascular risk. A high LDL level may be a necessary precursor for atherogenesis, but much of the damage may be due to oxidative modification of the LDL, making it more atherogenic (see Gotto and Pownall 1999). **VLDL,** another "bad" cholesterol, is carried in the **triglyceride fraction.**

Assessment

A variety of index measures have been proposed to assess the need for intervention and to monitor the success of preventive measures.

TC Level. Some screening programs measure only the TC level. In adults without known atherosclerotic disease, a level under 200 mg/dL does not suggest the need for action, although the level should be checked every 5 years. A level between 200 and 239 mg/dL is considered borderline high, and a fasting lipid profile is recommended, with action determined as below. If the TC level is 240 mg/dL or higher, diagnosis based on a fasting lipid profile is urgently needed, and dietary and life-style changes should be initiated; in addition, lipid-lowering therapy should be considered (see National Cholesterol Education Program 1994; Centers for Disease Control and Prevention 2000).

HDL Level. The higher the HDL level is, the better it is. The minimum acceptable HDL level is 50 mg/dL in women or 35 mg/dL in men. An HDL level under 35 mg/dL is of special concern if the LDL level or the triglyceride level is high (see below).

LDL Level. In an adult without known atherosclerotic disease, an LDL level of less than 130 mg/dL is considered acceptable, and another lipid profile is recommended within 5 years. If the LDL is borderline elevated (130–159 mg/dL) and the individual is without other risk factors, the lipid profile may be repeated within 1 year. However, if two or more other risk factors are present, dietary and life-style changes should be recommended. If the LDL level is 160 mg/dL or above, dietary and life-style changes should be recommended and lipid-lowering therapy considered.

In the presence of demonstrated atherosclerotic disease, the criteria are tightened, and an LDL level of greater than 100 mg/dL should lead to institution of dietary and life-style changes and to treatment with lipid-lowering medications. Some specialists pay special attention to the ratio of the TC level to the HDL level (see National Cholesterol Education Program 1994; Gotto and Pownall 1999).

Triglyceride Level. The preferred level of triglycerides is under 150 mg/dL. Levels over 200 mg/dL are reason for concern.

VLDL Level. The VLDL can be determined by dividing the triglyceride level by 5.

Total Non-HDL Cholesterol Level. Frick et al. (1987) have defined primary dyslipidemia as the presence of a non-HDL cholesterol level equal to or greater than 200 mg/dL in two successive measurements. This index is useful because it looks at the total contribution of cholesterol fractions currently considered harmful, and it would seem that minimizing the harmful types of cholesterol is a reasonable treatment goal (see Gotto and Pownall 1999).

TC/HDL Ratio. Some investigators monitor the ratio of TC to HDL. Using this approach, Arntzenius et al. (1985) reported that angiograms in patients with a TC/HDL ratio of greater than 6.9 showed progression of coronary atherosclerosis during the study time, whereas angiograms in patients with a lower TC/HDL ratio did not show progression. Currently, a ratio of less than 4.5 is recommended if atherosclerotic disease is absent, while a ratio of less than 3.5 is recommended if atherosclerotic disease is present (see Gotto and Pownall 1999).

Triglyceride-HDL Relationship. Research suggests that the combination of an HDL level below 35 mg/dL and a triglyceride level above 200 mg/dL places an individual at high risk for coronary artery disease, and the possibility of a genetic hyperlipidemia should be considered (see Consensus Development Conference 1992). This pattern is commonly associated with insulin resistance.

Homocysteine Level. The hypothesis that an elevated homocysteine level increases the risk of atherogenesis is supported by a number of observational studies. Although some experts have recommended the use of dietary supplements of folic acid, pyridoxine, or vitamin B_{12} to lower homocysteine levels, no clinical trials have been conducted to determine the therapeutic benefit of these measures. Some believe that homocysteine is merely a marker for the true culprit, perhaps a low level of folic acid (see Gotto and Pownall 1999).

Therapy and Symptomatic Stage Prevention

Any primary care physician must be able to treat patients with a moderately elevated TC level or abnormal lipid level and should be aware of the therapeutic options. Persons with severe lipid abnormalities, however, probably should be treated by specialists.

In the primary prevention of coronary artery disease, a trial of life-style modifications (dietary changes, increased exercise, and smoking cessation) should usually be attempted before a lipid-lowering medication, such as an HMG-CoA reductase inhibitor ("statin" drug), is prescribed. When coronary artery disease becomes symptomatic, life-style modifications and drug treatment should both be started as soon as possible.

Hypertension

According to the Joint National Committee on Prevention, Detection, Evaluation, and Treatment of High Blood Pressure, hypertension is defined as an average systolic blood pressure of 140 mm Hg or higher or an average diastolic blood pressure of 90 mm Hg or higher after blood pressure is measured on three different occasions in a person who is not

acutely ill and not taking antihypertensive medications (see National Institutes of Health 1997). These are the levels that are high enough for treatment to bring proven benefits. Based on this definition, more than 50 million people in the USA have hypertension. Among the groups at increased risk are pregnant women, women taking estrogens or oral contraceptives, and African-Americans. Children are also at risk for hypertension.

Assessment

Hypertension may be detected by community or occupational screening, by individual case finding (e.g., when a person seeks care for dental problems or for medical problems that are unrelated to hypertension), or when a person develops one or more common complications of hypertension, such as visual problems, early renal failure, congestive heart failure, stroke, or myocardial infarction. Over the last 20 years, the risk of mortality from coronary artery disease and stroke in hypertensive individuals has dropped by 50% or more as a result of early detection and improved management of high blood pressure.

Table 18–1 provides information regarding the evaluation and staging of hypertension, based on average systolic and diastolic blood pressures. In addition to listing the ranges for optimal, normal, and high normal pressures, the table shows the ranges for three stages of hypertension.

Therapy and Symptomatic Stage Prevention

After the stage of hypertension has been determined, the Joint National Committee on Prevention, Detec-

TABLE 18–1 Evaluation of Blood Pressure and Staging of Hypertension, Based on Average Systolic and Diastolic Blood Pressures in Persons Who Are Not Acutely Ill and Are Not Taking Antihypertensive Medications*

Systolic Blood Pressure (mm Hg)	Diastolic Blood Pressure (mm Hg)	Interpretation
< 120	< 80	Optimal blood pressure
120–129	80–84	Normal blood pressure
130–139	85–89	High normal blood pressure
140–159	90–99	Stage 1 (mild) hypertension
160–179	100–109	Stage 2 (moderate) hypertension
≥ 180	≥ 110	Stage 3 (severe) hypertension

Source of data: National Institutes of Health. The Sixth Report of the Joint National Committee on Prevention, Detection, Evaluation, and Treatment of High Blood Pressure. Publication No. (NIH)98-4080. Bethesda, Md., National Institutes of Health, 1997.
*The highest stage for which either part of the blood pressure qualifies is taken as the stage of hypertension. For example, if the systolic blood pressure is 165 mm Hg and the diastolic blood pressure is 115 mm Hg, the stage is 3 (severe).

tion, Evaluation, and Treatment of High Blood Pressure recommends the following actions: Individuals with **optimal or normal blood pressure** should be monitored at 2-year intervals. Those with **high normal blood pressure** should be counseled about life-style changes and monitored at 1-year intervals. In those with **stage 1 (mild) hypertension,** counseling should be given and the blood pressure confirmed within 2 months; also within this period, treatment, if indicated, should be instituted. In those with **stage 2 (moderate) hypertension,** evaluation and treatment should be instituted within 1 month. In those with **stage 3 (severe) hypertension,** evaluation and treatment should be instituted immediately or within 1 week, based on clinical judgment. During evaluation, the presence or absence of target organ damage should be noted, because any stage of hypertension is more severe if there is evidence of such damage.

Most hypertension is classified as **essential hypertension,** meaning that no known underlying specific cause exists. **Nonessential hypertension** is due to specific, treatable causes, such as renal artery stenosis or tumors of the adrenal medulla. The specific causes of hypertension should be ruled out before measures to reduce hypertension are started.

Symptomatic stage prevention and therapy are aimed at reducing the systolic blood pressure to under 140 mm Hg, reducing the diastolic blood pressure to under 90 mm Hg, and monitoring patients to make sure that these levels are maintained. The goal is to prevent damage to the organs at risk from hypertension. For patients with any stage of hypertension, the following life-style modifications are indicated: weight reduction, increased physical activity, and institution of a healthy diet. In the Dietary Approaches to Stop Hypertension (DASH) trials, investigators found that instituting a diet that was rich in fruits, vegetables, grains, and nonfat dairy products was associated with a reduction in systolic blood pressure, especially if sodium intake was restricted to no more than 1200 mg per day (see Svetkey et al. 1999). Other dietary measures to reduce blood pressure include the moderation of alcohol intake and the institution of an increase in the intake of potassium, calcium, and magnesium. Smokers should be encouraged to stop smoking, not because it directly influences the blood pressure but because smoking cessation will reduce the risk of damage to many of the same target organs that hypertension can damage.

For patients whose blood pressure levels remain high despite these life-style modifications, use of one or more antihypertensive medications is indicated. Because most hypertension is asymptomatic, patients must be made aware of the importance of taking medications and the risks of stopping treatment. Many of the antihypertensive medications prescribed in the past caused dizziness (because of suppression of vasal reflexes), impotence, and other side effects that discouraged patients from using them. Fortunately, current medications have fewer side effects than previous medications and are more convenient to use (e.g., need only be taken once a day).

Among the major classes of effective antihypertensive agents are diuretics, beta blockers, angiotensin-converting enzyme (ACE) inhibitors, angiotensin receptor blockers, calcium channel blockers, alpha blockers, and vasodilators. The wide range of choice should be used to develop a treatment plan that is satisfactory to the patient.

In controlled clinical trials, thiazide diuretics and beta blockers have been shown to reduce cardiovascular disease by reducing blood pressure, so there is an argument for starting treatment of hypertension with one of these types of drugs. Thiazide diuretics are a good choice for most adults but should be used with caution in the elderly. Beta blockers may be a good choice for patients who have a history of myocardial infarction or angina pectoris but no history of a conduction abnormality. The use of beta blockers is contraindicated, however, in patients with conduction abnormalities, asthma, or chronic obstructive pulmonary disease. In the Heart Outcomes Prevention Evaluation (HOPE) trials, investigators found clear evidence that the use of ACE inhibitors can prevent deaths caused by myocardial infarction and stroke and can reduce the overall rate of mortality in many groups of high-risk cardiac patients (see Yusuf et al. 2000). ACE inhibitors should not, however, be used in patients who might become pregnant or in patients who have renal artery stenosis.

Diabetes Mellitus

In the USA, about 700,000 people have **type I diabetes mellitus,** a disease that requires lifelong treatment with insulin and places them at higher risk for a variety of cardiovascular, renal, and other serious complications. Up to 20 million people now have **type II diabetes mellitus,** and the number of persons with this milder form of diabetes continues to rise. Type II diabetes is often found in association with obesity and **insulin resistance.**

Much can be done to prevent target organ damage from diabetes, as was demonstrated in the Diabetes Control and Complications Trial (DCCT) and the United Kingdom Prospective Diabetes Study (UKPDS). In patients with type I diabetes, the DCCT showed that improved control of blood glucose levels significantly reduced the incidence of microvascular disease (retinopathy, nephropathy, and neuropathy) and also reduced the incidence of macrovascular disease (atherosclerosis of large blood vessels, myocardial infarction, angina pectoris, strokes, aneurysms, and amputations of the distal lower extremity) (see DCCT Research Group 1993; Santiago 1993). Similarly, in patients with type II diabetes, the UKPDS found that in general the lower the average glycemic level was in patients, the fewer the complications that the patients experienced (Stratton et al. 2000).

Members of the DCCT intervention group had to self-monitor their blood glucose levels, keep detailed records of insulin dosages and glucose levels, regulate their dietary intake and level of insulin based on the results of self-monitoring, and be actively involved in other aspects of their own care, with the supervision and support of physicians and other professionals. Although the risk of hypoglycemic episodes was 3 times as high in the intervention group as in the control group, no serious sequelae of hypoglycemia occurred in the intervention group, whereas one death from hypoglycemia occurred in the control group. Weight gain was a common side effect of tight diabetic control.

Based on the results of the DCCT, tight control (defined as control as good as that obtained in the DCCT) may be beneficial for patients who are willing to participate actively in their own care. Tight control should be supplemented with frequent examination of the eyegrounds and with laser treatment of microvascular lesions when indicated. The use of ACE inhibitors has proved valuable not only in controlling hypertension but also in reducing the incidence of microalbuminuria and delaying the onset of diabetes-induced renal failure.

All patients with type I or type II diabetes should be advised of the need for moderate to high levels of physical activity and should receive individual counseling about nutrition. In addition, they should be informed of the common complications of diabetes and the importance of contacting their physician if they note early symptoms of any of these complications.

An area of increasing focus is the possibility of using some of the newer oral hypoglycemic agents to treat insulin resistance before it develops into frank type II diabetes. Current interest centers particularly on biguanides and thiazolidinediones, which are more effective when used in combination than when used alone. Moreover, there is now some evidence that ACE inhibitors may retard the progression from insulin resistance to diabetes. This approach to preventing type II diabetes is developing rapidly.

■ REHABILITATION

Rehabilitation, occurring as it does after disease has already caused damage, may seem to take place when there is nothing left to prevent. However, as mentioned at the beginning of the chapter, the goal of rehabilitation is to reduce the social disability produced by a given level of impairment, both by strengthening the patient's remaining functions and by helping the patient learn to function in alternative ways.

General Approach to Rehabilitation

Rehabilitation must begin in the early phases of treatment if it is to be maximally effective. For example, in patients who have suffered a stroke, head injury, hip fracture, or other problem that makes them temporarily immobile, it is important to keep joints flexible from the beginning of the illness or injury, so that weakened but recovering muscles do not have to overcome stiffened joints. Beginning rehabilitation efforts early also tends to increase the cooperation of patients and their family members by convincing them that improvement is expected.

The most effective rehabilitation program is one tailored to meet the physical, emotional, and occupational needs of the individual patient. There is often a **rehabilitation counselor** to coordinate the efforts of a team of specialists. **Physical therapists** work to strengthen weakened muscles, to increase joint movement and flexibility, and to teach patients ways of accomplishing routine tasks despite their disabilities. These tasks, referred to as **activities of daily living,** include feeding oneself, transferring from bed to chair and back, grooming, controlling the bladder and bowels, bathing, dressing, walking on a level surface, and going up and down stairs. **Speech therapists** seek to improve the ability of patients to articulate their thoughts following a stroke or head injury that produces aphasia. **Occupational therapists** evaluate the occupational abilities of patients, counsel them regarding suitable types of work, provide them with job training or retraining, and assist them in obtaining a suitable job. Usually, the most cost-effective efforts are those designed to help a patient return to his or her previous place of employment and obtain a new or modified job there. **Psychiatric or emotional counseling** may be important, as may **spiritual counseling** by a minister, priest, or rabbi.

Categories of Disability

Disability is a socially defined concept, but it has very practical implications in terms of financial support. There are several categories used in most states for reimbursement of workers who have job-related injuries or illnesses covered under a workers' compensation program: (1) **permanent total disability,** e.g., the loss of two limbs or of vision in both eyes; (2) **permanent partial disability,** e.g., the loss of one limb or of vision in one eye; (3) **temporary total disability,** e.g., a fractured arm in a truck driver; (4) **temporary partial disability,** e.g., a fractured arm in an elementary school teacher; and (5) **death.** In these categories, benefits for disabled persons (or for their surviving family in the case of death) are usually set by law according to a fixed schedule. Less well defined illnesses and injuries, such as repetitive motion or back injuries, are usually compensated by a mixture of financial and vocational rehabilitation benefits, including counseling, retraining, and even job placement (see LaDou 1997).

A disability is temporary if it is expected that a person will return to his or her job within a time period defined by statute. If the disability is job-related, the person will be partially reimbursed for lost wages and fully reimbursed for the costs of medical care from the state workers' compensation fund (see Chapters 19 and 21).

A person with a permanent disability is reimbursed at a fixed rate for the rest of his or her life or for a defined period of time. The rate varies from state to state (as stipulated by law) but is based on the type of disability and degree of function lost (as determined by a physician).

■ SUMMARY

The goal of tertiary prevention is to limit the physical and social consequences of an injury or disease after it has occurred or become symptomatic. The two major categories of tertiary prevention are disability limitation and rehabilitation.

Methods of disability limitation include therapy, which seeks to undo the threat or damage from an existing disease, and symptomatic stage prevention, which attempts to halt or limit the future progression of disease. The strategies of symptomatic stage prevention are taken both from primary prevention (e.g., modification of diet, behavior, and environment) and from secondary prevention (e.g., frequent screening for incipient complications, followed by treatment when complications are discovered). The effective management of chronic diseases such as coronary artery disease, hyperlipidemia, hypertension, and diabetes mellitus requires a combination of therapy and symptomatic stage prevention. This approach can also be used in the management of many other diseases, including stroke, chronic obstructive pulmonary disease, arthritis, and some cancers and infectious diseases.

Rehabilitation should begin in the early stages of treatment. Depending on the needs of the patient, the rehabilitation team may include a rehabilitation counselor, physical therapist, speech therapist, occupational therapist, and psychiatric, emotional, or spiritual counselor. Under most state laws concerning workers' compensation, several categories of job-related illnesses or injuries are recognized: permanent total disability, permanent partial disability, temporary total disability, temporary partial disability, and death. The goal of rehabilitation for workers, whether their impairment is temporary or permanent, is to minimize the social and occupational consequences of the impairment.

Although it might seem that the opportunity for prevention is lost when a disease appears or an injury occurs, this is often not the case. The appearance of symptoms or the threat of severe complications may lead patients to take an active interest in their health status, seek the health care that they need, and make positive changes in their environment, diet, and life-style.

■ QUESTIONS

Directions (Items 1–10). Each of the numbered items or incomplete statements in this section is followed by answers or by completions of the statement. Select the ONE lettered answer or completion that is BEST in each case. Correct answers and explanations are given at the end of the chapter.

1. Which of the following is an example of tertiary prevention?
   - (A) Hospice care
   - (B) Occupational therapy following a stroke (cerebrovascular accident)
   - (C) Postexposure prophylaxis for rabies
   - (D) The treatment of essential hypertension
   - (E) The use of nasal decongestants

2. Under what circumstances can primary and tertiary prevention be achieved concurrently?
   - (A) Never, because primary and tertiary prevention are mutually exclusive
   - (B) When a patient is treated for a hip fracture
   - (C) When a patient is treated for active tuberculosis
   - (D) When a patient is treated for cystitis
   - (E) When a patient is treated for myocardial infarction

3. How much higher is the age-specific risk of myocardial infarction in smokers than in nonsmokers?
   - (A) 2 times as high
   - (B) 3 times as high
   - (C) 4 times as high
   - (D) 5 times as high
   - (E) 7 times as high

4. The desirable level of low-density lipoprotein (LDL) cholesterol varies according to
   - (A) age
   - (B) gender
   - (C) the body mass index
   - (D) the level of high-density lipoprotein (HDL) cholesterol
   - (E) the presence or absence of symptomatic coronary artery disease

5. A disadvantage of using only the total cholesterol level to predict the risk of cardiovascular disease is that
   - (A) high-density lipoprotein (HDL) is included in the measure
   - (B) the ratio of low-density lipoprotein (LDL) to very low density lipoprotein (VLDL) is unknown
   - (C) total cholesterol levels are estimated rather than measured
   - (D) total cholesterol levels do not correlate with risk
   - (E) unlike triglyceride levels, total cholesterol levels vary with meals

6. Dietary intake of which of the following substances is inversely associated with blood pressure?
   - (A) Alcohol
   - (B) Calcium
   - (C) Insoluble fiber
   - (D) Polyunsaturated fat
   - (E) Sodium

7. Which of the following antihypertensive medications has been shown to reduce the risk of cardiovascular disease?
   (A) Alpha blockers
   (B) Angiotensin receptor blockers
   (C) Calcium channel blockers
   (D) Thiazide diuretics
   (E) Vasodilators

8. The Diabetes Control and Complications Trial demonstrated that
   (A) microvascular complications of diabetes are independent of glycemic control
   (B) monitoring the urine glucose level is more cost-effective than monitoring the blood glucose level
   (C) only macrovascular complications of diabetes are preventable
   (D) the risk of hypoglycemia outweighs the benefit of tight glycemic control
   (E) tight glycemic control delays the onset of microvascular complications

9. Microalbuminuria of diabetes is best treated with
   (A) a sulfonylurea
   (B) an angiotensin-converting enzyme (ACE) inhibitor
   (C) dialysis
   (D) insulin
   (E) life-style modifications

10. In the USA, preventive care for cerebrovascular accidents
    (A) includes the restoration of functional ability through physical therapy
    (B) is generally ineffective, as the incidence is rising
    (C) is generally ineffective, because risk factors for cerebrovascular accidents are largely unknown
    (D) relies predominantly on pharmacotherapy for hyperlipidemia
    (E) relies predominantly on screening for carotid stenosis

■ ANSWERS AND EXPLANATIONS

1. **The answer is B: occupational therapy following a stroke (cerebrovascular accident).** Tertiary prevention is the prevention of disease progression and complications that might result in further impairment, and it is also rehabilitation to reverse impairment and disability. Occupational therapy is a form of rehabilitation directed at preventing disability and is therefore an example of tertiary prevention. The treatment of essential hypertension is best considered a form of secondary prevention, although one might argue that it constitutes primary prevention of ischemic heart disease or cardiomyopathy. Postexposure prophylaxis for rabies is secondary prevention. The use of nasal decongestants is a way of treating symptoms and not truly a preventive measure, although it may play a role in preventing sinusitis. Hospice care is intended to provide comfort during the late stages of terminal illness and does not specifically have the goal of preventing disease progression.

2. **The answer is C: when a patient is treated for active tuberculosis.** The management of communicable diseases, such as tuberculosis, offers a unique opportunity for prevention. When the patient with active disease is treated, the progression of disease and impairment are prevented in the patient; this is tertiary prevention. At the same time, the spread of disease to the patient's various social contacts is prevented; this is primary prevention.

3. **The answer is A: 2 times as high.** Multiple data sources suggest that smoking raises the risk of age-specific cardiovascular mortality by a factor of approximately 2 (see Bartecchi, Mackenzie, and Schrier 1994). Cigarette smoking is generally considered the most important cause of preventable death and disease in the USA.

4. **The answer is E: the presence or absence of symptomatic coronary artery disease.** According to a report issued by the National Cholesterol Education Program (1994), low-density lipoprotein (LDL) levels should be below 160 mg/dL in all adults, even in the absence of other risk factors for coronary artery disease. In those without coronary disease but with two or more other risk factors, LDL levels should be maintained below 130 mg/dL. In those with coronary disease, LDL levels should be maintained below 100 mg/dL.

5. **The answer is A: high-density lipoprotein (HDL) is included in the measure.** HDL levels are inversely associated with the risk of cardiovascular disease. All other moieties contributing to the total cholesterol level are associated directly, to varying degrees, with this risk. Therefore, the total cholesterol level includes several positive correlates and one negative correlate of heart disease risk, and this reduces its utility. The ratio of total cholesterol to HDL "purifies" the measure, so that a positive correlate of cardiovascular disease risk is produced (see National Cholesterol Education Program 1994).

6. **The answer is B: calcium.** The intake of alcohol and sodium is positively associated with hypertension, but the intake of insoluble fiber and polyunsaturated fat does not seem to have any appreciable association with the disease. The intake of calcium has been inversely associated with hypertension in some studies, as has the intake of potassium, magnesium, and soluble fiber (Stamler et al. 1987; National High Blood Pressure Education Program Working Group 1993).

7. **The answer is D: thiazide diuretics.** Three classes of antihypertensive medication have been shown to reduce the rate of cardiovascular and cerebrovascular morbidity and mortality: thiazide diuretics, beta blockers, and angiotensin-converting enzyme inhibitors. Of these, only thiazide diuretics appear among the choices for this question. The other medications listed (alpha blockers, angiotensin receptor blockers, calcium channel blockers, and vasodilators) are effective in treating hypertension but have not been shown in clinical trials to reduce complications and mortality rates. In 1995, there was a discussion in the lay press regarding an association between the use of short-acting dihydropyridine calcium channel blockers and increased mortality rates (Altman 1995; Furberg, Psaty, and Meyer 1995). However, there is no evidence of such an association with the longer-acting calcium channel blockers generally preferred in the management of hypertension.

8. **The answer is E: tight glycemic control delays the onset of microvascular complications.** In the 1990s, the Diabetes Control and Complications Trial was designed specifically to test the hypothesis that tight glycemic control could forestall microvascular complications of diabetes. The trial demonstrated that the closer to normal that serum glucose and glycohemoglobin levels were maintained, the less progression there was in such microvascular complications as retinopathy and nephropathy (see Diabetes Control and Complications Trial Research Group 1993). Greater effort is now devoted to achieving nearly normal control of serum glucose levels whenever this is feasible, although the risk of hypoglycemia is raised by such an effort.

9. **The answer is B: an angiotensin-converting enzyme (ACE) inhibitor.** Before renal function begins to decline as a result of diabetic nephropathy, there is a period during which glomerular filtration actually increases because a high osmotic load is delivered to the glomerulus. The renal hyperfunction is associated with microalbuminuria (microscopic albumin spillage in urine) and presages a decline in creatinine clearance. Evidence is now substantial that ACE inhibitors attenuate renal hyperfunction in diabetes, mitigate the associated microscopic proteinuria, and slow the subsequent decline in glomerular filtration (Lewis et al. 1993; Ravid et al. 1993; Viberti et al. 1994). Sulfonylureas and insulin may indirectly slow the progression of nephropathy by providing tight glycemic control. Dialysis is life-sustaining once renal failure has occurred. Life-style modification may contribute to better glycemic control and thereby indirectly help in the preservation of renal function in diabetes.

10. **The answer is A: includes the restoration of functional ability through physical therapy.** As noted at the beginning of the chapter, tertiary prevention consists of rehabilitation and efforts to prevent disease progression. Physical therapy is a form of rehabilitation and a means of preventing further impairment and disability. In the USA, the incidence of cardiovascular accidents has been falling for several decades, largely owing to improved treatment of hypertension. Risk factors for cerebrovascular disease are known and discussed in the chapter; hypertension is the most important. Pharmacotherapy for hyperlipidemia appears to reduce the risk of a cardiovascular accident, but it is unlikely to be as important as the control of hypertension (DiMascio, Marchioli, and Tognoni 2000). Screening for carotid stenosis remains controversial, although evidence is available to support case-finding efforts (Hill 1998; Longstreth et al. 1998).

References Cited

Altman, L. K. Agency issues warning for drug widely used for heart disease. New York Times, September 1, 1995.

Arntzenius, A. C., et al. Diet, lipoproteins, and the progression of coronary atherosclerosis: the Leiden Intervention Trial. New England Journal of Medicine 312:805–811, 1985.

Bartecchi, C. E., T. D. Mackenzie, and R. W. Schrier. The human costs of tobacco use. New England Journal of Medicine 330:907–914, 1994.

Breslow, L. Risk factor intervention for health maintenance. Science 200:908–912, 1978.

Centers for Disease Control and Prevention. National cholesterol education month: September 2000. Morbidity and Mortality Weekly Report 49:749–750, 2000.

Consensus Development Conference. Triglyceride, High-Density Lipoprotein, and Coronary Heart Disease. Bethesda, Md., National Institutes of Health, 1992.

Dawber, T. R., G. F. Meadors, and F. E. Moore, Jr. Epidemiologic approaches to heart disease: the Framingham Study. American Journal of Public Health 41:279–286, 1951.

Diabetes Control and Complications Trial (DCCT) Research Group. The Diabetes Control and Complications Trial. New England Journal of Medicine 329:683–689, 1993.

DiMascio, R., R. Marchioli, and G. Tognoni. Cholesterol reduction and stroke occurrence: an overview of randomized clinical trials. Cerebrovascular Diseases 10:85–92, 2000.

Frick, M. H., et al. Helsinki Heart Study: primary prevention trial with gemfibrozil in middle-aged men with dyslipidemia. New England Journal of Medicine 317:1237–1245, 1987.

Furberg, C. D., B. M. Psaty, and J. V. Meyer. Nifedipine: dose-related increase in mortality in patients with coronary heart disease. Circulation 92:1326–1331, 1995.

Gotto, A. M., and H. J. Pownall. Manual of Lipid Disorders, 2nd ed. Baltimore, Williams & Wilkins, 1999.

Hill, A. B. Should patients be screened for asymptomatic carotid artery stenosis? Canadian Journal of Surgery 41:208–213, 1998.

LaDou, J. Occupational and Environmental Medicine, 2nd ed. Stamford, Conn., Appleton and Lange, 1997.

Leavell, H. R., and E. G. Clark. Preventive Medicine for the Doctor in His Community, 3rd ed. New York, McGraw-Hill Book Company, 1965.

Lewis, E. J., et al. The effect of angiotensin-converting enzyme inhibition on diabetic nephropathy. New England Journal of Medicine 329:1456–1462, 1993.

Lissner, L., et al. Variability of body weight and health outcomes in the Framingham population. New England Journal of Medicine 324:1839–1844, 1991.

Longstreth, W. T., Jr., et al. Asymptomatic internal carotid artery stenosis defined by ultrasound and the risk of subsequent stroke in the elderly: the Cardiovascular Health Study. Stroke 29:2371–2376, 1998.

National Cholesterol Education Program. The second report of the Expert Panel on Detection, Evaluation, and Treatment of High Blood Cholesterol in Adults (Adult Treatment Panel II). Circulation 89:1329–1445, 1994.

National High Blood Pressure Education Program Working Group. Primary prevention of hypertension. Archives of Internal Medicine 153:186–208, 1993.

National Institutes of Health. The Sixth Report of the Joint National Committee on Prevention, Detection, Evaluation, and Treatment of High Blood Pressure. Publication No. (NIH)98-4080. Bethesda, Md., National Institutes of Health, 1997.

Ravid, M., et al. Long-term stabilizing effect of angiotensin-converting enzyme inhibition on plasma creatinine and on proteinuria in normotensive type II diabetic patients. Annals of Internal Medicine 118:577–581, 1993.

Santiago, J. V. Lessons from the Diabetes Control and Complications Trial. Diabetes 42:1549–1554, 1993.

Stamler, R., et al. Nutritional therapy for high blood pressure: final report of a four-year randomized controlled trial, the Hypertension Control Program. Journal of the American Medical Association 257:1484–1491, 1987.

Stratton, I. M., et al. Association of glycaemia with macrovascular and microvascular complications of type II diabetes: prospective observational study. British Medical Journal 321:405–412, 2000.

Svetkey, L. P., et al. The DASH diet, sodium intake, and blood pressure trial (DASH-sodium): rationale and design. Journal of the American Dietetic Association 99(supplement 8):96–104, 1999.

Viberti, G., et al. Effect of captopril on progression to clinical proteinuria in patients with insulin-dependent diabetes mellitus and microalbuminuria. Journal of the American Medical Association 271:275–279, 1994.

Wing, R. R., R. W. Jeffery, and W. L. Hellerstedt. A prospective study of effects of weight cycling on cardiovascular risk factors. Archives of Internal Medicine 155:1416–1422, 1995.

Yusuf, S., et al. Effects of an angiotensin-converting enzyme inhibitor, ramipril, on cardiovascular events in high-risk patients. New England Journal of Medicine 342:145–153, 2000.

Selected Readings

American Heart Association. Primer in Preventive Cardiology. Dallas, American Heart Association, 1994.

Brownson, R. C., P. L. Remington, and J. R. Davis. Chronic Disease Epidemiology and Control, 2nd ed. Washington, D. C., American Public Health Association, 1998.

Diabetes Control and Complications Trial (DCCT) Research Group. The Diabetes Control and Complications Trial. New England Journal of Medicine 329:683–689, 1993.

Gotto, A. M., and H. J. Pownall. Manual of Lipid Disorders, 2nd ed. Baltimore, Williams & Wilkins, 1999.

LaDou, J. Occupational and Environmental Medicine, 2nd ed. Stamford, Conn., Appleton and Lange, 1997.

National Cholesterol Education Program. The second report of the Expert Panel on Detection, Evaluation, and Treatment of High Blood Cholesterol in Adults (Adult Treatment Panel II). Circulation 89:1329–1445, 1994.

National Institutes of Health. The Sixth Report of the Joint National Committee on Prevention, Detection, Evaluation, and Treatment of High Blood Pressure. Publication No. (NIH)98-4080. Bethesda, Md., National Institutes of Health, 1997.

19 Selected Topics in Prevention

■ MATERNAL AND CHILD HEALTH

Although efforts to prevent diseases and injuries are important throughout life, perhaps the most opportune periods for prevention are the reproductive years, infancy, and early childhood. Unfortunately, the youngest members of society act somewhat like the canaries taken into mines: they provide early warnings of health problems involving the environment, nutrition, and human behavior that ultimately will be hazardous to adults as well. This is one reason that the rates of infant mortality and deaths of children under the age of 5 years can be valuable indicators of health conditions in the general population. It is not surprising, therefore, that the first clinical spe-

cialties to emphasize preventive medicine were obstetrics and gynecology and pediatrics.

Family Planning

The opportunities for prevention begin in the preconception stage, when primary health care workers can answer questions and provide information about contraception to those who wish to plan the number of children and timing of childbirth (see Barnes 1978). The preconception period is also the time to ensure that potential mothers are in good health, are eating a healthy diet, and are taking folic acid supplements to reduce the risk for neural tube defects in the fetus (see Chapter 15).

Family planning efforts can be considered health promotion, by enabling good spacing of children, but because of the technical medical aspects of contraception, it can also be considered specific protection. Family planning is intended to enable families to meet their reproductive goals; therefore, even if family planning was perfect, it would not achieve population control (such as a zero growth rate) in a country unless the number of children desired by the people of the country was sufficiently low. For this reason, family planning should not be equated with population control, even though family planning may contribute to population control. Such control is achieved in a country only when the policy goals of that country are in agreement with the fertility goals of its people.

Prenatal Care

Prenatal care is an accepted part of good medical care (see Institute of Medicine 1988a). The benefits of prenatal care, although real, are difficult to assess because the content and the quality of prenatal care vary greatly from place to place (Klerman 1990). Ideally, prenatal care is aimed at primary, secondary, and tertiary prevention (see Barnes 1978 for guidelines).

Primary prevention includes counseling to promote good nutrition and healthful behavior, as well as referral to appropriate programs and specialists if necessary. Some women may be referred, for example, to the Women, Infants, and Children (WIC) Program, which provides food vouchers to those with low income. Others may require referral for specific programs concerning cigarette smoking, alcohol use, illegal drug use, or other behaviors that affect the health of the pregnant woman and her fetus. Good prenatal care includes the monitoring of pregnancy-related weight gain and the prescription or provision of vitamin and mineral supplements. Unfortunately, for folic acid to be of benefit, a woman must be taking this vitamin before conception and during the first weeks following conception; therefore, even the first prenatal visit is too late to begin folic acid supplements.

Secondary prevention includes screening pregnant women for syphilis, human immunodeficiency virus (HIV), and other infectious diseases, followed by confirmatory diagnosis and treatment. Although in its 1996 report the US Preventive Services Task Force (USPSTF) indicates that there is "insufficient evidence" to recommend for or against routine screening for gestational diabetes, many physicians believe that screening for this disease is worthwhile. The prevention of isoimmunization and erythroblastosis fetalis is now possible by screening for maternal antibodies to Rh (D) proteins on the fetal red blood cells, followed by the timely use of Rh (D) immune globulin when levels of these antibodies begin to rise.

Tertiary prevention includes the control of existing disease (e.g., heart disease, hypertension, and diabetes) and the control of toxemia during pregnancy.

Labor and Delivery Care

Many complications of pregnancy and delivery that can cause death or long-term damage to mother or fetus can be treated at the time of labor and delivery by expert obstetric and pediatric management. In addition, infants who are unwell at birth or whose mothers had significant risk factors can be monitored for a time and treated when necessary in a newborn special care nursery. These measures have proved their value in minimizing neonatal morbidity and mortality. While the use of technology and more invasive types of procedures (such as fetal monitoring and cesarean sections) is beneficial under some circumstances, the debate continues about whether such procedures are being overused and causing unnecessary morbidity for the mother and child.

Well Child Care

Primary prevention in well child care includes immunizations (see Chapter 16 and Table 16–2) and review and counseling regarding the child's nutrition, growth, and development.

Secondary prevention includes screening for visual and hearing problems. According to the USPSTF, 2–5% of children in the USA have amblyopia ("lazy eye") and strabismus (ocular misalignment), and many have refractive errors by the time they are 16 years old. Children should be screened for these before entering school, preferably between 3 and 4 years of age, usually by their primary care physi-

cians. Although neonates should be screened for hearing problems, the USPSTF does not recommend routine screening of schoolchildren for hearing defects (see US Preventive Services Task Force 1996).

Day-Care and Preschool Programs

Day-care and preschool programs offer many children the opportunity to learn social skills, interact with other children and adults, and receive stimulation outside the home environment. For children enrolled in Headstart programs, there is the added benefit of involvement in a medical screening program called Healthstart, which can supplement well child visits.

Most states have regulations to promote health and safety in day-care facilities, including regulations concerning environmental sanitation, the qualifications of personnel caring for children, and the ratio of personnel to children. Specific protection as applied to day care includes the requirement that children have up-to-date immunizations and be monitored carefully for infectious diseases.

School Health

Schools can promote health by offering health education courses and programs involving a variety of participants, including teachers in the school system and representatives of the local health department and other health agencies.

Health promotion in children requires that the school setting be regularly inspected to ensure a safe water supply, sanitary food service facilities, and compliance with fire safety regulations. Specific protection is achieved through laws that make evidence of adequate immunization a prerequisite for enrolling in schools in the USA. This has helped to reduce the spread of some infections through school classrooms and from schools to younger children at home.

Secondary prevention in the school setting has historically included screening examinations of schoolchildren. These are seldom performed on a mass basis today, because of accumulated evidence that the examinations usually were not performed well and were not very productive. The emphasis now is to encourage parents to choose a primary care physician and to have their children visit the physician on a regular basis (see Well Child Care, above).

A relatively new role for schools in health is to provide school-based health centers that offer counseling, immunizations, and illness care. Some centers also make information about family planning available, and some offer counseling about violence, which is an increasingly important health concern both inside and outside of school. For example, one study of urban adolescent girls found that 67% met the formal criteria for having posttraumatic stress disorder in association with episodes of violence that they had seen or experienced (Horowitz, Weine, and Jekel 1995). Many students, particularly those in junior high and high school, feel more comfortable visiting school-based facilities than going to a practitioner or clinic outside the school. Although these centers have not been fully evaluated, the information so far has been encouraging.

■ ACQUIRED IMMUNODEFICIENCY SYNDROME (AIDS)

No new disease in modern times has had as severe a worldwide impact as acquired immunodeficiency syndrome (AIDS), which is caused by the human immunodeficiency virus (HIV). Worldwide, at the end of 2000, the number of persons living with HIV infection was approximately 36.1 million. During 2000, the number of persons newly infected was over 5 million, and the number of deaths caused by the disease was 3 million. In the USA, the estimated prevalence and incidence rates for 2000 were 850,000 and 40,000, respectively (see Centers for Disease Control and Prevention 2000). Although HIV transmission and management are of major concern in the USA, the situation is more serious in Southeast Asia, South America, and Russia and on the Indian subcontinent. It is catastrophic in central Africa, where in many countries over 25% of the adults are infected, death rates in the most productive age groups are extremely high, and many children are becoming orphans. The methods for managing HIV infection continue to improve, with recent drugs proving capable of producing long asymptomatic periods in some patients and perhaps even eliminating infection in others. However, these drugs are extremely expensive and entirely out of reach at this time for patients in the poorer countries of the world, where the highest rates of HIV infection are found. At present, the most cost-effective approach may be to reduce the vertical transmission of the virus from mothers to their unborn children by the use of prenatal antiretroviral drugs.

The Spread of HIV Infection

HIV is spread primarily by sexual contact (both heterosexual and homosexual) and by intravenous drug use (IVDU). The spread of HIV among drug users is due to the sharing of the equipment ("works") for injecting drugs. These works include needles, syringes, cookers (for heating the drug to dissolve it), cottons (to filter the drug to be injected), and water (used for mixing the drug and cleaning the needle and syringe). HIV can also be spread by transfusions of blood and blood products, although with modern testing, this risk is vanishingly small where all of the tests are done and done correctly. Rarely, HIV is spread by accidental punctures of the skin with contaminated needles or other medical equipment. HIV is not spread by ordinary household contact that does not involve one of the above risk behaviors.

HIV is often spread from an infected pregnant woman to her fetus. After delivery, HIV can be spread to the newborn via breast-feeding if viremia in the mother is not controlled. These modes of vertical transmission can be prevented by treatment with antiretroviral drugs, as discussed above.

In the USA, among men, the first and second most frequent routes of infection are homosexual intercourse and IVDU, respectively. Among women, the most frequent route of infection is heterosexual intercourse. In some countries with high rates of IVDU, sharing of drug equipment is the leading route of spread. In central Africa and Southeast Asia, however, heterosexual intercourse is the predominant route of spread. Where the rates of new HIV infections are approximately equal between men and women, heterosexual intercourse is the most important route of spread. Where the prevalence and new infections involve far more men than women, either homosexual intercourse or IVDU is likely to be the dominant route.

Primary, Secondary, and Tertiary Prevention of HIV Infection and AIDS

The best ways to prevent the spread of AIDS have been known since soon after the syndrome was discovered, even before the responsible microorganism was identified. They consist of restricting sexual activity to a monogamous relationship and avoiding IVDU. If these two practices were followed, exposure to HIV would be limited to extremely rare events, such as might occasionally happen from a blood transfusion.

If a person chooses to have multiple sexual partners, the next best prevention is to use condoms for every act of sexual intercourse. Condoms are far from foolproof, but if used consistently, they will reduce the risk of exposure considerably. If a person chooses to use intravenous drugs, exposure can be prevented if only new, clean "works" are used for every injection. Sharing any part of the "works" with another intravenous drug user is extremely hazardous. Needle-exchange programs have been shown to reduce the rate of spread of HIV in urban areas (Kaplan 1992), but they do not eliminate it.

Infected persons may change their behaviors to protect others if they know they are infected with HIV. For this reason, HIV testing centers have been established in most parts of the USA and allow individuals to be tested anonymously.

Other than behavioral changes, the primary means of preventing the spread of AIDS are (1) testing donated blood for HIV antibodies and discarding units that are infected and (2) treating HIV-positive pregnant women with antiretroviral drugs, a practice that reduces the proportion of infants who will be infected. Ironically, while there are no definite cures for AIDS and few effective technical means of preventing the spread of HIV, the infection could be largely eliminated over time by behavioral changes alone.

■ TUBERCULOSIS

Before the process of industrialization and urbanization transformed Western civilization, tuberculosis was a known problem, but it was not a scourge in Europe and the USA. During the 19th century, however, tuberculosis became the leading cause of death in the industrialized nations. The disease killed people of all ages (but especially adolescents and young adults) and in all socioeconomic circumstances. Although it was predominantly spread within the home, it also was frequently spread in crowded working conditions. For the treatment of patients with tuberculosis, physicians prescribed rest (often in sanatoriums), exposure to fresh air, and, in some cases, lung collapse therapy or the more permanent thoracoplasty.

Despite the lack of any specific medical prevention or therapy, the tuberculosis mortality rates began to decline in the late 19th century and continued to decline steadily until the end of World War II. Dubos (1959) claimed that a crucial factor in the decline was biologic selection. Adolescents and young adults, who were particularly susceptible to infection from *Mycobacterium tuberculosis,* tended to die young from the disease, before they could produce many children. As a result, the surviving world populations in which tuberculosis was common became far more resistant to tuberculosis than other populations were. Dubos also claimed that improvements in socioeconomic conditions, including better nutrition, less crowding in homes and worksites, and improved sanitation, were important factors in the steady decline of tuberculosis in the industrialized nations.

Although control of tuberculosis was far advanced by the late 1940s, it was improved further with the introduction of streptomycin as a treatment for tuberculosis, with the subsequent discovery of the therapeutic value of isoniazid (INH) and para-amino salicylic acid (PAS), and with the availability of additional antimicrobial agents, such as rifampin, ethambutol, and pyrazinamide.

In the USA, the incidence of tuberculosis continued to decline until the mid-1980s. In 1985, the decline stopped, and a resurgence of tuberculosis was noted. Although the incidence has dropped somewhat since 1993, tuberculosis still represents a formidable threat, especially in immunocompromised patients.

As the 21st century began, a number of reports documented the truly global nature of the tuberculosis problem (see, for example, Horsburgh 2000). According to the World Health Organization, *M. tuberculosis* still causes about 2 million deaths per year in the world, which is more deaths than are caused by any other single bacterial species. Most worrisome are the organism's widespread resistance to multiple antibiotics and the fact that tuberculosis frequently occurs in HIV-infected individuals. These problems are stimulating new research and control efforts throughout the world, and they have led experts in the USA to recommend a new US commitment to the elimination of tuberculosis (see Centers for Disease Control and Prevention 1999).

Stages and Natural History of Tuberculosis

The natural history of mycobacterial infection makes the control of tuberculosis considerably more complex than the control of other bacterial diseases.

The manifestations of tuberculosis vary greatly among patients. In a small percentage of individuals who are newly infected with mycobacteria, the infection proceeds fairly rapidly either to invade lung tissue or to cause a generalized systemic disease such as miliary tuberculosis. In most persons with normal immune systems, however, lesions develop in the lung and become contained as cell-mediated immunity develops. The presence of cell-mediated immunity is revealed by a positive reaction in the tuberculin skin test using purified protein derivative (PPD).

The initial infection with tuberculosis, when it is successfully resolved, is called **primary tuberculosis,** and it often leaves a telltale radiographic picture called a primary (Ghon) complex. The resolved primary infection, however, is not necessarily the end of the story, because the mycobacteria remain alive—albeit isolated—in the body of the infected person. This person, therefore, is more correctly considered to have **inactive tuberculosis** than to be completely healed.

The inactive tuberculosis, which is noninfectious, will ultimately take one of three possible courses: (1) The tuberculosis may remain inactive for the rest of the infected person's life. In Europe and the USA, this is by far the most common course. (2) The infected person's own disease may reactivate later in life to become **active tuberculosis.** This occurs in 4–8% of infected persons and is called **reactivation tuberculosis or endogenous** ("from within") tuberculosis. Reactivation tuberculosis is usually infectious. (3) The infected person may be exposed to a new tuberculosis infection, which may or may not become active infectious pulmonary tuberculosis. If a new exposure results in active disease, it is called **reinfection tuberculosis** or exogenous ("from without") tuberculosis.

The Incidence of Tuberculosis in the USA

From the 1960s to the mid-1980s, most new active cases of tuberculosis in the USA were due to endogenous tuberculosis, the reactivation of long-standing infection. During this period, the central goal for the US Public Health Service tuberculosis program was to minimize the spread of tuberculosis from the older population to the younger population. If this could be accomplished, over time the older people, many of whom had been infected while young, would die out, leaving the US population largely uninfected. Because of its central goal, the program was called the "child-centered" program to prevent tuberculosis (see Centers for Disease Control 1965).

The US program pursued several measures to accomplish its goal. First, school-age children were tested, and those with positive results in the tuberculin skin test were treated prophylactically with INH. Those with negative results were retested periodically. Second, efforts were made to trace the contacts of children whose skin test results recently converted from negative to positive (skin test converters) and the contacts of persons with newly discovered active tuberculosis. People who were identified as being actual sources of infection were treated to reduce the spread of mycobacteria. People who were identified as being at risk for infection were tested, and those whose results showed a recent conversion from negative to positive were given INH prophylaxis if they were under 35 years old. This age limit was imposed because of the discovery that INH use in older individuals posed a threat of severe liver damage.

The incidence of tuberculosis (often called the new active case rate) declined at approximately 5% per year from the 1950s to the mid-1980s. Indeed, by the 1970s, the proportion of schoolchildren with positive skin test results had dropped to such a low level that it was no longer cost-effective to continue skin testing in most schoolchildren. The search for the contacts of active cases continued, as did the use of INH prophylaxis for newly discovered skin test converters.

In 1985, the incidence of tuberculosis leveled off and then began to rise. Two factors appeared to be responsible for the resurgence of tuberculosis. First, an increasing proportion of newly discovered cases of tuberculosis were resistant to more than one antimicrobial agent. Much of the reason for this **multiple drug–resistant tuberculosis** (MDRTB) appears to be that infected persons started, but did not complete, the prescribed course of antituberculosis treatment. This allowed the mycobacteria to develop resistance to antimicrobial agents. Second, the patterns of tuberculosis were affected by the presence of human immunodeficiency virus (HIV) infection. In HIV-positive individuals, tuberculosis is frequently the first sign of acquired immunodeficiency syndrome, or AIDS (Selwyn et al. 1992). When HIV-positive individuals are exposed to mycobacteria, the result is often severe and sometimes overwhelming tuberculosis. Reactivation of inactive tuberculosis in HIV-positive persons tends to occur as immune deficiency progresses. Moreover, persons with HIV infection are often in a position to give their infections to other persons with immunodeficiency, thus continuing the cycle.

The problem of MDRTB has been especially severe in three types of institutions: prisons, general hospitals, and homeless shelters. Prisons and general hospitals are often overcrowded, partly because of the rise of illegal drug use, and have become important sites for the spread of tuberculosis (Bellin, Fletcher, and Safyer 1993; Edlin et al. 1992). The use of "crack" cocaine and other illegal drugs has contributed to homelessness (as has the "deinstitutionalization" of the mentally ill), and homeless shelters have become

sources of spread of tuberculosis (see Centers for Disease Control 1991; Brudney and Dobkin 1991). In addition, tuberculosis has been shown to spread in other public settings, such as on commercial aircraft, on occasion (see Centers for Disease Control and Prevention 1995).

Primary, Secondary, and Tertiary Prevention of Tuberculosis

The control of tuberculosis has been assisted by the discovery of methods for primary, secondary, and tertiary prevention.

The first discovery was a vaccine derived from a live, attenuated mycobacterium and called the bacillus Calmette-Guérin (BCG) vaccine after its developers. When the BCG vaccine is applied to a scratch in the skin of a previously uninfected child or adult, it stimulates the production of cell-mediated immunity, which provides some protection against a first infection with *M. tuberculosis*. Immunization with BCG can be considered a method of primary prevention. It is the least expensive approach to tuberculosis control, and although there has been considerable debate regarding its efficacy (see Clemens, Chuong, and Feinstein 1983), it is widely used in developing nations that have high rates of tuberculosis. In the USA, BCG vaccine is recommended only for children who are likely to be exposed to tuberculosis in an environment in which cooperation with diagnosis and treatment efforts is unlikely.

The second discovery was that a 6-month course of isoniazid (INH) could reduce the risk of endogenous (reactivation) tuberculosis by more than 50% in people with inactive primary tuberculosis (Mount and Ferebee 1961). INH use can therefore be considered secondary prevention. The US Public Health Service chose not to recommend the use of BCG vaccine but instead to emphasize the identification of those who had positive results in the tuberculin skin test (particularly recent skin test converters) and the use of INH to reduce their risk of reactivation tuberculosis if they are under 35 years old.

Subsequent discoveries have led to new strategies of secondary and tertiary prevention. Increasingly, tuberculosis control depends on the early identification and appropriate treatment of patients with MDRTB, immunodeficiency, or both. Patients with MDRTB must be treated with a combination of antituberculosis agents. To ensure compliance, therapy is given in a setting in which patients can be directly observed while taking these agents. Although this approach is expensive in terms of personnel time, preliminary evidence indicates that directly observed therapy (DOT) can be effective in reducing the incidence of tuberculosis if it is followed consistently (Frieden et al. 1995). In addition, some hospitals have developed special negative-pressure rooms in which patients with suspected MDRTB can be tested and treated without risking the spread of drug-resistant infection to other patients and to hospital staff (Bellin, Fletcher, and Safyer 1993).

In the presence of immunodeficiency, the tuberculin skin test using PPD often yields false-negative results (Selwyn et al. 1992). To prevent this problem in an individual who might be immunodeficient, the PPD skin test can be performed on one arm while an anergy panel is tested on the other arm. The anergy panel consists of a number of common allergens, at least one of which will elicit a delayed-type hypersensitivity reaction if the immune system is not impaired. Immunodeficient patients, however, may show no reaction, which tells the clinician that a negative result in the PPD skin test cannot be used to exclude the presence of tuberculosis.

In institutions, a variety of special precautions must be taken to prevent the spread of tuberculosis. Methods of primary prevention include the avoidance of overcrowding, the use of improved ventilation, and, when possible, the introduction of ultraviolet radiation, which kills mycobacteria in the air. Methods of secondary prevention include chest x-rays and tuberculin skin testing. Methods of tertiary prevention include combination therapy, DOT therapy, and use of negative-pressure rooms.

To prevent the spread of MDRTB, the World Health Organization now advocates that all countries follow a strategy called directly observed therapy, short-course (DOTS). This strategy includes a commitment to the following practices: identifying patients (case finding) through sputum microscopy; maintaining a continuous supply of the drugs needed to treat MDRTB; providing treatment that follows a specific schedule, is directly observed, and includes multiple antibiotics; and using a standard reporting system to monitor the outcome of treatment (see World Health Organization 1997).

■ CHEMICAL SUBSTANCE ABUSE

Several chemical substances are frequently used to alter the mind, to elevate the mood, to modify the feelings (especially about oneself), and sometimes to improve performance temporarily. Because the chemical substances used for these purposes may cause problems even before all of the criteria for addiction are met, the broader terms "chemical dependency" and "substance abuse" have come into general use. They imply both physical dependence (including tolerance) and psychologic dependence on the use of chemicals to modify mood and performance and to escape from anxiety.

Abuse of alcohol and abuse of illegal drugs are discussed below. Cigarette smoking, which is discussed in other chapters, is also properly considered a form of chemical dependency or substance abuse, because once the use of nicotine has become regular, withdrawal symptoms occur when the substance is withdrawn for any period of time.

Abuse of Alcohol

The most commonly abused substance is alcohol. In comparison with nondrinkers, heavy drinkers are at increased risk of a number of health problems. Among persons who are heavy drinkers (including alcoholics), the median estimate of the relative risk for cirrhosis is almost 8. For suicides, accidents, and cancer of the upper digestive and respiratory tracts, it is about 4. For stroke, it is about 1. The overall relative risk for mortality is slightly over 2.

The combination of a high rate of alcohol use and a relatively low rate of alcoholism in some European wine-producing countries has led some investigators to postulate that alcohol is best controlled if it is integrated into the normal pattern of food consumption and socialization. The view of alcoholism in the USA is based on the disease model: for genetic and other reasons, a portion of the members of society cannot adapt successfully to alcohol use, and their failure to adapt makes them "diseased" or at least a problem to be treated.

Because alcohol abuse not only damages the body of the drinker but also affects his or her performance of tasks, it often places others at risk for serious injuries, including those suffered in automobile crashes. Alcohol abuse often has devastating effects on the affected person's family, with high rates of spouse abuse, child abuse, divorce, and related problems. A variety of methods of primary, secondary, and tertiary prevention have been suggested to reduce the risk of alcohol-related diseases and injuries.

Primary Prevention of Alcohol Abuse

The social environment in which one is raised is probably important for the primary prevention of alcohol abuse. If an individual grows up without using alcohol, he or she may avoid its use for life. The promotion of healthy life-styles in which alcohol use is avoided or controlled is largely a function of families and other social groups to which a person belongs, such as churches.

Reducing legal accessibility of young people to alcohol tends to reduce alcohol use, but this probably is less effective than are family values. Limiting the promotion of alcohol in the media may decrease the desire of young people to start using alcohol. Raising the tax on liquor reduces the amount of alcohol purchased, but it is not clear that it reduces rates of alcoholism.

Secondary and Tertiary Prevention of Alcohol Abuse

The goals of secondary and tertiary prevention are the early detection and the early treatment of alcohol problems. For early detection in their patients, primary care physicians can use the so-called CAGE instrument, which consists of the four questions outlined in Table 19–1. If a patient answers "yes" to two or more of the questions, the likelihood that he or she meets the criteria for alcohol dependence is greater than 90%. Screening is important because, unfortunately, many patients do not seek help for their drinking problems until some untoward event occurs, such as injuring someone while drinking and

TABLE 19–1   The CAGE Instrument to Detect Alcoholism*

The so-called CAGE instrument consists of four questions:

C: Have you ever felt that you ought to Cut down on drinking?
A: Have people Annoyed you by criticizing your drinking?
G: Have you ever felt bad or Guilty about your drinking?
E: Have you ever had a drink first thing in the morning (as an Eye opener) to steady your nerves or get rid of a hangover?

Sources of data: (1) Ewing, J. A. Detection of alcoholism: the CAGE questionnaire. Journal of the American Medical Association 252:1905–1907, 1984. (2) US Preventive Services Task Force (USPSTF). Guide to Clinical Preventive Services, 2nd ed. Baltimore, Williams & Williams, 1996.
*If a person answers "yes" to two or more of the questions, the likelihood that he or she meets the criteria for alcohol dependence is greater than 90%.

driving. The long-term treatment of people who are alcohol abusers is difficult. There are good medications for treating the acute effects of withdrawal, but long-term success often depends on a lifetime commitment to treatment, such as is encouraged in the 12-step program of Alcoholics Anonymous. For some alcoholics, a major change in personal commitment, such as a religious conversion, may be effective.

Abuse of Illegal Drugs

The effects of psychoactive drugs such as cocaine and heroin are due as much to the rate at which the blood level of the drug is increased as they are to the blood level finally achieved (Zahler et al. 1982). A route of administration that causes a rapid rise in the blood level of a euphoria-producing drug causes more euphoria than one that delivers the same amount of drug slowly to the bloodstream. Moreover, a drug will have more psychic effect at any blood level while the level is rising than while it is falling.

An upsurge of violence began in the USA in 1986 as a result of the influx of a new form of cocaine, free-base cocaine, called "crack" because of the crackling sounds it makes when being manufactured or smoked (Allen and Jekel 1991). Crack, the most dangerous form of cocaine, is inhaled while it is heated. Inhaled crack is absorbed very rapidly, causes a strong euphoria, and is rapidly addictive.

In contrast to heroin addicts, crack addicts are at least as dangerous to others when they are high on the drug as when they are seeking money to get high. This is because crack is a stimulant, whereas heroin is a sedative. While high on crack, a user may have strong feelings of paranoia and may be in physical danger of myocardial infarction, stroke, or seizures.

Powdered cocaine (the hydrochloride) may be mixed with heroin before intravenous injection; this is an extremely dangerous mixture called a "speedball." To some extent, the stimulant effect of cocaine is counteracted by the depressant effect of heroin, but in high doses, both depress respiration.

During the 1990s, the use of heroin and cocaine generally leveled off in all segments of US society. However, the use of marijuana, amphet-

amines, and amphetamine derivatives (particularly 3,4-methylenedioxymethamphetamine, which is also called MDMA or ecstasy) increased significantly among teenagers, and amphetamines were especially a problem in the western USA. Near the end of the millennium, there was a dramatic increase in seizures of clandestine amphetamine laboratories. In 2000, a committee of experts in the USA issued a report that includes evidence-based principles for substance abuse prevention and is called the National Drug Control Strategy (see Office of Drug Control Policy 2000).

Primary Prevention of Drug Abuse

Some experts believe that human beings have an inborn need for euphoria, whereas others believe that the desire for drugs is a learned desire for pleasure or escape. It is known that young people who smoke cigarettes are more likely to experiment with drugs and eventually become drug abusers. Children are more likely to take up illegal drug use if illegal drugs are used at home. Children from religious homes have a lower risk of illegal drug use. The cost of drugs also appears to influence the rate of subsequent drug use: the cheaper a drug, the more people will use it.

To be effective, a national illegal drug control program must be multifaceted and not rely on only one strategy. In general, one might consider the broad strategies of demand reduction, supply reduction, and the elimination of money laundering (Jekel et al. 1994). Demand reduction not only involves educating people to make them aware of the dangers of drugs but also involves the treatment of drug abusers. Supply reduction implies the reduction of the amount of drug imported, as well as the control of selling drugs on the street. It appears that scattered drug "pushers" at isolated locations are less dangerous than are organized drug "bazaars," so that one police strategy might be to keep the selling of drugs a scattered business. It is more difficult to market large amounts of drugs if banking practices and export regulations make it problematic to "launder" the cash obtained from drug deals. In at least one experience, the use of broad strategies to reduce demand and supply and to eliminate money laundering resulted in a marked decrease in the abuse of crack cocaine following a nationwide epidemic (Jekel et al. 1994).

Secondary and Tertiary Prevention of Drug Abuse

As with alcohol abuse, with drug abuse the goals of secondary and tertiary prevention are early detection and early treatment of the problem. The treatment for illegal drug abuse may be thought of in four stages: assessment, abstinence initiation, relapse prevention, and follow-up. A careful assessment is necessary to provide the proper treatment. Abstinence initiation often involves individual psychotherapy as well as medications that suppress craving. Relapse prevention is best achieved with the help of group therapy. Long-term success depends on the individual's joining support groups and developing new habit patterns. For some drug abusers, the 12-step approach to treatment, as embodied in Narcotics Anonymous, is helpful. A reorientation of the abuser's life, as with religious conversion, increases the likelihood of success.

■ MENTAL HEALTH

In the USA, the most direct evidence of an increase in mental health problems is seen in the rapidly rising rates of major depression. Based on their own studies and those of others, Klerman and Weissman (1989) noted that an increasing proportion of people in the USA have had one or more episodes of major depression in their lives and that the increase is occurring in younger birth cohorts. For example, 40% of the people born after 1955 have suffered from at least one episode of major depression by the age of 20 years. This represents a considerably greater incidence rate than for any prior birth cohort. The reasons for this increase are uncertain, but Klerman and Weissman suggested the following: increasing urbanization, mobility, and social anomie; changes in family structure (e.g., increases in the number of divorces and single-parent families); changing gender roles in employment and families; and increasing use of drugs and alcohol.

Although a discussion of the methods to detect and treat mental illness is beyond the scope of this book, it is important to note that a variety of methods of primary prevention have been developed with the goal of promoting mental health and providing education and emotional support during times of stress. Today, there are support groups for the families of patients with various physical, psychologic, and mental health problems, including cancer, Alzheimer's disease, alcoholism, eating disorders, and child abuse, to name only a few. There are also informal groups to provide counseling and support to new mothers, widows, widowers, retirees, and others going through major changes in life, as well as telephone "hotlines" to help people who are in a crisis and need advice about where to turn for professional help. Matthews, Larson, and Barry (1993) have reviewed the available scientific literature showing that religious belief and practice are consistently associated with better health, particularly mental health. Although more work needs to be done in this area because of the possibility of selection and detection biases, the consistency of the findings is impressive.

■ INJURIES

Injuries can be categorized as follows: automobile crashes; home incidents (falls, burns, poisonings, electrocutions, drownings, etc.); occupational incidents; homicides; suicides; and miscellaneous injuries (plane and train crashes, building collapses, etc.).

The impact of injuries is often described in terms of **years of potential life lost** (YPLL). In the USA,

injuries are the leading cause of YPLL before the age of 65.

This section of the chapter discusses automobile crashes and home incidents, and a later section on occupational health discusses worksite incidents. Specialists in the field of injury prevention do not refer to injuries sustained from automobile crashes or incidents in the home or worksite as "accidents," because the word carries the connotation that they are not predictable. In fact, these injury-producing events are fairly predictable and therefore are preventable.

Automobile Crashes

Haddon (1972), a founder of the field of automobile injury epidemiology, developed a detailed approach to injury prevention. This approach, now called the **Haddon matrix,** classifies the phases of injury and the factors involved (see Christoffel and Gallagher 1999). The Haddon matrix is followed here, with the **phases** classified as preinjury, injury, and postinjury and with the **risk factors** involved in automobile injuries classified as human, vehicle, physical environment, and social environment.

Risk Factors in the Preinjury Phase

Human Factors. New drivers, young drivers, and drivers suffering from alcohol intoxication, drug intoxication, fatigue, or a combination of these factors are at increased risk for automobile crashes.

In new drivers, the excess risk of automobile crashes is related to the inability to anticipate and prevent developing hazards, as well as the inability to recognize existing hazards and respond to them quickly and appropriately. For example, new drivers often do not anticipate the dangers of taking curves at high speeds, particularly when roads are wet, and they often have difficulties coordinating manual actions, such as steering and braking, when it is necessary to respond to urgent driving demands. New drivers are at increased risk, regardless of the age at which they begin driving, but the excess risk decreases to zero over a few years of driving.

People who start driving during their teenage years may be at increased risk not only because of their driving inexperience but also because of several "immaturity factors" commonly associated with adolescence: a sense of invulnerability, a refusal to be warned about hazards, and a tendency to let the mind wander and act less cautiously (including taking the eyes off the road) when friends are nearby. In the USA, the high rates of serious injuries per mile of driving for young drivers are generally attributed to a combination of inexperience and immaturity factors. However, in Canada, at least one study did not find an increased immaturity risk when the number of years of driving was controlled for in the analysis (Pierce 1977). It is not clear what factors are responsible for the differences noted between teenage drivers in the USA and those in other nations. In the USA, a newly emerging risk factor is the use of cell phones when driving. This practice tends to distract drivers, and it reduces the number of hands available to react quickly in an emergency. In some areas, authorities have begun to ban handheld cell phone use while a vehicle is moving.

New proposals to reduce the injury problems from teenage driving have been advanced (see Insurance Institute for Highway Safety 1994). Among them are "graduated licensing," which would require each new teenage driver to graduate from a provisional or beginner's license to one or more intermediate licenses before receiving an unrestricted license. The major provisions of the restrictive licenses limit how late the driver can operate a vehicle (i.e., they impose various kinds of curfews). Restrictive licenses have proved to be effective in Oregon, for example (James 1994).

Driving while intoxicated (DWI) with alcohol or drugs interacts with other factors, such as fatigue, and reduces sensory input to increase the risks late at night. This is one reason for considering a curfew of 11:00 PM or midnight for new teenage drivers, who are responsible for an excess number of fatal crashes, particularly single-vehicle crashes, in the USA (Williams et al. 1995).

Although some groups have advocated driver education programs in all US high schools, Robertson and Zador (1978) showed that the rates of teenage crashes and injuries in counties where in-school driver education was given to students were as high as or higher than the rates in counties where in-school driver education was not given. The reason appeared to be that the in-school driver education programs put significant numbers of young drivers on the road at an earlier age.

Laws concerning DWI are already in place in the USA, as are regulations concerning the number of hours that professional drivers can operate trucks, buses, and other vehicles on the road per day and per week. Dozing and fatigue have been found responsible for numerous vehicle crashes, including those involving trucks. Many roads now have "rumble strips" in the breakdown lanes to awaken dozing drivers who veer off the primary lanes.

Vehicle Factors. The ability of vehicles to brake and other aspects of vehicle construction and maintenance may influence the risk of injuries. Similarly, vehicle design may play a role. For example, research has demonstrated that a tail light pattern involving two lower red lights at the sides, plus one higher red light in the center of the vehicle, catches the attention of drivers best and reduces rear-end collisions. All new vehicles sold in the USA now have this tail light pattern.

Environmental Factors. Drivers should slow down during periods of rain, snow, or poor visibility, but they do not always do so. Poor design and maintenance of roads and highways also increase the risk of vehicle crashes.

Risk Factors in the Injury Phase

Human Factors. The ability of human beings to resist injury is influenced by the use of specific protection devices, such as seat belts in automobiles and helmets for motorcycle and bicycle riders. For children between the ages of 3 and 9 years, the risk of injury is increased if a booster seat is not used. It is also increased if the shoulder strap of the seat belt is placed behind the child's back.

Vehicle Factors. Vehicle design has been steadily improving under the influence of federal regulations. Vehicle safety features include collapsible steering columns, energy-absorbing construction, in-door side protection, seat belts and air bags, and protected gasoline tanks. The need for further improvements in the design of vehicles and their accessories was nevertheless underscored in 2000 by reports about the tendency of sports utility vehicles (SUVs) to roll over because of their high center of gravity and the use of defective tires.

Environmental Factors. The object into which a vehicle crashes affects the seriousness of the crash. Energy-absorbing barriers on the shoulder of the road reduce the risk that vehicles will go off the road, and median strip barriers reduce injuries from head-on collisions.

Risk Factors in the Postinjury Phase

Human Factors. The fate of crash victims may be influenced greatly by the ability of individuals at the crash scene to act quickly in summoning medical help and preventing other vehicles from becoming involved in the crash.

Vehicle Factors. The construction of a vehicle, including the extent to which it absorbs energy in a crash while maintaining the integrity of the passenger cage, may determine whether or not passengers survive a crash.

Environmental Factors. The extent of injury is influenced by the rapidity and quality of the emergency response. Advanced life support (ALS) ambulance teams seek to stabilize the condition of injured persons at the crash scene before transport. Helicopter ambulance systems appear to improve outcomes, in part because they carry injured persons to trauma centers rather than to the nearest emergency room, which may not be adequately equipped for serious trauma.

Surveillance and Prevention of Injuries

One of the most important factors in prevention is improved data on the nature of injuries, the rate at which they occur, and the circumstances under which they occur. The Fatal Accident Reporting System was developed by the National Highway Traffic Safety Administration and provides valuable epidemiologic data. Other injury surveillance systems depend on the use of the E-codes in the *International Classification of Diseases* (ICD) and the use of hospital emergency department and admission diagnoses.

A variety of methods of primary, secondary, and tertiary prevention have been devised to prevent serious injuries from automobile crashes. Examples of primary prevention include improvements in driver training, special tests and training for older persons, the passage and enforcement of laws concerning driving under the influence of alcohol or drugs, the construction and maintenance of good roads and highways, and the modification of automobiles to make them easier to control under hazardous conditions and to optimize passenger safety in the event of a crash. Examples of secondary prevention include testing of each driver's skill and vision before a license is issued. Examples of tertiary prevention include developing and using effective methods of transporting and caring for victims of automobile crashes so as to limit the degree of impairment they suffer.

Because prevention focuses on human factors, as well as vehicle and environmental factors, it requires an understanding of human behavior and of the kinds of behavioral interventions that do and do not work. Regulations regarding automobile construction have had a positive effect in reducing injuries from automobile crashes. Laws regarding human behavior, such as those requiring seat belt use, have been somewhat less successful, but they have still helped to move behavior in this direction. When lack of conforming behavior is easier to detect, as it is with lack of helmet use by motorcycle riders, conforming behavior tends to be higher, but in some states laws such as the helmet law have been challenged and overturned by referendum. It is not always clear when efforts to reduce injuries and their associated costs necessitate restrictions on behavioral freedoms. As medical care costs continue to rise, the balance may gradually shift in the direction of greater controls on behavior, especially on driving while intoxicated, as shown by efforts to reduce the allowable blood alcohol level to 0.08%.

Common Injuries in the Home

Among the many types of preventable injuries in the home are poisoning, fires, falls, and drowning.

The victims of **poisoning** are usually toddlers and preschool children, who experiment with tasting or swallowing substances that they encounter while exploring. Much has been accomplished in recent decades by developing child-proof caps for containers of medicines and household products; by counseling parents to keep cleaning solutions, pesticides, medicines, and other hazardous substances out of the reach of their children; and by establishing poison control centers and "hot lines."

Some reduction in the risk of **fires** has been achieved by tightening building codes, particularly the requirement for hard-wired smoke alarms in houses. Nevertheless, many older buildings are not retrofitted with these devices. The reduction in the prevalence of cigarette smoking has reduced one source of fires, but arson is still common, either for insurance or for revenge.

Although people of all ages can be the victims of **falls,** older people are at greater risk of serious injuries, such as hip fractures. A significant reduction in the incidence of hip fractures has been achieved by having high-risk elderly individuals wear padded hip protectors. In younger persons, falls are likely to be associated with activities such as climbing ladders, shoveling snow, or walking on a surface covered with ice. Among older people, falls are frequently due to failing vision, loss of equilibrium or physical strength, or use of medications that decrease stability (Tinetti, Speechley, and Ginter 1988). Architectural modifications, such as the provision of handrails in hallways and on stairs, can reduce the incidence of falls in the elderly.

Drowning occurs most often among school-age children, especially boys. Swimming lessons and water safety instruction at an early age may reduce the number of deaths and injuries associated with activities that occur in and near pools and other bodies of water.

■ OCCUPATIONAL HEALTH

The occupational environment is well suited for the practice of preventive medicine. There are two appropriate goals for occupational health: (1) the prevention of work-related injuries and diseases and (2) health promotion in the workplace. Occupational health is most likely to succeed when these health goals can be clearly shown to produce economic benefits for the company by increasing the productivity of its employees and reducing costs.

Surveillance of Occupational Injuries and Diseases

The surveillance of occupational injuries and diseases is as critical to their prevention as is the surveillance of infectious diseases. Federal efforts in this area were advanced when the Occupational Safety and Health Administration (OSHA) and the National Institute for Occupational Safety and Health (NIOSH) were established in 1970. Basically, OSHA is responsible for monitoring occupational injuries and diseases and enforcing laws regarding a safe workplace, while NIOSH is responsible for research in occupational injury and disease prevention. Unfortunately, the surveillance of occupational diseases is far from being as adequate or as well understood as the surveillance of infectious diseases (see Centers for Disease Control 1990). There are many reasons for this, including the difficulty of recognizing many occupational diseases and an incomplete understanding by many physicians of their reporting role in occupational illness.

Surveillance of occupational diseases serves the same functions as does the surveillance of other diseases: establishing a background rate, determining significant increases in disease, setting disease control priorities, and so forth (see Chapter 3). Currently, the majority of states have mandatory reporting requirements for occupational injuries and diseases, although these requirements, including the types of conditions that must be reported, vary somewhat from state to state.

Other sources of reporting certain occupational conditions include laboratories, workers' compensation programs, some industries, and, occasionally, death certificates. Of course, a physician may report a suspected occupational health problem directly to OSHA or to a state department of health, which will then investigate the report to determine if a problem exists and to enforce any federal regulations that may have been violated.

An important surveillance concept that has been applied to the occupational health field is the idea of **sentinel health events** (Rutstein et al. 1983). An occupational sentinel health event is a preventable event (death, disease, or impairment) that can be used to identify a problem in the system of prevention, detection, or treatment of occupational health problems.

Work-Related Injuries

While some jobs are associated with more risks than others, no job is completely free of risks for work-related injuries. Collisions are a common risk to truck drivers, taxi drivers, and other vehicle operators; falling objects represent a frequent threat to construction workers, longshoremen, and movers; the loss of limbs or digits is a risk of working with agricultural or manufacturing machines; and explosions, fires, and discharge of firearms are threats faced by miners, firemen, and police, respectively. Of the 2 million occupational injuries that occur each year in the USA, the number that resulted in death in 1997 was over 6200 (see Centers for Disease Control and Prevention and National Institute for Occupational Safety and Health 2000). The yearly number of deaths from occupational injuries and diseases combined may be as high as 100,000. Estimates of the yearly number of disabilities caused by occupational injuries and illnesses range as high as 400,000 (Levy and Wegman 1988; LaDou 1997).

Less striking, but becoming increasingly common, are repetitive motion injuries and back injuries. Repetitive motion injuries, such as carpal tunnel syndrome, can affect musicians, typists, assembly line workers, and people in various other jobs. Back injuries are a risk not only to employees whose jobs require lifting and other forms of intense physical labor but even to employees with sedentary office jobs.

Physicians who treat what is definitely or possibly an occupation-related injury or disease should report their findings. Ordinarily, they would report them to the state workers' compensation system, and the data would become available for surveillance purposes, as discussed above. However, if a physician believes that the injury or disease needs to be reported immediately, he or she should contact the state occupational medicine program if such a program exists or, alternatively, should contact the OSHA office in the federal region in which the patient works.

Work-Related Diseases

Skin Diseases

Skin trauma and diseases are the most frequent type of occupational health problem, causing 23–35% of occupational injuries and 34–50% of occupational diseases (Levy and Wegman 1988). Among the causes are exposure to chemicals, microorganisms, and physical agents (heat, cold, vibration, etc.). A predisposing skin condition makes an occupational skin disease more likely.

According to Rosenstock and Cullen (1986), 80% of occupational skin diseases are due to exposure to chemicals. Either direct irritation or an allergic reaction to a chemical can result in contact dermatitis. Oils and greases frequently irritate the skin, causing lesions to become infected. Exposure to bacteria or fungi is a frequent cause of occupational skin diseases in persons who work with animals, fish, food, or soil. Phototoxic dermatitis and photosensitization are problems that sometimes occur in people who work outdoors without protection from the sun.

Exposure to severe cold or severe vibration may result in Raynaud's phenomenon (white finger disease), and exposure to temperature extremes may also result in burns, frostbite, trenchfoot, or dermatitis. The skin is frequently abraded, penetrated, or cut by physical injury from falls or the use of tools.

Lung Diseases

Like the skin, the lung is a frequent site of work-related diseases. Occupational exposure to dusts, gases, fumes, mists, or vapors may cause acute or chronic disease, depending on factors such as the number, duration, and intensity (level) of exposures.

Obstructive Lung Disease. According to Chen-Yeung and Malo (1995), the most prevalent occupational lung disease in developed countries is occupational asthma. There is a distinction between work-aggravated asthma and occupational asthma. The former is found in people with preexisting asthma, while the latter refers to asthma caused strictly by occupational exposure. When there is no latent period (delay between exposure and disease onset) in occupational asthma, it is relatively easy to determine the occupational origin of disease. It is more difficult to determine the causative agent if asthma has its onset months or years after the occupational exposure.

Among the many agents that can cause occupational asthma are animal products, plant products, wood dusts, metal dusts, soldering fluxes, drugs, and organic chemicals. Isocyanates, which are used in the manufacture of polyurethane and in many paints, are one of the most common categories of causative agent and are frequently responsible for occupational asthma in automobile painters.

Byssinosis is a respiratory disease caused by the dust formed during the processing of cotton. Although it is characterized by bronchoconstriction, with chest tightness and shortness of breath, it is not typical asthma. The symptoms are thought to be due to a toxic effect on the bronchi, rather than to an immunologic reaction; one reason for this supposition is that byssinosis can occur the first time a person is exposed to cotton dust. The symptoms of byssinosis are especially severe after a period of time away from the dust, such as after a vacation or even after a weekend, but they abate somewhat upon continued exposure during the week. Byssinosis may not result in permanent lung damage if the duration and intensity of exposure are limited. It can, however, cause severe disability in people with long-term exposure, particularly those who smoke or have chronic bronchitis. A disease similar to byssinosis sometimes occurs in workers who process flax or hemp.

Interstitial Lung Disease. Asbestosis, silicosis, and coal worker's pneumoconiosis are examples of interstitial lung diseases associated with the inhalation of dusts. Chronic inhalation of asbestos or free silica causes the gradual development of fibrosis in the lung. Inhaled asbestos can also produce two highly fatal cancers, lung cancer and mesothelioma. Coal worker's pneumoconiosis (black lung disease) can cause a massive, diffuse fibrosis, the major symptom of which is progressive shortness of breath. The degree of disease and rate of progression are related to the type of dust and to the intensity and duration of exposure.

Hypersensitivity Pneumonitis. Hypersensitivity pneumonitis is an inflammatory response of the lungs to inhaled organic agents (usually bacteria or fungi) found in a variety of work settings. One example is farmer's lung, which is associated with inhaling moldy hay dust. The names of many types of hypersensitivity pneumonitis indicate the occupation at risk (cheese handler's lung, grain handler's lung, pigeon breeder's lung, etc.). Hypersensitivity pneumonitis affects the alveoli and respiratory bronchioles, rather than the bronchi, and usually wheezing is not prominent. In the early stages, removal of the affected person from the organic agent usually results in complete resolution. Chronic exposure, however, may lead to permanent lung damage.

Granuloma. The most prominent occupational disease characterized by lung granuloma is berylliosis, which can be impossible to distinguish from sarcoidosis without measuring tissue levels of beryllium or performing other specialized tests.

Liver and Kidney Diseases

Because the liver is heavily involved in detoxifying absorbed substances, particularly non–water-soluble chemicals absorbed through the gastrointestinal tract, the liver is often the site of damage. Occupational exposure to chemicals such as chlorinated hydrocarbons, halogenated aromatics, nitroaromatics, ethanol, vinyl chloride, and epoxy resins can cause acute or subacute toxic hepatitis or fibrosis. Occupational exposure to hepatitis virus, as sometimes occurs in health care workers, can cause viral hepatitis.

The kidneys are frequently damaged by water-soluble toxins and metals because of their role in the excretion of water-soluble wastes. Acute tubular necrosis can occur as a result of acute exposure to divalent metals (e.g., mercury, cadmium, and chromium), halogenated hydrocarbons, other hydrocarbons, arsine, and other compounds. Most cases of work-related chronic renal disease are caused by long-term exposure to metals (especially mercury, lead, and cadmium).

Eye Damage and Hearing Loss

Most occupational eye damage is due to chemical burns, radiation effects, or mechanical injuries, including lacerations, contusions, and damage to the eye from fractures to surrounding skull bones. Cataracts or corneal damage can result from ionizing radiation (especially to the lid) and from ultraviolet radiation. Workers exposed to the sun a great deal, such as those in the fishing trade, have an increased risk of cataracts.

Loud noise on the job may cause loss of high tone hearing, with considerable functional deafness in later life. Chronic exposure to noise at a level of 85 dB frequently results in hearing problems, and many workers are regularly exposed to a level higher than 85 dB at work. The decibel (dB) scale is a logarithmic scale of sound pressure levels; according to this scale, normal human hearing goes from near 0 to about 120 dB. The greatest hearing loss tends to occur at a frequency of 3000–4000 Hz, which is a crucial range for hearing the consonants of human speech (for example, f, p, s, and t) and therefore for understanding speech.

Prevention of Occupational Injuries and Diseases

Safety in the workplace demands control over the environment, including providing a drug-free workplace, protective equipment (safety goggles, hard hats, ear protection devices, etc.), tools and equipment in good working order, proper training for workers, and adequate rest periods. As research in the field of **ergonomics** has indicated, prevention of many occupational health problems, including repetitive motion injuries and back injuries, can be accomplished by adjusting the occupational environment to the needs of the workers. In offices, the use of properly designed computer keyboards and the correct placement of screens for each worker can reduce the risk of repetitive motion injuries. In factory warehouses, safe lifting of manufactured goods requires the proper training of individual workers, but well-designed aids to lifting, such as sturdy handles on objects to be lifted, can also help prevent back injuries. In 2000, prodded by the fact that an estimated 1.8 million US workers suffer from orthopedic injuries caused by repetitive strain, OSHA recommended an ergonomics regulation. This regulation would require almost all US employers to create programs to help protect workers from the causes of repetitive stress and strain in the workplace.

The prevention of occupational skin diseases usually can be accomplished by eliminating the causative biologic, physical, or chemical agent or by providing barrier protection (e.g., gloves or protective uniforms) so that the causative agent does not touch the skin. Prevention of a variety of occupational diseases, including those affecting the skin, lung, liver, and kidney, requires preventing or minimizing exposures to toxic agents, including those listed in Table 19–2 and discussed below (see Exposure to Toxins).

In health care workers, the prevention of some infectious diseases, such as hepatitis, can be accomplished by the use of vaccines (see Chapter 16). If no vaccine exists, as is the case for the human immunodeficiency virus (HIV), then appropriate training and equipment for the prevention of contact with the virus should be provided to the workers.

Health Promotion in the Workplace

Workers in a company tend to be concentrated at certain places and, with the support of the company, industry, or agency, the workers can be reached for education, prevention, and health-promoting services. By the time most people reach working age, they have relatively little contact with the medical profession, except for women with fertility control needs or with pregnancies, so health promotion activities provided in the workplace are usually found to be helpful.

Activities designed to promote good health in employees often include health education about nutrition, exercise, smoking cessation, and weight reduction. In some cases, companies offer fitness programs and the use of a fitness center; limit the areas in which employees can smoke on the premises; provide immunizations (e.g., influenza and hepatitis B vaccines); and sponsor specific screening programs (e.g., for hypertension or high cholesterol levels) or the more comprehensive health risk assessments (see Chapter 17).

Mental health, including freedom from alcohol and drug abuse, is becoming increasingly important for companies. Random screening programs for alcohol or illegal drug abuse are sometimes introduced for certain critical employees, such as pilots, air traffic controllers, or railroad engineers, but it is difficult to justify such activity for all employees.

Fearing the supposedly endless costs of mental health and substance abuse treatment, some companies have developed **employee assistance programs** (EAPs) within the company or have entered a contract with an outside agency to provide employee assistance in the form of counseling and treatment services for emotional problems and substance abuse. The advantage of these programs is that they are free

to the workers and usually have a high degree of confidentiality guaranteed. Their goal is to increase the attendance and productivity of the workers.

Company Support for Preventive Activities

If preventive activities can be shown to be cost-effective for a company, especially in terms of reducing worker turnover, days missed from work, and medical care costs, the company often will pay for the activities. If health promotion and disease prevention activities are sought by the workers and if provision of these activities contributes to their morale and to company loyalty, such services are more likely to be provided by companies.

There are other advantages of preventive services in the occupational setting. The health information and good health habits learned in the workplace may be carried home to improve the health of an entire family.

Occupational Health Regulations

The Occupational Safety and Health Administration (OSHA) establishes federal standards for exposure to occupational hazards, investigates complaints or reports of problems in the workplace, and enforces the federal standards and regulations in the workplace. OSHA has the right to issue fines or citations when it finds violations of federal laws.

Most states have occupational health units in their state health departments or elsewhere in the state government. These have the obligation to receive and investigate complaints and disease reports and, within the limits prescribed by state laws, to enforce workplace changes.

Workers' Compensation

Workers' Compensation, a mandatory insurance program in each state in the USA, provides for medical care and partial replacement of wages for workers with occupational diseases or injuries. Companies, agencies, and businesses are required to purchase a policy or to deposit premiums into a fund. For a given company, the size of the premiums is based on the amount of claims paid in recent years from Workers' Compensation to employees from that company. By this mechanism, the companies are liable without fault being assigned to the company or to the worker, and the worker's ability to sue for further damages is markedly limited.

The benefits are paid according to the severity and duration of the illness or injury, which is usually defined by law (see Chapter 18 for a discussion of the major categories of disability). Physicians play an important role in defining the level of impairment resulting from the occupational injury or disease.

Medical ("Health") Insurance

In the USA, most persons under the age of 65 obtain medical insurance through their place of work. For

TABLE 19–2   Routes and Effects of Exposure to Toxins That Are Often Found in the Workplace

Toxin	Routes and Effects of Exposure
Metals*	
Arsenic	May enter via the lungs, skin, or gastrointestinal tract. Arsenic compounds are used as insecticides and weed killers. Cause respiratory and gastrointestinal symptoms and, in high doses, can cause death. Can cause lung cancer.
Beryllium	Usually enters via the lungs. Causes granulomas in the lungs; lesions appear similar to those in sarcoidosis.
Cadmium	Usually enters via the lungs. Displaces zinc in enzyme systems, often damaging the renal tubules. Causes metal fume fever.
Lead	Usually enters via the gastrointestinal tract or lungs. Displaces calcium in chemical reactions. Inorganic form of lead causes gastrointestinal and neurologic symptoms. Organic compounds of lead cause diffuse neurologic symptoms.
Mercury	May enter via the lungs, skin, or gastrointestinal tract. Used in the past by hatmakers to make felt for hats. Chronic exposure damages the central nervous system, with the elemental form of mercury tending to cause tremors ("hatter's shakes") and the organic forms tending to cause psychiatric symptoms ("mad as a hatter") and even dementia. Mercury also damages the kidneys.
Zinc	Usually enters via the lungs. Inhaling zinc oxide causes metal fume fever (a disorder that also can be caused by other metal fumes).
Insecticides, Herbicides, and Fungicides	
Organophosphates	Usually enter via the skin from handling, but can enter via the lungs. Block acetylcholinesterase and produce both central nervous system and peripheral nerve damage.
Pentachlorophenol	Usually enters via the skin. Used as a wood preservative. Interferes with cellular respiration. Causes anorexia and respiratory symptoms and, in high doses, can cause coma and death.
Polychlorinated biphenyls	Enter via the skin or lungs. Are teratogens and possibly also carcinogens.
Hydrocarbon Solvents†	
Benzene	Absorbed through the lungs and skin. Is a lipid-soluble aromatic solvent that is used widely in industry. Chronic exposure can result in suppression of the bone marrow, with a possible end result of aplastic anemia.
Carbon tetrachloride	Absorbed readily through the lungs. Is a lipid-soluble chlorinated hydrocarbon that is not used much in industry because it is extremely toxic to kidneys and liver, but it is the prototype of this class of chemical. Damage to either the kidneys or the liver can predominate. Renal tubular necrosis may follow acute exposures, and hepatic centrilobular necrosis tends to predominate in chronic exposure, especially in the presence of ethanol or following hepatic damage by ethanol.
Toluene	Usually inhaled. Is a lipid-soluble aromatic solvent found in products such as glue. Primarily causes central nervous system effects, including hallucinations (which is why glue is sometimes sniffed).
Asphyxiants‡	
Carbon dioxide	Enters the body via the lungs and stimulates the respiratory center. Is a nonreactive asphyxiant. Begins to produce symptoms of rapid breathing when concentration reaches about 3% in the air. In high concentrations, causes coma and death.
Carbon monoxide	Enters the body via the lungs. Is a chemical asphyxiant that is ubiquitous in urban society (a product of automobile exhausts and sometimes of poorly ventilated space heaters). Combines with hemoglobin to form carboxyhemoglobin; when 50% or more of the hemoglobin is in the form of carboxyhemoglobin, fainting and death are likely. Smokers may inhale some carbon monoxide from smoking.
Hydrogen cyanide	Enters the body via the lungs or gastrointestinal tract. Is a chemical asphyxiant. Toxicity is retained in cyanide salts, because it is the reactive cyanide moiety that interferes with cytochrome oxidase. Causes headaches, rapid breathing, and, frequently, death.
Hydrogen sulfide	Absorbed through the lungs. Is a chemical asphyxiant that is as dangerous as hydrogen cyanide, but its smell tends to give warning of its presence before hazardous levels develop. Causes symptoms and effects similar to those of hydrogen cyanide.
Methane	Enters the body via the lungs. Is a nonreactive asphyxiant that is mainly a problem in mines, causing severe respiratory symptoms. The greater danger now is from explosion.
Nitrogen	Enters the body via the lungs. Is a nonreactive asphyxiant that used to be a problem in mines but now presents a hazard primarily to deep sea divers. Divers accumulate nitrogen in the fatty tissues during dives at high pressure. As divers approach the surface, nitrogen reenters their blood, and if the pressure is reduced too fast, it forms small bubbles in the blood, which interfere with circulation, especially to the brain. This process causes the "bends."
Miscellaneous Organic Compounds	
Resins	Usually enter via the skin, although may enter via the lungs. Produce asthma, irritation and allergic sensitization of the skin, and irritation of the eyes.
Vinyl chloride	Absorbed through the lungs and skin. Is ubiquitous in industry because it is used to make plastics. Can cause sclerodermatous skin lesions, Raynaud's phenomenon, and bone lesions in the hand, in addition to liver damage. The monomer form causes hemangiosarcoma of the liver in a small proportion of persons who are exposed.

*Metals often cause toxicity by interfering with the action of other metals as cofactors in enzyme reactions.
†Lipid-soluble hydrocarbon solvents build up in the body in tissues with high levels of lipids (e.g., the central nervous system), and they all have narcotic effects. Their central nervous system effects are exacerbated by alcohol. Exposure to more than one solvent may result in complex interactions.
‡Asphyxiants can be divided into two groups. The first group consists of gases that have no direct toxic effect but can reduce the partial pressure of oxygen in the lungs to dangerous levels; these gases are often called simple or nonreactive asphyxiants. The second group consists of gases that interfere with respiration at the cellular level; these are called chemical or reactive asphyxiants.

decades, the medical insurance was a tax-free benefit to workers and, hence, was partly subsidized by the federal government. As the costs of workers' medical insurance outstrip the inflation rate, companies are increasingly demanding limits on their costs for such insurance. As a result, more and more companies are (1) requiring managed care plans (see Chapter 21); (2) requiring workers to pay a part of the costs of the insurance; or (3) not even offering health insurance. The strategy of not offering health insurance is frequently used by small businesses, especially those that have a rapid turnover of workers (such as restaurants) or operate on a slim profit margin. In the USA, an estimated 44 million people are without medical insurance because of unemployment or the lack of work-related medical insurance plans.

Diagnosis and Treatment of Occupational Health Problems

Traditionally, large companies had in-house physicians who, although doing some strictly preventive work, spent most of their time diagnosing and treating work-related injuries and illnesses in the company setting. These physicians were frequently in the difficult ethical position of depending on the company for their salary but believing that they were ethically responsible to advocate for the welfare of their patients. Supporting patients' claims that their illnesses were work-related could increase costs for the company and create tensions for the company physicians.

Today, many companies send their workers to outside occupational medicine practices, whose physicians can be somewhat more objective in their clinical evaluations.

■ EXPOSURE TO TOXINS

Forms of Toxins

The word "toxin" makes most people think of liquid chemicals, but toxins can be solids (such as plastics), particulate matter (such as dusts, fumes, or fibers), gases (including vapors or mists), or liquids. A **dust** consists of very fine solid particles of a larger solid (e.g., a rock or piece of coal or wood) and is created by crushing or sanding mechanisms. A **fume** consists of solid particles that develop by condensation from the gases given off by heated metals or plastics. A **gas** is a chemical that normally exists in the gaseous state at room temperature (such as oxygen or helium). A **vapor** is a gas from the evaporation of a liquid such as gasoline. A **mist** is formed when a liquid is aerosolized, as with an atomizer, forming fine droplets of the liquid.

Table 19–2 lists some of the more important toxins. Many of these are found primarily in the workplace, but some, such as carbon monoxide, are commonly encountered in everyday life. Not listed are substances that are toxic primarily if they pollute drinking water (such as gasoline, which can leak from

a storage tank in a filling station and enter a nearby aquifer).

Primary Prevention of Toxic Exposure

The prevention of toxic effects from a substance found in the environment or the workplace requires knowledge about what levels of the substance are considered safe, both for acute, short-term exposure and for chronic, long-term exposure. It also requires accurate measurement and surveillance of environmental or workplace levels of the substance. If the levels approach the threshold for harm, the options are (1) to reduce production or use (e.g., dry cleaners have tended to switch from using carbon tetrachloride to using less toxic solvents such as tetrachloroethylene); (2) to contain the substances within the industrial processes; (3) to remove the substances quickly from the working or living environment (e.g., by ventilation) before they can cause injury; or (4) to protect workers with special equipment (such as ventilatory masks).

Increasing knowledge of the risks of environmental exposures, particularly the possibility of fetal damage, has raised new ethical and legal liability questions. Is a company free of liability if a worker chooses to work in a potentially hazardous area and becomes ill from it? In particular, can a company prohibit pregnant women from working in an area where they might be exposed to a substance (such as lead) that could damage their fetuses? Recent court decisions have tended to say that such exclusion would be discrimination. It is not clear whether a company that initially sought to exclude pregnant women from doing certain jobs and was prohibited by law from doing so would later be liable if fetal injury occurred. The company would, however, still be liable for any violations of the Occupational Safety and Health Administration (OSHA) regulations.

Recent national laws have required that companies make public the potentially toxic substances used in the workplace. These laws have made the process of identification and control within a given area somewhat easier.

Secondary and Tertiary Prevention of Toxic Exposure

If there is any possibility that an injury or disease being treated is related to occupation, the physician should take a careful occupational history. It is not common for workers to be screened for asymptomatic diseases referable to the environment. Nevertheless, if there is a known possible exposure and a reliable screening test, then screening makes sense. Examples include periodic follow-up tuberculin skin tests for health care workers with negative results in the initial tuberculin test; periodic chest x-rays for health care workers with positive results in the tuberculin test; periodic pure tone audiograms to detect hearing loss in workers exposed to high levels of noise; and screening for lead in the serum of workers with unavoidable exposure to lead.

Radiation-sensitive badges for workers in x-ray units or nuclear power stations are more analogous to screening for a risk factor than for a disease.

The symptoms of toxic injury and methods of treatment vary, depending on the level of exposure and the type of toxic substance to which the injured person was exposed. For persons with high-level acute exposures, emergency treatment may be necessary. For workers who have symptoms of disease and are exposed daily to toxic substances, it is important to have well-trained physicians perform a thorough evaluation and provide appropriate treatment and follow-up care. In addition, the occupational exposure should be reported, so that interventions may be made in the workplace before others are injured or poisoned.

DENTAL HEALTH

The two areas of health in which the population is least adequately protected by insurance are dental health and mental health. In the USA, physicians tend to know less about dentistry than dentists know about medicine. This is unfortunate, since the field of dentistry has an early and strong record on the prevention of dental health problems. For example, dentistry consistently supported one of the most widespread community health promotion efforts in US history—namely, the effort to add fluoride to the water, thereby increasing the hardness of the dental enamel and making it more resistant to dental caries (tooth decay or cavities). In areas with fluoridated water, the rate of decayed, missing, and filled teeth (the DMF rate) among children has consistently decreased, and the benefits of strong teeth have continued into the adult years. Claims by opponents of fluoridation that areas with fluoridated water have higher rates of cancer or other diseases have not been supported by careful scientific examination.

Primary prevention in dentistry means more than fluoridation. New efforts in the promotion of dental health include covering teeth with sealants to make the teeth more resistant to decay, and continued efforts focus on attention to the gums as well as the teeth. In the USA, tooth loss occurs more frequently because of gum disease than because of dental caries. Regular dental visits focus chiefly on removing the buildup of calculus (tartar) at the gum line. This procedure can be considered a form of specific protection because it is designed to prevent gingivitis and subsequent periodontitis and tooth loss. If the calculus is not removed, the gums tend to recede from the teeth, causing pockets of inflammation to develop and deepen. If the inflammation spreads to the underlying supporting ligaments and bone, tooth support is weakened. The teeth then become loose and fall out or must be extracted. Both dental caries and gingivitis can be slowed by regular brushing and flossing of teeth, but periodic cleaning by dentists or dental hygienists is still essential to the preservation of teeth and underlying bone.

Secondary prevention in dentistry occurs with regular dental visits to screen for early signs of tooth and gum problems, as well as signs of local or systemic disease, including oral cancer. For all children, but particularly for those who do not have regular dental checkups, a visit to the physician should prompt a look inside the mouth, with special attention paid to the integrity of the 6-year molars. These teeth, which are the first permanent molars to come in, form the foundation of the dental arch. If they are lost as a result of decay or if they are malpositioned, a lifetime of dental problems may ensue. Problems with these molars should be referred for dental treatment immediately.

Tertiary prevention is common in dentistry and includes restorations for dental caries, crowns on more extensively damaged teeth, root canals to enable infected teeth to remain in place, bridges to retain proper tooth spacing when teeth are lost, orthodontic therapy to restore the proper relationship of the teeth to one another, periodontal surgery to treat gingivitis and save the underlying teeth, and implants or dentures to replace lost teeth.

GENETICS IN PREVENTIVE MEDICINE AND PUBLIC HEALTH

No field relevant to health promotion and disease prevention is growing more rapidly than human genetics. The Human Genome Project, an attempt to identify all of the 80,000 or so genes in the human genome (among the approximately 3 billion base pairs), is moving rapidly and probably will be completed well before its official target of 2003 (Collins 1999). In June 2000, scientists announced the completion of the "working draft" of the human genome, containing over 90% of the letters in the human genome sequence. This is an essential first step in identifying individual genes and in determining what they do and how they can be screened and possibly modified for the purpose of treating or preventing human disease.

Screening for Genetic Abnormalities

In the near future, the most important advance in genetic research is likely to be the ability to perform rapid screening for genetic abnormalities or tendencies. It is already possible to screen for several hundred gene abnormalities. Within years or decades, the use of screening "chips" should make it possible to evaluate a person's complete genome for abnormalities that are linked with serious health problems.

This screening potential is exciting for its prevention possibilities, but it is also worrisome in terms of its feasibility, costs, interpretation of results, and ethical implications. Indeed, it should be emphasized that the distinction between "good genes" and "bad genes" is a matter of interpretation, especially when considered in historical context. For example, the genes responsible for hemoglobinopathies (such as sickle cell disease and Mediterranean anemia) and for altered glucose metabolism have historically provided particular groups of people with survival advantages. The sickle cell trait has protected heterozygote carriers from dying from severe forms of falciparum malaria, and altered glucose metabolism may have helped protect Native Americans in the southwestern USA from periodic starvation. The historically beneficial effects are now overshadowed by the negative effects that these genetic differences have on people living in the USA and other countries where malaria is no longer endemic and food is usually abundant year round.

In pursuing the possibilities of genetic screening, an important question is whether individuals really want to know the potentially worrisome truths about their genetic makeup. For example, family members of patients with Huntington's disease can now be screened for this autosomal dominant disorder, which is characterized by the gradual progression of chorea and dementia in mid-adulthood. Although there is still no effective treatment for the disease, the mere fact that its genetic detection is possible places family members under considerable stress when deciding whether to undergo screening. Will there also be social and medical pressures on them to be tested and to use the results in deciding whether to marry and have children? If the results of testing become part of their medical file, what effect will this have on their insurability?

Because of issues and questions such as these, areas that must advance in step with genetic research include medical ethics, genetic counseling, and the development of health promotion methods (modification of nutrition, environment, and behavior) and specific protection methods (drug treatments) that are tailored to the needs of individuals.

To date, single-gene abnormalities provide the most dramatic examples of using the knowledge gained from genetic research to modify the nutrition, environment, or life-style of an affected individual and thereby prevent a negative outcome. In the case of phenylketonuria, for example, early modification of the patient's diet can prevent mental retardation. The impact on the patient is therefore substantial. However, the impact on public health in general would be small, since a single-gene abnormality such as this tends to affect only a small number of individuals.

The greatest impact that genetic research will have on public health will be its impact on diseases that have multiple gene causation, are found in a large number of individuals, and can be prevented or arrested in their early stages via screening and preventive intervention. Experience suggests, for example, that the general public is more likely to accept screening for the presence of the following: (1) genes whose effects can be attenuated by modifying nutrition (e.g., genes associated with hypercholesterolemia and diabetes); (2) genes whose effects can be attenuated by modifying the environment or life-style (e.g., genes associated with allergies and with increased sensitivity to ultraviolet radiation); (3) genes whose presence is considered a marker for a life-threatening but potentially curable disease (e.g., *BRCA1* and *BRCA2* genes, which are markers for breast and ovarian cancer); and (4) genes whose presence affects whether treatment with a specific drug is likely to be effective (e.g., estrogen receptor genes, which increase the probability of responding to treatment with tamoxifen).

In addition to identifying genetic abnormalities, screening techniques may help determine which persons can or cannot tolerate particular environmental or occupational exposures (Hamadeh and Afshari 2000). Genomic knowledge applied to pharmacology (**pharmacogenomics**) may also help determine which therapies for a nongenetic or genetic disease will be the most effective and cause the fewest adverse effects in a given individual (Collins 1999). Using genetic techniques, scientists have already produced over 50 drugs and biologic agents, including human insulin, erythropoietin, and nerve growth factor.

Genetic Counseling

If in the future individuals or potential marriage partners were able to obtain a complete report of their genetic makeup, then genetic counselors would need to be able to answer questions such as the following: What are the health implications of each gene, in both the heterozygous and the homozygous state? Which genes can be altered favorably with gene therapy, and what are the risks and benefits? What is the probability that an adult couple will produce a phenotypically abnormal child if a particular gene is abnormal in one of the adults, and what is the probability if it is abnormal in both of the adults?

Because scientists are likely to be able to screen for a particular gene long before they are able to answer the above questions concerning that gene, genetic counselors are likely to find themselves in the awkward position of not knowing the answers to many questions they are commonly asked. Issues of gene penetrance, severity, and so forth are likely to become the focus of much attention, and genetic counseling is likely to become an increasingly important field, both for physicians and for specifically trained paraprofessionals.

Not to be ignored is the extent to which the self-identity or self-confidence of individuals is affected by their knowledge of genetic weaknesses that are detected through screening. An individual's response to screening results will probably be an important area to be addressed by genetic counselors. A related issue is the possibility that individuals will want to use genetic information to help them produce what might be called designer babies, children whose genetic structure has been modified in advance to produce a desired type of person. This issue, too, must be considered in historical context.

The word **eugenics** (meaning "good genes" in Greek) has terrible connotations today because of the misuse to which the idea has been put in the past. Before World War II, a social movement advocating eugenics had many supporters in numerous countries. The thrust and goals of these supporters varied: some factions promoted the mixing of ethnic groups, while others discouraged it; some factions recommended that genetic counseling be based on knowledge of or inferences about phenotypes and genotypes; and some advocated that individuals with certain characteristics be prevented from marrying and having children. Tragically, in Nazi Germany, Hitler's ideas about eugenics led to the Holocaust.

Today, experts in the fields of genetic and medical ethics are exploring and debating the difficult issues that must be dealt with to ensure that history does not repeat itself. With respect to screening and genetic counseling, there is the potential for some parents to want to test and then either accept or reject (by abortion) a fetus based on the perceived quality of its genome. There is also the potential for some individuals to want to remake themselves or their children via the use of gene therapy. Although so far what some call the "new eugenics" consists of increasingly putting the power of detection and decision in the hands of parents, the time might come when government bodies would begin to enforce detection and perhaps also solutions. In the USA, most states currently require the screening of newborns for phenylketonuria and certain other metabolic errors for which treatment is available. Will states in the future require a complete postnatal genogram of infants, and if so, what therapeutic measures will be required? Or will screening be prohibited unless sufficient information is available for meaningful genetic counseling and unless something can be done to ameliorate the effects of abnormal genes? Will genograms be required of the fetus, and if so, to what end will the information be used?

Ethical and Legal Issues Concerning Advances in Genetic Research

When the Human Genome Project was founded, 5% of its annual research budget was set aside for the study of the ethical, legal, and social implications of the developing field of genetics (Collins 1999). Several of these implications are explored in the discussions of screening and genetic counseling, above.

Many types of screening measures are expensive, particularly in their early years of development, and their use may lead to costly dietary, environmental, and behavioral modifications, as well as costly drug therapy. At a time when a significant proportion of the US population is uninsured or underinsured, this raises the question of whether advances in genetic research and technology will increase the disparities in health that are already evident among socioeconomic groups in the USA. If insurance companies and health maintenance organizations fail to pay for genetic screening and associated medical care, then genetic screening may become a benefit only for the reasonably wealthy.

Confidentiality issues worry many people. To whom is it ethical and legal to release genetic information that has been acquired? Some of the most difficult questions concern the circumstances under which genetic information is released to a medical care insurer. One of the problems of getting reimbursed for genetic testing and counseling is that a request for reimbursement would alert the insurer to the fact that genetic testing was done. The insurer may want to know the results and would claim that it has the right to know because it paid for the tests. Would the results jeopardize an individual's current and future insurance coverage? If the individual personally paid for his or her genetic screening and kept the results from the insurer, would that jeopardize his or her insurance coverage at a later date?

Particularly difficult issues about confidentiality of medical results might arise with respect to couples who are already married or are contemplating marriage. In the case of a married couple, if genetic information is shared with a spouse and the information causes the spouse to unilaterally decide against having children or to file for a divorce, what is the ethical and legal liability? On the other hand, if genetic information is withheld from the spouse (perhaps because the partner would not give permission for the medical system to release the results) and if a child with severe medical problems is born to the couple, will one of the parents be able to demand care for the child and take legal action against the spouse, the physician who ordered the screening tests, the medical authority who performed the screening, the institution that withheld the genetic information, or others? In the case of unmarried individuals, should a medical institution release genetic information to a potential spouse, to enable that person to make a good marital decision? What liability risks would be entailed, particularly if there were an error in a critical test?

The rapid advances in genetic research have led many people to question the profit and patent rights of those involved. Much of the work involved in developing the genetic map has been done by private enterprises, and they expect a reasonable return on their investment. To what extent is it legitimate for private companies and individuals to gain financially from genetic research? If an individual or company used private funds to identify a specific gene, does that individual or company "own" the rights to that gene? If identification of the particular gene allowed other companies to develop diagnostic tests to detect it or to develop therapeutic agents to treat genetic diseases associated with the gene, does the individual or company who identified the gene have the right to a share of the profits from these tests and therapeutic agents?

While these and similar questions are currently being explored, new questions arise with each new advance in genetic research.

Public Health Responsibilities Concerning Advances in Genetic Research

In its report entitled *The Future of Public Health*, the Institute of Medicine (1988b) proposed that the core responsibilities of government in public health were threefold: assessment, policy development, and assurance. All three of these areas of responsibility are applicable to developments in the field of genetics.

Assessment and assurance often go together. The government health establishment will need to assess the accuracy of all proposed genetic tests, based on scientific data, and to ensure that those who do the testing are reliable, based on licensing and regular monitoring. This may require the development of a new branch of the Food and Drug Administration (FDA) or a parallel agency for genetic issues. Similarly, the government health establishment will need to assess the knowledge base for genetic counseling and to ensure the competence of genetic counselors as well as the safety and effectiveness of genetic interventions. The issue of public health responsibility for adequate medical care is discussed more in Chapter 21.

Ultimately, it will become a public health responsibility to define the policies that guide genetic research in the USA and that determine how this research will be applied to public and private medical care practices, with attention to the funding of medical care, to confidentiality issues, and to equity of care for Americans.

■ SUMMARY

In the area of maternal and child health, efforts to promote health and well-being begin with family planning and proceed through the stages of prenatal care, labor and delivery care, and well child care. Opportunities for the prevention of injury and disease continue in day-care, preschool, and school facilities, as well as in homes and worksites.

In the area of infectious diseases, efforts to prevent the spread of the human immunodeficiency virus (HIV) and *Mycobacterium tuberculosis*, the agents responsible for acquired immunodeficiency syndrome (AIDS) and tuberculosis, have helped stabilize the situation regarding these diseases in the highly industrialized countries. However, they have not been of much benefit to the developing countries, where the spread of AIDS remains unchecked and multiple drug–resistant tuberculosis continues to be inadequately treated.

Mental health efforts continue to be under-

funded. Although most forms of chemical substance abuse have stabilized in the USA, the use of amphetamine and amphetamine derivatives has recently increased among teenagers. Injuries continue to be the leading cause of years of life lost before the age of 65. In occupational health, increasing attention is being paid to ergonomic issues and the prevention of repetitive motion injuries, such as carpal tunnel syndrome. Dental health continues to make strides in efforts to prevent dental caries and periodontal disease. And the rising star in prevention appears to be human genetics, with its great potential for diagnosing genetic weaknesses and correcting them by various means, including the modification of nutrition, environment, and life-style, the provision of medications, and (perhaps considerably in the future) direct intervention in the genetic code.

■ QUESTIONS

Directions (Items 1–9). Each of the numbered items or incomplete statements in this section is followed by answers or by completions of the statement. Select the ONE lettered answer or completion that is BEST in each case. Correct answers and explanations are given at the end of the chapter.

1. Folic acid supplementation is important in the prevention of
   - (A) byssinosis
   - (B) intrauterine growth retardation
   - (C) neural tube defects
   - (D) pellagra
   - (E) preeclampsia

2. Which of the following interventions constitutes secondary prevention as a component of prenatal care?
   - (A) Performing a nonstress test prior to parturition
   - (B) Performing pelvic ultrasound examination during the second trimester of pregnancy
   - (C) Providing food vouchers through the Women, Infants, and Children (WIC) Program
   - (D) Screening for and treating gestational diabetes
   - (E) Screening for rubella antibodies

3. Worldwide, the number of people infected with human immunodeficiency virus (HIV) is thought to be approximately
   - (A) 200,000
   - (B) 2 million
   - (C) 5 million
   - (D) 36 million
   - (E) 200 million

4. Worldwide, by the beginning of the 21st century, the number of people dying each year of ac-

quired immunodeficiency syndrome (AIDS) was expected to be approximately

(A) 20,000–30,000
(B) 150,000–200,000
(C) 500,000–700,000
(D) 3 million
(E) 15 million

5. In central Africa and Southeast Asia, the spread of human immunodeficiency virus (HIV) infection is principally the result of

(A) a contaminated blood supply
(B) arthropod vectors
(C) heterosexual intercourse
(D) homosexual intercourse
(E) intravenous drug use

6. During the 19th century, the leading cause of death in industrialized nations was

(A) dropsy
(B) industrial accidents
(C) influenza
(D) malaria
(E) tuberculosis

7. In the USA, the incidence of tuberculosis has shown which of the following patterns?

(A) A decline from the end of the 19th century until 1985, then a rise until 1993, and then another decline
(B) A decline from the middle of the 19th century until the 1940s, then a sharp rise until 1985, and then another decline
(C) A rise from the middle of the 19th century until the 1940s and then a decline
(D) A steady decline since the end of the 19th century
(E) A steady rise since the middle of the 19th century

8. On chest x-rays, the finding of Ghon complexes is evidence of

(A) active tuberculosis
(B) anergy
(C) immunodeficiency
(D) latent tuberculosis
(E) reactivation of primary tuberculosis

9. In the presence of immunodeficiency, tuberculin skin testing with purified protein derivative (PPD) may produce

(A) a false-negative result
(B) a false-positive result
(C) a rash with pruritus
(D) primary tuberculosis
(E) reactivation of latent tuberculosis

■ **ANSWERS AND EXPLANATIONS**

1. **The answer is C: neural tube defects.** It is now well established that supplemental folic acid (fo-late) taken at the time of conception and during early embryogenesis substantially reduces the risk of neural tube defects (Daly et al. 1995). The only other choice specifically related to a micronutrient is pellagra, which is a result of niacin deficiency.

2. **The answer is D: screening for and treating gestational diabetes.** Secondary prevention is the early detection of generally asymptomatic disease and the prevention of adverse sequelae. When gestational diabetes is detected, the disease is already present, so primary prevention is not feasible. Meticulous treatment to maintain a nearly normal serum glucose level at all times prevents adverse consequences of the condition; this is an example of secondary prevention. The provision of food vouchers through the Woman, Infants, and Children (WIC) Program is primary prevention. The process of screening for rubella antibodies and immunizing nonpregnant women who lack them is another example of primary prevention. Routine pelvic ultrasound studies performed during the second trimester may be informative but have not been shown to alter the outcome (Ewigman et al. 1993). Performing a nonstress test prior to parturition helps the obstetrician predict and manage the course of labor and delivery.

3. **The answer is D: 36 million.** Data for 2000 suggest that approximately 36 million people worldwide are infected with human immunodeficiency virus. The quality of data from certain parts of the world is dubious, however. The incidence rate is falling in the USA but is rising steadily in parts of Southeast Asia and sub-Saharan Africa.

4. **The answer is D: 3 million.** If current data are inaccurate, either because of underreporting in certain parts of the world or for other reasons, the mortality estimate is likely to be low. However, with recent advances in drug treatment, if all infected persons were to receive optimum treatment, the mortality rates would decline in the future.

5. **The answer is C: heterosexual intercourse.** In the USA, AIDS is spread by homosexual and heterosexual intercourse and by the use of intravenous drugs. The sharing of contaminated equipment for injecting drugs is beginning to be the predominant manner in which the disease is spread. In parts of the world where the prevalence of HIV infection is similar in men and women, unprotected heterosexual intercourse is the predominant manner in which the disease is spread.

6. **The answer is E: tuberculosis.** *Mycobacterium tuberculosis* has been a human pathogen for cen-

turies but became a scourge in Europe only at the time of the industrial revolution during the 19th century. Contributing factors were thought to include population density, poor sanitation, and crowded working conditions.

7. **The answer is A: a decline from the end of the 19th century until 1985, then a rise until 1993, and then another decline.** The surge in incidence rates of tuberculosis during the 19th century has been ascribed to the industrial revolution and related factors discussed in the chapter. Improvements in sanitation toward the end of the 19th century, as well as some degree of acquired resistance to tuberculosis, caused the incidence rate to begin falling before the start of the 20th century. The rate fell at a variable pace until 1985, when immunodeficiency associated with HIV infection began to facilitate the transmission of tuberculosis. The incidence rate of tuberculosis rose in the USA between 1985 and 1993, and this rate included an alarming rise in the transmission of multiple drug–resistant serotypes. The implementation of more aggressive control and surveillance measures may be responsible for a decline in the incidence rate after 1993.

8. **The answer is D: latent tuberculosis.** On chest x-rays, Ghon complexes appear as calcified granulomas in the periphery of the lower two-thirds of the lungs. These complexes, which develop following containment of primary tuberculosis infection by the cell-mediated immune system, are evidence of infection in a latent state. Latent disease may reactivate as a result of immunosuppression caused by illnesses, use of immunosuppressive drugs, aging, and environmental stresses.

9. **The answer is A: a false-negative result.** In the most common skin test for tuberculosis, the dermis is injected with purified protein derivative (PPD). In individuals who have been exposed to *Mycobacterium tuberculosis,* this test generally elicits an immune reaction (induration of the skin). However, in immunosuppressed or immunocompromised individuals (e.g., patients with acquired immunodeficiency disease), the immune system may be incapable of mounting a reaction, even when exposure to *M. tuberculosis* has occurred. Consequently, those individuals most likely to be infected with tuberculosis are also those most likely to have a false-negative reaction to skin testing. To clarify exposure status in these individuals, an anergy panel, which tests the ability of the immune system to react to any antigen, is used. Several antigens to which exposure is nearly universal are tested on one arm at the same time as PPD is tested on the other arm. A positive reaction to any of the control antigens and a negative reaction to PPD may be interpreted as a true-negative reaction for tuberculosis. If the anergy panel fails to elicit a reaction, a negative result in the PPD test must be considered unreliable, and a chest x-ray is generally indicated.

References Cited

Allen, D. F., and J. F. Jekel. Crack: The Broken Promise. London, Macmillan Academic and Professional, Ltd., 1991.

Barnes, F. E., ed. Ambulatory Maternal Health Care and Family Planning Services: Policies, Principles, Practices. Washington, D. C., American Public Health Association, 1978.

Bellin, E. Y., D. D. Fletcher, and S. M. Safyer. Association of tuberculosis infection with increased time in or admission to the New York City jail system. Journal of the American Medical Association 269:2228–2231, 1993.

Brudney, K., and J. Dobkin. Resurgent tuberculosis in New York City: human immunodeficiency virus, homelessness, and the decline of tuberculosis programs. American Review of Respiratory Diseases 144:745–749, 1991.

Centers for Disease Control. A Child-Centered Program to Prevent Tuberculosis. Publication No. (PHS) 1280. Washington, D. C., Government Printing Office, March 1965.

Centers for Disease Control. Mandatory reporting of occupational diseases by clinicians. Morbidity and Mortality Weekly Report 39:19–28, 1990.

Centers for Disease Control. Tuberculosis among homeless shelter residents. Morbidity and Mortality Weekly Report 40:869–877, 1991.

Centers for Disease Control and Prevention. Exposure of passengers and flight crew to *Mycobacterium tuberculosis* on commercial aircraft, 1992–1995. Morbidity and Mortality Weekly Report 44:137–140, 1995.

Centers for Disease Control and Prevention. Tuberculosis elimination revisited: obstacles, opportunities, and a renewed commitment. Morbidity and Mortality Weekly Report 48:1–13 (RR-9), 1999.

Centers for Disease Control and Prevention. World AIDS Day: December 1, 2000. Morbidity and Mortality Weekly Report 49:1061, 2000.

Centers for Disease Control and Prevention and National Institute for Occupational Safety and Health. Worker Health Chart Book 2000. Department of Health and Human Services (DHHS) Publication No. 2000-127. Washington, D. C., Public Health Service, 2000.

Chen-Yeung, M., and J.-L. Malo. Occupational asthma. New England Journal of Medicine 333:107–112, 1995.

Christoffel, T., and S. S. Gallagher. Injury Prevention and Public Health. Gaithersburg, Md., Aspen Publishers, 1999.

Clemens, J. D., J. J. Chuong, and A. R. Feinstein. The BCG controversy: a methodological and statistical reappraisal. Journal of the American Medical Association 249:2362–2368, 1983.

Collins, F. S. Shattuck lecture: medical and societal consequences of the Human Genome Project. New England Journal of Medicine 341:28–37, 1999.

Daly, L. E., et al. Folate levels and neural tube defects: implications for prevention. Journal of the American Medical Association 274:1698–1702, 1995.

Dubos, R. Mirage of Health: Utopias, Progress, and Biological Change. New York, Harper and Row, 1959.

Edlin, B. R., et al. An outbreak of multidrug-resistant tuberculosis among hospitalized patients with the acquired immunodeficiency syndrome. New England Journal of Medicine 326:1514–1521, 1992.

Ewigman, B. G., et al. Effect of prenatal ultrasound screening on perinatal outcome. New England Journal of Medicine 329:821–827, 1993.

Frieden, T. R., et al. Tuberculosis in New York City: turning the tide. New England Journal of Medicine 333:229–233, 1995.

Haddon, W., Jr. A logical framework for categorizing highway safety phenomena and activity. Journal of Trauma 12:197–207, 1972.

Hamadeh, H., and C. A. Afshari. Gene chips and functional genomics. American Scientist 88:508–515, 2000.

Horowitz, K., S. Weine, and J. F. Jekel. Posttraumatic stress disorder symptoms in urban adolescent girls: compounded community trauma. Journal of Child and Adolescent Psychiatry 34:1353–1361, 1995.

Horsburgh, C. R., Jr. The global problem of multidrug-resistant tuberculosis: the genie is out of the bottle. Journal of the American Medical Association 283:2575–2576, 2000.

Institute of Medicine. Prenatal Care: Reaching Mothers, Reaching Infants. Washington, D. C., National Academy Press, 1988a.

Institute of Medicine. The Future of Public Health. Washington, D. C., National Academy Press, 1988b.

Insurance Institute for Highway Safety (IIFHS). Status Report: Slower Graduation to Full Licensing Means Fewer Teenage Deaths. Arlington, Va., IIFHS, 1994.

Jekel, J. F., et al. Nine years of the freebase cocaine epidemic in the Bahamas. American Journal on Addictions 3:14–24, 1994.

Jones, B. The effect of provisional licensing in Oregon: an analysis of traffic safety benefits. Accident Analysis and Prevention 25:33–46, 1994.

Kaplan, E. Evaluating needle-exchange programs via syringe tracking and testing (STT). AIDS and Public Policy Journal 6:109–115, 1992.

Klerman, G. L., and M. M. Weissman. Increasing rates of depression. Journal of the American Medical Association 261:2229–2235, 1989.

Klerman, L. V. The need for a new perspective on prenatal care. In Merkatz, I. R., et al., eds. New Perspectives on Prenatal Care. New York, Elsevier, 1990.

LaDou, J., ed. Occupational and Environmental Medicine, 2nd ed. Stamford, Conn., Appleton and Lange, 1997.

Levy, B. S., and D. H. Wegman, eds. Occupational Health: Recognizing and Preventing Work-Related Diseases, 2nd ed. Boston, Little, Brown, and Company, 1988.

Matthews, D. A., D. B. Larson, and C. P. Barry. The Faith Factor: An Annotated Bibliography of Clinical Research on Spiritual Subjects. Rockville, Md., National Institute for Healthcare Research, 1993.

Mount, F. W., and S. H. Ferebee. Preventive effects of isoniazid in the treatment of primary tuberculosis in children. New England Journal of Medicine 265:713, 1961.

Office of Drug Control Policy. The National Drug Control Strategy: 2000 Annual Report. Washington, D. C., Government Printing Office, 2000.

Pierce, J. A. Drivers First Licensed in Ontario, October 1969 to October 1975. Toronto, Ontario Ministry of Transportation and Communication, 1977.

Robertson, L. S., and P. L. Zador. Driver education and crash involvement of teenaged drivers. American Journal of Public Health 68:959–965, 1978.

Rosenstock, L., and M. R. Cullen. Clinical Occupational Medicine. Philadelphia, W. B. Saunders Company, 1986.

Rutstein, D. D., et al. Sentinel health events (occupational): a basis for physician recognition and public health surveillance. American Journal of Public Health 73:1054–1062, 1983.

Selwyn, P. A., et al. High risk of active tuberculosis in HIV-infected drug users with cutaneous anergy. Journal of the American Medical Association 268:504–509, 1992.

Tinetti, M. E., M. Speechley, and S. F. Ginter. Risk factors for falls among elderly persons living in the community. New England Journal of Medicine 319:1701–1707, 1988.

US Preventive Services Task Force. Guide to Clinical Preventive Services, 2nd ed. Baltimore, Williams & Wilkins, 1996.

Williams, A. F., et al. Characteristics of Fatal Crashes of Sixteen-Year-Old Drivers. Arlington, Va., Insurance Institute for Highway Safety, January 1995.

World Health Organization (WHO), Global Tuberculosis Programme. Treatment of Tuberculosis: Guidelines for National Programmes, 2nd ed. Geneva, WHO, 1997.

Zahler, P., et al. Kinetics of drug effect by distributed lags analysis: an application to cocaine. Clinical Pharmacology and Therapeutics 31:775–782, 1982.

Selected Readings

American Academy of Pediatrics (AAP). 2000 Red Book: Report of the Committee on Infectious Diseases. Elk Grove Village, Ill., AAP, 2000. [Maternal and child health.]

American Academy of Pediatrics (AAP) and American College of Obstetricians and Gynecologists (ACOG). Guidelines for Perinatal Care, 4th ed. Elk Grove Village, Ill., and Washington, D. C., AAP and ACOG, 1997. [Maternal and child health.]

Christoffel, T., and S. S. Gallagher. Injury Prevention and Public Health. Gaithersburg, Md., Aspen Publishers, 1999. [Injuries.]

Collins, F. S. Shattuck lecture: medical and societal consequences of the Human Genome Project. New England Journal of Medicine 341:28–37, 1999. [Genetics.]

Institute of Medicine. The Future of Public Health. Washington, D. C., National Academy Press, 1988. [Public health.]

Khoury, M. J., W. Burke, and E. J. Thomson. Genetics and Public Health in the 21st Century. New York, Oxford University Press, 2000. [Genetics.]

LaDou, J., ed. Occupational and Environmental Medicine, 2nd ed. Stamford, Conn., Appleton and Lange, 1997. [Occupational health.]

Levy, B. S., and D. H. Wegman, eds. Occupational Health: Recognizing and Preventing Work-Related Disease, 2nd ed. Boston, Little, Brown, and Company, 1988. [Occupational health.]

Office of Drug Control Policy. The National Drug Control Strategy: 2000 Annual Report. Washington, D. C., Government Printing Office, 2000. [Chemical substance abuse.]

Robertson, L. S. Injury Epidemiology, 2nd ed. New York, Oxford University Press, 1998. [Injuries.]

Rosenstock, L., and M. R. Cullen. Clinical Occupational Medicine. Philadelphia, W. B. Saunders Company, 1986. [Occupational health.]

Seashore, M. R., and R. S. Wappner. Genetics in Primary Care and Clinical Medicine. Stamford, Conn., Appleton and Lange, 1996. [Genetics.]

Wallace, H. M., G. Ryan, Jr., and A. C. Oglesby. Maternal and Child Health Practices, 3rd ed. Oakland, Calif., Third Party Publishing Company, 1988. [Maternal and child health.]

Weeks, J. L., B. S. Levy, and G. R. Wagner. Preventing Occupational Disease and Injury. Washington, D. C., American Public Health Association, 1991. [Occupational health.]

20 The Public Health System: Structure and Function

■ DEFINITION OF PUBLIC HEALTH

The term "public health" has two meanings. The first refers to the health status of the public—that is, of a defined population. Chapter 2 provided some tools for estimating the health of a population, and Chapter 14 gave several definitions of health, including a discussion of their limitations. The second meaning, which is the focus of Chapters 20 and 21, refers to the organized social efforts made to preserve and improve the health of a defined population.

The best-known definition of public health in terms of this second meaning was written in 1920 by C.-E. A. Winslow and is still remarkably current:

Public health is the science and art of preventing disease, prolonging life, and promoting physical health and efficiency through organized community efforts for the sanitation of the environment, the control of community infections, the education of the individual in principles of personal hygiene, the organization of medical and nursing service for the early diagnosis and preventive treatment of disease, and the development of the social machinery which will ensure to every individual in the community a standard of living adequate for the maintenance of health.

This definition is profound in many ways. First, it states the central emphasis of all public health work—namely, promoting health and preventing disease. Second, it emphasizes the diverse strategies that are required to bring this about, including environmental sanitation, specific disease control efforts, health education, medical care, and an adequate standard of living. Third, it makes clear that for these goals to be achieved, organized social action is required. This action is largely expressed in the policies of the federal, state, and local government bodies and in the activities of the agencies designed to promote and protect the health of the public. As the Institute of Medicine indicated in its 1988 report entitled *The Future of Public Health,* "Public health is what we, as a society, do collectively to assure the conditions in which people can be healthy."

■ ADMINISTRATION OF PUBLIC HEALTH
Responsibilities of the Federal Government

In theory, the public health responsibility of the federal government in the USA is rather limited. In practice, the federal government bases its role in health on two clauses from Article 1, Section 8, of the US Constitution. One is the interstate commerce clause, which gives the federal government the right "to regulate Commerce with foreign Nations, and among the several States, and with the Indian Tribes." The other is the general welfare clause, which states that "the Congress shall have Power to lay and collect Taxes . . . for the common Defense and general Welfare of the United States." Federal responsibility is also inferred from statements about Congress having the authority to create and support a military and the authority to deal with Indian tribes and other special groups.

Regulation of Commerce

The regulation of commerce involves controlling the entry of people and products into the USA, as well as regulating commercial relationships among the states.

People who may be excluded from entry to the USA include those with particular health problems such as active tuberculosis. Products excluded from entry include fruits and vegetables that are infested with certain organisms (e.g., the Mediterranean fruit fly) or have been treated with prohibited insecticides or fungicides.

The regulation of commercial relationships between states has increased over time and caused some dissent in the USA. Contaminated food products that cross state lines are considered to be "interstate commerce" in harmful microorganisms. Therefore, the federal government takes the responsibility for inspection of all milk, meat, and other food products at their site of production and processing. (In contrast, the state or local government is responsible for inspection of restaurants and food stores.) Likewise, polluted air and polluted water that may flow from state to state are deemed to be "interstate commerce" in polluting agents and therefore come under federal regulation.

Taxation for the General Welfare

The power to "tax for the general welfare" is the constitutional basis for the federal government's development of most of its public health programs and agencies, including the Centers for Disease Control and Prevention (CDC) and the Occupational Safety and Health Administration (OSHA); for research programs, such as those of the National Institutes of Health (NIH); and for the payment for medical care, such as Medicare and Medicaid (see Chapter 21).

Provision of Care for Special Groups

The federal government has taken special responsibility for providing health services to active military personnel through military hospitals; to the families of military personnel through military hospitals or the Civilian Health and Medical Program of the Uniformed Services (CHAMPUS); to veterans through the Veterans' Administration hospital system; and to Native Americans and Alaska natives through the Indian Health Service of the US Public Health Service.

Coordination of Federal Agencies

In the USA, the major federal department most concerned with health is the **Department of Health and Human Services (DHHS).** As outlined in Table 20–1, the DHHS has four major operating units, most of which are called "administrations."

Administration on Aging (AOA). This agency provides advice to the Secretary of the DHHS on issues and policies regarding aging persons in the USA. It also administers certain grant programs for the benefit of the aging population.

Administration for Children and Families (ACF). This agency is responsible for administering child welfare

TABLE 20–1 Major Operating Units and Subunits of the US Department of Health and Human Services

Administration on Aging
Administration for Children and Families
Health Care Financing Administration
  Medicaid
  Medicare
  Quality Assurance
Public Health Service
  Agency for Healthcare Research and Quality
  Agency for Toxic Substances and Disease Registry
  Centers for Disease Control and Prevention
    Epidemiology Program Office
    National Center for Chronic Disease Prevention and Health Promotion
    National Center for Environmental Health
    National Center for Health Statistics
    National Center for Human Immunodeficiency Virus, Sexually Transmitted Disease, and Tuberculosis Prevention
    National Center for Infectious Diseases
    National Center for Injury Prevention and Control
    National Immunization Program
    National Institute for Occupational Safety and Health
    Office of Global Health
    Public Health Practice Program Office
  Food and Drug Administration
  Health Resources and Services Administration
  Indian Health Service
  National Institutes of Health
    Fogarty International Center
    National Cancer Institute
    National Center for Human Genome Research
    National Eye Institute
    National Heart, Lung, and Blood Institute
    National Institute on Aging
    National Institute of Alcohol Abuse and Alcoholism
    National Institute of Allergy and Infectious Diseases
    National Institute of Arthritis and Musculoskeletal and Skin Diseases
    National Institute of Child Health and Human Development
    National Institute on Deafness and Other Communication Disorders
    National Institute of Dental Research
    National Institute of Diabetes and Digestive and Kidney Diseases
    National Institute on Drug Abuse
    National Institute of Environmental Health Sciences
    National Institute of General Medical Sciences
    National Institute of Mental Health
    National Institute of Neurological Disorders and Stroke
    National Institute of Nursing Research
    National Library of Medicine
  Substance Abuse and Mental Health Services Administration
    Center for Mental Health Services
    Center for Substance Abuse Prevention
    Center for Substance Abuse Treatment

Sources of data: (1) Office of the Federal Register, National Archives and Records Administration. United States Government Manual 1998/1999. Washington, D. C., Government Printing Office, 1998. (2) Department of Health and Human Services and Centers for Disease Control and Prevention. About the CDC. Washington, D. C., Government Printing Office, 1999.

programs through the states, Head Start programs, child abuse prevention and treatment programs, foster care, adoption assistance, developmental disabilities programs, and child support enforcement.

Health Care Financing Administration (HCFA). This agency is responsible for administering two major programs from the Social Security Act: (1) **Medicare,** which is covered under **Title 18** and pays for medical care for the elderly; and (2) **Medicaid,** which is covered under **Title 19** and which, in cooperation with the states, pays for medical and nursing home care for the poor (see Chapter 21). The agency's duties include setting standards for programs and institutions that provide medical care, developing payment policies, contracting for third-party payers to pay the bills, and monitoring the quality of care provided. The HCFA is also a major supporter of graduate medical education residency programs that provide care for persons who qualify for services under Medicare or Medicaid.

Public Health Service (PHS). The PHS has eight constituent agencies.

(1) The **Agency for Healthcare Research and Quality (AHRQ)** is the main federal agency for research and policy development in the area of medical care organization, financing, and quality assessment. In 2000, the emphasis on medical care quality increased.

(2) The **Agency for Toxic Substances and Disease Registry (ATSDR)** provides leadership and direction to programs designed to protect workers and the public from exposure to and adverse health effects of hazardous substances that are kept in storage sites or are released by fire, explosion, or accident.

(3) The **Centers for Disease Control and Prevention (CDC)** has the responsibility for "protecting the public health of the Nation by providing leadership and direction in the prevention and control of diseases and other preventable conditions and responding to public health emergencies" (see Office of the Federal Register 1998). The CDC directs and enforces federal quarantine activities, works with states in disease surveillance and control activities, develops immunization and other preventive programs, is involved in research and training, works to promote environmental and occupational health and safety, provides consultation to other nations in the control of preventable diseases, and participates with international agencies in the eradication and control of diseases around the world. The CDC has 11 major operating components, as shown in Table 20–1.

(4) The **Food and Drug Administration (FDA)** is the primary agency for regulating the safety and effectiveness of drugs for use in humans and animals; vaccines and other biologic products; diagnostic tests; and medical devices, including ionizing and nonionizing radiation–emitting electronic products. The FDA is also responsible for the safety, quality, and labeling of cosmetics, foods, and food additives and colorings.

(5) The **Health Resources and Services Administration (HRSA)** is responsible for developing the human resources and methods to improve access to health services and improve the equity and quality of health care. Its emphasis is on promoting primary medical care. The HRSA also supports training grants and training programs in preventive medicine and public health.

(6) The **Indian Health Service (IHS)** promotes the health of and provides medical care for Native Americans and Alaska natives.

(7) The **National Institutes of Health (NIH)** consists of the 18 institutes listed in Table 20–1, plus the Fogarty International Center, the National Library of Medicine, a clinical center, and certain other support divisions. The 18 institutes perform intramural (in-house) research on particular diseases or organ systems, sponsor extramural research through competitive grant programs, and are responsible for some disease control programs and public and professional education.

(8) The **Substance Abuse and Mental Health Services Administration (SAMHSA)** provides national leadership in the prevention and treatment of addictive and mental disorders, based on up-to-date science and practices. Its three major operating divisions are the Center for Mental Health Services, the Center for Substance Abuse Prevention, and the Center for Substance Abuse Treatment.

Responsibilities of States

In the USA, the fundamental responsibility for the health of the public lies with the states. This authority is clarified in the Tenth Amendment to the US Constitution: "The powers not delegated to the United States by the Constitution, nor prohibited by it to the States, are reserved to the States respectively, or to the people."

In each state, there is a state health department to oversee the implementation of the **public health code,** a compilation of the state laws and regulations regarding public health and safety. (While laws must be passed by the legislature, regulations are technical rules added later by an empowered body with specific expertise, such as a state or local board of health.) Mental health services in some states are the responsibility of the health department and in other states are the responsibility of a separate department of mental health services. As a part of its duty to ensure the health of the public, every state licenses medical and other health-related practitioners, as well as medical care institutions such as hospitals, nursing homes, and home care programs.

Responsibilities of Municipalities and Counties

Although the states have the fundamental police power regarding health, they delegate much of this authority to chartered municipalities, such as cities or other incorporated areas. These municipalities accept public health responsibilities in return for a considerable degree of independence from the state in running their affairs, including matters concerning property ownership and tax levies. In this respect, they differ from counties, which are bureaucratic subdivisions of the state created for the purpose of administering (with varying degrees of local control) state responsibilities such as courts of law, educational programs, highway construction and maintenance, police and fire protection, and health services.

Local public health departments usually are administrative divisions of municipalities or counties, and their policy is established by a city or county board of health. These boards of health have the right to establish public health laws and regulations, provided that they are at least as strict as similar laws and regulations in the state public health code and that they are "reasonable." Anything that is too strict can be challenged in the courts as being "unreasonable."

The courts have generally upheld local and state health department laws and regulations when they have to do with the control of communicable diseases. For example, laws relating to safe water and subsurface sewage disposal, immunization, regulation of restaurants and food stores, quarantine or treatment of persons with an infectious disease, investigation and control of acute disease outbreaks, and abatement of complaints relating to the spread of infectious disease (e.g., via possibly rabid animals) have generally been upheld by the courts.

Neither legislatures nor courts, however, have been as supportive of laws and regulations that control human behavior when communicable diseases are not involved. For example, laws requiring motorcyclists and bicyclists to wear helmets often fail to be enacted into law or are repealed following passage, despite abundant evidence of their benefits (see Centers for Disease Control and Prevention 1995). However, if an individual risk factor for disease can be shown to have a negative public impact, such as passive smoke inhalation, legislatures usually support controls.

Responsibilities of Local Public Health Departments

Beginning in the 1920s, the Committee on Administrative Practices of the American Public Health Association studied the role of local health departments and issued a series of statements about their mission (Jekel 1991). The most famous of these statements emerged in 1940, when six primary responsibilities were defined: (1) vital statistics, (2) communicable disease control, (3) maternal and child health, (4) environmental health, (5) health education, and (6) public health laboratories. These responsibilities, which came to be known as the "basic six" functions of local health departments, have continued to influence the direction of local departments, despite the many changes in the nature of public health problems since 1940.

Because the "basic six" functions are not adequate to deal with some of the recent public health problems, such as environmental pollution, occupational toxins and safety hazards, and the increased incidence of chronic degenerative diseases, public health leaders continue to debate the proper functions and responsibilities of health departments at both the local and state level (see, for example, Hanlon 1973 and Terris 1976). Table 20–2 lists functions and essential services that are now considered appropriate for local health departments.

The ability to carry out public health responsibilities depends, of course, on the allocation of funds by legislative bodies. From the 1950s to the early 1970s, the danger of infectious diseases appeared to be waning. Despite occasional warnings that communicable

TABLE 20–2   The Current US Position on the Missions, Functions, and Ten Essential Public Health Services of Public Health Agencies

Missions of Public Health
(1) Promote physical and mental health
(2) Prevent disease, injury, and disability

Functions of Public Health
(1) Prevent epidemics and the spread of disease
(2) Protect against environmental hazards
(3) Prevent injuries
(4) Promote and encourage healthy behaviors
(5) Respond to disasters and assist communities in recovery
(6) Ensure the quality and accessibility of health services

The Ten Essential Public Health Services
(1) Monitor health status to identify and solve community problems
(2) Diagnose and investigate health problems and health hazards in the community
(3) Inform, educate, and empower people about health issues
(4) Mobilize community partnerships and action to identify and solve health problems
(5) Develop policies and plans that support individual and community health efforts
(6) Enforce laws and regulations that protect health and ensure safety
(7) Link people to needed personal health services
(8) Ensure a competent public and personal health care workforce
(9) Evaluate effectiveness, accessibility, and quality of personal and population-based health services
(10) Promote research for new insights and innovative solutions to health problems

Source of data on missions and functions: Public Health Functions Steering Committee, Public Health Functions Team, Office of Disease Prevention and Health Promotion, US Department of Health and Human Services. Public Health in America (pamphlet). Washington, D. C., Government Printing Office, 1994. Source of data on essential services: Centers for Disease Control and Prevention. National Public Health Performance Standards Program (pamphlet). Washington, D. C., Government Printing Office, 1999.

diseases were still major threats (see, for example, Jekel 1972), legislatures saw infectious diseases as a diminishing threat and were not generous with resources for public health agencies. The appearance of legionnaires' disease and Lyme disease in the mid-1970s was soon followed by toxic shock syndrome, acquired immunodeficiency syndrome (AIDS), multiple drug–resistant tuberculosis, and the resurgence of other infectious diseases (see Institute of Medicine 1992 and Garrett 1994). Unfortunately, by the time society began to awaken to the problem of the emerging public health diseases, the Institute of Medicine and others considered the public health system to be in "disarray" (Institute of Medicine 1988; Garrett 2000). It is ironic that because of the resurgence of infectious diseases, the supposedly outdated "basic six" functions have reappeared as the most important functions of local health departments.

Despite the problems that public health agencies have always had in obtaining enough popular and government support to do an effective job of promoting health and preventing disease, the achievements of public health efforts, in conjunction with laboratory research, clinical medicine, and sanitary and safety engineering, are many. Table 20–3 lists what the CDC considers to be the 10 greatest public health achievements of the 20th century.

The Mission of Public Health

In its 1988 committee report, the Institute of Medicine called for a new definition of the role of public health agencies: "The committee defines the mission of public health as fulfilling society's interest in assuring conditions in which people can be healthy." According to the committee, the "core functions of public health agencies at all levels of government are assessment, policy development, and assurance" (Institute of Medicine 1988).

The **assessment** role requires that "every public health agency regularly and systematically collect, assemble, analyze, and make available information on the health of the community, including statistics on health status, community health needs, and epidemiologic and other studies of health problems." The **policy development** role requires that "every public health agency exercise its responsibility to serve the public interest in the development of comprehensive public health policies by promoting the use of the scientific knowledge base in decision-making about public health, . . . by leading in developing public health policy, [and by taking] a strategic approach, developed on the basis of a positive appreciation for the democratic political process." The **assurance** role requires that "public health agencies assure their constituents that services necessary to achieve agreed upon goals are provided, either by encouraging action by other entities (private or public sector), by requiring such action through regulation, or by providing services directly" (Institute of Medicine 1988).

The Institute of Medicine's report has been generally accepted as the broad directive for government functioning in public health in the USA, although it is not viewed as very helpful regarding specifics. Administrators and others involved in the field of public health have been struggling to define how the mission and core functions can best be fulfilled. As indicated in the statement concerning the assurance role, considerable latitude is allowed for public health agencies: they do not have to provide all of (or even

most of) the services required. They are, however, expected to use all their authority and resources to make sure that needed policies, laws, regulations, and services exist.

It should be noted that the current view of "public health policy" in the USA is narrower than that in the world public health scene. For example, according to the Ottawa Charter for Health Promotion (1986), which guides much of the international work in this area, health promotion requires that all policies be reviewed for their health impact and adjusted to strengthen, rather than hinder, the effort to achieve good health:

> Health promotion goes beyond health care. It puts health on the agenda of policy makers in all sectors and at all levels, directing them to be aware of the health consequences of their decisions and to accept their responsibilities for health.
>
> Health promotion policy combines diverse but complementary approaches including legislation, fiscal measures, taxation and organizational change. It is coordinated action that leads to health, income and social policies that foster greater equity. Joint action contributes to ensuring safer and healthier goods and services, healthier public services, and cleaner, more enjoyable environments.
>
> Health promotion policy requires identification of obstacles to the adoption of healthy public policies in non-health sectors, and ways of removing them. The aim must be to make the healthier choice the easier choice for policy makers as well.

An Intersectoral Approach to Public Health

Although this chapter has thus far emphasized the role of specific US public health agencies at the federal, state, and local level, many duties with public health implications are carried out by government agencies that are not usually considered health agencies (as was also emphasized by the Ottawa Charter). For example, departments of agriculture may be responsible for monitoring the safety of milk, meat, and other agricultural products, as well as controlling zoonoses (animal diseases that can be spread to human beings). Departments of parks and recreation are responsible for the safety of water and sewage disposal in their facilities. Highway departments are responsible for the safe design and maintenance of roads and highways. Education departments have the responsibility for health education, as well as for providing a safe and healthful environment in which to learn. Government departments that have to do with promoting a healthy economy are critical, because when an economy is failing, the health of the people will falter as well.

The USA is home to many voluntary health agencies, whose focus is to prevent or control certain diseases, either those of one organ system (e.g., the American Heart Association and the American Lung Association) or a related group of diseases (e.g., the American Cancer Society). Cigarette smoking is a ma-

---

TABLE 20–3 **The Ten Greatest Public Health Achievements of the 20th Century, According to the Centers for Disease Control and Prevention**

(1) Immunization
(2) Motor vehicle safety
(3) Improvements in workplace safety
(4) Control of infectious diseases
(5) Decline in deaths from coronary heart disease and stroke
(6) Safer and healthier foods
(7) Healthier mothers and babies
(8) Family planning
(9) Fluoridation of drinking water
(10) Recognition of tobacco use as a health hazard

Source of data: Centers for Disease Control and Prevention. Morbidity and Mortality Weekly Report, various issues of volume 48, 1998 and 1999.

jor risk factor for heart disease, lung disease, and cancer, so these three agencies may work together to curtail smoking. Indeed, there are voluntary health agencies that focus on almost every organ system in the body and major disease type. These organizations raise money for research, public education, and preventive programs and often for direct patient care as well.

An important conclusion from this is that health is the result of the entire fabric of the environment and life of a population. Therefore, a true public health approach must be intersectoral—that is, it must consider the health impact of policies in every sector of a society and government, not just in the health sector or medical care sector.

The perspectives of the Ottawa Charter and intersectoral policy analysis are foundations for the broader, more community action–oriented approach to public health that currently is being emphasized in Europe and many other places. This approach is sometimes called "the new public health" (see Ashton 1988) or the "healthy communities" approach. In the USA, the healthy communities movement continues to grow (see Duhl and Lee 2000).

■ GOALS OF PUBLIC HEALTH

Overview

During the 1970s, representatives from many public health and scientific organizations began to develop national health promotion and disease prevention objectives. Their efforts resulted in the publication of *Healthy People 2000* (see US Department of Health and Human Services 1990). Although the federal government acted as coordinator and facilitator of these efforts and supported the goals and objectives outlined in the publication, the document itself was "not intended as a statement of federal standards or requirements." It was, however, a national consensus strategy of the government, public health organizations, and public-spirited citizens, and it has had a major impact on the way government and other institutions in the USA are directing their resources in public health.

Healthy People 2010: Understanding and Improving Health

Healthy People 2000 has recently been updated to set goals for 2010. The two **broad goals** listed in the new publication, entitled *Healthy People 2010: Understanding and Improving Health,* are (1) to increase the quality and years of healthy life and (2) to eliminate health disparities (see US Department of Health and Human Services 2000). These goals are to be met by achieving measurable objectives in the focus areas outlined in Table 20–4.

Many public health experts argue that the list of **focus areas,** which increased from 21 in *Healthy People 2000* to 28 in *Healthy People 2010,* has become a "laundry list" of all major areas of health concern. As shown in Table 20–4, the list consists of a mixture of diseases (e.g., cancer, diabetes, and heart disease and

TABLE 20–4   Twenty-Eight Focus Areas Listed in Alphabetical Order in *Healthy People 2010*

(1) Access to quality health services
(2) Arthritis, osteoporosis, and chronic back conditions
(3) Cancer
(4) Chronic kidney disease
(5) Diabetes
(6) Disability and secondary conditions
(7) Educational and community-based programs
(8) Environmental health
(9) Family planning
(10) Food safety
(11) Health communication
(12) Heart disease and stroke
(13) Human immunodeficiency virus (HIV)
(14) Immunization and infectious diseases
(15) Injury and violence prevention
(16) Maternal, infant, and child health
(17) Medical product safety
(18) Mental health and mental disorders
(19) Nutrition and overweight
(20) Occupational safety and health
(21) Oral health
(22) Physical activity and fitness
(23) Public health infrastructure
(24) Respiratory diseases
(25) Sexually transmitted diseases
(26) Substance abuse
(27) Tobacco use
(28) Vision and hearing

Source of data: US Department of Health and Human Services. Healthy People 2010: Understanding and Improving Health. Washington, D. C., Government Printing Office, 2000.

stroke), behaviors (e.g., nutrition and tobacco use), methods of prevention (e.g., immunization), concerns about specific groups (e.g., maternal, infant, and child health), and concerns about the health system (e.g., access to quality health services and public health infrastructure). In *Healthy People 2000,* the 21 objectives had been grouped under three categories: health promotion, health protection, and preventive health services. In the draft version of *Healthy People 2010* (see US Department of Health and Human Services 1998), the objectives had been subdivided into four categories of goals: promote healthy behaviors, promote healthy and safe communities, improve systems for personal and public health, and prevent and reduce diseases and disorders. In the final version of *Healthy People 2010,* however, the categories were eliminated in favor of using an alphabetical listing. Because there is little sense of organization or priorities among the 28 focus areas listed in *Healthy People 2010,* this document will probably not help greatly in the two most difficult tasks faced by policy makers— namely, the tasks of developing health policy and allocating resources. Nevertheless, in each of the 28 focus areas, the document includes measurable indicators of progress, which should prove helpful in tracking progress or documenting the lack of progress.

There is one area in which *Healthy People 2010* breaks with tradition in defining a new set of **leading health indicators.** Heretofore, such measures as the infant mortality rate, life expectancy at birth, and years of potential life lost before age 65 were considered leading health indicators. The new approach takes seriously the perspective set forth by McGinnis and Foege (1993), who have pointed out that the "real" killers are not heart disease, cancer, and stroke but are instead the environmental, behavioral, and nutritional factors that make these organ-based diseases common. Thus, the 10 leading health indicators outlined in *Healthy People 2010* reflect "the major public health concerns" in the USA and were chosen based on "their ability to motivate action, the availability of data to measure their progress, and their relevance as broad public health issues" (see US Department of Health and Human Services 2000). Table 20–5 lists the 10 indicators. Because many of them overlap with the 28 focus areas shown in Table 20–4, their inclusion in the list may have represented a way for the more public health–oriented members of the committee who wrote the document to keep a prevention-focused agenda before the public and to set forth a set of priorities.

For each of the 28 focus areas included in *Healthy People 2010,* an objective is described and appropriate background information is provided. If the focus area is occupational safety and health, for example, the information includes the number of people potentially affected by occupational injuries and diseases, the costs attributable to these health problems, and the amount of progress made toward the earlier (year 2000) goals concerning these problems. Each focus area objective is broken into many subobjectives, and each of these has baseline values and target values for subgroups of the population (age, gender, ethnic, and other subgroups). In occupational safety and health, for example, in addition to baseline values and target values concerning death rates for workers 16 years of age and older in all industries, there are baseline and target values concerning workers in four special high-risk areas (mining; construction; transportation; and agriculture, forestry, and fishing). For each focus area, there are a glossary of terminology specific to the area, a listing of related objectives from other focus areas, and some references. *Healthy People 2010* is a large, two-volume book, and the specific information it provides will undoubtedly be helpful to people working in a focus area, even if it is less helpful to policy makers.

TABLE 20–5 **The Ten Leading Health Indicators**

(1) Physical activity
(2) Overweight and obesity
(3) Tobacco use
(4) Substance abuse
(5) Responsible sexual behavior
(6) Mental health
(7) Injury and violence
(8) Environmental quality
(9) Immunization
(10) Access to health care

Source of data: US Department of Health and Human Services. Healthy People 2010: Understanding and Improving Health. Washington, D. C., Government Printing Office, 2000.

Guide to Community Preventive Services

Chapter 17 discusses the US Preventive Services Task Force and its most recent edition of the *Guide to Clinical Preventive Services,* which was published in 1996. The development of this guide led to a much more rigorous, evidence-based examination of **clinical preventive services** than had been carried out in the past. It also revealed that much of what had been assumed to be good prevention practice lacked adequate evidence to support it or, in some cases, actually had good evidence to show that it was ineffective (see McGinnis and Foege 2000).

The parallel development of *Healthy People 2000,* along with its measures of effectiveness and data bases required for application in the companion planning tool entitled *Healthy Communities 2000,* suggested to public health leaders that there should be an evidence-based examination of **community preventive services** and a resulting document that would parallel in approach and methods the *Guide to Clinical Preventive Services.* There has been considerable enthusiasm for this effort, but there has also been an awareness that communities tend to differ from one another in their response to programs far more than individual persons tend to differ in their response to standard medications, for example. What works clinically in one study group at one time and place will very likely work in a similar manner among similar individuals at other times and places. The same cannot be said of different communities. Health program evaluators have long known that a particular program may be an outstanding success with one community when it is carried out with a certain set of clinicians and program staff during one period and yet may fail miserably in another community or even in the same community during another period, with its different political, social, and economic climate, its different demographic and cultural patterns, and its different program initiators. Thus, most of the people involved in developing the *Guide to Community Preventive Services,* which is scheduled to be published in 2001, have been aware from the onset that their task will be difficult (see McGinnis and Foege 2000). Nevertheless, there is much evidence that can be applied to community preventive services. The goal is to promote evidence-based public health policies and practices. It is one of the more exciting developments in community health services in the past decade.

■ ORGANIZATIONS AND TRAINING IN PREVENTIVE MEDICINE

Organizations

The largest public health organization in the USA is the **American Public Health Association (APHA).** Annual meetings typically bring together from 12,000 to 15,000 people, with all of the excitement and confusion that a large convention can produce. The APHA has gradually changed from being an organization focusing on science and the practice of public health to being an organization focusing primarily on influencing national public health and medical care policy, although some sections within it still emphasize science or practice. This transition was evidenced by the moving of the APHA home offices from New York City to Washington, D. C., decades ago. The APHA welcomes as members anyone who is trained in, working in, or just interested in public health. Its address is 800 I St., NW, Washington, DC 20001.

Physicians who have obtained board certification in preventive medicine and public health are eligible to apply for membership in the **American College of Preventive Medicine (ACPM).** This organization seeks to improve standards of training in preventive medicine residency programs; create and evaluate board examinations in the clinical subspecialties of preventive medicine; and support research and political action to increase the visibility and importance of health promotion and disease prevention. Along with the Association of Teachers of Preventive Medicine (see below), the ACPM copublishes the *American Journal of Preventive Medicine* and cosponsors a yearly conference on prevention science. The address of the ACPM is 1660 L St., NW, Suite 206, Washington, DC 20036.

Members of the **Association of Teachers of Preventive Medicine (ATPM)** include university faculty, preventive medicine residency program directors and faculty, and others interested in teaching health promotion and disease prevention in schools of medicine, public health, and other health professions. The goal of the ATPM is to improve research, training, and practice in preventive medicine and to support the funding for training programs. In many areas, the ATPM works closely with the ACPM because of the similarity of goals and a considerable overlap in membership. The address of the ATPM is 1660 L St., NW, Suite 208, Washington, DC 20036.

Medical Specialty Training

Physicians desiring to become board certified as specialists in preventive medicine may seek postgraduate residency training in a program approved for preventive medicine training by the **Accreditation Council for Graduate Medical Education (ACGME).** These ACGME-approved programs are listed in the American Medical Association "green book" (see American Medical Association 1999).

Certification in preventive medicine must be in one of the following three **subspecialty areas:** (1) general preventive medicine and public health; (2) occupational medicine; or (3) aerospace medicine. Occasionally, a physician will be certified in two subspecialties (most commonly, the first and second areas listed). A number of medical residency programs offer a combined residency in a clinical specialty (such as internal medicine) and preventive medicine. In the residency directory, the residency programs in medical toxicology are listed as related to preventive medicine, but they do not constitute a

fourth subspecialty of preventive medicine. It appears that the residency review committee for preventive medicine is responsible for this subspecialty field, which can be added to a number of clinical residencies.

Certification in preventive medicine requires 3 years of residency. The first year (PGY 1) is called the clinical year. It consists of an internship with substantial patient care responsibility, usually in internal medicine, family practice, or pediatrics, although other areas will be acceptable if they provide sufficient patient care responsibility. The internship may be done in any accredited PGY 1 residency program. A few preventive medicine residency programs offer the PGY 1, but most do not. The second year (PGY 2) is called the academic year and consists of taking courses to obtain the master of public health (MPH) degree or its equivalent. The course work may be pursued in any accredited MPH program and need not be done in a formal preventive medicine residency program, although there are some advantages for doing so. The third year (PGY 3) is called the practicum year, and it must be completed in an accredited preventive medicine residency program. It consists of a year of supervised practice of the subspecialty in varied rotation sites, and it is tailored to fit an individual resident's needs. It typically includes clinical practice of the subspecialty; experience in program planning, development, administration, and evaluation; analysis and solution of problems (such as those related to epidemics); and research and teaching.

The certification examination has two parts: a core examination and a subspecialty examination. The core examination is the same for all three subspecialties and covers topics such as epidemiology, biostatistics, environmental health, health policy and financing, social science as applied to public health, and general clinical preventive medicine. Physicians in training who wish to explore the field further should contact the ACPM at the address listed above.

■ SUMMARY

Public health services in the USA are provided by the federal, state, and local levels of government, although the primary authority for health lies with the states. The federal government becomes involved in health mostly by regulating international and interstate commerce and by its power to tax for the general welfare. Local governments become involved in health as the states delegate authority for health to them. The fundamental health responsibilities have expanded greatly from the "basic six" minimum functions, which were outlined during a time when infectious diseases were the big concern, to a large and diverse set of functions that now include the control of chronic diseases, injuries, and environmental toxins. Administrators and others involved in public health services are currently moving toward a set of goals that are delineated in *Healthy People 2010*. This document emphasizes the improvements in nutrition, behavior, the environment, and clinical preventive services that are needed in 28 focus areas in order to promote health and prevent disease in the US population.

Among the many organizations that have a strong interest in preventive medicine and public health are the American Public Health Association, the American College of Preventive Medicine, and the Association of Teachers of Preventive Medicine. Many members of these organizations are actively involved in specialty medical board training in preventive medicine.

■ QUESTIONS

Directions (Items 1–4). Each of the numbered items or incomplete statements in this section is followed by answers or by completions of the statement. Select the ONE lettered answer or completion that is BEST in each case. Correct answers and explanations are given at the end of the chapter.

1. The authority of the US federal government to inspect food and regulate air pollutants derives from
   - (A)   the Department of Agriculture
   - (B)   the Environmental Protection Agency
   - (C)   the Food and Drug Administration
   - (D)   the interstate commerce clause
   - (E)   the tax law

2. The Food and Drug Administration and the Centers for Disease Control and Prevention are appropriately categorized as
   - (A)   agencies that are independent of the federal government
   - (B)   agencies that are subject to state law
   - (C)   constituent agencies of the Public Health Service
   - (D)   major operating units of the Department of Health and Human Services
   - (E)   major operating units of the Environmental Protection Agency

3. A requirement of public health laws established by city or county boards is that they
   - (A)   be approved by referendum
   - (B)   be approved by the federal government
   - (C)   be at least as strict as regulations in the state public health code
   - (D)   be revised annually
   - (E)   pertain to communicable diseases

4. The basic responsibilities of local health departments exclude
   - (A)   collating vital statistics
   - (B)   controlling communicable diseases
   - (C)   providing health education
   - (D)   providing maternal and child health services
   - (E)   setting radiation exposure standards

Directions (Items 5–13). Each set of matching questions in this section consists of a list of lettered options followed by several numbered items. For each numbered item, select the ONE lettered option that is most closely associated with it. To avoid spending too much time on matching sets with large numbers of options, begin each set by reading the list of options. Then, for each item in the list, try to generate the correct answer and locate it in the option list, rather than evaluating each option individually. Each lettered option may be selected once, more than once, or not at all.

Items 5–13

- (A)   Administration on Aging (AOA)
- (B)   Administration for Children and Families (ACF)
- (C)   Centers for Disease Control and Prevention (CDC)
- (D)   Department of Health and Human Services (DHHS)
- (E)   Environmental Protection Agency (EPA)
- (F)   Food and Drug Administration (FDA)
- (G)   Health Care Financing Administration (HCFA)
- (H)   Health Resources and Services Administration (HRSA)
- (I)   Institute of Medicine (IOM)
- (J)   National Center for Health Statistics (NCHS)
- (K)   National Institute of Environmental Health Sciences (NIEHS)
- (L)   National Institute for Occupational Safety and Health (NIOSH)
- (M)   National Institutes of Health (NIH)
- (N)   Occupational Safety and Health Administration (OSHA)
- (O)   Social Security Administration (SSA)
- (P)   US Preventive Services Task Force (USPSTF)

Match the administrative body with the corresponding definition or description.

5. This body oversees Medicare and Medicaid.
6. This body is responsible for disease surveillance.
7. This body is responsible for the funding of biomedical research.
8. This body generates and provides numerator data for US population statistics.
9. This body enforces workplace standards.
10. This body provides evidence-based recommendations for screening and counseling.
11. This body oversees the Behavioral Risk Factor Surveillance System.
12. This body is responsible for promoting access and equity in health care.
13. This body is responsible for regulating the safety and effectiveness of vaccines.

■ ANSWERS AND EXPLANATIONS

1. **The answer is D: the interstate commerce clause.** Most of the responsibility for protecting the public health resides with the states. Factors

that influence health but cross state lines often fall under federal jurisdiction. Contaminated food products and air pollutants are apt to cross state lines and are therefore considered a form of (undesirable) interstate commerce. As such, their regulation is a federal responsibility under the interstate commerce clause of the US Constitution.

2. **The answer is C: constituent agencies of the Public Health Service.** The Centers for Disease Control and Prevention (CDC) is responsible for the investigation and control of communicable diseases and other public health threats. The Food and Drug Administration (FDA) is responsible for regulating the safety and effectiveness of drugs and additives to the food supply. The CDC and FDA, along with six other agencies, are incorporated within the Public Health Service (see Table 20–1).

3. **The answer is C: be at least as strict as regulations in the state public health code.** City and county boards of health are delegated their authority by the state government, which has the fundamental responsibility for protecting the public health. These boards may generate local policy regulations that comply with statewide standards. Local regulations that are stricter than state laws must be deemed "reasonable," or they may be challenged in court.

4. **The answer is E: setting radiation exposure standards.** Collating vital statistics, controlling communicable diseases, providing health education, and providing maternal and child health services are all included in the "basic six" functions of local health departments, which were first espoused in 1940. The list of local health department responsibilities has expanded but does not include setting standards for occupational and environmental exposures. Depending on the situation, this is either a state or a federal responsibility.

5. **The answer is G: Health Care Financing Administration (HCFA).** Medicare pays for medical care for the elderly, and Medicaid provides health care coverage for the indigent and certain other groups. Although these programs were created under Title 18 and Title 19, respectively, of the Social Security Act, they are overseen by the HCFA. The Social Security Administration (SSA) does not oversee health care programs; it administers retirement payments for social security program recipients and disability payments for the disabled.

6. **The answer is C: Centers for Disease Control and Prevention (CDC).** While much disease surveillance is actually conducted at the level of local health departments, responsibility for surveillance in the country as a whole rests with the CDC.

7. **The answer is M: National Institutes of Health (NIH).** The NIH is largely responsible for the funding of biomedical research.

8. **The answer is J: National Center for Health Statistics (NCHS).** The NCHS generates and provides numerator data for population statistics in the USA.

9. **The answer is N: Occupational Safety and Health Administration (OSHA).** Workplace standards are recommended by the National Institute for Occupational Safety and Health (NIOSH), and they are enforced by OSHA.

10. **The answer is P: US Preventive Services Task Force (USPSTF).** The USPSTF was convened by the US government specifically to provide guidelines for the periodic health examination, health screening, and counseling. The Institute of Medicine (IOM) serves as an expert panel in the generation of other health policy guidelines in the USA.

11. **The answer is C: Centers for Disease Control and Prevention (CDC).** The Behavioral Risk Factor Surveillance System (BRFSS) is an ongoing survey of behavioral risk factors for chronic disease. The assessment of these risk factors falls within the purview of the CDC, which is charged with disease surveillance.

12. **The answer is H: Health Resources and Services Administration (HRSA).** The HRSA is responsible for the oversight of health system resource allocations and for the promotion of access and equity in health care.

13. **The answer is F: Food and Drug Administration (FDA).** The FDA is the primary agency for regulating the safety and effectiveness of drugs, vaccines and other biologic products, diagnostic tests, and medical devices. It is also responsible for the safety and labeling of cosmetics, foods, and food additives and colorings.

References Cited

American Medical Association. Graduate Medical Education Directory 1999–2000. Chicago, American Medical Association, 1999.

Ashton, J. The New Public Health. Buckingham, UK, Open University Press, 1988.

Centers for Disease Control and Prevention. Injury control recommendations: bicycle helmets. Morbidity and Mortality Weekly Report 44:1–17, 1995.

Duhl, L. J., and P. R. Lee, eds. Focus on Healthy Communities. Public Health Reports 115(2 and 3):114–289, 2000. [Special issues of Public Health Reports.]

Garrett, L. Betrayal of Trust: The Collapse of Global Public Health. New York, Hyperion, 2000.

Garrett, L. The Coming Plague. New York, Farrar, Straus, and Giroux, 1994.

Hanlon, J. J. Is there a future for local health departments? Health Services Reports 88:898–901, 1973.

Institute of Medicine. Emerging Infections: Microbial Threats to Health in the United States. Washington, D. C., National Academy Press, 1992.

Institute of Medicine. The Future of Public Health. Washington, D. C., National Academy Press, 1988.

Jekel, J. F. Communicable disease control in the 1970s: hot war, cold war, or peaceful coexistence? American Journal of Public Health 62:1578–1585, 1972.

Jekel, J. F. Health departments in the US, 1920–1988: statements of mission with special reference to the role of C.-E. A. Winslow. Yale Journal of Biology and Medicine 64:467–479, 1991.

McGinnis, J. M., and W. H. Foege. Actual causes of death in the United States. Journal of the American Medical Association 270: 2207–2212, 1993.

McGinnis, J. M., and W. H. Foege. Guide to Community Preventive Services: harnessing the science. American Journal of Preventive Medicine 18(supplement 1):1–2, 2000. [Introduction to a special issue on community preventive services; see the entire issue, pp. 1–140.]

Office of the Federal Register, National Archives and Records Administration. United States Government Manual 1994/1995. Washington, D. C., Government Printing Office, 1994.

Ottawa Charter for Health Promotion. Report of an International Conference on Health Promotion, Sponsored by the World Health Organization, Health and Welfare Canada, and the Canadian Public Health Association, Ottawa, Ontario, Canada, November 17–21, 1986.

Terris, M. The epidemiologic revolution, national health insurance, and the role of health departments. American Journal of Public Health 66:1155–1164, 1976.

US Department of Health and Human Services. Healthy Communities 2000. Washington, D. C., Government Printing Office, 1990.

US Department of Health and Human Services. Healthy People 2000: National Health Promotion and Disease Prevention Objectives. Washington, D. C., Government Printing Office, 1990.

US Department of Health and Human Services. Healthy People 2010 Objectives: Draft for Public Comment. Washington, D. C., Government Printing Office, 1998.

US Department of Health and Human Services. Healthy People 2010: Understanding and Improving Health. Washington, D. C., Government Printing Office, 2000.

US Preventive Services Task Force. Guide to Clinical Preventive Services, 2nd ed. Baltimore, Williams & Wilkins, 1996.

Winslow, C.-E. A. The untilled fields of public health. Science 51: 22–23, 1920.

Selected Readings

Ashton, J. The New Public Health. Buckingham, UK, Open University Press, 1988.

Duhl, L. J., and P. R. Lee, eds. Focus on Healthy Communities. Public Health Reports 115(2 and 3):114–289, 2000. [Special issues of Public Health Reports.]

Garrett, L. Betrayal of Trust: The Collapse of Global Public Health. New York, Hyperion, 2000.

McGinnis, J. M., and W. H. Foege. Actual causes of death in the United States. Journal of the American Medical Association 270: 2207–2212, 1993.

McGinnis, J. M., and W. H. Foege. Guide to Community Preventive Services: harnessing the science. American Journal of Preventive Medicine 18(supplement 1):1–2, 2000. [Introduction to a special issue on community preventive services; see the entire issue, pp. 1–140.]

Novick, L. F., and G. P. Mays. Public Health Administration. Gaithersburg, Md., Aspen Publishers, 2001.

US Department of Health and Human Services. Healthy People 2010: Understanding and Improving Health. Washington, D. C., Government Printing Office, 2000.

■ A FRAMEWORK FOR UNDERSTANDING MEDICAL CARE SYSTEMS

Is the physician's role primarily that of master of medical technology, or is it a broad healing role, involving the physician in the lives of patients, their families, their environment and employment, and their communities? In the modern era, is the physician responsible only for giving the best possible care to individual patients, or do all physicians have an obligation to make the system in which they work operate fairly, effectively, and efficiently for everyone? What obligations do physicians owe to society beyond providing competent and ethical medical care to individuals?

Those working in preventive medicine and public health in the USA are convinced that physicians must assume a broad role of caring for individuals and that physicians are at least partly responsible for bringing about and maintaining a fair and efficient system of medical care for everyone. The first step in accepting some responsibility for the current medical care system is to understand how it functions and in what ways it currently fails to serve both the American people and the medical profession itself.

Unresolved Tensions

In the USA, there are many unresolved tensions concerning the ways in which medical care is or should be organized and financed. Different systems of care and financing emphasize different responses to the questions listed below.

(1) Should the emphasis be on prevention or cure? In general, for an insurance program or health maintenance organization to be willing to provide significant preventive services beyond immunizations, some short-term cost savings need to be demonstrated (see Chapter 14).

(2) Within prevention, should the emphasis be on health promotion or disease prevention? In general, insurance programs and medical care systems are more willing to pay for disease prevention methods (e.g., vaccines, antibiotic prophylaxis, and screening) than for health promotion programs that emphasize the improvement of nutrition, health-related behavior, and the environment. Part of the hesitancy to support health promotion comes from uncertainty about the economic benefits that health promotion will bring to the insurance programs, and part may derive from a belief that such broad concerns are not the responsibility of an insurance company or the medical care system (see Chapters 15–17).

(3) What type of practice should be emphasized in medical education: primary care or specialty practice? The increasing complexity of technology and the greater financial rewards for specialty practice have encouraged specialization in medicine. The bulk of the need for medical care, however, is better served by primary care physicians.

(4) Should hospitals, health maintenance organizations, and group practices focus exclusively on the people who enter their institutions, or should they be actively involved in promoting the health of the entire community?

(5) To what extent should (and, indeed, to what extent can) physicians share medical decision-making with their patients?

(6) To what extent is there a tension between low cost and high quality in the care process? Depending on the circumstances, there may be no tension between these factors. The best medical care is usually the least amount of medical care that gives a good outcome. For example, the elimination of unnecessary surgery and unneeded medical procedures reduces costs and also improves care. It should be less costly to prevent hospital infections and drug errors than to pay for their negative consequences. A large proportion of medical care dollars go to caring for hopelessly ill people near the end of their lives, but there are ethical problems in knowing when to stop maximum medical effort. Nevertheless, there is no question that sometimes the best care is very costly; for example, coronary artery bypass grafts are costly but frequently improve the length and quality of life.

Terminology in Health Care

Health care policies and financing are influenced by distinctions between concepts such as disease and illness, impairment and disability, and needs and demands.

A **disease** is a medically definable process, in terms of pathophysiology and pathology, whereas **illness** is what the patient experiences. Several different diseases might produce similar illness experiences. For example, amebiasis, salmonellosis, shigellosis, and various other diseases can cause dysentery, which patients typically experience as gastrointestinal pain and diarrhea. On the other hand, the same basic disease process, such as diabetes mellitus, can produce different illness experiences in different patients. For example, one patient with diabetes mellitus may have a cerebrovascular accident, another may have a myocardial infarction, another may lose vision or kidney function, another may have circulatory problems in the feet, and another may experience no serious end-organ damage at all.

Impairment is defined as a limitation of capacity or functional ability, usually as determined by a licensed physician. In contrast, **disability** is a social definition of limitation, based on the degree of impairment. Disability is defined by society in laws dealing with social benefits (such as Social Security benefits) and rights for the handicapped. A physician will determine whether there is impairment in a person's eyesight, and then society determines whether or not this impairment is severe enough to prohibit a person from flying an airplane or driving a car or a bus. For purposes of social benefits, there are several categories of disability, including the following: (1) **temporary partial disability** (e.g., a fractured arm); (2) **temporary total disability** (e.g., a broken back without paralysis); (3) **permanent partial disability** (e.g., permanent loss of one eye or one limb); and (4) **permanent total disability** (e.g., permanent loss of two eyes, two limbs, or an eye and a limb).

The **need for medical care** is usually considered a professional judgment. Although the term **felt need** is sometimes used to describe a patient's judgment about the need for care, more commonly what is actually studied is the **demand for medical care.** Demand has both a medical and an economic definition. The medical definition of demand is the amount of care people would use if there were no barriers to care. The problem with this definition is that there almost always are barriers to care: cost, convenience, fear, lack of real availability because of distance to the care settings or because of the limited times they are open, and so forth. The economic definition of demand is the quantity of care that is purchased at a given price. For this economic definition to work, there must be an assumption of price elasticity—i.e., an assumption that as demand falls, the price for a given amount of care will also fall. This assumption often proves false in medical care economics.

Because of the difficulties of measuring demand, what is usually studied is the effective (realized) demand, which is **utilization.** Utilization is usually less than need, so the concept of unmet need was developed. **Unmet need** can be defined by the following equation:

$$\text{Unmet need} = \text{Need} - \text{Utilization}$$

Factors Influencing Need and Demand

Demographic factors are among the most important influences on the need and demand for medical care. Foremost among these is the **age of the population,** which is defined either as the median age of persons in the population or as the percentage of persons over a certain age, such as 65 years. The median age and the percentage over 65 are both determined more by **fertility patterns** than by **mortality rates.** As the birth rate falls, the population ages because fewer young people are born to counteract the continual aging of those already in the population. The US crude birth rate (the number of births per 1000 population) and the US general fertility rate (the number of children born to women aged 15–44 divided by the population of women aged 15–44) declined during most of the past century. The exception to this was the period immediately after World War II (the postwar "baby boom" period), when the birth rates were high. A rather sudden decline in birth rates occurred around 1970, when induced abortion became legally available. The process of aging of the population, which had been occurring somewhat gradually, accelerated after 1970, although immigration has moderated the process to some extent.

While the reduction in the rate of children born has reduced the demand for pediatricians and, to a lesser extent, has reduced the demand for obstetrician-gynecologists, the aging of the population has increased the proportionate use of hospitals and other sources of medical care by older persons. Currently, more than 50% of the patients hospitalized at any point in time are likely to be 65 years or older, whereas only 13–14% of the population is likely to be in this age group.

Fertility levels continue to be low. The long-term result of lowered fertility may be an extended period in which the proportion of workers in the US population will be the smallest in history. This period is expected to begin around 2015, when large numbers of "baby boom" children will enter retirement age. A major concern is whether the smaller number of workers will be able to support the large older population with such benefits as Medicare (see below) and Social Security retirement funds. The expected shortage of workers will put upward pressure on wages, making medical care and nursing home care more expensive than they already are. Chronic diseases among the elderly, with their high demand for medical and nursing home care, will be common.

Among the other factors that influence medical needs and demands are the **advances in medical technology,** especially genetic technology. As new methods of prevention, diagnosis, and treatment become available and are found to be useful, more physicians and more patients will view the use of this technology as necessary and desirable.

One might expect that the greatest unmet need for medical care would exist among the poorest members of society, but that is not always true. People below some percentage of the **poverty line** (often 125%) are eligible for Medicaid under Title 19 of the Social Security Act (see Medicaid, below). In addition to providing medical care insurance, Medicaid provides coverage for nursing home stays for poor people. People whose incomes are too high to be eligible for Medicaid, who do not receive medical insurance in their jobs, and who are not able to pay for individual medical care insurance policies are known as **medically indigent.** They may be able to support themselves until a medical catastrophe strikes, but then they are unable to pay their bills. Many of the **medically uninsured** (i.e., those who have no health insurance) and **medically underinsured** (those who have some but inadequate health insurance) are medically indigent. They are not on welfare, but they cannot financially tolerate major medical bills. In the USA, about 44 million people (17% of the US population) were uninsured in 2000.

■ THE MEDICAL CARE SYSTEM
Goals of Medical Care

Different societies and different eras in a given society may emphasize one goal or another for a medical care system. Usually considered among the important goals or functions of medical care are the following (not necessarily listed in order of priority): (1) to increase the length of life, (2) to improve the function of individuals, (3) to increase the comfort of ill persons and their families, (4) to explain medical problems to patients and their families, (5) to provide a prognosis for the patient, and (6) to provide support and care for patients and their families. These goals are not always fully compatible. For example, extending biological life to the maximum may increase pain and anxiety for the patient and family.

Basic Requirements for Good Medical Care

The basic requirements for good medical care can be summarized by a list of terms called the 7 A's and the 3 C's.

Availability of medical care means that care can be obtained during the hours and days when people need it. If care is available only 5 days a week between the hours of 9 AM and 5 PM, many working people will not receive good medical care. Only if providers are available in the evenings and on weekends does care meet this criterion.

Adequacy is a sufficient volume of care to meet the need and demand of a community. In some inner-city areas, as well as in some rural areas, the limited numbers of physicians and hospital emergency departments are not adequate to keep pace with the demand.

Accessibility refers to geographic, physical (e.g., for handicapped persons), and financial accessibility. Facilities that cannot be reached easily by public transportation and facilities that limit or deny care to those without adequate insurance or financial resources are inaccessible.

Acceptability of care depends on a variety of factors, such as whether the providers can communicate well with their patients (including whether they can speak the patients' languages), whether the care is seen as warm and humane and concerned with the whole person, and whether the patients believe in the confidentiality and privacy of information shared with their providers.

Appropriateness of care means that the procedures being performed are properly selected and carried out by trained personnel in the proper setting. Performing open heart surgery in a small rural hospital is probably not appropriate, since complicated procedures such as this require the resources of a major medical center where many similar operations are done each year.

Assessability means that the medical care can be readily evaluated. Care can be assessed more efficiently if the medical records are complete and if basic care information is available in linked computer data bases, allowing the facility to produce timely analyses.

Accountability has to do with public accountability. Is there public representation on the board of directors of the health care institution or facility? Are the financial records regularly reviewed by certified public accountants? Is there appropriate public disclosure of financial records and of quality of care studies?

Completeness of care requires adequate attention to all aspects of a medical problem. Complete care includes health promotion, disease prevention, early detection of diseases, and appropriate diagnostic and treatment measures, including follow-up care and rehabilitation.

Comprehensiveness of care means that care is provided for all types of health problems, including dental and mental health problems. If there are major exclusions, such as for psychiatric or substance abuse care, the coverage cannot be considered comprehensive.

Continuity of care requires that the management of a patient's care over time be coordinated among providers. Is there one physician or other provider who is basically in charge of a patient's care, who sees the patient regularly and makes sure that there are no major omissions or redundancies in the care? This has become a larger issue with the increase in specialists and referrals for high-technology procedures. Continuity of care influences quality, efficiency, and acceptability. Lack of continuity and the resultant disruption of the physician-patient relationship are thought to be significant factors in the frequency of malpractice litigation.

■ THE ORGANIZATION OF MEDICAL CARE
Historical Overview

In the late 1800s, most medical care was ambulatory care or care in the home, with local practitioners paid on a fee-for-service basis. The hospital tended to be viewed as a death house and a place for the sick poor, often supported by the church or other benevolent organizations. Those who could not pay for treatment at home were relegated to the hospital.

In the early 1900s, as medicine became more scientific and efficacious, the hospital came to be seen as the doctors' workshop. The technology and ancillary personnel and services were usually provided at no charge to the doctors, and these helped the doctors practice their craft. In turn, the doctors brought patients to the hospitals to keep the hospitals economically solvent. Thus, a mutually profitable relationship was established between hospital and physician.

Acute, general hospitals, however, did not usually offer care to the mentally ill. If mentally ill or retarded persons could not be cared for at home, they tended to be cared for in large hospitals run by the state. Mental hospitals generally were dismal facilities, usually built in sparsely populated areas. Eventually, the development of psychoactive medications enabled many patients with mental disorders to be treated in community settings, and state mental hospitals were progressively closed in the late 1960s and early 1970s. Unfortunately, this **deinstitutionalization** occurred without the concomitant development of adequate community resources to receive the large numbers of mentally ill patients being discharged. Some of these patients benefited from treatment in an outpatient setting. Others, however, could not function well in society. As a result, many discharged patients became poverty-stricken and homeless, particularly if they forgot or refused to take their medications.

General hospitals in the past usually did not offer care to patients with tuberculosis. These patients were treated in special, state-run tuberculosis hospitals until after World War II, when the development of antibiotics permitted them to be treated in general hospitals or at home.

The downsizing of mental hospitals and the closing of tuberculosis hospitals considerably reduced the costs to the states for these types of medical care. However, other medical care expenses of the states increased, notably their share of Medicaid costs, particularly payments for nursing home care for the elderly.

With the founding of the National Institutes of Health in 1948 came a push for improved biomedical technology. The research done since that time has made the practice of medicine much more effective but also far more complex and costly. The increased complexity has not only resulted in increasing specialization of physicians and other health care workers but has also required an increasing rationalization of the levels of care to make the complexity of care and the resulting costs appropriate to each patient's needs.

Levels of Medical Care

In an effort to maximize the effectiveness and efficiency of the medical care process, health care professionals have proposed an integrated system of graded levels of care. As shown in Table 21–1, the levels range from treatment in a tertiary medical center (the most complex level of care) to treatment in the patient's home (the least complex level). A patient is initially assigned to an appropriate level of care and is reassigned to another level whenever there is an improvement or setback in the patient's condition. Although the movement from one level to another should be easy, rapid, and smooth, often this is not the case.

At the top of the scale of complexity are three types of **acute, general hospital facilities.** The first type is the **tertiary medical center,** which has most or all of the latest technology and which usually participates

TABLE 21–1 Levels of the Medical Care System from the Most Complex (Top) to the Least Complex (Bottom)

(1) Acute, general hospital facilities
    (a) Tertiary medical center (with most or all of the latest technology)
    (b) Intermediate hospital (medium to large community hospital with a considerable amount of the latest technology)
    (c) Local community hospital
(2) Rehabilitation or convalescent care facilities
    (a) Special unit in a regular hospital
    (b) Rehabilitation hospital
(3) Extended care facilities (ECFs)
    (a) Skilled nursing facility (SNF, or "nursing home")
    (b) Intermediate care facility (ICF)
    (c) Hospice
(4) Organized home care
    (a) Public agencies (local health departments or visiting nurse associations)
    (b) Private organizations
(5) Self-care in the home

actively in medical education and clinical research. Within this facility there are different units offering different levels of care, including intensive care units, special units for observation of patients, and standard units for the care of patients. The second type is the **intermediate hospital,** which is a medium to large community hospital that has a considerable amount of the latest technology but less research and investigational activity. The intermediate hospital may support cardiac bypass surgery, for example, but not necessarily organ transplantation. The third type is the **local community hospital,** which provides services such as routine diagnosis, treatment, and surgery but which lacks the personnel and facilities for many complex procedures.

Next on the scale of complexity are two types of **rehabilitation or convalescent care facilities.** The first type is a **special unit in a regular hospital,** and the second type is a **rehabilitation hospital.** In particular, patients recovering from trauma or from neurologic diseases or surgery may benefit from physical therapy, occupational therapy, and other methods of tertiary prevention (see Chapters 14 and 18).

If patients are not discharged from the hospital directly to their homes, they are most likely to be discharged to one of three different types of **extended care facilities** (ECFs). The first type is the **skilled nursing facility** (SNF), which is often called a nursing home. It provides 24-hour nursing care and special kinds of care, such as intravenous fluids, medicines, and rehabilitation. The second type is the **intermediate care facility** (ICF), which is suitable if the patient's primary need is for help with the activities of daily living (eating, bathing, grooming, transferring, toileting, and so forth). Unlike an SNF, an ICF is not required to have a registered (skilled) nurse on duty at all times. Some nursing homes provide both skilled and intermediate levels of care. The third type is the **hospice,** a nursing home that specializes in providing terminal care, especially for patients with cancer or acquired immunodeficiency syndrome (AIDS).

Organized home care may be necessary for patients who are discharged from the hospital to the home, where they continue to receive treatment or follow-up procedures that require specialized skills. Examples include the placement and monitoring of intravenous lines for therapy and the drawing of blood for tests. In the past, most home care was provided by not-for-profit community groups such as visiting nurse associations or by public health nurses from local health departments. More recently, many hospitals have organized their own home care teams, which help ensure smooth transitions for patients discharged to their homes. In addition, there are a number of proprietary (for-profit) home care organizations, many of which operate nationwide.

As shown in Table 21–1, the least complex level of medical care is **self-care** in the home. In fact, the majority of medical care decisions are not made by professionals but instead are made by people for themselves, for friends, or for members of their families. Many home diagnostic tools, such as blood pressure cuffs and blood glucose testing equipment, have given patients greater power to monitor their own health status. One advantage of this has been improved self-care. For example, diabetic patients can monitor their blood glucose levels and more easily see for themselves the immediate results of stress and dietary indiscretions.

Some modern movements have included emphasis on the importance of people taking more control over decisions that affect their lives and bodies. Many medications that used to be available only by prescription are now sold over the counter. Although at one time Dr. Spock's book on infant and child care was practically the only available self-help book on a health care subject, now there are whole medical and health sections in bookstores, providing patients with considerably more information about (and therefore more control over) their own health and illnesses. The tremendous amount of health information now available on the Internet has been a major force for empowering people regarding their own health. However, this information is usually not "peer reviewed" and may contain incorrect or misleading statements.

Medical Care Institutions
Hospitals

While the term "hospital" is generally thought to refer to an institution providing acute, general care to persons with a wide range of health problems, there are, in fact, a variety of types of hospitals. Some focus on a special group of patients (e.g., a children's hospital), while others focus on a special type of medical problem (e.g., a psychiatric hospital) or a particular type of service (e.g., a rehabilitation hospital).

Hospitals may be for-profit or not-for-profit. A for-profit hospital may be independent or part of a for-profit chain of hospitals. Not-for-profit hospitals may be sponsored by (1) the community in which they are located; (2) a church or other religious group; (3) a charitable organization (e.g., Shriners' hospitals for children); (4) a city, county, or state government; or (5) the federal government (e.g., Veterans Administration Hospitals).

Ambulatory Primary Care Systems

Solo Medical Practices. Historically, most US physicians were in solo medical practice, although they might share night and weekend coverage with other solo practitioners. This type of practice could be quite rewarding, but frequently it was exhausting.

Partnerships. Gradually, US physicians began to develop practice partnerships, partly to solve the problem of sharing weekend and nighttime coverage and partly to achieve efficiencies and economies by sharing the cost of office space, equipment, and staff.

Group Practices. A logical extension of the partnership was the formation of a group practice consisting of three or more (often many more) physicians. This increased the efficiencies of sharing office space and staff and increased the free time available to physicians. It also had the advantage of providing built-in consultation with other physicians concerning complex cases.

Group practices could be of either the single-specialty or the multiple-specialty type. The physicians in some single-specialty group practices were primary care physicians (e.g., internists or pediatricians), while those in other group practices were specialists (e.g., neurosurgeons). Although most group practices initially operated on a fee-for-service basis, some began to develop the concept of prepaid group practice—a concept that goes at least as far back as the final report of the Committee on the Costs of Medical Care (1932). On the West Coast, the Kaiser Corporation set up its own multispecialty group practice before World War II to care for its workers, but membership has since been opened to the general public, and it is now known as Kaiser Permanente. This was the first example of a large prepaid group practice in the USA.

Health Maintenance Organizations. Prepaid group practices that met certain standards and contractual arrangements were named health maintenance organizations (HMOs) by the Nixon administration. The national HMO law was passed in 1973, and it encouraged the large-scale development of HMOs.

People who enrolled in an HMO were usually part of some economic group, such as workers in a company or industry, but their enrollment had to be voluntary. They paid a fixed monthly fee, which varied depending on the size of the group. In return, the HMO had the contractual obligation to provide the types of medical care specified in the contract (rather than to provide financial reimbursement, as in the case of an insurance company) or at least to ensure that the stipulated care was provided. The HMO assumed some of the risk when income was less than expenses and made a profit when income was greater than expenses.

Structurally, there are three main parts to an HMO: (1) the legal and fiscal entity that develops contracts and handles financial transactions, (2) the physicians, and (3) the hospitals and ancillary service providers. The HMO is defined by the organization that collects prepaid capitation (per head) premiums for medical services provided to its enrollees, monitors the service pattern, and approves and pays bills for services from physicians, hospitals, and others. The HMO either employs physicians directly or contracts with legal entities that represent the physicians, hospitals, and ancillary service providers. Unlike the early HMOs (see Luft 1981), today's HMOs have a variety of organizational and service components. Current discussions of HMOs are so riddled with acronyms for these components (IPA, PHO, PPO, POS, and so forth) that the acronyms will be included and defined in the discussions here.

Functionally, an HMO must have a defined set of preventive and curative services that it promises to provide to its enrollees for an established periodic (usually monthly) capitation premium. The HMO provides services using an organized system of providers, which includes primary care physicians, specialist physicians, hospitals, and ancillary services (such as laboratory and x-ray services). The variations on this theme resist clear categorization, but the terms commonly used for the main types of HMO, from the most structured to the least structured, are staff models, group models, network models, and independent practice associations (Rognehaugh 1998).

In the **staff model HMO,** most of the physicians are salaried, full-time employees who either work exclusively in the health plan or (as is typical in Kaiser Permanente) belong to a physician group that contracts to provide all of the medical services in the health plan. Some specialists may be contracted on a part-time basis to provide services by referral from the HMO's primary care physicians. A staff model HMO may own its hospitals (as does Kaiser Permanente); however, in most cases, the HMO contracts with one or more local hospitals for all hospital care. In the staff model, the full-time physicians' time and effort are directed mainly or exclusively toward care of the HMO patients, and these physicians serve as the **gatekeepers,** coordinating care to patients and controlling referrals to specialists. In theory, every patient must see a primary care physician before obtaining a referral to a specialist, although this may be relaxed for certain specialties, such as obstetrics and gynecology, ophthalmology, and dermatology.

A **group model HMO** provides the physician services through contracts with one or more organized groups of physicians. The HMO also contracts with one or more area hospitals for hospital services.

A **network model HMO** is similar to a group model HMO but is looser in structure. The network model HMO has contracts with many physician groups (single-specialty and multispecialty groups) and sometimes also with individual physicians. It may have a contract with one hospital but usually has contracts with more than one. Currently, the goal of these HMOs seems to be to recruit as many providers in a geographic area as possible. This makes the HMO attractive to patients because they are usually able to choose their preferred physicians and hospitals.

An **independent practice association** (IPA) is a legal entity, usually an organization of physicians, that solicits enrollees and their premiums (from HMO payers or companies) and also contracts with office-based fee-for-service physicians in private practice to provide the promised care, at a discounted fee rate. In addition, the IPA contracts with hospitals to provide inpatient care. (The **physician-hospital organization,** or PHO, is a variant type of IPA that is associated with a single hospital, which usually does the administrative work.) In IPAs, the practitioners are supposed to perform the gatekeeper function (although they are usually less effective in controlling costs than are practitioners in other HMOs), and the IPA monitors utilization for appropriateness. The enrollees must receive their care from an IPA-affiliated hospital and from members of the IPA's **panel** (primary care physicians and specialists who have a contractual arrangement with the IPA). In addition to providing care to enrollees in a particular IPA, a physician who is included in the panel may provide care to patients who are not enrolled in or covered by the IPA. Moreover, a physician may be a member of the panel of several IPAs, which makes the referral process quite confusing. Indeed, in some cases, the cry of the vendor at the ball game tends to hold true: You can't tell the players without a program. The "players" for a particular IPA consist of the panel of approved physicians and specialists. The patients must refer to the list of panel members ("program") to find out whom they can select for primary care, and the primary care physicians must consult the list before referring a patient for specialty care.

A **preferred provider organization** (PPO) is a variation on the IPA theme, but it is not usually approved as a federally qualified HMO, because it does not have tight cost-control procedures. A PPO is formed when a third-party payer (e.g., an insurance plan or company) establishes a network of contracts with independent practitioners. Like the standard IPA, the PPO has a panel of physicians who have contracted to provide services at agreed (reduced) rates. A major difference between the standard IPA and a PPO, however, is that the patients in a PPO can see physicians who are not on the PPO panel, although they will have to pay an extra amount to do so. This option of seeing other physicians, which is called a **point of service plan** (POS plan), is increasingly being required of HMOs by the government. If an HMO offers a POS plan, it is called an **open HMO.** If it does not, it is called a **closed HMO.**

Some HMOs offer more than one of the above models of care, depending on which client group they are serving. For example, a managed care plan may have a staff model facility and also offer a POS plan. This is called a **mixed model or a hybrid HMO or managed care plan.**

One of the primary ways an HMO reduces costs is to negotiate a reduced fee for services from hospitals and from physician groups. A hospital will lose patients if it does not accept all of the HMO plans available to individuals within in its geographic area. However, HMOs will lose enrollees if they do not cover care in a popular local hospital. The hospitals and HMOs are well aware of these facts. Therefore, the contract negotiations with hospitals can be difficult and protracted, but essentially every HMO obtains hospital care at a discounted price. To persuade physicians in private or group practices to join the HMO, the HMO must not only offer fees that are reasonable (though they are usually less than advertised fees) but also offer physicians a minimum of paperwork, a minimum of administrative rules controlling their practices, and the rapid payment of bills.

Hospital Outpatient Clinics. Traditionally, many hospital outpatient clinics have served people who are poor and may not be well insured. The patients receive treatment (although often following a long wait) in return for being cared for by physicians in training, with proper supervision. Increasingly, these clinics are becoming organized into primary care centers or even HMOs. In addition, many medical schools now have group practice arrangements for the physicians on their clinical faculty to practice medicine and augment both their income and the income of the medical school.

Hospital Emergency Departments. Emergency departments are becoming increasingly complex, and because of the heavy patient loads, their staff may triage nonurgent patients to a satellite convenience clinic.

Community or Neighborhood Health Centers. Federal health programs in the 1960s and 1970s encouraged the development of community health centers. Many of these centers were supported partly through federal and state grants, and most were placed in underserved areas in big cities or rural locations.

Surgicenters. Freestanding outpatient surgical centers have become increasingly popular and may be owned by hospitals or group practice associations.

Urgent Care Centers. Urgent care centers are freestanding clinics that are conveniently located (e.g., often in shopping centers) and allow ambulatory patients to be seen on a drop-in basis not only during the usual weekday hours but also during evenings and on weekends. Most of the urgent care centers are proprietary, and many specialize in evaluating and treating injured workers promptly in order to get them back to work.

■ PAYMENT FOR MEDICAL CARE

A century ago, physicians were paid directly by patients for their services. If times were tight, practitioners might get paid in food or other commodities, rather than in cash. As medicine became more scientific and technical, often requiring long hospital stays, the out-of-pocket payment method became inadequate. Patients became frustrated with large bills they could not pay, and hospitals and physicians were frustrated at not being reimbursed. Today, it is not unusual for a very sick patient to be charged $2000 or more per day for a hospital stay, even if no surgery or major procedures are done. One solution to the cost problem was to create a **third-party payer,** such as an insurance company. The third-party payer collected money regularly from a large population in the form of medical insurance premiums and paid the hospitals and physicians when care was required.

Physician Payments

Physicians today are usually paid in one of three ways: by the fee-for-service method, capitation, or salary.

In the **fee-for-service method,** physicians are paid for each major item of service provided. Charges are established on the basis of the type and complexity of service (complete workup, follow-up visit, hospital visit, major surgical procedure, etc.). The amount charged by a physician may exceed the amount that a third-party payer is willing to reimburse, in which case the patient is expected to pay the difference between the charges and the third-party payment. With HMOs, discounted fee-for-service payments are now increasingly common. The physician or physician group contracts to provide services at a reduced fee and to adhere to certain cost-containment strategies for the advantage of being on the HMO's panel of physicians.

Sometimes primary care physicians are paid on a **capitation basis,** meaning on a "per head" basis. Regardless of the number of services needed by a patient, the physician receives the same amount of money per year. This method of payment has much lower administrative costs, and it is thought to promote physicians' efforts in preventive care. It may lead to poor gatekeeping, however, because it may be easier to refer a patient than to provide a service. This payment method is sometimes used in the USA to pay practitioners working in HMOs and is commonly used in Britain to pay general practitioners.

The third method of payment is a **salary.** Physicians who work full-time for HMOs, hospitals, universities, companies, or some group practices may be paid this way. Productivity bonuses are sometimes added to the salary. Physicians who provide care on a part-time basis often receive a stipulated amount per clinic session.

Insurance and Third-Party Payers

About 4000 years ago, wealthy people in China were paying doctors to keep them well, and this sort of arrangement can be viewed as an early form of health insurance. However, in the Chinese system, a physician's payments ceased if the patron became sick, and the penalties if the patron died were strict, sometimes including the death of the physician (Prussin and Woods 1975).

Modern US hospital insurance had its foundation in Dallas, Texas, where a group of schoolteachers entered into a contract with Baylor University Hospital in 1929. The teachers paid the hospital 50 cents per person per month and, in turn, the hospital promised to cover 21 consecutive days in the hospital in a semiprivate room, along with medications, laboratory studies, the use of operating rooms, and so forth. This led to the development of Blue Cross, which is a form of insurance that covers only hospital care. Later, in response to recommendations from physicians and others, Blue Shield was developed as a parallel organization to enable prepayment of physician services.

To understand how insurance companies work, it is necessary to review a few concepts concerning benefits. If an insurance policy covers **indemnity benefits,** this means that the insurance company (carrier) will reimburse the insured patient a fixed number of dollars per service, regardless of the actual charges incurred for the service. If the insurance policy states that the carrier will pay up to $400 per day toward a semiprivate hospital room and the room actually costs $600 per day, the patient must pay the difference, unless he or she has other (supplemental) insurance. In contrast, if an insurance policy covers **service benefits,** the carrier will be responsible for the full amount of the contracted payment for the needed services, regardless of their costs.

Actuaries, the statisticians who estimate risks and establish premiums for insurance companies, have a standard set of **actuarial principles** that guide the process of underwriting (insuring) medical and other risks. Actuaries make sure that an insurance carrier does not collapse financially. Originally, insurance was designed to pool the risk from large groups to protect individuals from rare but devastating losses, such as those resulting from fires. The actuarial principles developed to accomplish this objective do not adapt well to medical care for two reasons. First, medical care involves frequent and fairly predictable costs as well as rare and catastrophic costs. Second, those at greatest risk of ill health and hospitalization can least afford the cost of insurance, although according to actuarial principles they should be charged the most. Therefore, other solutions are required to have a just and equitable system for financing medical care.

So far, one of the primary solutions applied to this dilemma in health care has been the concept of **pooling risk.** If all of the people in a large, natural community (i.e., a community consisting of people of various ages and degrees of health) were to be insured by the same carrier and were to pay the same monthly premium rate, then the law of averages would work so as to protect the carrier from excessive loss except, perhaps, in times of disaster. In effect, the low-risk people in the population would be helping to pay the premiums for the high-risk people, because the risk would be averaged according to the "experience rating" of the entire group. This is not a complete solution, because the poor still may not be able to pay the established premium, and the plan may not be offered where they work.

Insurance companies prefer to insure groups, particularly working groups. There are several reasons. First, group insurance requires less sales effort and paperwork. Second, by insuring a large group of people, a carrier is less likely to insure a high percentage of bad risks (i.e., people who will probably require a lot of medical care). Third, by insuring a working group, the carrier benefits from the **healthy worker effect.** Because people with jobs must be in reasonably good health to work in the first place, they have a lower risk of death and illness than the population as a whole. Fourth, the medical care costs for injuries and illnesses that are clearly job-related will probably be covered by a workers' compensation program and will thus save the insurer money. Unfortunately, many of the individuals who need the most medical care are unemployed, and this leaves them with the multiple problems of being unable to purchase insurance because they represent undesirable risks to an insurance company, being unable to pay for the health care they need because they have little earning power, and remaining in a poor state of health that keeps them from finding employment.

Initially, the Blue Cross plans began to cover large segments of communities, and the community pooling of risk appeared to work fairly well. However, many insurance carriers sought to attract the business of low-risk individuals and low-risk companies by offering lower premiums. As the people with low risks were removed from the community pool (a process called "cream skimming"), the people remaining in the pool were, on the average, at higher risk, so they had to be charged a higher premium, making the community pool still less attractive.

Some insurance companies have sought to use epidemiologic information to undersell the Blue Plans (Blue Cross and Blue Shield). These companies offer low-cost medical insurance to individuals with low epidemiologic risk profiles, usually those who do not drink alcohol or smoke. Some justify this approach as an appropriate reward for good health behavior.

The insurance world is complex. Most Blue Cross plans cover the first several thousand dollars of their liability, but they insure themselves against disastrous medical care liability by **reinsurance.** They pay a fee to another (reinsurance) company, which then assumes the liability for Blue Cross commitments above a certain agreed-upon amount.

In order for patients to be covered for huge medical costs, many plans also include a premium for **major medical insurance.** This insurance usually pays 80% of the amount by which a hospital bill exceeds the Blue Cross maximum, and the patient is obligated to pay the other 20% of the bill for major expenses. The patient's portion is called a **copayment,** because the patient and the insurance company are sharing the total cost. The copayment is also seen as a means to enlist the patient or the family in the effort to get the patient out of the hospital as soon as possible.

Social Insurance

Compulsory insurance for a population group is often called social or public insurance. Most people employed in the USA must make payments into the Social Security Trust Fund for two national social insurance programs: Medicare and retirement benefits.

Medicare is authorized under Title 18 of the Social Security Act and is administered by the federal government, although it uses insurance carriers as fiscal intermediaries. The people eligible for Medicare include most individuals who are 65 years or older and most individuals who receive Social Security benefits because of disability. Medicare has not covered prescription medications, but there is increasing political pressure for it to do so.

Part A and Part B of Medicare provide partial coverage for hospital expenses and physician expenses, respectively. Although Social Security beneficiaries do not pay premiums for Part A coverage after the age of 65, they do pay premiums on a regular basis if they elect to have Part B coverage. Medicare also will pay for a certain amount of home care or nursing home care for a medical problem that follows directly from a Medicare-covered hospitalization.

Since Medicare does not cover all hospital expenses, patients are billed for the portion of charges not covered by Medicare. Therefore, insurance plans have developed **Medicare supplemental insurance policies,** sometimes called **Medigap policies,** so that patients have few, if any, bills after a hospital admission.

To control Medicare costs, the federal government has also promoted **Medicare managed care plans** (MMC plans). In essence, Medicare pays an HMO to include the Medicare recipient. For some patients, this plan is attractive because there are essentially no costs other than paying the monthly Medicare Part B premiums for physician services. What is less attractive to patients are the limits to physician access that tend to come with HMOs. HMOs are finding that MMC plans can cause them to lose money, and the considerably reduced hospital payments from MMC plans have caused major losses for numerous hospitals.

Many children in the USA have not been covered by health insurance. Therefore, Congress passed a bill in 1977 to supply federal matching funds to the states to help them provide health care coverage to uninsured children from low-income families. To receive the matching funds, each state has the option of expanding Medicaid, establishing a state **children's health insurance program** (CHIP), or doing both.

By 1948, all states in the USA had some sort of **workers' compensation program.** Workers' compensation laws stipulate that people with a job-related injury or illness have their medical and rehabilitation expenses paid and also receive a certain amount of cash payments in lieu of wages while they are recuperating. Depending on the state, companies may have the option to self-insure, to enter an agreement to insure through a private third-party carrier, or to deposit premiums into a state fund. Regardless of the method used, the size of a company's premiums depends on that company's **experience rating,** which is the amount of claims paid in recent years. This serves as a stimulus for companies to invest in safety on the job. The level of benefits that workers receive varies considerably from state to state.

Social Welfare

Medicaid is authorized under Title 19 of the Social Security Act. Unlike Medicare recipients, Medicaid recipients have not previously paid money into a trust fund. Therefore, the benefits of Medicaid are considered to be social welfare, instead of social insurance. Medicaid is paid from general tax revenues of the federal and state governments.

The people covered by Medicaid are poor and usually receive additional types of welfare assistance, such as Aid to Families with Dependent Children (AFDC). In contrast to Medicare, which is entirely federally administered, Medicaid is administered by the states, which share the costs of the program with the federal government. Although the federal government usually reimburses a state for approximately half of its Medicaid costs for a given year, poorer states get slightly more. The eligibility criteria for Medicaid, as well as the size of the benefits, are set by the states and therefore vary from state to state.

Medicaid basically covers two things. First, it pays for medical care expenses, including both hospital and physician bills. The amount of reimbursement is usually far below the customary charges of physicians, making the program unpopular with many physicians. Second, Medicaid pays for long-term nursing home care, but only after people have largely exhausted their personal resources, a process called spend-down (see Long-Term Care, below).

■ COST CONTAINMENT AND QUALITY
Historical Overview

The recent history of the struggle of organized medicine in the USA has some resemblance to the Battle of Chancellorsville, which occurred in May 1863, during the American Civil War. In the town of Chancellorsville, the Union army, under General Joseph Hooker, was braced for Confederate attacks on the left flank and center, but its right flank was weak, almost unprotected. Confederate General Jackson took half of the Confederate army on a secret march around to the Union army's right flank and overwhelmed the troops that were there.

In like manner, organized medicine (especially the American Medical Association) has lived in fear of attacks on the primacy of private, fee-for-service medical practice from the political left flank, in the form of government programs or controls. Organized medicine spent vast amounts of money fighting government-provided medicine, national health insurance, and any form of change that would increase government control or regulation of the practice of medicine. What organized medicine did not notice was that it was entirely exposed on the political and economic right (entrepreneurial) flank.

Since the 1970s, for-profit hospitals, hospital chains, nursing homes, and insurance companies have rapidly gained control of the organization and financing of medical practice and have instituted managed care to achieve cost control. The forces of organized medicine did not recognize this threat from the right until it was too late to mount a well-organized resistance. Now the managed care forces are controlling the practice of medicine as much as or more than organized medicine ever thought big government would. By guarding only its left flank, organized medicine, like General Hooker, left its right flank unprotected. As Gray and Field (1989) stated:

With great speed and relatively little public awareness, a significant change has occurred in the way some decisions are made about a patient's medical care. Decisions that were once the exclusive province of the doctor and patient now may be examined in advance by an external reviewer—someone accountable to an employer, insurer, health maintenance organization, or other entity responsible for all or most of the cost of care. Depending upon the circumstances, this outside party may be involved in discussions about where care will occur, how treatment will be provided, and even whether some treatments are appropriate at all.

Reasons for the Rapid Increase in the Cost of Medical Care

Many of the controls over medical practice that were developed over the last half century were largely to limit the costs of medical care. These costs were increasing much faster than the general inflation rate and in 1994 represented about 14% of the gross domestic product. Although managed care was able to reduce the rate of medical care inflation for a while, the inflation rose to double digits again toward the end of the century. Among the reasons for this rapid increase in costs were the following: increases in the demand for care, increases in the wages for personnel, reliance on complex but only partially effective medical technology, underutilization of facilities, inadequate insurance, and planning failures.

The increasing effectiveness of medical care has led to an **increased demand for care,** thereby increasing the total costs. As noted above, demographic changes, particularly the increase in the number and proportion of older persons, are one of the major reasons for increased demand.

Several decades ago, the **wages of health care workers,** particularly nursing and related personnel, fell behind the wages of workers in many other sectors of the economy. As shortages in the supply of nurses developed, hospitals and other medical care institutions had to offer better wages to lure nurses (mostly women) out of retirement to fill the needs. Nursing wages have generally kept pace with other wage increases since then. The number and wages of administrators have also increased (Woolhandler, Himmelstein, and Lewontin 1993).

Medical costs have been and continue to be increased by the use of complex but only **partially effective technology** for the diagnosis and treatment of disease. Before polio vaccines were developed, for example, iron lungs were used to extend the lives of paralytic poliomyelitis victims. In contrast to the polio immunization program, which has proved to be highly cost-effective, the iron lung was an expensive and ineffective ("halfway") technology.

As medical care increasingly is dependent on technology, the cost of medical education also increases.

This in turn forces new physicians to move to geographic areas and pursue specialties that will enable them to live reasonably well while paying off their large educational debts. Medical education is now so expensive that many new physicians begin practice with more than $100,000 of educational debt.

Medical care facilities need to be properly used to be efficient and effective. **Underutilization of hospitals,** in particular, hurts the financial stability of the institutions. Hospitals need to have a steady bed occupancy rate of greater than 80% to remain solvent over the long run. Many hospitals, especially in rural areas, have closed in recent years because of low occupancy rates.

Not providing medical insurance for everyone is more costly than providing it. **Lack of insurance** leads to inappropriate utilization of emergency departments and to delayed care, with resulting increased expense because disease is found at a later and less treatable stage and in a more costly setting. The costs of this care eventually must be borne by society, and often this is done by shifting the costs in some hidden fashion from those who cannot pay to those who can.

Planning failures have contributed to the problem of increasing costs of medical care. One could argue that health care planning began with the Hill-Burton Act of 1946, which encouraged hospital construction. Beginning in the mid-1960s and continuing for almost 20 years, the federal government supported official health planning strategies, largely in an effort to control costs. Among the primary strategies it supported were the appointment of rate-setting authorities within states and the issuance of certificates of need (CON) for the construction of new hospitals or purchase of expensive equipment in particular locales.

Because many of the planning efforts were underfunded or difficult to enforce, they were often ineffective in preventing the duplication of facilities and expensive equipment. In some areas, however, the regulatory efforts were reasonably effective. For example, research has shown that Medicare hospital admission and readmission rates for given diseases are considerably lower in New Haven, Connecticut, than in Boston, Massachusetts, despite similar medical outcomes (Wennberg, Freeman, and Culp 1987; Fisher et al. 1994). The number of beds per 1000 population is considerably lower in Connecticut as a result of decades of aggressive state regulatory efforts at cost control. If there is an empty hospital bed, there will be an attempt to fill it.

To ensure that cost-cutting efforts did not decrease the quality of care, regulations were instituted to control the medical care institutions and the process of care. The effects of these regulations on quality is uncertain, but they added considerably to the costs of care by increasing all of the following: the amount of paperwork to be completed, the complexity of the administrative process, and the number of managers and administrators required. Sweet (1993) predicted that if the present trends in health care management and utilization continued, by the year 2026 there would be over two million administrators and no patients.

Because all of the methods noted above have either added to the costs of medical care or failed to contain the rising costs, there has been increasing use of new cost-containment strategies, many of which are lumped under the general term "managed care" (see below). Managed care has so changed the practice of medicine during the past two decades that no physician is adequately prepared to enter residency, to say nothing of medical practice, without a basic understanding of it. Managed care techniques will be around in one form or another for the foreseeable future.

Older Cost-Containment Strategies

The cost of medical care has been a topic of concern for a long time in the USA. The first committee focusing on this topic was established in 1929 and was called the Committee on the Costs of Medical Care. In 1932, it published its landmark report in which it recommended the development of prepaid group practices (the forerunners of HMOs) as the most effective and efficient means to provide and finance medical care. Until recent decades, the most common forms of cost containment were simple and straightforward.

The first and most basic method of discouraging the overuse of medical care was to create **deductibles,** which are out-of-pocket payments made by the patient, often at the beginning of the care process. Medical deductibles work in much the same way as current automobile or home insurance deductibles: they discourage the use of insurance for "unimportant" problems and reduce the amount of paperwork for the insurance companies. Deductibles could be applied for an entire year (the patient might have to pay the first $500 of yearly costs) or to each physician visit (the patient might have to pay $5 or $10 for each visit), with the insurance company paying the remainder of the eligible charges. In general, physicians have worried that deductibles might discourage patients from coming in for early symptoms of serious disease. Most HMOs have not had deductibles.

The second basic cost-control method was **copayments,** as discussed in the section entitled Insurance and Third-Party Payers (see above). Copayments were thought to "discourage" patients from staying in hospitals longer than necessary.

The third common method was **exclusions** in the insurance. Some insurance policies totally excluded psychiatric care and dental care from coverage, while others severely restricted the reimbursement for these types of care. Psychiatric care, in particular, was perceived by third-party payers as a potentially bottomless pit that could consume large amounts of money in endless visits. Even in Medicare Part A (hospital insurance), inpatient mental health care coverage in a psychiatric facility has been limited to 190 days in a lifetime (see Health Care Financing Administration 1999).

For many years, there has been considerable discussion about **health care markets,** based on assumptions of the free market economic model. Such a model requires many things to be true that are untrue in the world of medical care. First, there must be many sellers and many buyers for the buyers to have free choice. Second, the buyers must have good information regarding the products from which they choose. Third, there must not be monopolies; that is, no seller and no buyer should be able to dominate the market (Kropf 1990). The health care market usually does not meet any of these characteristics. First, in many areas, there are few choices of provider, either physician or hospital, and the federal government is often the dominant purchaser of care in the market. Second, patients usually do not have enough information about the quality and cost of medical care for them to make a valid market-based decision concerning their medical needs. Third, increasingly large market forces, such as hospital chains or huge HMOs, dominate the market in their primary regions. Market forces are inadequate to maximize efficiency and control the costs of medical care, because of the complexity of the care.

Current Cost-Containment Strategies

If resources for medical care are inadequate to meet demand, there are three basic methods of responding: (1) increase resources; (2) decrease demand (or at least utilization); and (3) increase efficiency. Although efforts are generally made in all three areas, the recent emphasis is on decreasing demand and increasing efficiency through two cost-containment strategies. One is the prospective payment system based on diagnosis-related groups, and the other is managed care.

Prospective Payment System Based on Diagnosis-Related Groups

Developed in the 1970s but first applied nationally in the USA to Medicare reimbursement in 1983, the prospective payment system (PPS) based on diagnosis-related groups (DRGs) has changed the way hospitals are reimbursed and the way hospitals and physicians think about the provision of care. Each hospital admission is classified into one of 23 major diagnostic categories based on organ systems (as outlined in the *International Classification of Diseases,* or ICD), and then these diagnostic categories are further subdivided into DRGs. A DRG may consist of a single diagnosis or procedure, or it may consist of several diagnoses or procedures that, on average, have similar hospital costs per admission. An uncomplicated delivery of an infant, for example, is coded as DRG #313, and a nonradical hysterectomy in a woman who is under the age of 70 and has no complicating condition is coded as DRG #355.

DRGs were first developed to enable hospitals to look for cost "outliers." For example, hospitals could analyze and identify those physicians who regularly generated greater than average costs for care coded as DRG #313. The hospitals could then try to find out why these physicians generated excess costs and to devise methods to control these costs in the future. The federal government, however, decided to use the DRG system to pay hospitals on the basis of a prospectively determined average cost for each of the more than 470 DRGs. This system began to be used in the treatment of Medicare patients in October 1983. Although there is no federal requirement that hospital payers other than Medicare use the DRG system for reimbursement, several states requested and received federal permission to incorporate DRGs into their own prospectively determined rate-setting programs. When this happened, all third-party payers in the state had to conform to the same prospectively determined rates. This is referred to as an **all-payer system.**

Note that the hospital is actually reimbursed *after* a specific type of care is given; however, the amount of payment for the specific type of care is decided prospectively (in advance). The average cost for each of the more than 470 DRGs is set prospectively for each region of the country. Although extra amounts are added for tertiary hospitals and for hospitals engaged in medical education, these adjustments do not always fully cover the costs of providing care to the indigent and paying for hospital-based medical education. Medicare reimburses hospitals with the predetermined fixed amount for the entire hospital stay of a Medicare patient, based on his or her DRG, regardless of whether it actually cost the hospital more or less than the prospectively determined DRG-specific payment to provide that care. If a hospital can find a way to reduce the costs and provide the care for less than the amount reimbursed by the PPS, it can retain the excess amount. If a hospital is inefficient and has higher than average costs for a hospital admission, it will lose money on that admission. Because hospitals with the strongest administrative teams and data systems are best able to keep costs below PPS reimbursements, there is a tendency for the strong hospitals to get stronger and the weak hospitals to get weaker.

There have been some good results from the PPS. For example, there are now more and better data than before, and hospitals have a greater ability than before to find unnecessary costs. Initially, because of efficiencies introduced in response to the PPS and because of the more rapid discharge of some patients, the PPS reduced hospital utilization (and therefore costs) considerably. After a period of reduced costs, however, the upward pressure on the cost of medical care has resumed.

The full impact of the PPS on the quality of medical care has not been determined. There is evidence that some patients are being discharged sooner than desirable, but no major change in medical care quality has been clearly discernible. Often, early discharge merely passes the medical care problems (and therefore costs) down the line to the care institutions that receive the patients from the hospital: the home, home care agencies, and skilled nursing facilities.

The PPS added urgency to an already-growing trend to move as much medical care as possible out of acute, general hospitals and into ambulatory surgery and diagnostic centers. Because the PPS does not apply to ambulatory procedures, providers in ambulatory settings could set their own rates. In addition, many hospitals and staff model HMOs began to develop infirmaries, where patients who did not need acute, intensive care could be given moderate supervision and some treatment at a much lower cost than if they were in hospitals.

Ambulatory Care Financing

For more than a decade, the US government has supported research to develop an improved system to pay for ambulatory care, particularly to reduce the tendency to overpay for procedures and underpay for quality primary care. The first result of this research was the **resource-based relative value scale** (RBRVS), which sought to reimburse physicians more equitably for outpatient care, based on their time spent on this care, their years of training, their level of skill, and their office equipment costs. At the same time, the government has been supporting research to determine how the general method used to develop DRGs could be applied to outpatient care. The result was the development of **ambulatory patient groups** (APGs) of conditions that require similar resources, based on the RBRVS. Thus, the two lines of research were combined with elements from the inpatient and outpatient care classification systems to produce the current **ambulatory payment classification system** (APC system). This federally mandated **outpatient prospective payment system** (outpatient PPS) is now being used by the federal government to reimburse for ambulatory care under Medicare.

Managed Care

In an analysis of the social structure of medical care, Freidson (1970) claimed that the characteristic that uniquely defines the "professions," including medicine, is autonomy in practice. With the advent of managed care, also known as **utilization management,** the trend is away from physician autonomy in some aspects of medical practice, such as deciding which patients can be admitted to the hospital, how long they may remain there, and what care must be done for them while they are hospitalized. These determinations are variously referred to as **clinical pathways, medical protocols, best practices, practice guidelines,** or **clinical algorithms** (see American College of Physicians 1992). Managed care is a system of administrative controls, the goal of which is to reduce the costs of medical care. According to Gray and Field (1989),

Such "utilization management" is part of a complex balancing act created by society's struggles with two important questions. First, how do we ensure that people get needed medical care without spending so much that we compromise other important social objectives? Second, how do we discourage unnecessary and inappropriate medical services without jeopardizing necessary high-quality care?

Managed care, which consists of some combination of the strategies that are discussed in this section, is thought to reduce medical care costs to the payer (usually a third-party payer) over the short run.

Preadmission Review and Certification. Some designated person in the managed care office (often a specially trained nurse) must approve a nonemergent hospital admission before the admission occurs. Otherwise, the hospital is not guaranteed payment from the patient's third-party payer. Using the emergency department for a nonemergent condition is not a way to bypass preadmission certification, as can be seen below.

Emergency Department Admission Review. An admission from the emergency department must have a case review within a day to be sure it is a justified admission. If the reviewer does not consider the admission justified, the hospital will not be paid, so the patient will receive the bill.

Concurrent (Continued Stay) Review. The attending physician must justify keeping a patient in the hospital longer than the number of days expected for that patient's DRG.

Discharge Planning. To avoid discharging patients to inappropriate places for their needs and to avoid delays in outplacement, planning for discharge should begin the day the patient is admitted to the hospital.

Second Opinions. A second physician's opinion concerning the patient's need for surgery must be obtained before a major elective invasive procedure is performed. Requiring a second opinion markedly reduces the rates for certain types of surgery, such as hysterectomy.

Gatekeepers. Many managed care plans, particularly staff model HMOs, require that all referrals to specialists be approved by the patient's primary care practitioner. In this role, the primary care practitioners are functioning as gatekeepers.

High-Cost Case Management. If the hospital care for a particular patient is costing or potentially will cost the third-party payer a large amount of money, an administrator is appointed to look hard for a less costly alternative, such as ambulatory care or home care. This strategy tends to work best in cases in which the patient has complex or multiple medical problems.

Benefit Design. Every benefit plan offered by a third-party payer, including HMOs of various types, seeks provisions to attract the patients they want to recruit to the plan while at the same time limiting the financial exposure of the insurer. First, the plan may try to reduce premiums and costs by enlisting the patients themselves in reducing costs through such traditional methods as deductibles and copayments. Second, a common practice is to exclude or at least limit the amount of certain benefits from the policy. As mentioned above, plans frequently limit or exclude mental health and dental health benefits. A serious problem for many patients forced to change insurers is that the insurer may refuse to cover the cost of certain **preexisting conditions,** thus limiting the company's financial exposure for many chronic diseases and disorders. Legislation is attempting to control these loopholes but has not been very effective. The worry increases as the potential to diagnose genetic diseases increases.

Financial Incentives for Physicians. If physicians are paid on a salary or capitation basis rather than on a fee-for-service basis, they have no incentive to provide unnecessary services to their patients. In theory, there should be an incentive for preventive measures when a physician or a health plan is paid on a capitation basis, because effective prevention may reduce the time and effort the physician must spend on the average patient. Another strategy that may be pursued to reduce unnecessary care is a system of bonuses for physicians if they use efficient practice techniques or if their group practice makes a sufficient profit in a given year. In fact, capitation has tended to increase the rate of referrals to specialists, because there is less incentive for the primary care practitioner to take extra time to care for a complex problem.

National Health Insurance

The financial problems created by "cream skimming" (see above) and other techniques for enticing low-risk populations into third-party payer networks could be reduced by taking any large natural population (either the entire US population or each state's population) as a risk pool. If this were done for the entire US population, it would be a form of nationwide (national) health insurance. National health insurance has been vigorously opposed by much of organized medicine, which still fears government control over medical practice as well as possible limitations of physician charges. The irony, as mentioned above, is that physicians now may be controlled as much or more from the "free enterprise" side of medical care than they probably would have been under national health insurance.

National health insurance is unlikely to be enacted unless a reliable way is found to control the costs of medical care. Given the rapid rise in these costs, some members of Congress tend to view the passage of national health insurance as equivalent to writing a blank check. In light of the Congress members' experiences with the rapidly rising cost of the Medicare program, which really is a federally administered national health insurance for the beneficiaries of Social Security, Congress is not likely to want to undertake a much larger version of it.

The prospects for the foreseeable future are for continuing reform from within the medical care system. Strategies for reform include (1) efforts by the states to create their own state solutions; (2) efforts by the federal government to modify Medicare, Medicaid, and third-party insurance; (3) efforts to develop some form of national health insurance for pregnant women and young children; and (4) efforts to obtain some form of federally sponsored assistance for prescription drug coverage.

Long-Term Care

A fairly high proportion (about 43%) of people who reach the age of 65 years eventually will spend some time in a nursing home (Kemper and Murtaugh 1991). Medicare (Title 18) will cover nursing home costs for a limited period (up to 100 days, with complete coverage for only the first 20 days), but it will do this only if two conditions are met: the patient is released from a hospital directly to the nursing home, and this immediate posthospital nursing home care is considered likely to improve the patient's condition. Medicare will not pay for nursing home care beyond the 100 days after discharge from a hospital. Medicare will not pay for nursing home care if a nonhospitalized person requires nursing home care because of failing strength or inability to care for himself or herself in the activities of daily living.

After Medicare coverage of nursing home (or home care) services is used up, the patient must assume the costs for these services until his or her financial resources have been "spent down" to a prescribed level (e.g., ownership of a home may be maintained as long as a spouse or dependent survives, and up to about $4000 in personal resources may be maintained). When the spend-down is complete, Medicaid (Title 19) begins to cover the costs, and in essence the patient is a welfare recipient.

Because part of the Medicaid costs are borne by the state in which the patient enters a nursing home, the state could put a lien on the patient's house and property, although it would not be taken until the patient's spouse had died. Some elderly people, suspecting that they will need a long stay in a nursing home soon, give their wealth to their children to avoid having their property and savings used to pay nursing home costs. For this reason, state governments have stipulated that if the gift giver is placed in a nursing home and requires Medicaid within a certain number of years of giving the gift, the gift recipient must reimburse the state for the nursing home costs, up to an amount equal to the gift.

A number of experiments with long-term care insurance have been initiated. Long-term care insurance will pay all or part of the costs of a nursing home but will not pay for an acute hospitalization or for physicians' charges. This type of insurance tends to be very costly and has not gained general acceptance thus far. Long-term care insurance is expensive because good nursing home care now costs more than $1000 per week in many areas of the USA and the need for nursing home care can extend for many years.

Assessment of the Quality of Medical Care

The quality of medical practice has been a major concern since early in this century. In 1910, for example, the Flexner Report was especially concerned with the need to improve medical education. Quality of medical care became a bigger issue after World War II, when Donabedian and other investigators began to define more clearly the dimensions of quality. In 1969, Donabedian indicated that quality should be examined in terms of **structure** (the physical resources and human resources that a hospital or HMO possessed for providing care), **process** (the way in which the physical and human resources were joined in the activities of physicians and other health care providers), and **outcome** (the end results of care, such as whether the patients actually did as well as would be expected, given the severity of their problems).

State accreditation of facilities usually focuses on structural issues, with some evaluation of process. Quality review programs of the past, including the programs of professional review organizations (PROs), tended to focus on particular aspects of process called **procedural end points** and offered a detailed review of the methods of care provided and an analysis of how well certain disease-specific criteria were met. Current efforts toward quality improvement emphasize quality monitoring, and this is focused more on outcomes of care than in the past. One of the primary national data sets on quality of care focuses on the services provided by managed care organizations (MCOs), with particular attention to prevention and health maintenance aspects of their health plans. This data set, which is called the Healthplan Employer Data and Information Set (HEDIS), includes such prevention items as providing immunizations; counseling patients to quit smoking; screening for breast cancer, cervical cancer, hypercholesterolemia, and *Chlamydia* infections; providing prenatal and postpartum care; instituting measures to manage mental illness, menopause, and chronic conditions such as asthma, depression, diabetes, and hypertension; and counseling patients regarding the proper use of medications for several diseases.

Measuring the quality of medical outcomes in a fair manner is a significant methodologic problem. Unless outcomes are adjusted for the severity of the patients' illnesses, hospitals treating the sickest patients will be at an unfair disadvantage. The process of adjusting for the severity of illness is usually referred to as **case-mix adjustment.** Moreover, the question arises as to whose judgment of outcome— the judgment of patients or that of professionals— should be used to evaluate outcomes.

The federal government now rates hospitals by giving a **case-mix adjusted mortality rate** for each hospital. Although controversial, this process has generally provided reproducible results. Hospitals that have initiated measures to improve medical care have been successful in lowering their case-mix adjusted mortality rates.

One major concern about the current efforts to reduce costs is whether quality will be reduced as well. Clinicians and epidemiologists continue to address this question in ongoing studies. Concern for quality of care received a boost by the publication of the book *To Err Is Human: Building a Safer Health System* (Institute of Medicine 2000).

Trends in Medical Care

Because US companies are paying huge amounts for the medical care insurance they provide to their workers, they are exploring a variety of means to reduce their costs. These include self-insuring, repackaging their insurance policies, and requiring their employees to pay a portion of the medical care premiums. In many cases, cost-saving packages come through special financial arrangements with providers in a preferred provider organization (see above).

In the USA, current medical care policy is determined largely by what care is reimbursed. Because reimbursement regulations vary from state to state, from year to year, from insurance plan to insurance plan, and even from person to person depending on the type of coverage that a person has, medical care policy is always in flux. Care that is reimbursed by HMOs, insurance programs, federal government programs, or a combination of these sources is part of the medical care policy; what is not reimbursed is not policy.

Many of the current trends in medical care have evolved from efforts to reduce costs. One trend is the increasing use of ambulatory (outpatient) facilities for hernia repair, cataract removal, and a host of operative procedures that would have been unthinkable to perform on an outpatient basis a decade or two ago. Another trend is the increase in care provided by medical personnel other than physicians. Experiences with medical corpsmen in World War II led to the development of the **physician assistant,** who could provide some primary care and could monitor ongoing care of more complex diseases once the diagnosis and treatment had been established. Today, through intensive clinical programs, **nurse practitioners** are trained to provide primary care and to recognize when the care of a physician is needed. **Certified nurse midwives** are licensed to provide prenatal care, labor and delivery care, and postpartum care for uncomplicated pregnancies and deliveries.

Survey data indicate that the use of **complementary and alternative medicine** (CAM) is increasing in the USA, with preferential use by women and those with higher education (Eisenberg et al. 1998). Insurance plans and HMOs are rather timidly starting to cover certain CAM outpatient visits and procedures, and the survey data suggest that the total number of visits to CAM practitioners in the USA now exceeds the total number of primary care visits to allopathic (traditional medical) physicians.

CAM practitioners can no longer be ignored, even though everything about CAM is at least somewhat controversial. The boundaries of what constitutes CAM are not clearly defined. Some disciplines generally considered alternative, such as chiropractic and acupuncture, are increasingly embraced by allopathic medicine and may eventually become standard in the care of certain medical problems. Reimbursement for CAM by third-party payers is somewhat chaotic, but increasingly some payment is being provided for chiropractic care and acupuncture for specified complaints. Other controversies relate to nomenclature and scientific evidence. Neither "alternative" nor "complementary" is thought to be an optimal designation for the field, and actually the terms are contradictory. Concerns persist that much of CAM lacks a rigorous evidence base, but most authorities agree that the effectiveness of nearly half of conventional medical practice is similarly unsubstantiated by the modern standards of evidence. Whether CAM use improves outcomes, reduces or increases the costs of care, or improves patient satisfaction is largely uncertain. The budget for the National Center for Complementary and Alternative Medicine continues to grow, in testimony to the federal government's commitment to advancing this field and the evidence base underlying it. Currently, there are increasing efforts toward a creative and responsible synthesis of conventional medicine and CAM, which is often called **integrative medicine.**

For-profit, investor-owned hospital chains (e.g., the Hospital Corporation of America), nursing homes, diagnostic laboratories, radiologic facilities, home care programs, urgent care facilities, and renal hemodialysis units now represent a significant proportion of provider institutions. It is not always easy to distinguish for-profit from not-for-profit hospitals, because many not-for-profit community hospitals are becoming large multifaceted medical care corporations providing a complex mix of services, including home care, long-term care, HMOs, and even some for-profit ventures under holding companies. Arnold Relman, former editor of the *New England Journal of Medicine,* has strongly criticized the morality of the "new medical-industrial complex" that has resulted from an increasing intrusion of for-profit ventures into the world of medical care (Relman 1991).

■ THE PROBLEM OF THE "MEDICAL COMMONS"

In 1968, Garrett Hardin wrote "The Tragedy of the Commons," perhaps the most famous contribution to the population control debates of the 1960s. Pointing out that the shared resources of the earth (the commons) are limited, Hardin argued that the attempt by one individual or group to maximize its own welfare by using more than its fair share of the commons would necessarily diminish the good that others can derive from it. This logic can be applied to the use of medical resources in the USA. Unless Americans are able and willing to organize, finance, and regulate medical care in light of the needs of the entire population, then various individual groups (e.g., industries, hospitals, hospital chains, HMOs, insurance companies, nursing homes, and home care programs) will continue to seek to maximize their benefits (their share of the commons) at the expense of others.

Apportioning resources from the medical commons is not simple, but a satisfactory resolution will not be achieved by piecemeal approaches. It is tempting to postulate that a single-payer system will improve the ability to achieve an ethical and rational allocation, but this method also has hazards. Health promotion and disease prevention will help, but they are not panaceas either. Efficiency will play a role, but what is needed now is more medically directed efficiency and possibly less emphasis on managerial and cost efficiency. A close monitoring of quality is essential, or the result may be a loss of the benefits that all are striving to achieve.

■ SUMMARY

In the USA, the medical care system has developed without strong direction from the local, state, or federal government. The result is a confusing mix of ways in which services are organized and paid for. The per capita cost of medical care and the proportion of the gross domestic product used for medical care are higher in the USA than anywhere else in the world, yet approximately 17% of Americans still have no financial protection from the costs of medical care. Moreover, the inflation rate of medical care costs in the USA is one of the highest in the world.

Because of the high costs of medical care, a variety of cost-containment strategies have been developed. Two that are used extensively in the USA are the prospective payment system and managed care. In the prospective payment system, the third-party payer reimburses hospitals for care at a predetermined rate, depending on the average duration and complexity of the medical care provided for each condition. In managed care, hospitalizations will be reimbursed by a third-party payer only if the payer has approved the admission beforehand (preadmission review and certification). If a patient is admitted through the emergency department, the admission is reviewed the next day and if not approved by the third-party payer, reimbursement may not be paid (emergency department admission review). Once a patient is in the hospital, the length of stay is closely monitored, and the patient may be discharged from the hospital as soon as possible (concurrent review and discharge planning). Other aspects of managed care include second opinions before elective surgery; use of primary care physicians as gatekeepers; high-cost case management; benefit design; and the provision of financial incentives for physicians to practice economically.

The medical care system in the USA has many costly inefficiencies, and correcting these may require major changes, such as national or regional health insurance, a single-payer system, or a combination of both. Nevertheless, the high initial costs of shifting to a new system, the uncertainty of its benefits, and the complex political compromises that would be necessary suggest that in the immediate future, no major, rapid change will take place in the organization or financing of medical care in the USA.

■ QUESTIONS

Directions (Items 1–4). The set of matching questions in this section consists of a list of lettered options followed by several numbered items. For each numbered item, select the ONE lettered option that is most closely associated with it. To avoid spending too much time on matching sets with large numbers of options, begin by reading the list of options. Then, for each item in the set, try to generate the correct answer and locate it in the option list, rather than evaluating each option individually. Each lettered option may be selected once, more than once, or not at all. Correct answers and explanations are given at the end of the chapter.

(A) Disability
(B) Disease
(C) Illness
(D) Impairment

Match the term with the appropriate definition.
1. Medically defined pathophysiology
2. Subjective experience of a pathologic process
3. Limitation of functional ability as defined by a physician
4. Social definition of physical limitations

Directions (Items 5–9). Each of the numbered items or incomplete statements in this section is followed by answers or by completions of the statement. Select the ONE lettered answer or completion that is BEST in each case.

5. The median age of a population is determined principally by
   (A) genetic factors
   (B) the age-adjusted mortality rate
   (C) the birth rate
   (D) the crude mortality rate
   (E) the prevalence of chronic disease

6. Which one of the following best reflects the relationship between the "need" for medical care and the "demand" for medical care?
   (A) They are always the same
   (B) They are different because "need" is professionally defined and "demand" is patient generated
   (C) They are different because "need" takes cost into consideration
   (D) They are different because patients "need" care but physicians "demand" it
   (E) They are the same when barriers to care are minimal

7. Which one of the following is true regarding the utilization of medical resources?
   (A) It is dependent on price elasticity
   (B) It is equal to demand
   (C) It is equal to need
   (D) It is greater than need
   (E) It is influenced by unmet need

8. The medically indigent population is composed of
   (A) individuals receiving Medicaid
   (B) individuals receiving Medicare
   (C) individuals receiving welfare benefits
   (D) individuals with limited or no medical insurance and too much income to qualify for Medicaid
   (E) unemployed women with young children

9. In the year 2000, what percentage of the US population lacked medical insurance?
   (A) 5%
   (B) 17%
   (C) 21%
   (D) 25%
   (E) 37%

■ ANSWERS AND EXPLANATIONS

1. **The answer is B: disease.** A disease is a medically defined pathologic process. The process may occur with or without symptoms. If a disease is asymptomatic, the physician might regard it more seriously than does the patient. For example, aortic root dilatation caused by Marfan's syndrome (a disorder of connective tissue) might become life-threatening before symptoms are present, and a patient who feels well might need to be convinced of the need for cardiac surgery. The need to manage a disease must be balanced with the need to care for the patient, whose experience of the disease may differ markedly from that of the physician.

2. **The answer is C: illness.** On the one hand, an individual may feel ill without having a disease. On the other hand, as discussed in the answer to question 1, above, an individual may harbor serious disease yet feel well. Illness is a subjective experience of a pathologic process.

3. **The answer is D: impairment.** Impairment is a limitation of functional ability, as defined by the physician. Impairment refers to a reduction in physical function resulting from illness or injury. The degree to which an individual can compensate for impairment determines the extent of the resultant disability.

4. **The answer is A: disability.** Disability is the loss of ability. It is the consequence of impairment. Disability is defined on the basis of what functions an individual can and cannot perform following illness or injury, as compared with the status of these functions before the impairment

was acquired. Disability is a socially defined concept, based largely on a person's capacity to perform employment duties before and after an injury or illness. Disability can be partial or total, and it can be temporary or permanent.

5. **The answer is C: the birth rate.** The birth rate varies from country to country far more than does either the crude death rate or the life expectancy rate. A high birth rate can rapidly bring down the median age of a population, even if the death rate is low among the elderly. A low birth rate will cause the median age of the population to climb steadily, even if life expectancy is relatively low by world standards and age-adjusted death rates are high. Often, a low birth rate and a low age-adjusted death rate occur together, as in Scandinavia, where the median age of the population is consequently high.

6. **The answer is B: they are different because "need" is professionally defined and "demand" is patient generated.** A patient with a common cold, or viral upper respiratory tract infection, may demand medical care that the physician considers unnecessary (i.e., unneeded). Conversely, a patient using intravenous drugs may refuse help that the physician or other provider considers essential (i.e., needed). The need for medical care is professionally defined as the health care for which medical intervention is indicated in a given population. Demand is the amount of care sought by the public under varying assumptions about the cost of care.

7. **The answer is E: it is influenced by unmet need.** Utilization of health care resources is effective demand, the overlap between the desire for care and the delivery of care. Both demand and need tend to be greater than utilization. The difference between need and utilization is unmet need. The greater is the utilization of available resources, the smaller is the disparity between utilization and need, and the smaller the unmet need is likely to become.

8. **The answer is D: individuals with limited or no medical insurance and too much income to qualify for Medicaid.** In the USA, persons with no financial resources often receive medical care under Medicaid, Title 19 of the Social Security Act. These persons have limited ability to pay medical bills and are not expected to do so. In contrast, individuals whose incomes are too high to allow them to qualify for Medicaid are expected to pay for their care. Many of these individuals are either medically uninsured or underinsured and can be financially destroyed by an illness or injury. In the absence of guaranteed health care insurance for all US citizens, the number of medically indigent will continue to grow.

9. **The answer is B: 17%.** In the USA, about 44 million people (17% of the US population) lacked medical insurance in the year 2000. The number of uninsured and underinsured adults is rising annually. Most members of this group are one health crisis away from poverty and are therefore considered medically indigent.

References Cited

American College of Physicians (ACP). Clinical Practice Guidelines Approved by the American College of Physicians. Philadelphia, ACP, 1992.

Committee on the Costs of Medical Care. Medical Care for the American People. Chicago, University of Chicago Press, 1932.

Donabedian, A. A Guide to Medical Care Administration. Vol. 2, Medical Care Appraisal. New York, American Public Health Association, 1969.

Eisenberg, D. M., et al. Trends in alternative medicine use in the United States, 1990–1997. Journal of the American Medical Association 280:1569–1575, 1998.

Fisher, E. S., et al. Hospital readmission rates for cohorts of Medicare beneficiaries in Boston and New Haven. New England Journal of Medicine 331:989–995, 1994.

Flexner, A. Medical Education in the United States and Canada: A Report to the Carnegie Foundation for the Advancement of Teaching. Buffalo, N. Y., Heritage Press, 1910.

Freidson, E. Professional Dominance: The Social Structure of Medical Care. New York, Atherton Press, 1970.

Gray, B. H., and M. J. Field, eds. Controlling Costs and Changing Patient Care? The Role of Utilization Management. Washington, D. C., National Academy Press, 1989.

Hardin, G. The tragedy of the commons. Science 162:1243–1248, 1968.

Health Care Financing Administration. Medicare and You: 2000. Department of Health and Human Services (DHHS) Publication No. 10050. Washington, D. C., Public Health Service, 1999.

Institute of Medicine. To Err Is Human: Building a Safer Health System. Washington, D. C., National Academy Press, 2000.

Kemper, P., and C. M. Murtaugh. Lifetime use of nursing home care. New England Journal of Medicine 324:595–600, 1991.

Kropf, R. Planning for health services. In Kovner, A. R., ed. Health Care Delivery in the United States, 4th ed. New York, Springer Publishing Company, 1990.

Luft, H. S. Health Maintenance Organizations. New York, John Wiley and Sons, 1981.

Prussin, J. A., and J. C. Woods. Development of Health Insurance. Topics in Health Care Financing 2:1–12, 1975.

Relman, A. S. The health care industry: where is it taking us? New England Journal of Medicine 325:854–859, 1991.

Rognehaugh, R. The Managed Health Care Dictionary, 2nd ed. Gaithersburg, Md., Aspen Publishers, 1998.

Sweet, V. Letter to the editor. New England Journal of Medicine 329:1655, 1993.

Wennberg, J. E., J. L. Freeman, and W. J. Culp. Are hospital services rationed in New Haven or overutilized in Boston? Lancet 1:1185–1189, 1987.

Woolhandler, S., D. U. Himmelstein, and J. P. Lewontin. Administrative costs in US hospitals. New England Journal of Medicine 329:400–403, 1993.

Selected Readings

Bodenheimer, T. S., and K. Grumbach. Understanding Health Policy: A Clinical Approach. Norwalk, Conn., Appleton and Lange, 1995.

Institute of Medicine. To Err Is Human: Building a Safer Health System. Washington, D. C., National Academy Press, 2000.

Kovner, A. R., and S. Jonas. Health Care Delivery in the United States, 6th ed. New York, Springer Publishing Company, 1999.

Rognehaugh, R. The Managed Health Care Dictionary, 2nd ed. Gaithersburg, Md., Aspen Publishers, 1998.

Comprehensive Examination

■ QUESTIONS

Directions (Items 1–38). Each of the numbered items or incomplete statements in this section is followed by answers or by completions of the statement. Select the ONE lettered answer or completion that is BEST in each case. Correct answers and explanations are given at the end of the examination.

1. When a 2×2 table is used, the probability of disease in a patient with a negative test result is expressed as
   - (A) $a/(a+c)$
   - (B) $c/(a+c)$
   - (C) $c/(c+d)$
   - (D) $d/(c+d)$
   - (E) d

2. You wish to determine the proportion of myocardial infarctions that are fatal within 24 hours of their occurrence. You decide to examine the records of all local emergency departments and physicians' offices. You will then calculate the proportion of the reported myocardial infarctions that resulted in death 24 hours or less after the patient was initially seen. You briefly discuss your plan with a friendly neighborhood biostatistician, who immediately points out that your study is particularly subject to which one of the following forms of bias?
   - (A) Late look bias
   - (B) Lead-time bias
   - (C) Measurement bias
   - (D) Observer bias
   - (E) Selection bias

3. Two of your colleagues are trying to determine whether medical screening programs that use chest x-rays to detect lung cancer will improve the survival time of the persons screened. They look at the most recent year's data in the Connecticut Tumor Registry and discover that the median survival time following the diagnosis of lung cancer is 6 months. They then perform a chest x-ray screening program in shopping centers and bowling alleys. They find that in persons screened by this program, the median time from diagnosis to death is 9 months for the 95 cases of lung cancer discovered. The survival time difference is statistically significant. They conclude that the screening program and subsequent treatment are adding an average of 3 months to the lives of lung cancer patients. You disagree with their conclusion because their study is particularly subject to which one of the following forms of bias?
   - (A) Late look bias
   - (B) Lead-time bias
   - (C) Measurement bias
   - (D) Observer bias
   - (E) Selection bias

4. A company was concerned about productivity that was lost because of health problems, so it instituted an intensive medical treatment and support program for the 10% of its workers who missed the most work because of illness during a certain year. The treated group had much better attendance and productivity the next year. You know that the intensive program used was actually ineffective, and you believe that the most likely explanation for the outcome is
   - (A) effect modification
   - (B) excessive power
   - (C) random error
   - (D) the statistical regression effect
   - (E) type II error

5. A screening test is applied to a population of 1000 in which the prevalence of disease Y is 10%. The sensitivity of this test is 96%, and the specificity is 92%. The diagnostic workup for each person found to have a positive result in the screening test will cost $50. A newer screening test has the same sensitivity but has a specificity of 96% and costs $0.50 more per test than the older screening test. How much money would be saved or lost by choosing the newer test?
   - (A) $500 lost
   - (B) $500 saved
   - (C) $1300 lost
   - (D) $1300 saved
   - (E) $1800 saved

6. You have just completed a history and physical examination of a patient for whom you consider the diagnosis of systemic lupus erythematosus (SLE) possible but not very likely. You order a battery of six different tests for the disease. The results of four are positive, and the results of two are negative. To determine the probability of SLE at this point, you would need to know

(A) the incidence of SLE and the predictive value of each test
(B) the incidence, prevalence, and natural history of SLE
(C) the patient's risk factor profile, the family history, and the predictive value of each test
(D) the prior probability of SLE and the sensitivity and specificity of each test
(E) the relative risk of SLE in this patient

7. At a given level of alpha, the z value associated with a one-tailed test is smaller than the z value associated with a two-tailed test because

(A) the entire rejection region is on one side of the mean with a one-tailed test
(B) the entire rejection region is on one side of the mean with a two-tailed test
(C) the rejection region is smaller for a one-tailed test
(D) the rejection region is smaller for a two-tailed test
(E) there is 1 less degree of freedom with a one-tailed test

8. A clinical trial of an antihypertensive agent is performed by administering the drug or a placebo, with a "washout period" in between, to each study subject. The treatments are administered in random order, and each subject serves as his or her own control. The trial is double-blind. The appropriate significance test for the change in blood pressure with drug versus placebo is

(A) analysis of variance (ANOVA)
(B) chi-square analysis
(C) the logrank test
(D) the paired t-test
(E) the Pearson correlation coefficient

9. A preferred provider organization (PPO) is most similar to

(A) a DRG
(B) a staff model HMO
(C) an ICF
(D) an IPA
(E) solo practice

10. The figure at the bottom of the page depicts the epidemic threshold for

(A) influenza
(B) measles
(C) pertussis
(D) rubella
(E) varicella

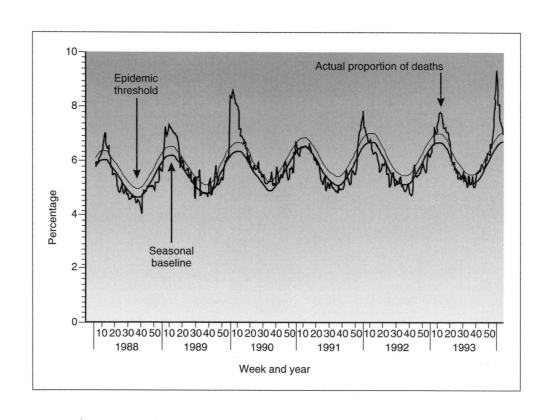

Items 11–12

The following unpublished data concern the relationship between preventive treatment with chicken soup and the frequency with which colds develop. Assume that the data are from a randomized, double-blind trial of chicken soup versus placebo (e.g., gazpacho) over the course of 1 school year.

		OUTCOME		
		Colds	No Colds	Total
TREATMENT	Chicken Soup	36	21	57
	Placebo	35	11	46
	Total	71	32	103

11. When you begin to analyze the table, you decide to use percentages. Which of the following sets of percentages represents a correct and meaningful representation of the data above and provides a basis for making the comparison of interest?

(A)   5% and 95%
(B)   10% and 14%
(C)   52% and 57%
(D)   63% and 76%
(E)   65% and 51%

12. For these data, the appropriate significance test is

(A)   chi-square analysis
(B)   the logrank test
(C)   the paired t-test
(D)   the Pearson correlation coefficient
(E)   the Student's t-test

Items 13–17

A new test for the detection of baldness is devised. It is applied to a population of 200 men who live in the USA and insist that they have hair. Based on a gold standard—namely, asking the subjects to remove their hats—20 of the 200 men are actually bald. The new test detects 12 cases of baldness, of which 8 are positive by the gold standard and 4 are negative.

13. Based on these data, the sensitivity of the new test is

(A)   8%
(B)   12%
(C)   40%
(D)   80%
(E)   92%

14. The specificity of the new test is

(A)   1%
(B)   12%
(C)   40%
(D)   66%
(E)   98%

15. The positive predictive value of the new test in this population is

(A)   1%
(B)   12%
(C)   40%
(D)   67%
(E)   98%

16. The negative predictive value of the new test is approximately

(A)   1%
(B)   12%
(C)   67%
(D)   94%
(E)   98%

17. The likelihood ratio positive for the data is

(A)   2
(B)   8
(C)   12
(D)   18
(E)   42

Items 18–19

Assume that the sensitivity and specificity of the new test for baldness in questions 13–17 remain unchanged. This time, however, the gold standard is a consultant from Topknot Toupee, Inc., who decides that there are actually 150 cases of baldness instead of 20 cases.

18. The positive predictive value is now

(A)   1%
(B)   12%
(C)   67%
(D)   94%
(E)   98%

19. The negative predictive value, given the revised prevalence, is

(A)   1%
(B)   12%
(C)   35%
(D)   67%
(E)   98%

Item 20

Two radiologists independently review 200 mammograms. Based on their readings, radiologist A recommends biopsies in 40 patients, and radiologist B recommends biopsies in 32 patients. The distribution of their readings is shown in the table at the top of the next page.

		RADIOLOGIST B		
		Positive	Negative	Total
RADIOLOGIST A	Positive	28	12	40
	Negative	4	156	160
	Total	32	168	200

20. The kappa test ratio for this table is
   - (A) 0.18
   - (B) 0.50
   - (C) 0.64
   - (D) 0.73
   - (E) 0.88

Items 21–24

You are the medical director of a company that manufactures little plastic caps for the ends of shoe-laces, a position to which you have aspired from early childhood. You wish to screen the workers for the dreaded *capus plasticus pedo-reversilosus*, a condition that causes the worker to place caps for the laces of the right shoe on the laces of the left, and vice versa. The condition can be treated effectively with ice-water immersion and concomitant hypnosis if it is detected early. From the literature on the subject, you determine that the sensitivity of the screening test is 94% and that the specificity is 90%. You estimate the prevalence of the condition in the workers to be 5%.

21. What percentage of positive screening test results will be false-positive results?
   - (A) 18%
   - (B) 23%
   - (C) 48%
   - (D) 67%
   - (E) 81%

22. What is the positive predictive value of the screening test?
   - (A) 28%
   - (B) 33%
   - (C) 48%
   - (D) 67%
   - (E) 81%

23. How many cases of the disease will be missed if 1000 workers are screened?
   - (A) 3
   - (B) 8
   - (C) 16
   - (D) 47
   - (E) 95

24. Which of the following facts would be the most important to establish before deciding whether or not to implement the screening test?
   - (A) The cost of screening, follow-up, and treatment

   - (B) The genetic risk factors for the disease
   - (C) The incidence of the disease
   - (D) The prevalence of other diseases in the population
   - (E) The size of the population at risk

Items 25–28

A friend of yours thinks that she may be pregnant. She purchased a product to test for pregnancy and found the following data provided in the product brochure:

		PREGNANCY TEST RESULT		
		Positive	Negative	Total
TRUE STATUS	Pregnant	253	24	277
	Not Pregnant	8	93	101
	Total	261	117	378

25. Turning to you for advice, your friend asks, "If the test says that I am pregnant, what is the probability that I really am pregnant?" Your answer is
   - (A) 67%
   - (B) 79%
   - (C) 85%
   - (D) 97%
   - (E) 100%

26. Your friend then asks, "If the test says that I am not pregnant, what is the probability that I really am not?" Your answer is
   - (A) 67%
   - (B) 79%
   - (C) 85%
   - (D) 97%
   - (E) 100%

27. Your friend is convinced that you actually know what you are talking about, so she asks, "If I really am pregnant, what is the probability that the test will discover that fact?" You confidently reply
   - (A) 57%
   - (B) 79%
   - (C) 88%
   - (D) 91%
   - (E) 97%

28. You caution your friend that the numbers provided in the product brochure may not apply to her because
   - (A) the false-positive error rate of the test is high
   - (B) the prevalence in the population tested is unknown
   - (C) the prevalence in the population tested may not match her prior probability
   - (D) the test sensitivity is unknown
   - (E) the test specificity is unknown

Items 29–31

Assume that you are in charge of a state committee responsible for recommending whether or not to screen for congenital disease M, which is expected to be found in 1 per 10,000 births. If this disease is treated early, there will be a lifetime savings for the state of $250,000 per infant (discounted for inflation) because of reductions in the cost of institutionalizing the affected infants. You determine from the literature that the sensitivity of the screening test is 95%, the specificity is 99%, the cost per screening test is $10, and the cost to evaluate each infant with a positive screening test result is $100.

29. What percentage of the infants who have a positive screening test result will have disease M?

    (A)   1%
    (B)   5%
    (C)   9%
    (D)   20%
    (E)   68%

30. If 100,000 infants are born each year, what will be the approximate net yearly savings or loss to the state of screening for disease M?

    (A) $25,000 saved
    (B) $200,000 lost
    (C) $1.3 million saved
    (D) $1.5 million lost
    (E) $5 million saved

31. If disease M occurred once in each 1000 births, rather than once in each 10,000 births, approximately what percentage of the positive cases identified by screening would be diseased?

    (A)   1%
    (B)   5.3%
    (C)   8.7%
    (D)   20%
    (E)   68.8%

Items 32–33

The resting heart rates of 10 subjects are 70, 68, 84, 76, 88, 66, 56, 60, 80, and 70 beats per minute.

32. What is the variance of this data set?

    (A)   8.6
    (B)   10.2
    (C)   12.2
    (D)   86.6
    (E)   104.4

33. What is the standard deviation of this data set?

    (A)   8.6
    (B)   10.2
    (C)   12.2
    (D)   86.6
    (E)   104.4

Items 34–36

The following story is taken from the New King James Version of the Bible, Book of Daniel, Chapter 1, verses 1–16:

> Daniel said to the steward whom the chief of the eunuchs had set over Daniel, Hananiah, Mishael, and Azariah, "Please test your servants for ten days, and let them give us vegetables to eat and water to drink. Then let our countenances be examined before you, and the countenances of the young men who eat the portion of the king's delicacies; and as you see fit, so deal with your servants."
>
> So he consented with them in this matter, and tested them [i.e., the Israelites] for ten days. And at the end of ten days their countenance appeared better and fatter in flesh than all the young men who ate the portion of the king's delicacies. Thus, the steward took away their portion of delicacies and the wine that they were to drink, and gave them vegetables.

34. What type of study design is described?

    (A)   Case-control study
    (B)   Cross-sectional study
    (C)   Field trial
    (D)   Prospective cohort study
    (E)   Retrospective cohort study

35. Although this study is in some ways quite primitive, a strength it demonstrates is

    (A)   blinding
    (B)   matching
    (C)   random allocation
    (D)   random sampling
    (E)   use of controls

36. Although studies of this type are susceptible to numerous potential sources of error, they are able to avoid

    (A)   confounding
    (B)   measurement bias
    (C)   observer bias
    (D)   recall bias
    (E)   selection bias

Items 37–38

Two different groups of investigators perform clinical trials of the same therapy. The trials have approximately the same sample size. In the first trial, the investigators find more successes in the treatment group and report a p value of 0.04. Based on these results, the investigators recommend the therapy. In the second trial, the investigators find more successes in the treatment group but report a p value of 0.08. Based on these results, the investigators do not recommend the therapy.

37. After the clinician reviews the studies, which of the following statements could he or she make that would best describe the statistical significance of the data?

    (A) Data that are not statistically significant may nonetheless be clinically important
    (B) If the data achieve statistical significance, the studies will be clinically important
    (C) If the data do not achieve statistical significance, the studies cannot be clinically important
    (D) The reason that statistical significance has not been achieved is probably that alpha has been set too high
    (E) The reason that statistical significance has not been achieved is probably that beta has been set too low

38. An appropriate means for reconciling the conflicting recommendations would be to

    (A) conduct a case-control study
    (B) obtain expert opinion
    (C) perform "intention to treat" analysis
    (D) pool the data
    (E) use multivariable methods to analyze the data

Directions (Items 39–51). Each set of matching questions in this section consists of a list of lettered options followed by several numbered items. For each numbered item, select the ONE lettered option that is most closely associated with it. To avoid spending too much time on matching sets with large numbers of options, begin each set by reading the list of options. Then, for each item in the list, try to generate the correct answer and locate it in the option list, rather than evaluating each option individually. Each lettered option may be selected once, more than once, or not at all.

Items 39–42

(A) $a/(a + b)$
(B) $d/(c + d)$
(C) $(1 - \text{sensitivity})$
(D) $(1 - \text{specificity})$

Match the given rate or value with the correct formula.
39. False-negative error rate
40. False-positive error rate
41. Negative predictive value
42. Positive predictive value

Items 43–49

(A) Acceptability of medical care
(B) Accessibility of medical care
(C) Accountability of medical care
(D) Adequacy of medical care
(E) Appropriateness of medical care
(F) Assessability of medical care
(G) Availability of medical care

Match each of the criteria for high-quality health care with the corresponding definition or description.
43. The interventions are properly selected and performed by trained professionals.
44. There is public disclosure of financial records and quality standards.
45. There are no geographic or financial barriers to care.
46. The care provided is compatible with the patient's belief systems.
47. The quality of medical care can be professionally reviewed.
48. Care is provided during the times it is needed.
49. The amount of care provided is commensurate with the need, the demand, or both.

Items 50–51

(A) Case-control study
(B) Longitudinal ecologic study
(C) Prospective cohort study

Match the study design with the appropriate description.
50. Multiple disease outcomes can be studied, but only the risk factors defined and measured at the beginning of the study can be assessed.
51. Only one outcome can be studied, but many risk factors or exposures can be assessed.

Directions (Items 52–101). Each of the numbered items or incomplete statements in this section is followed by answers or by completions of the statement. Select the ONE lettered answer or completion that is BEST in each case.

52. You are preparing a before and after trial of the effects of a hypoglycemic agent in the management of type II diabetes mellitus. In the trial, each subject will serve as his or her own control. You plan to set a two-tailed alpha at 0.05, to look for a difference ($\overline{d}$) of 10 mg/dL in the serum glucose level, and to ignore beta. You select a standard deviation (s) of 22 mg/dL from prior studies. The total sample size needed for your study is best represented by which of the following formulas?

    (A) $N = \dfrac{(z_\alpha)^2 \cdot (s)^2}{(\overline{d})^2}$

    (B) $N = \dfrac{(z_\alpha)^2 \cdot 2 \cdot (s)^2}{(\overline{d})^2}$

    (C) $N = \dfrac{2 \cdot (z_\alpha)^2 \cdot 2 \cdot (s)^2}{(\overline{d})^2}$

    (D) $N = \dfrac{\sqrt{(z_\alpha - \overline{d})^2}}{s^2}$

(E) $N = \dfrac{(z_\alpha)^2 \cdot (\bar{d})^2}{s^2}$

53. Diagnosis-related groups (DRGs) are used to
    (A) assess the quality of subspecialty care in hospitals
    (B) assign patients to appropriate hospital wards
    (C) provide support for patients following hospital discharge
    (D) review interobserver agreement in radiology
    (E) stipulate prospective payment to hospitals

54. Epidemiology is best defined as the study of
    (A) causal factors in disease
    (B) disease outbreaks
    (C) factors that influence the occurrence and distribution of disease in human populations
    (D) the incidence of human disease
    (E) the transmission of infectious diseases and exposure to environmental toxins

55. The mosquito involved in the transmission of malaria assumes the role of
    (A) animal reservoir
    (B) commensal
    (C) parasite
    (D) surrogate host
    (E) vector

56. When the number of cancer cases diagnosed annually in the USA is compared with the number of cases expected to occur if the lowest rates applied, what is the result?
    (A) There are half as many cases as would be expected
    (B) There are 2 times as many cases as would be expected
    (C) There are 5 times as many cases as would be expected
    (D) There are 10 times as many cases as would be expected
    (E) This comparison is not valid

57. The bacterium responsible for legionnaires' disease usually replicates in and is spread from
    (A) drinking water
    (B) food, especially meat, cooked at inadequate temperatures
    (C) swimming pools
    (D) unpasteurized beer
    (E) warm water systems such as air-conditioning cooling towers

58. Mormons and Seventh-Day Adventists have lower than average age-adjusted death rates. The avoidance of alcohol and tobacco and the adherence to a healthful diet by members of these groups are factors that

(A) are associated with reduced mortality rates from cardiovascular disease but not from cancer
(B) are associated with the lower mortality rates but may not be causal factors
(C) are unrelated to age-adjusted death rates, which are largely influenced by the age distribution of the population
(D) are unrelated to mortality rates, because the rates are largely the result of genetic factors
(E) cause the lower mortality rates

59. Which of the following best describes the effect of vaccination against diphtheria when the disease was more common than it is currently?
    (A) Frequent exposure resulted in boosted immunity following immunization
    (B) Frequent exposure resulted in infection, against which vaccination was not protective
    (C) Susceptibility to severe infection redeveloped several years after vaccination
    (D) Vaccination resulted in hypersensitivity to the infectious agent
    (E) Vaccination resulted in unusually severe clinical disease when immunity was not achieved

60. The demographic gap refers to
    (A) disruption of the nuclear family
    (B) persons living below the poverty line in the USA
    (C) socioeconomic differences among countries
    (D) the difference between Medicare reimbursement and hospital charges
    (E) the difference between the birth rate and death rate of a society

61. Construction of the Aswan High Dam in Egypt resulted in increased transmission of which of the following diseases?
    (A) Leishmaniasis
    (B) Necrotizing fasciitis
    (C) Schistosomiasis
    (D) Tuberculosis
    (E) Yellow fever

62. Data reported for cases of relatively mild diseases, such as chickenpox, could generally be characterized as
    (A) highly accurate because of active surveillance
    (B) useful for establishing prevalence but not incidence
    (C) valuable for detecting changes in the pattern of a disease
    (D) valueless because mild diseases are underreported
    (E) valueless because most patients with mild diseases do not present for medical care

63. Which one of the following types of data does epidemiology derive directly from the US census?

    (A) Data for direct standardization
    (B) Data for indirect standardization
    (C) Denominator data for population-based studies
    (D) The standardized mortality ratio
    (E) Time trend data

64. What percentage of death certificate diagnoses are thought to be potentially inaccurate?

    (A) 5%
    (B) 15–20%
    (C) 30%
    (D) 50%
    (E) 80–85%

65. The number of cases of influenza in a population is divided by the population at the beginning of the observation period. This is reported as the "risk" of influenza. This measure could be characterized as

    (A) a rate, not a risk
    (B) an acceptable risk estimate, although the best denominator would be the midyear population at risk
    (C) an acceptable risk estimate, because the risk is similar to the rate when the disease is common
    (D) an acceptable risk estimate, even though the best denominator would include only subjects without protective immunity to influenza
    (E) an unacceptable estimate of risk, because too many cases of influenza go unreported

66. Rates are not synonymous with risks. In comparison with risks, rates

    (A) are based on a more accurate denominator
    (B) are generally lower
    (C) are significantly higher
    (D) better demonstrate the force of mortality
    (E) rely on more constant denominators

67. Which of the following is a valid rate?

    (A) Lung cancer in men in the USA
    (B) Poliomyelitis in elementary school children
    (C) Prostatitis in adults over 65 years of age
    (D) Rubella in pregnant women
    (E) Uterine cancer in the US population

68. A particularly useful measure of events that can occur repeatedly in individual subjects under observation is

    (A) the frequency
    (B) the incidence density
    (C) the incidence rate
    (D) the period prevalence
    (E) the risk

69. Obesity has been labeled an epidemic in the USA. This characterization is

    (A) correct, because current prevalence exceeds the historical baseline
    (B) correct, because obesity has a genetic component
    (C) correct, because one in three adults is considered obese
    (D) incorrect, because obesity is not a communicable disease
    (E) incorrect, because obesity takes years to develop

70. The following deaths are reported for a population of 2807 men, aged 35–68 years: 4 deaths in nonsmokers; 11 deaths in those smoking up to one-half pack of cigarettes per day; 18 deaths in those smoking one-half to one pack per day; and 43 deaths in those smoking over one pack per day. From this, one may conclude that

    (A) smoking increases mortality
    (B) the relationship between mortality rates and smoking is linear
    (C) there is a dose-response relationship between smoking and death
    (D) to interpret the data, the age at death is required for each case
    (E) to interpret the data, the information must be expressed as rates

71. Among elderly subjects who are physically fit, vigorous exercise reduces the risk of heart disease. Among elderly subjects who are physically unfit, the initiation of vigorous exercise might precipitate a myocardial infarction. Fitness may be considered

    (A) a confounder
    (B) a necessary cause
    (C) a risk factor
    (D) a sufficient cause
    (E) an effect modifier

72. In the relationship between obesity and cardiovascular disease, what are hyperlipidemia and hyperglycemia?

    (A) Confounders
    (B) Effect modifiers
    (C) Intervening variables
    (D) Necessary causes
    (E) Unrelated

73. When questioned years after an illness, individuals who served as cases reported more severe subjective symptoms than did those who served as controls. This is probably an example of

    (A) confounding
    (B) misclassification
    (C) random error
    (D) recall bias
    (E) spectrum bias

74. What is the relationship of asbestos to asbestosis?

    (A) Confounder
    (B) Effect modifier
    (C) Necessary cause
    (D) Sufficient cause
    (E) Synergism

75. The National Health and Nutrition Examination Surveys (NHANES) are conducted at intervals by the US government to establish trends in health-related behaviors and dietary practices. For example, NHANES III, Phase 1, conducted from 1988 to 1991, showed a decline in the population's mean fat intake from 37% of total calories to 34% of total calories. This type of research is an example of

    (A) a longitudinal cohort study
    (B) a randomized field trial
    (C) a repeated cross-sectional study
    (D) a retrospective cohort study
    (E) hypothesis testing

76. Which of the following examples might represent a retrospective cohort study?

    (A) Cases of lung cancer assessed for prior exposures
    (B) Subjects randomly assigned to active varicella vaccine versus placebo, followed for chickenpox
    (C) Subjects with current angina followed for the development of myocardial infarction
    (D) Subjects with prior radiation exposure followed for the development of lymphoproliferative cancers
    (E) Subjects with skin cancer assessed for life-long, cumulative sun exposure

77. The Physicians' Health Study was a randomized, double-blind, placebo-controlled trial that was designed to test the effects of aspirin and beta carotene on cardiovascular disease and cancer (Physicians' Health Study Steering Committee 1989). The participants in the trial consisted of approximately 22,000 male physicians who lived in the USA and were 40–75 years of age. The randomization of participants in the study was performed to help achieve which of the following?

    (A) Elimination of bias
    (B) External validity
    (C) Internal validity
    (D) Prevention of confounding by known and unknown factors
    (E) Statistical significance

78. In a cohort study, the groups are compared on the basis of

    (A) age
    (B) disease status
    (C) exclusion criteria
    (D) exposure status
    (E) inclusion criteria

Age Group (Years)	Population A		Population B	
	Size of Population	Number of Deaths	Size of Population	Number of Deaths
<30	13,000	13	4,000	3
30–65	15,000	45	15,000	30
>65	4,000	120	13,000	145

Items 79–88

For populations A and B, information about deaths in certain age groups is shown in the above table.

79. The crude death rate for population A is best expressed as

   (A) 0.005
   (B) 1.8 per 10,000
   (C) 5.6 per 1000
   (D) 60 per 100,000
   (E) 178

80. In selecting an answer for question 79, which of the following assumptions was made?

   (A) All deaths occurred during the period of interest
   (B) All deaths were due to chronic disease
   (C) Diagnostic criteria for the cause of death were consistent during the study period
   (D) The force of mortality was constant over the period of interest
   (E) The population figures were constant over time

81. The crude death rate for population B is

   (A) 0.005
   (B) 1.8 per 10,000
   (C) 5.6 per 1000
   (D) 60 per 100,000
   (E) 178

82. Crude death rates in populations are determined by

   (A) disease surveillance and reporting
   (B) seasonal variation in mortality rates and consistency in diagnostic criteria
   (C) the age distribution
   (D) the causes of death
   (E) the size of the population and the total number of deaths

83. The age-specific death rate for those over 65 years of age in population A is

   (A) 3%
   (B) 3 per 1000
   (C) 120
   (D) always less than the crude rate
   (E) dependent upon the size of the standard population

84. Direct standardization is needed to compare the mortality rates of populations A and B because

   (A) the age distributions are different
   (B) the causes of death are different
   (C) the force of mortality is variable
   (D) the numerators are not comparable
   (E) the period of observation is unknown

85. Which of the following would be inappropriate to use as a reference population in calculating standardized mortality rates by the direct method?

   (A) A population of nursing home residents
   (B) The population of a country other than the USA
   (C) The population of the USA
   (D) The sum of populations A and B
   (E) The sum of populations A and B in each age group

86. The standardized mortality rate for population A is

   (A) 0.003
   (B) 0.034
   (C) 5.1 per 1000
   (D) 9.64 per 1000
   (E) 17

87. The standardized mortality rate for population B is

   (A) 0.007
   (B) 0.023
   (C) 4.06 per 1000
   (D) 9.64 per 1000
   (E) exactly 1%

88. The standardized mortality rate for population A differs from that for population B because

   (A) population A is smaller
   (B) population B has lower age-specific death rates
   (C) population B is dying sooner
   (D) the crude rates are the same
   (E) the crude rates differ

Items 89–91

In the US population, approximately 50 million people have hypertension to varying degrees (see National Institutes of Health 1997). Hypertension is the most important risk factor for cerebrovascular disease, which accounted for 144,000 deaths in 1990 (McGinnis and Foege 1993). The relative risk for a cerebrovascular accident rises with the magnitude of hypertension and has ranged in published studies from slightly over 1 to nearly 50 (Fletcher and Bulpitt 1992). To answer the following items, assume that the annual number of deaths from a cerebrovascular accident is 150,000, that the total US population is 265 million, and that the rate of death caused by a cerebrovascular accident is 3.5 times as high in hypertensive individuals as it is in the general population.

89. Among the general population, how much of the total risk for death caused by a cerebrovascular accident is due to hypertension?

   (A) 1/8
   (B) 3.4 per 10,000 population
   (C) 5.7
   (D) 11.6 per 10,000 population
   (E) 12%

90. Among the general population, what percentage of the total risk for cerebrovascular accident mortality is due to hypertension?

   (A) 0%
   (B) 3.4%
   (C) 8.4%
   (D) 59.6%
   (E) 72%

91. The risk for cerebrovascular accident mortality that is attributable to hypertension is

   (A) 1.8 per 100,000

   (B) 3.1 per 10,000
   (C) 17.7 per 10,000
   (D) 28%
   (E) 32%

Items 92–93

You are conducting a study to determine the effects of chemotherapy on the survival of subjects with pancreatic carcinoma. Subjects are enrolled at diagnosis and treated immediately after staging. The study is conducted over a period of 4 years. You observe 10 subjects for an average of 6 months each before the occurrence of death, loss to follow-up, or study termination; 6 of these subjects die. You observe 30 subjects for an average of 4 months each, and 16 die. You observe 2 subjects for an average of 3 years each, and 1 dies.

92. What is the total observation period?

   (A) It cannot be determined from the available information
   (B) It is best expressed as 4 person-years
   (C) It is best expressed as 4 years
   (D) It is best expressed as 21 person-years
   (E) It is best expressed as 48 person-months

93. What is the mortality rate?

   (A) It cannot be determined, because of losses to follow-up
   (B) It is approximately 1.1 deaths per person-year of observation
   (C) It is approximately 5.8 deaths per person-month of observation
   (D) It is approximately 23 deaths per person-year of observation
   (E) It is 5.75 deaths per year of observation

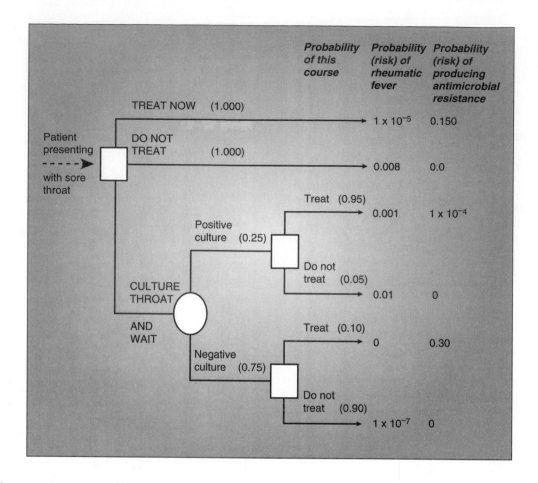

	Probability of this course	Probability (risk) of rheumatic fever	Probability (risk) of producing antimicrobial resistance

Items 94–98

Oropharyngeal infection with *Streptococcus pyogenes* (group A streptococcus) is a risk factor for rheumatic fever and may cause injury to the heart valves (carditis). Although the incidence of rheumatic fever declined in the USA from the early part of the 20th century up until the 1980s, there has been a subsequent resurgence of this disease (Bisno 1991). You are contemplating these facts when a patient shows up for a routine office visit and complains of a sore throat. The patient has no significant medical problems and no allergies to antibiotics. You are fearful of leaving "strep throat" untreated, but you are also concerned about the unnecessary use of antibiotics and the consequent propagation of antibiotic-resistant strains of bacteria. Suddenly overcome with uncertainty, you resort to the decision tree shown at the top of this page.

94. If you decide to treat your patient immediately, the risk of rheumatic fever is

    (A)   0.009
    (B)   0.150
    (C)   0.44
    (D) $1/10^5$
    (E) $1/10^7$

95. If you decide not to treat your patient, the risk of rheumatic fever is

    (A)   0.0063
    (B)   0.008

    (C)   0.011
    (D)   1
    (E)   8%

96. If you decide to obtain a throat culture and the result is positive and you then decide to treat your patient, the risk of rheumatic fever is

    (A)   0.001
    (B)   1%
    (C)   2.2%
    (D)   2.4/10,000
    (E)   9.5/10,000

97. If you decide to obtain a throat culture and the result is positive and you then decide to treat your patient, the risk of producing antimicrobial resistance is

    (A)   0
    (B) $1/10^4$
    (C) $1/10^5$
    (D) $1/10^7$
    (E)   9.5/10,000

98. The overall risk of rheumatic fever in all of the patients for whom a throat culture is obtained is

    (A)   0%
    (B) $1.25/10^4$
    (C) $2.375/10^4$
    (D) $3.6/10^4$
    (E) $6.75/10^8$

Items 99–101

In untreated patients, disease X causes death in 22% and serious complications in 1%. In treated patients, the mortality rate falls to 6%, but the rate of serious complications rises to 5%.

99. What is the number needed to treat (NNT) in this scenario?
    - (A) 2.8
    - (B) 6.25
    - (C) 8
    - (D) 15
    - (E) 30

100. What is the number needed to harm (NNH) in this scenario?
    - (A) 10
    - (B) 20
    - (C) 25
    - (D) 30
    - (E) 35

101. What will be the net result of intervention in this scenario?
    - (A) 0.5 patients harmed for each patient benefited
    - (B) 2 patients benefited for each patient harmed
    - (C) 4 patients benefited for each patient harmed
    - (D) 10 patients benefited for each patient harmed
    - (E) 30 patients harmed for each patient benefited

Directions (Items 102–108). Each set of matching questions in this section consists of a list of lettered options followed by several numbered items. For each numbered item, select the ONE lettered option that is most closely associated with it. To avoid spending too much time on matching sets with large numbers of options, begin each set by reading the list of options. Then, for each item in the list, try to generate the correct answer and locate it in the option list, rather than evaluating each option individually. Each lettered option may be selected once, more than once, or not at all.

Items 102–104

- (A) Double-blinding
- (B) Hypothesis testing
- (C) Increasing the sample size
- (D) Randomization
- (E) Statistical analysis

Match each of the terms related to study design and interpretation with the appropriate description.

102. This reduces confounding by both known and unknown factors.
103. This minimizes measurement bias.
104. This is required to compensate for the fact that in a prospective randomized trial, the two subject groups differ significantly with regard to several factors other than the intervention under investigation.

Items 105–108

(A) $N = \dfrac{(z_\alpha + z_\beta)^2 \cdot 2 \cdot \overline{p}(1 - \overline{p})}{(\overline{d})^2}$

(B) $N = \dfrac{(z_\alpha)^2 \cdot (s)^2}{(\overline{d})^2}$

(C) $N = \dfrac{(z_\alpha)^2 \cdot 2 \cdot (s)^2}{(\overline{d})^2}$

(D) $N = \dfrac{(z_\alpha + z_\beta)^2 \cdot 2 \cdot (s)^2}{(\overline{d})^2}$

Match the description of the trial with the appropriate formula for sample size.

105. A randomized controlled trial of the effects of chocolate versus placebo on the development of complete inner peace, with the outcome expressed as the proportion of subjects in each group
106. A randomized controlled trial of the effects of sautéed gravel (unpretentious, with a lingering crunch) versus placebo on serum cholesterol levels, with experimental and control groups of comparable size (sample size considers type I error but not type II error)
107. A before and after study, in one group of subjects, of the effects that watching reruns of "The Brady Bunch" has on IQ
108. A randomized controlled trial of soluble fiber and postprandial glycemia, with comparable control and experimental groups (sample size considers both type I error and type II error)

Directions (Items 109–150). Each of the numbered items or incomplete statements in this section is followed by answers or by completions of the statement. Select the ONE lettered answer or completion that is BEST in each case.

109. Which of the following measures is most useful in the generation of public health policy?
    - (A) Attributable risk, or AR
    - (B) Attributable risk percent in the exposed, or AR%(exposed)
    - (C) Odds ratio, or OR
    - (D) Population attributable risk percent, or PAR%
    - (E) Risk ratio, or RR

110. The square of the correlation coefficient, the r^2 value, represents
    (A) $(1 - \text{specificity})$
    (B) the covariance of y
    (C) the degrees of freedom associated with x
    (D) the risk ratio
    (E) the strength of the association between x and y

111. Linear regression would be an appropriate method for which of the following scenarios?
    (A) Calculating the probability of achieving remission of leukemia when the prior response to chemotherapy is known
    (B) Predicting blood pressure levels when the family history of the presence or absence of hypertension is known
    (C) Predicting serum cholesterol levels when dietary intake data are known
    (D) Predicting the blood type of a patient when the blood types of the parents are known
    (E) Predicting the peak air flow rates when the pack-years of cigarettes smoked are known

112. When the chi-square test for statistical analysis of a 2×2 contingency table is used, the null hypothesis is
    (A) that p is <0.05
    (B) that the row and column totals are the same
    (C) that the two means do not differ
    (D) that the two variables are independent of each other
    (E) that the two variances do not differ

113. Which of the following is most likely to contribute to a statistically significant but clinically meaningless outcome?
    (A) Obtaining a p value larger than alpha
    (B) Performing a two-tailed test instead of a one-tailed test
    (C) Performing subgroup analysis
    (D) Setting alpha at <0.05
    (E) Using a very large sample

114. The principal way in which the Kaplan-Meier life table method differs from the actuarial method is that the Kaplan-Meier method
    (A) can be used only if death is the outcome of interest
    (B) counts censored subjects as deaths
    (C) is not limited to dichotomous outcomes
    (D) requires a larger sample
    (E) uses uneven death-free intervals

115. An enormously successful hypertension screening campaign is repeated after 1 year in a retirement community. This time, the results are disappointing because very few new cases of hypertension are detected. The likely explanation for this outcome is
    (A) a decline in the prevalence of hypertension
    (B) a high rate of mortality among elderly individuals with hypertension
    (C) a new cutoff level for diagnosing hypertension
    (D) the fact that only incident cases are detected
    (E) the phenomenon of regression toward the mean

116. Patients may be more amenable to tertiary prevention than to either primary or secondary prevention because
    (A) only tertiary prevention limits disability in older age groups
    (B) only tertiary prevention occurs after the onset of disease
    (C) tertiary prevention is more cost-effective
    (D) tertiary prevention produces the greatest net benefit
    (E) the onset of symptoms may cause concern and raise motivation

117. The effect of obesity on the risk of cardiovascular disease is known to be related to
    (A) age
    (B) body fat distribution
    (C) cigarette smoking
    (D) family history
    (E) gender

118. Data from the Framingham Study suggest that risk factors for coronary artery disease are
    (A) additive
    (B) common only in men
    (C) synergistic
    (D) too common to justify screening
    (E) unimportant in women

119. The circulating level of which of the following lipid moieties is inversely related to the risk of myocardial infarction?
    (A) High-density lipoprotein
    (B) Low-density lipoprotein
    (C) Total cholesterol
    (D) Triglycerides
    (E) Very low density lipoprotein

120. Which class of drugs disrupts cholesterol biosynthesis in the liver?
    (A) Angiotensin-converting enzyme inhibitors
    (B) Bile acid sequestrants
    (C) Fibrates
    (D) HMG-CoA reductase inhibitors ("statins")
    (E) Selective serotonin reuptake inhibitors

121. According to the generally accepted definition of hypertension, approximately how many prevalent cases of hypertension are there in the USA?

(A)   500,000
(B)   5 million
(C)   10 million
(D)   25 million
(E)   50 million

122. The only routine screening programs for diabetes that are thought to be cost-effective are those in

(A)   elderly persons
(B)   neonates
(C)   obese persons
(D)   pregnant women
(E)   school-aged children

123. The difference between impairment and disability is that

(A)   disability is medically defined
(B)   disability is permanent
(C)   disability is socially defined
(D)   impairment is permanent
(E)   impairment is socially defined

124. The fundamental responsibility for the health of the US public lies with

(A)   the federal government
(B)   the Institute of Medicine
(C)   the local governments
(D)   the states
(E)   the Surgeon General

125. In contrast to the view of public health espoused in the USA, the Ottawa Charter (1906) emphasizes

(A)   consideration of the health impact of all public policy
(B)   corporate responsibility for health
(C)   individual responsibility for health
(D)   nuclear disarmament
(E)   population control and renewable energy sources

126. The current recommendation concerning dietary fat intake in adults is to reduce the intake to

(A)   1 g/kg of body weight per day
(B)   10% of total daily calories
(C)   20% of total daily calories
(D)   30% of total daily calories
(E)   80 g/d

127. A 42-year-old woman visits her physician for a routine examination. She has a family history of heart disease but not breast cancer. She smokes one pack of cigarettes daily and has done so for 24 years. She is sedentary and is about 16 kg (35 pounds) overweight. Her diet is of the "typical" North American variety, which means that her intake of dietary fat and sodium exceeds recommendations. Her systolic blood pressure is 146 mm Hg, and her diastolic blood pressure is 92 mm Hg. The physician's priority for this encounter with the patient should be to

(A)   encourage physical activity
(B)   encourage smoking cessation
(C)   initiate antihypertensive therapy
(D)   obtain a lipid profile
(E)   order a mammogram

128. In the USA, the year 2000 goal concerning deaths resulting from coronary artery disease was to reduce the annual age-adjusted death rate to

(A)   12 per 1000 persons
(B)   35 per 10,000 persons
(C)   35 per 100,000 persons
(D)   100 per 10,000 persons
(E)   100 per 100,000 persons

129. During a 3-month period, hantavirus pulmonary syndrome is reported in 9 individuals, and 3 of these individuals die. Which of the following calculations would be 33%?

(A)   The adjusted death rate
(B)   The attack rate
(C)   The case fatality ratio
(D)   The crude death rate
(E)   The standardized mortality ratio

130. Why does the epidemiologic year for hepatitis A run from January to January?

(A)   Fecal-oral transmission peaks in the summer
(B)   Hepatitis A is spread via respiratory droplets
(C)   The calendar year runs from January to January
(D)   The incidence of hepatitis A does not vary seasonally
(E)   The incidence rate of hepatitis A peaks in January

131. Surveillance in the USA is most sophisticated for which of the following?

(A)   Human immunodeficiency virus infection
(B)   Influenza
(C)   Measles
(D)   Syphilis
(E)   Varicella

132. What is the most appropriate sequence of action in an outbreak investigation?
    (A) Determine whether an epidemic exists; characterize the epidemic by time, place, and person; establish the diagnosis; and initiate control measures
    (B) Determine whether an epidemic exists; initiate control measures; characterize the epidemic by time, place, and person; and establish the diagnosis
    (C) Establish a diagnosis; conduct a case-control study; and initiate control measures
    (D) Establish the case definition; determine whether an epidemic exists; characterize the epidemic by time, place, and person; develop hypotheses regarding spread; and initiate control measures
    (E) Establish the case definition; test hypotheses; characterize the epidemic by time, place, and person; and establish the diagnosis

133. The most appropriate outcome measure in a cost-utility analysis usually is
    (A) accrued savings
    (B) dollars
    (C) marginal utility
    (D) quality-adjusted life years
    (E) years

134. The standardized mortality ratio indicates fewer deaths than expected when it is
    (A) between 0 and 1
    (B) less than 100
    (C) less than 1000
    (D) less than the crude death rate
    (E) negative

135. Which of the following would provide the best data to estimate the value of a health care screening program begun 15 years ago?
    (A) Average number of years of survival following screening
    (B) Cost of the program
    (C) Cost of the program and estimated years of life saved by screening
    (D) Cost of the program and number of patients admitted to the hospital for further workup
    (E) Cost of the program and number of patients screened

136. The adequacy of the health care system in a country is best measured by the
    (A) cause-specific death rate
    (B) crude birth rate
    (C) crude death rate
    (D) infant mortality rate
    (E) standardized mortality ratio

137. Which of the following characteristics is most important in a screening test that is used to rule out a diagnosis?
    (A) A high degree of sensitivity
    (B) A high degree of specificity
    (C) A low false-negative error rate
    (D) A reasonable cost
    (E) Precision

138. Which of the following is most likely to be the cause of asthma in an automobile painter?
    (A) Byssinosis
    (B) Isocyanates
    (C) Particulates
    (D) Pneumoconiosis
    (E) Solvents

139. Which of the following is true of risk age?
    (A) It is determined in part by behavioral risk factors and family history
    (B) It is greater than the chronologic age
    (C) It is increased by a healthy diet and physical activity
    (D) It is less than the chronologic age
    (E) It is the age at which an individual is likely to die

140. Which of the following is an accurate statement concerning the statistical power of a study?
    (A) It is low when the alpha error is high
    (B) It is low when the beta error is high
    (C) It is low when the beta error is low
    (D) It varies inversely with sample size
    (E) It varies with the degrees of freedom

Items 141–150

A study is conducted to determine the rates of iron deficiency anemia among 400 adult male manganese miners, some of whom use dental floss and some of whom do not. The following data are gathered:

		IRON DEFICIENCY ANEMIA	
		Positive	Negative
EXPOSURE TO DENTAL FLOSS	Positive	150	50
	Negative	20	180

141. What type of study is this?
    (A) Case-control study
    (B) Cohort trial
    (C) Ecologic study
    (D) Field trial
    (E) Randomized study

142. Which of the following can be determined from the data provided?
    (A) The incidence of anemia
    (B) The mean value for each population
    (C) The odds ratio
    (D) The prevalence
    (E) The relative risk

143. The number of subjects using dental floss and expected to have iron deficiency anemia is
    (A) 20
    (B) 50
    (C) 75
    (D) 85
    (E) 200

144. The number of subjects not using dental floss and expected to have iron deficiency anemia is
    (A) 20
    (B) 50
    (C) 75
    (D) 85
    (E) 200

145. The number of subjects not using dental floss and expected not to have iron deficiency anemia is
    (A) 26
    (B) 40
    (C) 115
    (D) 130
    (E) 230

146. The null hypothesis for this study is best expressed by which of the following?
    (A) Iron deficiency anemia is associated with both the mining of manganese and the use of dental floss
    (B) The mining of manganese and the use of dental floss are not associated
    (C) The mining of manganese causes iron deficiency anemia
    (D) The use of dental floss and iron deficiency anemia are not associated
    (E) The use of dental floss causes iron deficiency anemia

147. Cell c of the table represents
    (A) those with both the exposure and the outcome
    (B) those with neither the exposure nor the outcome
    (C) those with the exposure but not the outcome
    (D) those with the outcome but not the exposure
    (E) those with unknown exposure or outcome

148. The chi-square value for this table is
    (A) 0.125
    (B) 12.5
    (C) 16.4
    (D) 172.8
    (E) 400

149. How many degrees of freedom are associated with the chi-square value calculated in question 148?
    (A) 0
    (B) 1

    (C) 2
    (D) 3
    (E) 4

150. To determine the statistical significance of a given chi-square value, one must
    (A) determine the 95% confidence limits
    (B) determine the variance
    (C) find the corresponding p value in a chi-square table
    (D) perform power calculations
    (E) perform sample size calculations

■ ANSWERS AND EXPLANATIONS

1. **The answer is C: $c/(c + d)$.** When a test result is negative, the probability that disease is truly absent is the negative predictive value, or $d/(c+d)$. This question, however, asks for the probability that disease is present even though the test result is negative. A disease may be either present or absent when a test result is negative, so the probability that either one or the other of these options will be found is 1. The probability that a disease is present must be 1 minus the probability that the disease is absent. This is (1 – negative predictive value), or $1 - [d/(c+d)]$, which equals $c/(c+d)$. This question of probability is frequently asked in clinical medicine. A clinician orders a test on the basis of a suspicion that a disease is present. If the test result is negative, the clinician must decide whether to continue to suspect the diagnosis or to rule it out and suspect another diagnosis. This depends on the probability of the disease being present given the negative test result. Depending on the strength of the clinician's suspicion (i.e., the prior probability) and the operating characteristics of the test (i.e., the sensitivity and specificity), the probability of disease following a negative result may be reduced to nearly 0 or may remain high. See Chapter 7.

2. **The answer is A: late look bias.** Late look bias is a tendency to detect only those cases of a serious disease that were mild enough to be detected prior to death. Many cases of massive myocardial infarction result in death before a patient can reach a physician's office or emergency department. Consequently, the study might underestimate the probability of early death following infarction. Other errors, such as classification error, which is the result of inconsistency in the diagnosis of myocardial infarction, could create bias in the findings as well. Selection bias is a problem when subjects are recruited for study participation or assigned to treatment in a nonrandom manner, and neither of these conditions is operative here. Observer bias and measurement bias occur when there is distorted interpretation of the outcome in two

study groups. In this case, the outcome is death, which is not particularly subject to interpretive error. Lead-time bias is the detection of a disease by screening earlier in its natural history than it would have otherwise been detected, resulting in a longer survival time after diagnosis but no change in actual survival time. See Chapter 5.

3. **The answer is B: lead-time bias.** Screening for lung cancer with chest x-rays has proved ineffective, not because it fails to detect cases of lung cancer but, rather, because when it does detect cases, the natural history of the disease is the same as it would have been if the disease were found and treated after symptoms developed. Lead-time bias is the prolongation of survival time after diagnosis, which occurs not because death comes later but because diagnosis comes earlier. See Chapter 17.

4. **The answer is D: the statistical regression effect.** When subjects with the most extreme values for any measure are observed over time, the values tend to become less extreme. This is the statistical regression effect, or regression toward the mean. This would be the most likely reason to see that extreme absenteeism was curbed even though the treatment program was ineffective. See Chapter 12.

5. **The answer is D: $1300 saved.** Regardless of whether the old test or the new test is used, the entire population, or 1000 people, will be screened. We do not know the cost of the old test, but we know that the new test costs $0.50 more per application. Therefore, screening the population of 1000 will cost ($0.50 × 1000), or $500 more with the new test than with the old one. We know that the prevalence of disease Y is 10%, so 90% of the population, or 900 people, are disease-free. We also know that the specificity of the old test (i.e., 92%) is lower than the specificity of the new test (i.e., 96%). The old test will correctly identify 92%, or 828, of these 900 subjects, and there will be 72 false-positive results. The new test will correctly identify 96%, or 864, of the 900 subjects, and there will be 36 false-positive results. This means that there will be 36 fewer false-positive results with the new test than with the old one. The number of true-positive results remains unchanged because the sensitivity of the new test is the same as that of the old test (i.e., 96%). All of the subjects who test positive will require a $50 workup, and there will be 36 fewer of these with the new test. The savings resulting from not having to do the workups for 36 people is (36 × $50), or $1800. When the $500 in additional costs associated with the new test is subtracted from $1800, there is a net savings of $1300 if the new test is used. See Chapter 7.

6. **The answer is D: the prior probability of systemic lupus erythematosus (SLE) and the sensitivity and specificity of each test.** Bayes' theorem is in constant application in clinical medicine, whether or not clinicians are aware of it. After completing a history and physical examination, a physician has an impression of the patient's health status that may differ from the impression he or she had before the history and physical examination were taken or from the impression after the history was taken but before the physical examination was performed. What has happened? The initial impression is based on the small amount of information known about the patient before the medical history is obtained. This is a relatively nonspecific prior probability. Each answer to each question in the medical history may cause the physician to generate a posterior probability of disease and overall health that is different than the probability he or she was considering before the answer. When the examination is completed, the impression may be revised further. Tests that are ordered to pursue a diagnosis entertained after completing the history and physical examination are intended to modify the physician's estimate of the probability of the particular diagnosis in question. To use Bayes' theorem for this purpose, the prior probability of disease before each test as well as the sensitivity and specificity of each test must be known. The posterior probability after one test becomes the prior probability for the next test. Interestingly, we know little about the operating characteristics (sensitivity and specificity for different diagnoses) of the most sophisticated diagnostic instrument to which patients are exposed: the physician's brain. This same instrument makes the original estimation of disease probability upon which all subsequent testing is dependent. See Chapter 8.

7. **The answer is A: the entire rejection region is on one side of the mean with a one-tailed test.** The distinction between a one-tailed test and a two-tailed test of significance is illustrated in Fig. 10–1 and discussed in Box 10–6. The value of z represents the number of standard deviations between a data point and the mean for the sample. When alpha is 0.05 and the significance test is two-tailed, the rejection region must be divided evenly between the high end and the low end of the distribution, placing 0.025 of the total curve area in each rejection region. To deviate from the mean as far as a two-tailed alpha of 0.05, a data point must move past 0.475 of the curve area, since half the curve lies on either side of the mean. A dispersion of 0.475 of the total curve area from the mean is associated with a z value of 1.96. When a one-tailed test is performed, the entire rejection region, or 0.05 of the total curve area, is placed on one side of the

mean. To deviate from the mean that far requires that a data point be removed only 0.45 of the curve area from the mean. This smaller deviation from the mean is associated with a smaller value of z, or 1.645. Achieving statistical significance, therefore, is easier with a one-tailed test than with a two-tailed test, provided that the outcome occurs in the expected direction. See Chapter 10.

8. **The answer is D: the paired t-test.** Selecting the appropriate significance test is essential for ensuring valid data analysis. The choice of test is dependent on the study type and the nature of independent and dependent variables. The study described in the question is a before and after trial, so the data are paired. There are two groups (a drug treatment group and placebo group), so the independent variable is dichotomous. The outcome variable is blood pressure measurements, which are continuous data. The appropriate test for this situation is the paired t-test, as indicated in Table 11–1 and discussed in Chapter 10.

9. **The answer is D: an IPA.** A preferred provider organization (PPO) is formed when an insurer establishes a network of contracts with independent practitioners. A patient may see a physician on the approved panel and receive full insurance benefits, or the patient may consult a physician who is not on the panel and pay a surcharge. Like a PPO, an independent practice association (IPA) consists of providers associated by contract with an insurer. However, in an IPA, there are cost controls, and patients are not reimbursed for care outside of the network. A staff model health maintenance organization (staff model HMO) is a type of prepaid group practice. An intermediate care facility (ICF) is usually a type of nursing home. A diagnosis-related group (DRG) is a system of designating prepayment standards for hospital care. See Chapter 21.

10. **The answer is A: influenza.** The figure depicts the variable baseline in influenza incidence and the threshold above which an epidemic is defined (source of figure: Centers for Disease Control and Prevention 1994). The surveillance for influenza is more elaborate than the surveillance for any other infectious disease in the USA. This is largely because of the somewhat predictable seasonal variations in the disease, the characteristics of antigenic drift and shift, and the feasibility of producing a strain-specific vaccine on a yearly basis. See Chapter 3.

11. **The answer is D: 63% and 76%.** When data from a table are expressed as percentages, the percentage of the dependent variable is usually shown as a function of the independent vari-

able. For this table, the assignment to either chicken soup or placebo is the independent variable, and the frequency of colds is the dependent variable. To express the frequency of colds as a function of treatment assignment, the percentage of subjects who develop colds in each group can be shown. The percentage in the chicken soup group is 63%, and that in the placebo group is 76%. The only other meaningful facts that could be learned from the table are the percentages of subjects who did not develop colds in each group. These percentages, which are 37% in the chicken soup group and 24% in the placebo group, were not among the options provided in the question. See Chapter 11.

12. **The answer is A: chi-square analysis.** Chi-square analysis is the appropriate significance test for the comparison of two dichotomous data sets. The dichotomous outcome here is having a cold or not having a cold. The two groups are chicken soup and placebo. The chi-square value for this table is 1.985 at 1 degree of freedom and is not statistically significant at an alpha level of 0.05. Unlike chi-square analysis, t-tests are used for comparing means and require two groups of continuous data, rather than dichotomous data. The Pearson correlation coefficient is used to assess the strength of association between two continuous variables. The logrank test analyzes the significance of life table analysis. See Chapter 11.

13. **The answer is C: 40%.** Sensitivity is the proportion of positive cases that also have a positive test result. We have been told that there are 20 cases. Of these 20, 8 had positive test results with the new test. The sensitivity is 8/20, or 40%. The sensitivity can also be calculated by setting up the following 2 × 2 table:

TEST STATUS		TRUE STATUS		
		Positive	Negative	Total
	Positive	8	4	12
	Negative	12	176	188
	Total	20	180	200

The cells in the table contain the data we have been given. We know that there are 20 cases, so the total for the first column in the table, the disease (positive) column, must be 20. Cell a shows the positive cases detected by the test; we know that there are 8 of these. If cell a is 8 and column 1 adds to 20, cell c must be 12. We know that there are 12 positive test results, representing the total in row 1 of the table. If cell a is 8 and the row 1 total is 12, cell b must be 4. The total for the table must be 200. Cells a, b, and c

add to 24, so cell d must be 176. The sensitivity is $a/(a+c)$, or $8/(8+12)$, which is 40%, the same answer we obtained above. See Chapter 7.

14. **The answer is E: 98%.** The specificity of a test is the proportion of negative cases that the test identifies as negative cases. There are 180 negative cases in this population, according to the available gold standard. The test identifies 4 of these as positive and the remainder, or 176, as negative. The proportion of negative cases correctly identified as such by the test is 176/180, or approximately 98%. From the table provided in the explanation to question 13, above, the specificity is $d/(b+d)$, or $176/(4+176)$, which is 98%. See Chapter 7.

15. **The answer is D: 67%.** The positive predictive value is the probability that the condition is present given a positive test result. This is the proportion of all positive results (cell a plus cell b) that are true-positive results (cell a). The formula for the positive predictive value is therefore $a/(a+b)$. In this case, the calculation is $8/(8+4)$, or about 67%. Recall that the predictive value, which is calculated as a percentage of subjects with a particular test result, includes subjects with and without the condition and is therefore dependent on the prevalence. Neither sensitivity nor specificity is dependent on the prevalence. See Chapter 7.

16. **The answer is D: 94%.** The negative predictive value is the probability that the condition is absent given a negative test result. This is the proportion of all negative test results (cell c plus cell d) that are truly negative (cell d). The negative predictive value is therefore $d/(c+d)$, which here is $176/(12+176)$. This is 93.6%, or approximately 94%. The negative predictive value is much higher than the positive predictive value in this instance because there are few cases of the condition in the population (i.e., the prevalence is low). The probability that anyone in the population has the condition is only 20 out of 200, or 10%. Therefore, the probability that a negative test result is correct is fairly high because of the low prevalence and the high specificity of the test. See Chapter 7.

17. **The answer is D: 18.** The likelihood ratio positive (LR+) indicates how much more likely it is for a positive test result to be true than to be false. The LR+ is the sensitivity, or $a/(a+c)$, divided by the false-positive error rate, or $b/(b+d)$. This becomes 8/20 divided by 4/180, which equals 18. The likelihood (odds) that disease is present in a subject with a positive test result is 18 times as great as the likelihood that disease is, in fact, absent. See Chapter 7.

18. **The answer is E: 98%.** The positive predictive value is profoundly influenced by the prevalence, even when the operating characteristics of the test remain unchanged. The sensitivity of the new test is 40%, and the specificity is 98%. We have now been told that there are 150 actual cases in the study population. Cell a in a new 2×2 table shows the number of true-positive results, or the sensitivity multiplied by the prevalence. This is 0.40×150, or 60. The total for column 1, the positive cases, must be 150, so cell c is 90. The number of noncases is equal to the total population, or 200, minus the 150 cases, or 50. The number of true-negative cases is equal to the specificity, or 0.98, multiplied by the number of noncases, or 50. This is 49, and this number is placed in cell d. Cells b and d must add to 50, so cell b is 1. The table is as follows:

		TRUE STATUS		
		Positive	Negative	Total
TEST STATUS	Positive	60	1	61
	Negative	90	49	139
	Total	150	50	200

The positive predictive value is $a/(a+b)$, or $60/(60+1)$, which is slightly greater than 98%. See Chapter 7.

19. **The answer is C: 35%.** The negative predictive value, as discussed in the explanation to question 16, above, is $d/(c+d)$. This is $49/(90+49)$, or approximately 35%. The negative predictive value has fallen as the prevalence has risen. The probability that disease is absent given a negative test result declines as the overall probability of disease being absent declines. The extreme example of this would be the use of a very sensitive and specific test in a population in which the condition being studied was universal. Despite the high sensitivity of the test, any negative test result would be false. Cell d in the table would be 0, and the negative predictive value would also be 0. See Chapter 7.

20. **The answer is D: 0.73.** The kappa test ratio is a means of assessing the degree to which agreement in paired data exceeds what would be expected by chance. The formula for kappa is $(A_o - A_c)/(N - A_c)$, where A_o is the observed agreement, A_c is the agreement expected by chance, and N is the total sample. The observed agreement is equal to the sum of cell a, in which both radiologists recommend biopsy, and cell d, in which both recommend no biopsy. The agreement expected by chance is the sum of the expected values in cells a and d, which are derived as they would be for a chi-square value. The expected value in any cell is the row total multiplied by the column total, divided by the

sample total. The expected value for cell a is 40 multiplied by 32, divided by 200, or 6.4. The expected value for cell d is 160 multiplied by 168, divided by 200, or 134.4. When these figures are entered in the kappa formula, the following calculation can be made:

$$\text{kappa} = \frac{(28 + 156) - (6.4 + 134.4)}{200 - (6.4 + 134.4)}$$

$$= \frac{184 - 140.8}{200 - 140.8}$$

$$= \frac{43.2}{59.2}$$

$$= 0.73$$

A kappa ratio between 0.60 and 0.80 (60–80%) is usually considered good agreement, and a kappa ratio greater than 0.80 is considered excellent agreement. See Chapter 7.

21. **The answer is D: 67%.** The easiest approach to the question is to construct a 2×2 table based on an arbitrary sample size. The prevalence is 5%. If the sample size is 1000, then 50 workers will have the disease. The sensitivity of the test is 94%. Of the 50 workers, 94%, or 47, will be detected by the test. This is cell a. Cells a and c must add to the prevalence of 50, so cell c is 3. Of the 1000 workers, 950 are disease-free. Since the test specificity is 90%, the test will correctly identify 90%, or 855, of these workers; this is cell d. Cells b and d must add to 950, so cell b is 95. The table is drawn up as follows:

		DISEASE STATUS		
		Positive	Negative	Total
TEST STATUS	Positive	47	95	142
	Negative	3	855	858
	Total	50	950	1000

The percentage of positive test results (cells a and b) that are false-positive results (cell b) is $b/(a + b)$, or $95/(47 + 95)$. This is approximately 67%. The high percentage of false-positive results obtained despite the fairly good specificity of the test is the result of low prevalence. See Chapter 7.

22. **The answer is B: 33%.** The positive predictive value is $a/(a + b)$. Based on the table shown in the explanation to question 21, above, this is $47/(47 + 95)$, or approximately 33%. Note that the false-positive error rate (the probability that disease is absent when the test result is positive) calculated for question 21 and the positive predictive value (the probability that disease is present when the test result is positive) add to 100%, or 1. See Chapter 7.

23. **The answer is A: 3.** The prevalence of the disease is given as 5% of the population, and we are told that the population is 1000 workers. Therefore, we can expect 5% of 1000, or 50 persons, to have the disease. Of these 50 cases, 94%, or 47 cases, will be detected by our test. This is what sensitivity tells us. Therefore, the positive cases not detected, or the remaining 3 cases, are the false-negative cases. The number of false-negative cases is (1 – sensitivity) multiplied by the prevalence. In this example, that is $[(1 - 94\%) \times 50]$, or $(6\% \times 50)$, which is the 3 cases in cell c of the table. See Chapter 7.

24. **The answer is A: the cost of screening, follow-up, and treatment.** We have already been told that the disease described in the question can be treated. We also know the operating characteristics of our screening test. If the screening test is prohibitively expensive, we cannot implement it successfully. We need to consider the cost of follow-up testing, because 67% of our positive test results will be false-positive results and all of these subjects will need additional testing to demonstrate whether they do not, in fact, have the disease. The cost of treatment for the true-positive cases must not be prohibitive or it will not be possible to provide therapy. The prevalence of other diseases in the population is not critical information, although if other diseases are considered more important and more prevalent, they might be a higher company priority. The disease incidence would be an important consideration in deciding how often to repeat the screening test after the initial round of testing. Once the prevalent cases have been detected, only incident cases remain to be found at subsequent screenings. The size of the population might influence the overall cost of screening, but a greater concern is the cost-effectiveness of the program for the company (i.e., whether the company profits by treating the disease and improving the workforce). If the company profits, the size of the population will not be a limiting factor, and if the company loses money, the program will not be cost-effective in even a small population. Identifying a genetic risk factor is usually important only in an effort to prevent disease or to determine which persons are at increased risk for a disease. This issue is not important in a program of screening for established disease. See Chapter 17.

25. **The answer is D: 97%.** The question is asking for the positive predictive value of the test, or the probability that the condition is present if the test result is positive. The positive predictive value is equal to the true-positive results (cell a) divided by all the positive test results (usually cells a and b, but this table is shown with the

true disease status in rows rather than columns, and the data usually shown in cell *b* of a 2 × 2 table are in the position of cell *c* in this table). The positive predictive value is therefore 253/(253 + 8), or 253/261, which is approximately 97%. See Chapter 7.

26. **The answer is B: 79%.** The question calls for the negative predictive value, or the proportion of all negative test results (24 + 93) that are truly negative (93). In this case, 93/(24 + 93) yields a result of approximately 79%. See Chapter 7.

27. **The answer is D: 91%.** The probability that a test will detect a condition when it is actually present is the sensitivity. This is equal to the true-positive test results (253) divided by the true-positive cases (253 + 24), or 253/277, which is approximately 91%. See Chapter 7.

28. **The answer is C: the prevalence in the population tested may not match her prior probability.** The predictive values, both positive and negative, are dependent on the prevalence. In the case of an individual, the prevalence is not applicable, but the probability of the condition in the individual, or the prior probability, is analogous to the prevalence. Both indicate the probability of the condition before testing and influence the probability after testing. The data in the product brochure are derived from a population in which the prevalence of pregnancy is 277 out of 378 women, or about 73% of the population. If your friend is unlikely to be pregnant, perhaps because of consistent use of effective contraceptives, her prior probability of pregnancy may be much lower than 73%. If this were true, the estimates of positive and negative predictive value calculated above would not be applicable. All data should be assessed on the basis of both internal validity (i.e., correctness) and external validity (i.e., generalizability to people other than the study participants). The data reported in the pregnancy test brochure are most likely correct, but whether or not they pertain to your friend is uncertain. See Chapter 8.

29. **The answer is A: 1%.** A 2 × 2 table could be constructed to answer the question, but the information provided is more amenable to the use of Bayes' theorem. The sensitivity provided is 95%. The prevalence is 1 per 10,000, or 0.0001. The specificity provided is 99%; therefore, the false-positive error rate is 1%, or 0.01. The (1 – prevalence) is 0.9999. The calculation is as follows:

$$p(D+ \mid T+) = \frac{p(T+ \mid D+)p(D+)}{[p(T+ \mid D+)p(D+)] + [p(T+ \mid D-)p(D-)]}$$

$$= \frac{(\text{Sensitivity})(\text{Prevalence})}{[(\text{Sensitivity})(\text{Prevalence})] + [(\text{False-positive error rate})(1 - \text{Prevalence})]}$$

$$= \frac{(0.95)(0.0001)}{[(0.95)(0.0001)] + [(0.01)(0.9999)]}$$

$$= \frac{0.000095}{0.000095 + 0.009999}$$

$$= \frac{0.000095}{0.01}$$

$$= 0.0095, \text{ or approximately } 1\%$$

See Chapter 8.

30. **The answer is C: $1.3 million saved.** The cost per screening test is $10, so screening 100,000 newborn infants will cost $1 million. Given a prevalence of 1 case per 10,000, we can expect 10 cases of disease M in a population of 100,000. Of these 10 cases, 95%, or 9.5, will be detected. There will be 99,990 disease-free infants born, of whom our test will correctly identify 99%, or 98,990.1. The remainder of those without disease, or 999.9 infants, will be false-positive cases. The cost of evaluating each case with a positive test result, of which there are 9.5 true-positive and 999.9 false-positive results, for a total of 1009.4, is $100. The total evaluation costs, therefore, are $100,940. For each of the 9.5 true-positive test results, $250,000 will be saved, for a total savings of (9.5 × $250,000), or $2,375,000. Subtracting the cost of screening ($1 million) and the cost of evaluating ($100,940) from the gross savings yields the following: 2,375,000 – (1,000,000 + 100,940) = 1,274,060, or nearly $1.3 million in net savings. See Chapters 7 and 17.

31. **The answer is C: 8.7%.** This question is essentially the same as question 29, except that the prevalence of disease is different. When the formula for Bayes' theorem is used and the new prevalence of 0.001 is entered, the calculations are as follows:

$$p(D+ \mid T+) = \frac{p(T+ \mid D+)p(D+)}{[p(T+ \mid D+)p(D+)] + [p(T+ \mid D-)p(D-)]}$$

$$= \frac{(\text{Sensitivity})(\text{Prevalence})}{[(\text{Sensitivity})(\text{Prevalence})] + [(\text{False-positive error rate})(1 - \text{Prevalence})]}$$

$$= \frac{(0.95)(0.001)}{[(0.95)(0.001)] + [(0.01)(0.999)]}$$

$$= \frac{0.00095}{0.00095 + 0.00999}$$

$$= \frac{0.00095}{0.01094}$$

$$= 0.0868, \text{ or approximately } 8.7\%$$

See Chapter 8.

32. **The answer is E: 104.4.** Variance, a measure of dispersion in a data set, is the sum of the squared differences of each data point from the mean, divided by the sample size minus 1:

$$\text{Variance} = s^2 = \frac{\sum(x_i - \bar{x})^2}{N - 1}$$

The data set in the question consists of 10 values (i.e., 70, 68, 84, 76, 88, 66, 56, 60, 80, and 70 beats per minute). The mean for the data set is derived by adding the 10 values and dividing the sum by 10. The mean is therefore 71.8. The mean is then subtracted from each entry, and the difference is squared. The first entry is 70. Subtracting the mean of 71.8 from 70 yields 1.8. This number squared is 3.24. This calculation is repeated for each entry, and the 10 values obtained are summed, yielding 939.6. This number is divided by the sample size minus 1, which represents the degrees of freedom associated with the data set. This yields 939.6/9, or 104.4. This is the variance. See Chapter 9.

33. **The answer is B: 10.2.** The standard deviation is the square root of the variance. The variance for this data set was calculated for question 32, above, as 104.4. The square root of 104.4 is 10.2. See Chapter 9.

34. **The answer is D: prospective cohort study.** The groups of subjects are assembled on the basis of exposure. One group has been exposed to the king's delicacies, and the other has been exposed to vegetables. The groups, or cohorts, are followed over 10 days for the outcome, a change in countenance. This is a prospective cohort study. See Chapter 5.

35. **The answer is E: use of controls.** Two groups are followed over time. One group receives the active intervention (vegetables), while the other group, the control group, receives the placebo (the king's delicacies). The "investigator" might simply have followed a group eating vegetables for 10 days and reported some improvement in countenance, but the inclusion of a control group improves this study considerably (which is not to say it would be likely to be funded by the National Institutes of Health). The study is not blinded or randomized, and we have not been given any evidence that the cohorts are matched. See Chapter 5.

36. **The answer is D: recall bias.** Recall bias is introduced in retrospective studies, usually case-control studies, when one group is more likely than another group to remember a previous exposure to a disease. Recall bias is virtually never a factor in a prospective study. Selection bias is a likely source of error in this study. We know little, for example, about how subjects were chosen to participate and nothing about the appearance of their countenances at baseline. Measuring the quality of a countenance is a rather unscientific endeavor and likely to be performed differently each time, introducing measurement error. Observer bias would be introduced if the investigator assessed countenances differently for the two groups, a likely possibility. Factors other than diet may differ between the two groups, and the difference in outcome may be the result of one of these unstudied influences. If these unstudied influences were associated with both exposure and outcome, they would be confounders. See Chapter 4.

37. **The answer is A: data that are not statistically significant may nonetheless be clinically important.** When statistical significance is not achieved, the implication is that there is more than a 5% probability (if alpha is set at 0.05) that the outcome difference is due to chance. However, a *p* value of 0.08 still indicates a 92% probability that the outcome difference is not due to chance. In other words, failure to reject the null hypothesis does not mean that the null hypothesis is true. If a therapy is desperately needed and looks promising on the basis of trials that fail to show statistical significance, there are circumstances under which judicious use of the therapy would be appropriate. Certainly, with large samples, statistical significance may be achieved for outcomes that are not important clinically. Setting alpha high or setting beta low increases the probability of achieving statistical significance instead of decreasing it. See Chapter 10.

38. **The answer is D: pool the data.** The two studies show similar results, one with and one without statistical significance. If the studies are sufficiently similar, a quantitative meta-

analysis would be appropriate. Pooling data effectively increases the sample size, providing greater power to detect a significant outcome difference. An alternative would be to recruit more subjects, but this approach is obviously more expensive. The studies were perhaps both somewhat underfunded in the first place, resulting in restriction of sample size to the bare minimum. When sample sizes are small, power is reduced, and type II (false-negative) error increases. See Chapter 8.

39. **The answer is C: (1 − sensitivity).** In a 2×2 table, sensitivity is $a/(a + c)$. Sensitivity is the ability of a test to show a positive result when a condition is truly present. False-negative results occur when the test gives a negative result even though the condition is actually present. This is (1 − sensitivity), or $c/(a + c)$. See Chapter 7.

40. **The answer is D: (1 − specificity).** In a 2×2 table, specificity is $d/(b + d)$, or the number of true-negative test results. Specificity is the ability of a test to exclude a disease when it is truly absent. Test results for those who do not have a disease can be either negative (i.e., true-negative results) or positive (i.e., false-positive results). The (1 − specificity) is the number of negative cases remaining after the true-negative cases have been subtracted (i.e., the false-positive results). This is shown algebraically as $1 - [d/(b + d)] = b/(b + d)$. This is the false-positive error rate. See Chapter 7.

41. **The answer is B: $d/(c + d)$.** The negative predictive value is the probability of the absence of disease in a patient with a negative test result. This is the proportion of all patients with negative test results $(c + d)$ who truly do not have the disease (cell d), or $d/(c + d)$. See Chapter 7.

42. **The answer is A: $a/(a + b)$.** The positive predictive value is the probability of disease in a patient with a positive test result. This is the proportion of all patients with positive test results $(a + b)$ who truly have the condition (cell a), or $a/(a + b)$. See Chapter 7.

43. **The answer is E: appropriateness of medical care.** Care is appropriate when the right thing is done in the right way by the right person for the right reason. These are criteria for professional competency and comprehensiveness. Appropriateness is therefore defined by professional standards of care. See Chapter 21.

44. **The answer is C: accountability of medical care.** Accountability of care is the disclosure of standards of care to the public and an acceptance of responsibility by providers for the judgment of the public. See Chapter 21.

45. **The answer is B: accessibility of medical care.** Medical care may be available but not accessible if patients lack transportation to the site where care is given or lack the means to pay for care. Care is accessible when financial and geographic barriers are negligible. See Chapter 21.

46. **The answer is A: acceptability of medical care.** Care may be accessible and available but will not be utilized if it is unacceptable to patients. Acceptability requires that patients and providers can communicate in the same language, that care is delivered with compassion, and that cultural beliefs and practices of patients are respected. If the quantity of available care is commensurate with need but the care is unacceptable to patients in the community, the care provided cannot be considered adequate. See Chapter 21.

47. **The answer is F: assessability of medical care.** In contrast to accountability, assessability is contingent on professional scrutiny, rather than public scrutiny. The quality of medical care is assessable when it is open to review by impartial professionals. The care is accountable when the results of such a review are disclosed to the public. See Chapter 21.

48. **The answer is G: availability of medical care.** The provision of care does not necessarily make it available to the community. For people who cannot take time off from work to see a physician, care is available only if it is provided in the mornings or evenings or on weekends. The provision of care during the times it can be utilized by those in need of it is availability. See Chapter 21.

49. **The answer is D: adequacy of medical care.** Care is adequate in supply when it meets demand. In health care, need and demand differ. Demand is patient-generated, while need is a professional assessment of the requirement for health care services. Care may be adequate when it is less than the demand for it, provided that the need is met. See Chapter 21.

50. **The answer is C: prospective cohort study.** In a prospective cohort study, the cohort is assembled on the basis of risk factors or exposures defined and measured at the beginning of the study. Because these characteristics define the cohort, only these characteristics can be assessed. However, observed outcomes in the cohort can be assessed even if they were not the outcomes anticipated. The occurrence of an unanticipated outcome should serve as the basis for a new hypothesis. This hypothesis must be tested in another study. See Chapter 5.

51. **The answer is A: case-control study.** In a

case-control study, cases are the subjects who have the outcome of interest (e.g., a particular disease), and controls are those who do not have this outcome. Because the study groups are defined at entry on the basis of outcome, only this one outcome can be assessed. However, both groups can be evaluated for any number of past exposures or risk factors. See Chapter 5.

52. **The answer is A:**

$$N = \frac{(z_\alpha)^2 \cdot (s)^2}{(\bar{d})^2}$$

The smaller the alpha (and, therefore, the larger the z_α), the larger the sample size must be. The larger the variance, the larger the sample size must be. That is why z_α and s appear in the numerator of the sample size formula. The larger the difference the investigator is seeking, the easier it is to detect the difference and the smaller the necessary sample size will be. The difference sought is in the denominator. When only one group of subjects is required, the sample size calculation provides the total for the study. When one group is to be compared with another, the size of each group is doubled because of the introduction of more variance, and the total is doubled again to allow for two groups. These formulas are shown as options B and C, respectively. Options D and E are statistical gibberish. See Chapter 12.

53. **The answer is E: stipulate prospective payment to hospitals.** Diagnosis related groups (DRGs) represent categories of diagnosis for which a standard hospital stay and resultant cost of care are anticipated. Hospitals are paid by insurers such as Medicare on the basis of the diagnostic group, rather than the actual care delivered. Efficient care results in a profit for the hospital. Complications that cause hospital costs to exceed the DRG reimbursement will result in a financial loss for the hospital. See Chapter 21.

54. **The answer is C: factors that influence the occurrence and distribution of disease in human populations.** Epidemiology (from the Greek *epi*, meaning upon, and *dēmos*, meaning population) is the study of all factors influencing patterns of human health and disease. Epidemiology is not restricted to outbreaks. It also is the study of endemic, or prevailing, patterns of disease in populations. The science of epidemiology addresses many types of human health problems and is not restricted to infectious agents or environmental toxins. While causality is one area studied in epidemiology, it is not the sole focus of this science. See Chapter 1.

55. **The answer is E: vector.** A vector, which is usually an arthropod insect, facilitates contact between the pathogen of a human disease and the host. The vector is usually not affected by the pathogen. The vector does not serve as an animal reservoir, because the pathogen must have another definitive host in order to complete its life cycle. See Chapter 1.

56. **The answer is C: there are 5 times as many cases as would be expected.** To determine the number of preventable cases of a given disease in the US population, investigators would begin by identifying the population that has the lowest observed incidence rate of the disease. This rate becomes the standard. The actual rate in the USA is then compared with this standard, and the number of excess incident cases of the disease is noted. Since there are numerous types of cancer, this process would be followed for each type of cancer. Use of this method suggests that there are 5 times as many cancers in the USA as there would be if the lowest observed rates for each type of cancer could be achieved. See Chapter 1.

57. **The answer is E: warm water systems such as air-conditioning cooling towers.** The original outbreak of legionnaires' disease in 1976 was ultimately traced to the air-conditioning and ventilation systems of the hotel that was hosting a conference for legionnaires. The causative organism, *Legionella pneumophila*, thrives in warm water. Respiratory therapy equipment is a potential means of spreading this organism and must be thoroughly sterilized after it is used. See Chapter 1.

58. **The answer is B: are associated with the lower mortality rates but may not be causal factors.** Mormons and Seventh-Day Adventists are relatively strict about avoiding a number of potentially harmful substances and also about eating a diet that is rich in vegetables, fruits, and grains and low in processed foods and fat. These factors are thought to contribute to the exceptionally good health and low mortality rates of these groups. However, these lifestyle practices are only part of a larger context in which the family, work, and social environment often differs from that found in other populations in the USA. Other factors may therefore also contribute to the differences in age-adjusted death rates (Berkman and Breslow 1983). Health outcomes are usually multifactorial, and establishing direct causality is often difficult. See Chapter 1.

59. **The answer is A: frequent exposure resulted in boosted immunity following immunization.** Levels of protective antibody that develop following immunization often drop as time passes.

The levels eventually fall below the threshold required to prevent symptomatic infection, and susceptibility to the disease redevelops. This is true of diphtheria now that the disease is uncommon. In the past, frequent exposure to *Corynebacterium diphtheriae* resulted in periodic boosting of the antibody levels following the original immunization, so that protective immunity was preserved. The more effectively immunization programs prevent exposure to historically important pathogens, the greater is the potential susceptibility to these pathogens as time passes. The administration of periodic booster vaccines is recommended under such circumstances. The difficulty of immunizing a large population is compounded when immunization must be repeated over a period of time. See Chapter 1.

60. **The answer is E: the difference between the birth rate and the death rate of a society.** The demographic gap is the difference between the birth rate and the overall rate of death in a population and is used to specify the rate of population growth. See Chapter 1.

61. **The answer is C: schistosomiasis.** Schistosomes require snails to serve as hosts during a portion of their life cycle, and snails must have standing water in which to reproduce. Epidemiologists had predicted that the incidence of schistosomiasis would rise when the Aswan High Dam was constructed, and their prediction was fulfilled. Whenever ecologic systems are modified, changes in the pattern of human diseases are possible. See Chapter 1.

62. **The answer is C: valuable for detecting changes in the pattern of a disease.** Underreporting of common and mild diseases is substantial. Therefore, the number of cases of chickenpox that is reported represents only a portion of the total number of cases of this disease. If the proportion of patients who seek medical care is fairly constant and the proportion of cases that are reported is fairly constant, then a sudden change in the number of cases reported, even if this number is inaccurate, should reliably reflect an actual change in the pattern of disease. See Chapter 2.

63. **The answer is C: denominator data for population-based studies.** The US census, conducted every 10 years in years ending in 0, provides the best available estimate of the total US population and the populations of various subgroups. These data are used as the denominators in population-based epidemiologic studies. While rates based on census data may provide the basis for direct or indirect standardization, they do not derive directly from the census data. Similarly, census data may be put to use in studies of various time trends, but the data do not reveal these trends directly. See Chapter 2.

64. **The answer is B: 15–20%.** In death certificate diagnoses, inaccuracies may arise because of uncertainty about the immediate versus underlying cause of death, lack of familiarity with the deceased, or some combination of these, along with sleep deprivation of the reporting physician, who is often a house officer (Moriyama 1966). See Chapter 2.

65. **The answer is D: an acceptable risk estimate, even though the best denominator would include only subjects without protective immunity to influenza.** Risk is defined as the proportion of subjects who are unaffected at the beginning of the study period and undergo the risk event during the study period. The denominator should include only subjects at risk for the study event at the beginning of the study. In the case of an infectious disease, the at-risk subjects are those who lack protective immunity. However, since the immune status is generally not known, the population is often used as the denominator. See Chapter 2.

66. **The answer is D: better demonstrate the force of mortality.** The risk for a given event, such as death, will be reported as the same whether the deaths occur evenly throughout the study period or whether they occur all at the beginning or all at the end of the study period. The rate will vary with these changes and will be highest for the clustering of events at the beginning of the study period. When the event is death, the rate reveals the force of mortality on a population by rising when most of the deaths occur early. The denominator for a rate is the midperiod population. Rates are usually higher than risks, but not significantly higher. They may be virtually the same, depending on the distribution of events over the study period and on the proportion of subjects in the population considered to be at risk for the event. See Chapter 2.

67. **The answer is A: lung cancer in men in the USA.** For a rate to be valid, its numerator must represent events occurring in subjects from the denominator, and its denominator must represent those at risk for the numerator. In all of the choices except A, the denominators contain subjects not at risk for the event in the numerator. Poliomyelitis in elementary school children is not valid, because most children in US schools have been immunized and are therefore not susceptible to poliovirus. Prostatitis in adults over 65 years of age is not valid, because only men in this group are at risk. Rubella in pregnant women is not valid, because only the unimmunized are at risk. Uterine cancer in the US population is not valid, because the US pop-

ulation includes men, who are not at risk. Lung cancer in men is valid, as all men are potentially at risk for this disease. See Chapter 2.

68. **The answer is B: the incidence density.** The incidence density is the frequency of new events per person-time. The denominator is the cumulative time contributed by subjects under observation, rather than the number of subjects. Consequently, this measure is useful for characterizing the pattern of events that may recur in individuals. See Chapter 2.

69. **The answer is A: correct, because current prevalence exceeds the historical baseline.** By definition, an epidemic is the occurrence of any adverse health event within a population at a rate that exceeds either precedent or expectation. The current prevalence of obesity is greater than the historical precedent, and it defies the expectations of many in the weight control and nutrition fields, although it is not truly surprising given the life-style and dietary practices in the USA (Kuczmarski et al. 1994; Stamler 1993). Obesity has a complex etiology and is partly the result of genetic factors (Bennett 1995; Lindpainter 1995). Approximately one in three adults in the US population is considered obese, but it takes more than simple frequency to define an epidemic. For example, although most individuals suffer an occasional headache, headaches are not an epidemic; headaches are an endemic state, occurring at a predictably high frequency. If the high prevalence of obesity persists over time, obesity too may come to be recognized as an endemic state, with its current rise in prevalence recognized as a secular trend, rather than an epidemic. See Chapter 3.

70. **The answer is E: to interpret the data, the information must be expressed as rates.** The number of deaths associated with cigarette smoking at different levels (defined in terms of packs per day) cannot readily be interpreted, unless some information is provided about who in the population is smoking. Specifically, if a very large percentage of the population were smoking more than a pack of cigarettes per day, one would expect a comparably large percentage of all deaths in this group. If the older cohorts in the population were smoking more heavily than the younger cohorts, one would expect a higher percentage of deaths among the smokers because of the influence of age on mortality. The raw data in the question imply that smoking increases mortality, but they cannot be interpreted to demonstrate this. Conversion of the data to rates would facilitate interpretation. Of course, smoking does contribute to overall mortality rates, but this cannot be known from the information provided in the question. See Chapter 2.

71. **The answer is E: an effect modifier.** An effect modifier is a third variable that alters the relationship between an independent variable and a dependent (outcome) variable. For effect modification to occur, a true relationship must exist between the independent and dependent variables. In this case, vigorous exercise is the independent variable, myocardial infarction is the dependent variable, and physical fitness is the effect modifier. The effect modifier neither explains nor obscures the relationship between the causal factor of interest and the outcome; instead, it alters the relationship so that under differing conditions of the effect modifier, the relationship between independent and dependent variables changes in magnitude or, as in this case, changes in direction. See Chapter 4.

72. **The answer is C: intervening variables.** Obesity, particularly abdominal obesity, represents a risk for cardiovascular disease (Pi-Sunyer 1991). When obesity precedes cardiovascular disease, however, it is often (although not always) associated with hyperlipidemia and hyperglycemia, as well as hypertension. There is less evidence that obesity contributes to the incidence of heart disease when these other conditions do not develop. Therefore, obesity may increase the risk of cardiovascular disease only when it results in the development of other risk factors that intervene. Heart disease can develop in the absence of either hyperlipidemia or hyperglycemia, so neither is a necessary cause of heart disease. See Chapter 4.

73. **The answer is D: recall bias.** Once an adverse outcome has occurred, events in the past that may have contributed to it take on greater significance. These same events, when the adverse outcome does not occur, may be easily forgotten. The tendency to recall events preferentially when they are related to an adverse outcome is recall bias. See Chapter 4.

74. **The answer is C: necessary cause.** Asbestosis, a disease in which asbestos fibers in the lung disrupt the pulmonary architecture and impair respiratory capacity, can occur only with exposure to asbestos fibers. However, many individuals exposed to these fibers do not develop asbestosis. Therefore, asbestos is a necessary cause, but not a sufficient cause, of asbestosis. See Chapter 4.

75. **The answer is C: a repeated cross-sectional study.** The National Health and Nutrition Examination Surveys (NHANES) are cross-sectional surveys conducted at regular intervals to establish secular trends in health-related behaviors. See Chapter 5.

76. **The answer is D: subjects with prior radiation**

exposure followed for the development of lymphoproliferative cancers. A retrospective cohort study is performed when an exposure or risk factor is established at some time in the past, before the outcome in question has occurred. Subjects are then interviewed or assessed through chart review to identify cases of the outcome that occurred after the exposure or risk factor was recorded. If a radiation exposure occurred in the distant past and the subjects were followed for lymphoproliferative disease into the more recent past, this would be a retrospective cohort study. If the exposure were current and subjects were followed forward in time, as in option C (subjects with current angina followed for the development of myocardial infarction), the study would be a prospective cohort design. Retrospective cohort studies are usually cheaper and are certainly quicker to perform than are comparable prospective studies. Option A (cases of lung cancer assessed for prior exposures) and option E (subjects with skin cancer assessed for lifelong, cumulative sun exposure) are amenable to case-control studies. Option B (subjects randomly assigned to active varicella vaccine versus placebo, followed for chickenpox) is a randomized field trial. See Chapter 5.

77. **The answer is D: prevention of confounding by known and unknown factors.** The goal in an intervention trial is to compare two groups that differ only with regard to the intervention of interest. In animal research, this is achieved by using genetically homogeneous populations that are, for all relevant intents and purposes, identical. Clearly, human populations cannot be manipulated in this way. The only opportunity to study genetically identical humans is afforded by studies of monozygotic twins. Randomization is performed so that all of the factors contributing to human variability are equally likely to appear in the control group and the intervention group. When successful, this method results in groups that differ significantly only in terms of the intervention, although this is not ensured. Randomization, therefore, minimizes both known and unknown confounders. A study that successfully tests its principal hypothesis in an unbiased manner is internally valid; randomized, prospective, double-blind trials often meet this condition. However, measurement error is always possible. Therefore, the study design described does not ensure internal validity. Randomization ensures unbiased distribution of participants to control and intervention groups but does not ensure that the study population represents the general population, although there are methods to achieve this as well. The results of the Physicians' Health Study, whose subjects were restricted to male physicians in good health, may not be generalizable to other groups and there-

fore may not be externally valid. Although a large sample size increases the likelihood of detecting a statistically significant difference in the outcome measure, this is never ensured, particularly if no such difference exists. See Chapter 5.

78. **The answer is B: disease status.** In a cohort study, the group to be followed is assembled on the basis of inclusion and exclusion criteria; an age range is usually included among such criteria. These factors define the cohort. The exposure in question should be included among the eligibility criteria. Similar groups that differ with regard to the exposure in question should be assembled. The comparison to be made, however, is the rate at which a particular disease (or other outcome) occurs in those with and those without the exposure of interest. Therefore, disease status is the important comparison to be made at the conclusion of any cohort study. In contrast, in a case-control study, disease status is known at entry, and the exposure status of cases versus controls is compared. See Chapter 6.

79. **The answer is C: 5.6 per 1000.** The crude death rate is calculated by adding all of the deaths that occur in the studied population during the period of observation and then dividing by the midyear population. In population A, the total number of deaths is $120 + 45 + 13 = 178$. The total population is 32,000. The rate is therefore equal to 178/32,000, or 5.6/1000. The population figures provided are assumed to be the midperiod populations. See Chapter 2.

80. **The answer is A: all deaths occurred during the period of interest.** The crude death rate is equal to the total deaths in the study population during the period of observation, divided by the midperiod population. To derive the crude death rate from the data provided, one assumes that all deaths occurred during the observation period and that the population figures represent the midperiod population. The force of mortality, or the temporal distribution of deaths during the observation period, does not influence the crude death rate. Crude mortality rates are independent of the causes of death. See Chapter 2.

81. **The answer is C: 5.6 per 1000.** The crude death rates are the same for populations A and B. They are calculated in the same way, as described in the explanation for question 79, above. By convention, crude death rates are multiplied by a constant, in this case 1000, so that the rates are easier to manipulate and discuss. See Chapter 2.

82. **The answer is E: the size of the population and the total number of deaths.** The total number of

deaths, divided by the midperiod population, is the crude death rate. As these two terms define the rate, nothing else influences it directly. Causes of death may affect the force of mortality, with some causes producing rapid deaths and others producing slower deaths. Seasonal variation in mortality would also influence the force of mortality. Diagnostic consistency is necessary only to ensure that comparable numerators are compared when the cause of death is being considered. Disease surveillance and reporting do not affect the death rate, as few deaths are unregistered. The age distribution of a population will affect the crude death rate by influencing the total number of deaths that occur during a specified period. See Chapter 2.

83. **The answer is A: 3%.** The age-specific death rate (ASDR) is equal to the number of deaths in a particular age group, divided by the population in that age group. For subjects over 65 years of age in population A, the ASDR is 120 divided by 4000, which is 0.03, or 3%. See Chapter 2.

84. **The answer is A: the age distributions are different.** Crude death rates will be high in an elderly population, even if health care is excellent and longevity great. Crude death rates will usually be low in young populations, even if health care is poor and life expectancy limited. To make valid comparisons, the rates must be manipulated to answer this question: What would mortality rates be in these two populations if they had the same age distribution? See Chapter 2.

85. **The answer is A: a population of nursing home residents.** Whenever possible, direct standardization is used to compare the mortality rates of different populations; as discussed in the text, indirect standardization can be used when ASDRs are not known for one or more of the populations to be compared. In direct standardization, ASDRs must be calculated or provided for the populations being considered. Then a hypothetical age distribution is established, usually by finding the sum of the numbers in each age group of the study populations. The ASDRs are then applied to the new age distribution, generating an expected number of to-

tal deaths in that population. This is then divided by the total in the standard population (e.g., the total sum of the study populations). The resultant standardized mortality rates allow one to compare the populations as if they had the same age distribution. Any reference population with an adequate age distribution might be used. A population of nursing home residents would be unacceptable, because the entire population would be clustered in a narrow age range, and this would not permit calculation of standardized mortality rates for the younger groups in the study populations. See Chapter 2.

86. **The answer is D: 9.64 per 1000.** A table like the one shown below must be devised to make the calculations for questions 86–88. Each ASDR in this table was calculated by dividing the number of deaths in a particular age group by the population of that age group, as described in the explanation for question 83. A standard age distribution was created by obtaining the sum of populations A and B in each of the three age groups, as described in the explanation for question 85. The ASDRs were then applied to the standard population to generate the numbers of deaths that would be expected in each age group if populations A and B had the same age distribution. For population A, the expected numbers of deaths in the three age groups were added to produce the total number of expected deaths; this figure was then divided by the total standard population to produce the standardized mortality ratio for population A. For population B, the same procedure was followed. By convention, the results were converted to a number with one digit to the left of the decimal point by use of a constant multiplier. See Chapter 2.

87. **The answer is C: 4.06 per 1000.** Please refer to the explanation for question 86; the same discussion pertains in this case. Calculations are shown in the accompanying table.

88. **The answer is B: population B has lower age-specific death rates (ASDRs).** Because of different population ages, the crude mortality rates for two populations might be the same,

Age Group (Years)	Population A			Population B		
	Population Size	Age-Specific Death Rate	Expected Number of Deaths	Population Size	Age-Specific Death Rate	Expected Number of Deaths
<30	17,000	× 0.001	17	17,000	× 0.00075	12.75
30–65	30,000	× 0.003	90	30,000	× 0.002	60
>65	17,000	× 0.03	510	17,000	× 0.011	187
Total	64,000		617	64,000		259.75
Standardized Death Rate	617/64,000 = 9.64 per 1000			259.75/64,000 = 4.06 per 1000		

even when the ASDRs differ. The determinants of standardized rates are the ASDRs and the age distribution. In the example provided, populations A and B have the same crude death rate, 5.06 per 1000; this does not explain why the standardized rates differ. We know nothing about the timing of death in either population during the observation period. The size of the population does not influence the mortality rate, except that in a very small population, the rates might be unstable estimates because of random variation. The reason population B has less than half the standardized mortality rate of population A is that population B has lower ASDRs. If population B had the same age distribution as population A, the death rate would be much lower in population B; this is what the standardized rate tells us. See Chapter 2.

89. The answer is B: 3.4 per 10,000 population. Calculation of the population attributable risk (PAR) will tell us how much of the total risk for death caused by a cerebrovascular accident is due to hypertension. The PAR is calculated by subtracting the risk in the unexposed group from the risk in the total population. The question does not provide the risk in the unexposed group. To determine this, we must first calculate the risk in the total population and then in the exposed group. The total population risk for death due to a cerebrovascular accident is 150,000 per 265 million = 5.7 per 10,000. This represents the total population cause-specific death rate for cerebrovascular disease. We are told that the risk for death due to a cerebrovascular accident is 3.5 times as high in hypertensive individuals as it is in the general population, so the death rate in the exposed group is (3.5×5.7) per 10,000 = 20 per 10,000. Given 50 million individuals in the exposed group, a cerebrovascular accident death rate of 20 per 10,000 yields 100,000 deaths among the exposed. Subtracting deaths among the exposed from total deaths yields 50,000 deaths among the unexposed. The unexposed population is the 265 million US residents minus the 50 million in the exposed group, or 215 million. The PAR can now be calculated as follows:

$$PAR = Risk_{(total)} - Risk_{(unexposed)}$$

$$= (150,000/265 \text{ million}) -$$
$$(50,000/215 \text{ million})$$

$$= (5.7/10,000) - (2.3/10,000)$$

$$= 3.4/10,000$$

Out of every 5.7 deaths caused by a cerebrovascular accident in the general population, 3.4 may be attributed to hypertension. See Chapter 6.

90. The answer is D: 59.6%. Calculation of the population attributable risk percent (PAR%) will tell us what percentage of the total risk for cerebrovascular accident mortality is due to hypertension:

$$PAR\% = \frac{Risk_{(total)} - Risk_{(unexposed)}}{Risk_{(total)}} \times 100$$

$$= \frac{(5.7/10,000) - (2.3/10,000)}{(5.7/10,000)} \times 100$$

Because the total risk minus the risk in the unexposed is the same as the risk in the exposed, a more direct approach to the same calculation is as follows:

$$PAR\% = \frac{Risk_{(exposed)}}{Risk_{(total)}} \times 100$$

Either way, the calculation becomes:

$$PAR\% = \frac{3.4/10,000}{5.7/10,000} \times 100 = 0.596 \times 100 = 59.6\%$$

The answer, 59.6%, is the percentage of deaths from cerebrovascular disease in the general population that is attributable to hypertension.

Alternatively, the PAR% can be calculated using the following formula:

$$PAR\% = \frac{(Pe)(RR - 1)}{1 + (Pe)(RR - 1)} \times 100$$

where Pe is the proportion of the population with the exposure and RR is the risk ratio (relative risk). Here, Pe is 50 million per 265 million = 0.19. RR is the risk of death caused by a cerebrovascular accident in those with hypertension (20 per 10,000) divided by the risk in those without hypertension (2.3 per 10,000) = 8.7. The formula therefore becomes:

$$PAR\% = \frac{(0.19)(8.7 - 1)}{1 + (0.19)(8.7 - 1)} \times 100$$

$$= \frac{1.463}{2.463} \times 100 = 59.4\%$$

The slight discrepancy in answers (59.6% versus 59.4%) is due to the error introduced by rounding to the nearest decimal. See Chapter 6.

91. The answer is C: 17.7 per 10,000. Calculation of the attributable risk (AR) will tell us how much of the risk for cerebrovascular accident mortality is attributable to hypertension:

$$AR = Risk_{(exposed)} - Risk_{(unexposed)}$$

$$= (20/10,000) - (2.3/10,000)$$

$$= 17.7/10,000$$

See Chapter 6.

92. The answer is D: it is best expressed as 21

person-years. Person-time methods are useful in survival analyses, when the observation period varies from subject to subject. By adding each participant's experience to the total, regardless of outcome, the interpretable observation period is maximized. The total observation period need not be measured in years, but it generally is measured in years whenever this provides whole numbers. In the study described in the question, 10 subjects are under observation for 6 months, so they contribute 60 months, or 5 years, of observation. The 30 subjects who are observed for 4 months contribute 120 months, or 10 years, of observation. The remaining 2 subjects contribute 3 years each, or 6 years. The total is therefore 21 person-years. Subjects who are lost to follow-up contribute the time they were observed prior to leaving the study. See Chapter 11.

93. The answer is B: it is approximately 1.1 deaths per person-year of observation. As explained in the answer to question 92, the observation period in this study is best expressed as 21 person-years. A total of 23 deaths occurred during the observation period. The death rate for the study is simply total deaths divided by the units of observation, or 23 deaths per 21 person-years, which is approximately 1.1 deaths per person-year of observation. See Chapter 11.

94. The answer is D: $1/10^5$. Each branch of the decision tree represents the outcomes associated with a particular decision. If you decide to treat your patient immediately, the probability of treatment is 1 (100%). The risk of rheumatic fever in patients treated immediately is given as $1/10^5$; $1/10^5$ multiplied by 1 is $1/10^5$, the correct answer. See Chapter 8.

95. The answer is B: 0.008. The probability of not treating is 100%, or 1, once the decision not to treat is made. The risk of rheumatic fever in the patients for whom neither a culture is obtained nor treatment is given is 0.008. The answer is 0.008×1, or 0.008. See Chapter 8.

96. The answer is A: 0.001. To answer the question, you need only follow the branch of the decision tree that corresponds to the management of this patient and find the associated risk. The risk of rheumatic fever in patients treated on the basis of a positive culture is given as 0.001, or 1 per thousand; this is the correct answer. While the probability of a positive culture in patients who are cultured is only 1 in 4 (0.25) and the probability of treatment in patients with a positive culture is only 0.95, these numbers are not needed to answer the question, because we have been told that the patient's culture was positive and that the patient was then treated.

Therefore, in this scenario, the probability of a positive culture is 1, and the probability of treatment is 1. The answer, then, may be thought of as the probability of a positive culture multiplied by the probability of treatment multiplied by the risk of rheumatic fever in a patient given treatment after a positive culture, or $1 \times 1 \times 0.001$, which is 0.001. See Chapter 8.

97. The answer is B: $1/10^4$. As in question 96, the scenario described represents the end of a decision tree branch. Therefore, the risk is provided in the tree and does not require calculation. Start with the branch for obtaining a throat culture and waiting for the results. Follow it to the branch for positive cultures. Follow this to the branch for treatment. The risk of rheumatic fever in this group, 0.001, was the answer to question 96. The risk of antimicrobial resistance is provided as $1/10^4$, and this is the answer here. See Chapter 8.

98. The answer is D: $3.6/10^4$. The risk in all patients for whom a culture was ordered includes those with positive cultures (whether treated or not) and those with negative cultures (whether treated or not).

In the group of patients for whom a culture was ordered, the probability of the culture being positive is 0.25. In the group with positive cultures, the probability of being treated is 0.95. The risk of rheumatic fever associated with positive culture and treatment is 0.001. Therefore, of the patients for whom a culture was ordered, those who are treated on the basis of a positive culture contribute a risk of $(0.25 \times 0.95 \times 0.001)$, or $2.375/10^4$, to the overall risk in this group. Similarly, those who are not treated after a positive culture is obtained contribute a risk of $(0.25 \times 0.05 \times 0.01)$, or $1.25/10^4$, to the overall risk.

In the group of patients for whom a culture was ordered, the probability of the culture being negative is 0.75. In the group with negative cultures, the treated patients contribute $(0.75 \times 0.10 \times 0)$, or 0, to the overall risk; and the untreated patients contribute $[0.75 \times 0.90 \times (1/10^7)]$, or $6.75/10^8$, to the overall risk.

The risk of rheumatic fever in all cultured patients is the sum of these: $2.375/10^4 + 1.25/10^4 + 0 + 6.75/10^8 = 0.0003626$, or approximately $3.6/10^4$.

In actual practice, you would consider other characteristics in each patient when estimating the risk of rheumatic fever, and then you would follow the branches of the decision tree that would lead to the lowest risk of an adverse outcome for that individual. For example, the risk of treatment might be high in a patient with multiple antibiotic allergies, and this would indicate either that no treatment should be given or that it would be wise to obtain a culture and wait. In a patient known to have recurrent positive cultures for "strep throat" and a history of rheumatic fever, immediate treatment would be prudent. A decision, like a hammer, is a tool. A decision tree is neither necessary nor sufficient for building the foundation of a good decision, but like any appropriate tool used well, it helps improve the construction process and the product. See Chapter 8.

99. **The answer is B: 6.25.** In the scenario, the mortality rate is 22% in untreated patients and 6% in treated patients. The number needed to treat (NNT) is defined as the number of patients who would need to be treated, on average, in order for one of them to experience the benefit of treatment. The NNT is calculated as 1 divided by the absolute risk reduction (ARR). The ARR in this case is 22% minus 6%, or 16%. Dividing 1 by 0.16 yields 6.25. See Chapter 6.

100. **The answer is C: 25.** In the scenario, the rate of serious complications is 1% in untreated patients and 5% in treated patients. The number needed to harm (NNH) is defined as the number of patients who would need to be treated, on average, in order for one of them to experience the adverse effects of treatment. The NNH is calculated as 1 divided by the absolute risk increase (ARI). The ARI in this case is 5% minus 1%, or 4%. Dividing 1 by 0.04 yields 25. See Chapter 6.

101. **The answer is C: 4 patients benefited for each patient harmed.** If the NNH is greater than the NNT, more patients must be treated to cause harm to one than to provide benefit to one, so there is (at least numerically) net benefit. Conversely, if the NNH is less than the NNT, there is net harm. In this case, since 6.25 patients need to be treated for one to benefit and since 25 need to be treated for one to be harmed, then 4 patients (or 25 divided by 6.25) will benefit for each patient who is harmed. In the calculation of this ratio, the fact that the clinical impact of the benefit provided may be quantitatively different from the clinical impact of the harm done is not taken into account. See Chapter 6.

102. **The answer is D: randomization.** The process of randomization provides each study subject with an equal chance of entering each of the study groups. With a large enough sample, the characteristics of the subjects will be balanced among the study groups as a result of random distribution. This effect will influence the distribution of known confounders as well as factors not yet known to confound the association under investigation. The smaller the sample, the less likely it is that subject traits will be balanced among the study groups. Therefore, randomization cannot guarantee that the groups will be comparable in all ways but the intervention under study, and it cannot guarantee that confounding will be completely eliminated. However, randomization will at least reduce confounding by known and unknown factors. See Chapter 5.

103. **The answer is A: double-blinding.** In a double-blind study, neither the investigator nor the subject knows which intervention is being administered. While measurement error may occur, it will not be influenced by knowledge of the intervention and will therefore be random. Random error reduces the power of a study to detect a true difference between control and intervention groups, but it does not introduce bias. See Chapters 5 and 12.

104. **The answer is E: statistical analysis.** Randomization ensures that all participants in a trial will be assigned to the different groups with equal probability. However, particularly when groups are small, randomization cannot ensure that all relevant characteristics will be evenly distributed among the groups. Bias is removed from the assignment by a randomization technique, but residual confounding by unevenly distributed factors may remain. This residual confounding is controlled in the statistical analysis of the data. See Chapter 5.

105. **The answer is A:**

$$N = \frac{(z_\alpha + z_\beta)^2 \cdot 2 \cdot \overline{p}(1 - \overline{p})}{(\overline{d})^2}$$

The study described measures outcome as a proportion. The sample size formula for use with proportional data is shown above. The use of this formula is discussed in Chapter 12 and Box 12–4.

106. **The answer is C:**

$$N = \frac{(z_\alpha)^2 \cdot 2 \cdot (s)^2}{(\overline{d})^2}$$

The study described uses separate control and intervention groups. Therefore, the sample size formula has a 2 in the numerator to double N. The total sample size is $2N$. The use of this formula is discussed in Chapter 12 and Box 12–2.

107. **The answer is B:**

$$N = \frac{(z_\alpha)^2 \cdot (s)^2}{(\overline{d})^2}$$

This study described uses subjects as their own controls, thereby reducing the number of subjects needed. The use of this formula is discussed in Chapter 12 and Box 12–1.

108. The answer is D:

$$N = \frac{(z_\alpha + z_\beta)^2 \cdot 2 \cdot (s)^2}{(\bar{d})^2}$$

In a study using separate control and intervention groups and considering both alpha and beta error, the appropriate sample size formula is shown above. N is increased both by adjusting for beta error and by the need for separate controls. The formula provides the number of subjects needed for each group. In order to recruit adequately for both control and intervention subjects, the number of participants needed would be $2N$. The use of this formula is discussed in Chapter 12 and Box 12–3.

109. The answer is D: population attributable risk percent, or PAR%. The utility of attributable risk to health policy is its application to cost-benefit (cost-utility) analysis and cost-effectiveness analysis. The population attributable risk percent (PAR%) is useful in that it provides information about the impact of a particular exposure on the total population and about the degree to which that exposure influences total risk in the population. Of the measures listed in the question, the PAR% is of greatest interest to policy makers because it considers the aggregate population risk. The attributable risk (AR), attributable risk percent in the exposed (AR%$_{(exposed)}$), odds ratio (OR), or risk ratio (RR) might be very high if an exposure were highly correlated with an adverse outcome, even in a very small segment of the population. For example, the risk of death due to Ebola virus may be impressively high among the exposed, but the rate of exposure in the USA may be too low to warrant the allocation of financial resources to a program aimed at prevention of the disease. Of the choices, only the PAR% would reveal that the impact of Ebola virus on the US population is negligible, despite the virulence of the pathogen. See Chapters 6 and 14.

110. The answer is E: the strength of the association between x and y. The square of the correlation coefficient, r^2, is an expression of the proportion of variation in the dependent variable (generally, y) explained by the variation in the independent variable (generally, x). For example, if the correlation coefficient for a set of data displaying height (the independent variable) and weight (the dependent variable) were 0.90, the square of this, or 0.81, would represent the proportion of variation in weight explained by variation in height. The more the variation in the dependent variable is explained by the variation in the independent variable, the greater is the strength of the association between the two. See Chapter 11.

111. The answer is E: predicting the peak air flow rates when the pack-years of cigarettes smoked are known. Linear regression is a form of statistical modeling. The model is used to predict y, given x and information about the relationship between x and y (i.e., the slope and y-intercept). The quality of the model is determined by how closely the predicted values of y approximate the actual measured values. Linear regression is related to correlation and, like correlation, can be performed only when both the independent and dependent variables are continuous. In choice A (calculating the probability of achieving remission of leukemia when the prior response to chemotherapy is known) and choice B (predicting blood pressure levels when the family history of the presence or absence of hypertension is known), the independent variables are not continuous. In choice D (predicting the blood type of a patient when the blood types of the parents are known), neither the independent nor the dependent variable is continuous. In choice C (predicting serum cholesterol levels when dietary intake data are known), dietary intake data would provide multiple independent variables; linear regression analyzes the relationship between only one independent variable and one dependent variable. See Chapter 11.

112. The answer is D: that the two variables are independent of each other. A chi-square analysis of a 2×2 contingency table seeks evidence that the variation in one of the variables is due in part to variation in the other variable, rather than to chance. The data are dichotomous and therefore cannot be characterized by a mean. The expected values for each cell, calculated by methods discussed in Chapter 11, are the values expected if the null hypothesis is true (i.e., if the variation in the two variables is independent). The significance test associated with the chi-square value determines whether or not the variation in one variable is explained by the variation in the other variable to a greater degree than would be expected by chance alone, at a conventional alpha level of 0.05. See Chapter 11.

113. The answer is E: using a very large sample. When the sample size is sufficiently large, even trivial differences may achieve statistical significance. If, for example, a vaccine against Lyme disease were tested and found to reduce the rate of infection from 11.1 per 1000 among the unvaccinated to 10.9 per 1000 among the vaccinated (these figures are fictitious), the vaccine would be of virtually no clinical value. To prevent one case of Lyme disease with this vaccine, more than 5000 people would need to be vaccinated. If data were collected for many thousands of subjects over many years, even this trivial difference might be statistically significant. Statistical significance may be misleading when outcome differences are not clinically meaningful. See Chapter 10.

114. **The answer is E: uses uneven death-free intervals.** The principal difference between the actuarial method and the Kaplan-Meier method is that the Kaplan-Meier method begins a new observation interval with each death. Because deaths are generally not evenly distributed, the observation intervals (the so-called death-free intervals) are uneven. In comparison with the actuarial method approach, this approach compensates better for losses to follow-up and censored data when samples are small. The uneven intervals of the Kaplan-Meier method account for the uneven stairlike curves that result when the data are plotted. The actuarial method and the Kaplan-Meier method are both forms of life table analysis. While these methods are often used for survival analysis, the outcome of interest need not be death. For either method, however, the outcome variable must be a dichotomous variable. See Chapter 11.

115. **The answer is D: the fact that only incident cases are detected.** Whenever a new screening program is introduced, the number of cases detected includes new cases (incident cases) plus cases that have accumulated over time (prevalent cases). If the same program is repeated in the same population at relatively frequent intervals, only the much smaller number of incident cases remains to be detected. See Chapter 17.

116. **The answer is E: the onset of symptoms may cause concern and raise motivation.** Primary prevention occurs before the onset of disease, whereas both secondary prevention and tertiary prevention occur after the onset of disease. Most patients are much more willing to modify potentially dangerous life-styles after they have suffered some of the adverse consequences of pursuing such life-styles. This is the proverbial case of not knowing what you've got until it's gone. The adverse consequences heighten awareness of and interest in disease prevention and health promotion. Unfortunately, however, the restoration of health following serious illness is often incomplete and therefore inferior to the preservation of health in the first place. Tertiary prevention is generally less cost-effective than prevention at earlier stages, although this is not universally true. Illness may in fact limit compliance with medical advice, as might wellness, but this does not explain the greater influence of tertiary prevention. Tertiary prevention usually produces the least net benefit of all preventive strategies. See Chapter 18.

117. **The answer is B: body fat distribution.** Gender, age, family history, and cigarette smoking all influence the risk of cardiovascular disease whether or not obesity is present. Obesity is associated with an increased risk of cardiovascular disease, especially (and perhaps exclusively) when fat is distributed predominantly in the abdomen, rather than in the buttocks and lower extremities (Lemieux et al. 1993). The accumulation of adipose tissue in the upper body and abdomen has been labeled the android pattern because it predominates in men. This pattern may contribute to the higher risk of cardiovascular disease in men than in age-matched premenopausal women. The accumulation of adipose tissue in the buttocks and lower extremities has been labeled the gynecoid pattern. Neither pattern, of course, consistently respects the gender boundary. See Chapter 18.

118. **The answer is C: synergistic.** As risk factors for cardiovascular disease accumulate, the relative risk of the disease rises at a rate that is faster than the simple addition of the effects of each factor (see Table 5–2). The risk factors are therefore synergistic. Until recently, men have been preferentially selected as subjects in studies of heart disease. Cardiovascular disease is just as important in women, although the onset is later (Kuhn and Rackley 1993). See Chapter 18.

119. **The answer is A: high-density lipoprotein (HDL).** Total cholesterol (TC) includes high-density lipoprotein (HDL), low-density lipoprotein (LDL), and very low density lipoprotein (VLDL). LDLs (particularly small and dense LDL variants and oxidized LDLs) are considered the most atherogenic of lipid particles in the blood. Levels of TC, LDL, VLDL, and triglycerides correlate positively, to varying degrees, with the risk of coronary atherosclerosis. HDL functions in reverse cholesterol transport, removing atherogenic lipid particles from the circulation (for details, see Gordon and Rifkind 1989). Therefore, HDL levels are inversely correlated with the risk of coronary artery disease. The ratio of TC to HDL or the ratio of LDL to HDL is preferable to any of the measures used alone in the estimation of heart disease risk (National Cholesterol Education Program 1994). See Chapter 18.

120. **The answer is D: HMG-CoA reductase inhibitors ("statins").** HMG-CoA reductase inhibitors, bile acid sequestrants, and fibrates are drugs used in the treatment of hypercholesterolemia. HMG-CoA reductase is the rate-limiting enzyme in cholesterol biosynthesis in hepatocytes. The statins (which include atorvastatin, fluvastatin, lovastatin, pravastatin, and simvastatin) act by competitively inhibiting HMG-CoA reductase and thereby disrupting cholesterol biosynthesis. Studies indicate that the statins decrease the mortality rate when used as

secondary prevention (Scandinavian Simvastatin Survival Study Group 1994) or as primary prevention (Shepherd et al. 1995). Bile acid sequestrants, such as cholestyramine and colestipol, act by causing cholesterol to exit the enterohepatic circulation and be eliminated from the body in stool. Fibrates, such as gemfibrozil, act by interfering with the metabolism and transfer of triglycerides (National Cholesterol Education Program 1994). Angiotensin-converting enzyme inhibitors (ACE inhibitors) and selective serotonin reuptake inhibitors (SSRIs) are not used in the treatment of hypercholesterolemia. ACE inhibitors are antihypertensive drugs, and SSRIs are antidepressants. See Chapter 18.

121. **The answer is E: 50 million.** Hypertension is defined as an average systolic blood pressure of 140 mm Hg or higher or an average diastolic blood pressure of 90 mm Hg or higher in a person who is not acutely ill and not taking antihypertensive medications. By this definition, there are approximately 50 million prevalent cases in the USA (National Institutes of Health 1997). See Chapter 18.

122. **The answer is D: pregnant women.** The usefulness of any screening program is its ability to detect a disease that would otherwise go undetected (at least temporarily) and to thereby improve the outcome. While diabetes is common, screening for it is not considered cost-effective, because symptoms tend to unmask the disease early. The yield of screening for diabetes is generally low in completely asymptomatic individuals. The one exception to this is pregnant women who have not previously been diagnosed with diabetes; in these women, counter-regulatory hormones may unmask a susceptibility to the disease. Another factor that contributes to the cost-effectiveness of screening for diabetes in pregnant women is that the detection of gestational diabetes allows for the prevention of severe congenital deformities. These deformities can be completely prevented through the maintenance of normal serum glucose levels (euglycemia) during pregnancy. Recall that the cost-effectiveness of a screening program is determined by the cost of screening and by the number of individuals who would need to be screened in order to identify one case that would have gone undetected without screening. The cost-effectiveness of screening may change over time as less expensive diagnostic methods are developed, treatment options change, or prevalence varies. See Chapter 18.

123. **The answer is C: disability is socially defined.** The severity and chronicity of disability and impairment are variable. Impairment is a medically defined change in physical status following injury or illness. The resultant decline in functional status (disability) is defined socially in terms of what the patient can and cannot do. See Chapter 18.

124. **The answer is D: the states.** In the USA, the fundamental responsibility for the health of the public lies with the states, as clarified in the Tenth Amendment to the US Constitution: "The powers not delegated to the United States by the Constitution, nor prohibited by it to the States, are reserved to the States respectively, or to the people." The limited responsibility of the federal government for the administration of public health policy is predicated upon the interstate commerce clause and the general welfare clause from Article 1, Section 8, of the US Constitution. See Chapter 20.

125. **The answer is A: consideration of the health impact of all public policy.** The public health perspective in the USA may be considered narrow by world standards. The mission statement by the Institute of Medicine in 1988 placed emphasis on the responsibilities of all public health agencies in the promotion of the public well-being. In contrast, the Ottawa Charter for Health Promotion, released in Canada in 1986, considers the pursuit of well-being and health to be a universal responsibility. All public policy, according to the charter, is to be assessed for any potential impact on health and modified so as to promote health whenever possible. The notion of "healthy public policy" as public health policy is increasingly popular worldwide and is advocated by many in the USA. See Chapter 20.

126. **The answer is D: 30% of total daily calories.** The restriction of dietary fat to no more than 30% of total daily calories is the current official guideline in the USA and was included among the nutrition goals in *Healthy People 2000*. At the time of the second National Health and Nutrition Examination Survey (NHANES II), the mean fat intake for adults in the USA was estimated to be 37% of calories. In the more recent NHANES III, the estimate fell to 34%. Given the rising prevalence of obesity and the caloric density of fat (9 kcal/g), some nutrition experts question whether this trend reflects dietary changes or merely changes in the way people respond to dietary surveys. The 30% goal is not considered optimal but is the lower limit of what authorities considered a feasible goal for the year 2000. Most nutritionists agree that if fat intake were much lower than 30%, there would be additional health benefits for adults. See Chapter 15.

127. **The answer is B: encourage smoking cessation.** Smoking is considered the most important cause of preventable morbidity and mortality in the USA, and smoking cessation would be the

highest priority for the clinical encounter in the case described. In general, the treatment of any imminently dangerous condition is the first priority for any clinical encounter. The treatment of symptomatic but not necessarily dangerous conditions would be the second priority. Asymptomatic conditions that pose no immediate threat but require management to prevent adverse outcomes would be the third priority. Screening for additional risk factors is important but less so than managing the risk factors that are already apparent. Of the several risk factors for chronic disease revealed in this encounter, smoking is the single most important and might exacerbate other risk factors, such as the slightly elevated blood pressure. Of importance always are the patient's preferences. If this patient were interested in weight loss but not smoking cessation, it would be appropriate to encourage her to consider smoking cessation at a later date and then to give advice regarding diet and exercise to promote weight loss. Although it is difficult to make multiple life-style changes at one time, health-promoting behaviors are often interrelated. Interest in smoking cessation might arise after the initiation of an exercise program, for example, when the patient first becomes aware of activity-limiting dyspnea (breathlessness). See Chapter 20.

128. **The answer is E: 100 per 100,000 persons.** In 1987, the age-adjusted death rate from coronary artery disease in the USA was 135 per 100,000 persons. The goal for the year 2000 was to reduce this to 100 per 100,000 persons. See Chapter 20.

129. **The answer is C: the case fatality ratio.** The case fatality ratio is the percentage or proportion of cases of a particular disease that prove fatal. The attack rate is the proportion of exposed individuals who become ill. The crude death rate is not cause-specific and would not accurately be derived from so small a population. The standardized mortality ratio derives from indirect standardization of death rates and is not relevant. The adjusted death rate is the same as the standardized mortality rate and is not relevant. See Chapter 3.

130. **The answer is A: fecal-oral transmission peaks in the summer.** Hepatitis A is spread via the fecal-oral route. Diseases associated with this mode of transmission tend to show peak incidence rates in the summer, owing at least in part to proliferation of the organisms in contaminated water and food and in part to contamination by flies and other insects. The epidemiologic year is a plot of incident cases over a year and begins during the month of lowest incidence. The incidence of hepatitis A would reach its peak in the summer and would reach its nadir in the winter, perhaps in January for a

particular year. The epidemiologic year may mimic the calendar year but often does not. See Chapter 3.

131. **The answer is B: influenza.** Viral influenza A varies seasonally, with the peak incidence in the USA seen during the fall and winter. Because of this variation, because of the known propensity of the virus to undergo mutations (antigenic drift and shift), because of the extent of illness and death associated with the disease, and because of the availability of a protective vaccine against influenza, a sophisticated surveillance system has been established to facilitate the recognition and control of influenza outbreaks. See Chapter 3.

132. **The answer is D: establish the case definition; determine whether an epidemic exists; characterize the epidemic by time, place, and person; develop hypotheses regarding spread; and initiate control measures.** None of the options outlines all of the steps in an outbreak investigation. Of the options listed, only D shows the steps in the correct order. The initial action is to make a diagnosis, albeit a tentative one, which specifies the disease to be investigated. The next step is to establish a case definition, so that cases may be distinguished from noncases. Only after these steps have been taken can the number of cases be established and a judgment made as to whether a true epidemic exists. Once the determination has been made that an epidemic does exist, it must be characterized by time, place, and person. This leads to hypotheses regarding the source, type, and route of spread. The hypotheses must be tested, such as in case-control studies and laboratory assays. Control measures are then implemented, and follow-up surveillance is devised. In reality, some of these steps may take place concomitantly. This sequence, however, provides the theoretical model upon which any true outbreak investigation should be based. See Chapter 3.

133. **The answer is D: quality-adjusted life years.** The quality-adjusted life year (QALY) is used as an increment of health benefit, or utility, that can indicate how much is achieved with each dollar spent. A cost-benefit analysis requires that cost and benefit be measured in dollars. Health care providers have difficulty assigning a dollar value to years of life. The QALY, which incorporates both length and quality of life, is a preferable measure that is increasingly applied. In general, the measure assigns a value to a year of life as a fraction of perfect health (a fraction of 1) and then multiplies the fraction by the length of life to produce a measure of net gain. For example, 10 years of life at "half" the quality of perfect health would equal 10×0.5, or 5 QALYs. Marginal utility refers to incremental

benefit associated with the expansion of a service to more recipients. See Chapter 14.

134. The answer is B: less than 100. The standardized mortality ratio sets the reference standard at 100. The mortality rate of a study population is compared with the reference standard. If the study population has a lower mortality rate than the reference population, the standardized mortality ratio (based on age-standardized mortality) is less than 100. Conversely, if the study population has a higher mortality rate, the standardized mortality ratio is greater than 100. See Chapter 2.

135. The answer is C: cost of the program and estimated years of life saved by screening. The cost of a screening program is important, but it cannot be interpreted without consideration of the program's benefits. The number of patients screened and the number admitted to the hospital do not indicate the program benefits, while years of life saved clearly would. The average years of survival following screening may be unrelated to screening and is therefore an unreliable measure of benefit. See Chapter 14.

136. The answer is D: infant mortality rate. The infant mortality rate is calculated by dividing the number of deaths in infants under 1 year of age by the number of live births in the same population and then multiplying the result by 1000. Deaths in this age group are closely related to overall environmental conditions, sanitation, nutritional adequacy, and the adequacy of other basic health and human services. Thus, the infant mortality rate is considered a good index of the overall quality of the health care system of a country. See Chapter 2.

137. The answer is A: a high degree of sensitivity. A highly sensitive test will be positive in almost all cases of disease. Therefore, it will tend to be negative only if disease is truly absent. Thus, a negative result on a highly sensitive test is a reliable way of ruling out a disease. See Chapter 7.

138. The answer is B: isocyanates. Isocyanates are constituents of paint applied to automobiles. They are associated with airway irritation and bronchospasm, and they are considered to be the leading cause of occupational asthma. Particulates may cause airway irritation; solvents generally do not. Pneumoconiosis refers to any fibrosing lung disease that is related to inspired particles or fibers. Byssinosis is a form of obstructive pulmonary disease induced by the inspiration of cotton fibers. See Chapter 19.

139. The answer is A: it is determined in part by behavioral risk factors and family history. The risk age is determined by the use of a health risk assessment (HRA). A woman's risk age is higher than her actual (chronologic) age if on the basis of her behavioral or genetic risk factors her risk of dying is comparable to the risk in persons older than she is. If a person is in unusually good health for his or her age, the risk age would be lower than the chronologic age. See Chapter 17.

140. The answer is B: it is low when the beta error is high. Statistical power equals 1 minus beta error. Therefore, the larger the beta error, the lower is the power to detect a difference. See Chapter 12.

141. The answer is B: cohort trial. A cohort trial is defined by the assembly of one or more groups (cohorts) characterized by an exposure and followed for an outcome. The cohorts here are manganese miners who have or have not been exposed to the benefits (and hazards) of dental floss. The cohorts are then followed for the occurrence of the specified outcome, which is iron deficiency anemia. See Chapter 5.

142. The answer is E: the relative risk. Data from a cohort trial can be used to calculate the relative risk, whereas data from a case-control trial can be used only to estimate the relative risk by calculation of the odds ratio. The odds ratio is a good estimate of the risk ratio only when the disease under investigation is rare. The relative risk of iron deficiency anemia is the risk in those who floss, which is $150/(150 + 50)$, divided by the risk in those who do not floss, which is $20/(20 + 180)$, or 7.5. To calculate the incidence, we would need to know the specific period of time during which new cases of iron deficiency anemia developed in our population. To define the prevalence, we would need to know the number of cases of iron deficiency anemia present in our population at a given point in time. A dichotomous outcome is not characterized by a mean. See Chapters 5 and 6.

143. The answer is D: 85. The question refers to the expected count for cell *a*. To calculate the expected count (E) for any cell in a contingency table, you need to know the total for the row in which the cell is located (row total), the total for the column in which the cell is located (column total), and the total for the table (study total). For cell *a*, the row total is $150 + 50 = 200$; the column total is $150 + 20 = 170$; and the study total is $150 + 50 + 20 + 180 = 400$. The formula can be expressed as follows:

$$E = \frac{\text{Row total}}{\text{Study total}} \times \text{Column total}$$

The expected count is therefore $(200/400)(170) = 85$. Alternatively, the row total could be multiplied by the column total and then divided by the study total, and the expected count would be the same: $(200 \times 170)/400 = 85$. See Chapter 11.

144. **The answer is D: 85.** The question asks for the expected count in cell c of the contingency table. To calculate the expected count, the row total $(20 + 180)$ is multiplied by the column total $(150 + 20)$, and the product is divided by the total for the table, or 400. This becomes $(200 \times 170)/400$, or 85. See Chapter 11.

145. **The answer is C: 115.** The question asks for the expected count in cell d of the contingency table. The row total is $(20 + 180)$. The column total is $(50 + 180)$. The table total is 400. The expected count is $(200 \times 230)/400$, or 115. See Chapter 11.

146. **The answer is D: the use of dental floss and iron deficiency anemia are not associated.** The null hypothesis for a contingency table is that the variables of interest are independent. In a cohort study such as the one described, the independent variable is the exposure (in this case, use of dental floss). The dependent variable is the outcome (in this case, iron deficiency anemia). The null hypothesis stipulates that the exposure and outcome are independent, or that, in this case, the use of dental floss and the development of iron deficiency anemia are independent. See Chapter 11.

147. **The answer is D: those with the outcome but not the exposure.** Conceptual understanding of a contingency table requires identification of the type of data represented by each cell in the table. By convention, disease status is expressed in the columns of the table and exposure status in the rows, as is true of the example provided for this set of questions. Cell a represents subjects with both exposure and outcome; cell b represents subjects with exposure but not the outcome; cell d represents subjects with neither exposure nor outcome; and cell c, the correct answer, represents subjects with the outcome (column 1) but not the exposure (row 2). See Chapter 11.

148. **The answer is D: 172.8.** The chi-square value, $[(O - E)^2/E]$, is first calculated for each of the four cells in the table, and then the four values are summed. For cell a, the observed value is 150, and the expected value is 85. The expected value for each cell is the row total multiplied by the column total, with the product divided by the total for the study. For cell a, this is $[(150 + 50) \times (150 + 20)]/400$; this equals 85. The chi-square value for the cell is $(150 - 85)^2/85$, which is 49.7. The chi-square value for each of the other cells is determined in the same way. The expected value for cell b is 115; for cell c, 85; and for cell d, 115. You may be surprised that the expected values are the same for cells a and c

and for cells b and d. This will occur any time the sample is evenly divided into two groups, one with and one without the exposure. Because half of the sample is in row 1 and half in row 2, half of each column total is expected to occur in the top row and half in the bottom row. The chi-square value for cell b is 36.7; for cell c, 49.7; and for cell d, 36.7. The chi-square value for the table is therefore $49.7 + 36.7 + 49.7 + 36.7$, which is approximately 172.8. See Chapter 11.

149. **The answer is B: 1.** In any contingency table, there are $(R - 1) \times (C - 1)$ degrees of freedom, where R is the number of rows in the table and C is the number of columns. In a 2×2 table, therefore, there will always be $(2 - 1) \times (2 - 1)$, or 1, degree of freedom. The conceptual basis for this is uncomplicated. Given the total number of data points for the table and the totals for each of the rows and columns, how many of the cells are "free" to vary? In a 2×2 table, if we know the total for row 1 and fill in a value for cell a, cell b is no longer free to vary; cell a plus cell b must add up to the known total for row 1. Now that cells a and b are filled in, cells c and d become fixed, because cell a plus cell c must add up to the known total for column 1 and because cell b plus cell d must add up to the known total for column 2. Therefore, once one value is entered into a 2×2 table, the other counts become fixed and are not "free." The degrees of freedom specifies the number of cells in the table that are free to vary. See Chapter 11.

150. **The answer is C: find the corresponding p value in a chi-square table.** Once the chi-square value for the 2×2 table and the degrees of freedom have been established, no further calculation is necessary to determine the statistical significance of the model. A chi-square table is provided in the Appendix, as well as in most books of biostatistics. Across the top of the table are p values associated with a given value of chi-square, and running down the first column are the number of degrees of freedom. In this case, the corresponding p value is less than 0.0005, and this model is therefore highly statistically significant. Our conclusion from this study is that, at least in male manganese miners, the use of dental floss predisposes to iron deficiency anemia. We have learned nothing of the effects of flossing in other populations. See Chapter 11.

References Cited

Bennett, W. I., ed. Beyond overeating. New England Journal of Medicine 332:673–674, 1995.

Berkman, L. F., and L. Breslow. Health and Ways of Living: The Alameda County Study. New York, Oxford University Press, 1983.

Bisno, A. L. Group A streptococcal infections and acute rheumatic fever. New England Journal of Medicine 325:783–793, 1991.

Centers for Disease Control and Prevention. Update: influenza activity–United States and worldwide, 1993–1994 season, and composition of the 1994–1995 influenza vaccine. Morbidity and Mortality Weekly Report 43:179–183, 1994.

Fletcher, A. E., and C. J. Bulpitt. How far should blood pressure be lowered? New England Journal of Medicine 326:251–254, 1992.

Gordon, D. J., and B. M. Rifkind. High-density lipoprotein: the clinical implications of recent studies. New England Journal of Medicine 321:1311–1316, 1989.

Institute of Medicine. The Future of Public Health. Washington, D. C., National Academy Press, 1988.

Kuczmarski, R. J., et al. Increasing prevalence of overweight among US adults: the National Health and Nutrition Examination Surveys, 1960 to 1991. Journal of the American Medical Association 272:205–211, 1994.

Kuhn, F., and C. E. Rackley. Coronary artery disease in women: risk factors, evaluation, treatment, and prevention. Archives of Internal Medicine 153:2626–2636, 1993.

Lemieux, S., et al. Sex differences in the relation of visceral adipose tissue accumulation to total body fatness. American Journal of Clinical Nutrition 58:463–467, 1993.

Lindpainter, K. Finding an obesity gene: a tale of mice and men. New England Journal of Medicine 332:679–680, 1995.

McGinnis, J. M., and W. H. Foege. Actual causes of death in the United States. Journal of the American Medical Association 270:2207–2212, 1993.

Moriyama, I. M. Inquiring into the diagnostic evidence supporting medical certifications of death. *In* Lilienfeld, A. M., and A. J. Gifford, eds. Chronic Diseases and Public Health. Baltimore, Johns Hopkins University Press, 1966.

National Cholesterol Education Program. Second report of the expert panel on detection, evaluation, and treatment of high blood cholesterol in adults. Circulation 89:1329–1445, 1994.

National Institutes of Health. The Sixth Report of the Joint National Committee on Prevention, Detection, Evaluation, and Treatment of High Blood Pressure. Publication No. (NIH)98-4080. Bethesda, Md., National Institutes of Health, 1997.

Ottawa Charter for Health Promotion. Report of an International Conference on Health Promotion, Sponsored by the World Health Organization, Health and Welfare Canada, and the Canadian Public Health Association, Ottawa, Ontario, Canada, November 17–21, 1986.

Physicians' Health Study Steering Committee. Final report on the aspirin component of the ongoing Physicians' Health Study. New England Journal of Medicine 321:129–135, 1989.

Pi-Sunyer, F. X. Health implications of obesity. American Journal of Clinical Nutrition 53:1595S–1603S, 1991.

Scandinavian Simvastatin Survival Study Group. Randomised trial of cholesterol lowering in 4444 patients with coronary heart disease. Lancet 344:1383–1389, 1994.

Shepherd, J., et al. Prevention of coronary heart disease with pravastatin in men with hypercholesterolemia. New England Journal of Medicine 333:1301–1307, 1995.

Stamler, J., ed. Epidemic obesity in the United States. Archives of Internal Medicine 153:1040–1044, 1993.

Epidemiologic and Medical Glossary

Acceptability of medical care   A measure of the patients' satisfaction with available medical care. Acceptability is influenced by such factors as whether the health care professionals can communicate well with their patients, whether the care is seen as warm and humane and concerned with the whole person, and whether the patients believe in the confidentiality and privacy of information shared with their health care providers.

Accessibility of medical care   The degree to which patients can receive care without undue geographic or financial obstacles.

Accountability of medical care   The degree to which the health care system takes public responsibility for its actions. This involves public representation on the board of directors of the health care facility, regular review of financial records by certified public accountants, and appropriate public disclosure of financial records and of quality of care studies.

Accuracy   The ability of a test to obtain the correct measure, on average.

Acquired immunodeficiency syndrome (AIDS)   A state of severe immunocompromise resulting from infection with the human immunodeficiency virus (HIV).

Active immunity   Immunity conferred by exposure to an antigen that stimulates the host to produce antibody. Active immunity is far superior to passive immunity, because active immunity lasts longer (a lifetime in some cases) and is rapidly stimulated to high levels by a reexposure to the same antigen or closely related antigens.

Active surveillance   Occurs when public health officials initiate contact with physicians, laboratories, or hospitals to obtain information about diseases of interest.

Actuarial method of life table analysis   A method of life table analysis in which proportionate survival is assessed at fixed intervals, such as months, that have been established prior to data accrual. *See also* Life table analysis.

Acute and convalescent sera   Acute sera are the first serum samples collected soon after symptoms of an infectious disease occur. Convalescent sera are follow-up samples collected after a period of time that is sufficient to allow for antibody titers to rise. A significant increase in the titers is taken as proof of recent infection.

Acute tubular necrosis   Sudden severe injury to renal tubule cells, often resulting from transient hypoperfusion.

Adequacy of medical care   A sufficient volume of care to meet the needs of a community.

Adjusted rates   *Same as* Standardized rates.

Advanced life support (ALS)   Intervention protocols applied to resuscitate or stabilize the condition of critically ill or critically injured patients.

Air inversion   Occurs when cooler air settles close to the surface of the earth and warmer air rises above, so that the natural mixing of air does not occur and pollution is concentrated.

Alcohol abuse   *See* Chemical substance abuse.

Allostatic load   The ongoing level of demand for adaptation in an individual. An elevated level may be an important contributor to many chronic diseases.

Alpha error   *Same as* Type I error.

Alpha level   The maximum probability of making a false-positive error that the investigator is willing to accept.

Alternative hypothesis   The hypothesis that there is in fact a real (true) difference between means or proportions of groups being compared or that there is a real association between two variables. *Compare* Null hypothesis.

Ames test   A quick and frequently used test to estimate the mutagenic potential of a chemical substance.

Analysis of covariance (ANCOVA)   A method of significance testing based on the ratio of between-groups variance to within-groups variance. This method is used in multivariable analysis if the dependent variable is continuous, some of the independent variables are categorical (i.e., nominal, dichotomous, or ordinal), and some of the independent variables are continuous.

Analysis of variance (ANOVA)   A method of significance testing based on the ratio of between-groups variance to within-groups variance. This method is used in statistical analysis if the dependent variable is continuous and the independent variable or variables are all categorical (i.e., nominal, dichotomous, or ordinal). If there is only one independent variable, the method is called one-way ANOVA. If there is more than one independent variable, the method is called N-way ANOVA, with N representing the number of independent variables.

Anergy panel   A panel containing several prevalent antigens that are injected to assess immunocompetence. At least one of the antigens should elicit a reaction if the immune system is not impaired.

Angina pectoris   Chest pain resulting from periods of myocardial ischemia.

Antigenic drift   Relatively minor change in the surface antigens of a viral influenza strain.

Antigenic shift   Major change in the surface antigens of a viral influenza strain, with the potential to create worldwide epidemics (pandemics).

Appropriateness of medical care   The procedures being performed are properly selected and carried out by trained personnel in the proper setting.

Asbestosis   Pulmonary compromise resulting from an accumulation of asbestos fibers in the lungs and from the associated inflammatory response, ultimately leading to pulmonary fibrosis.

Assessability of medical care   Care can be readily evaluated.

Atherogenesis   The development and accumulation of atherosclerotic plaque in arteries.

Attack rate   The proportion of exposed persons who become ill. This is the customary measure used to establish the severity of a disease outbreak.

Attributable risk (AR)   Of the total risk for a particular outcome, the attributable risk is the proportion that is attributable to a particular exposure. *Same as* Risk difference.

Attributable risk percent in the exposed (AR%$_{(exposed)}$)   Answers the following question: Among those with the risk factor, what percentage of the total risk for the disease is due to the risk factor?

Availability of medical care   The provision of care during the hours and days when people need it.

Bacillus Calmette-Guérin (BCG) vaccine   A live bacterial antigen vaccine that gives partial immunity against *Mycobacterium tuberculosis* infection.

Bayes' theorem   Answers the two important questions that remain unanswered by sensitivity and specificity: (1) If the test results are positive, what is the probability that the patient has the disease? (2) If the test results are negative, what is the probability that the patient does not have the disease? The theorem stipulates that the probability of a given condition in an individual is related to the prevalence of that condition in the population of which the individual is a member.

Berylliosis   Poisoning by fumes or dust of the metal beryllium, usually resulting in pneumonitis.

Best estimate   Estimate achieved with the statistical model that produces the smallest sum of the squared error terms.

Beta error   *Same as* Type II error.

Between-groups mean square   *Same as* Between-groups variance.

Between-groups variance   Measurement of the variation between (or among) the means of more than one group, based on the independent variables under study.

Bias   The introduction of error that produces deviations or distortions of data that are predominantly in one direction, as opposed to random error. *Same as* Differential error.

Binary variables   *Same as* Dichotomous variables.

Biochemical oxygen demand   The quantity of oxygen that aerobic bacteria in sewage will deplete from the water.

Bivariate analysis   Analysis of the relationship between one independent variable and one dependent variable.

Black lung disease   *Same as* Coal worker's pneumoconiosis.

Bonferroni adjustment to alpha   A method for adjusting alpha when multiple hypotheses are being tested. To keep the risk of a false-positive finding in the entire study to no more than alpha (which is usually 0.05), the alpha level chosen for rejecting the null hypothesis is made more stringent by dividing alpha by the number of hypotheses being tested.

Botulism   Poisoning by a neurotoxin produced by the bacterium *Clostridium botulinum.* Botulism usually results from ingestion of improperly canned or prepared food.

Bronchitis   Inflammation of the bronchi, producing a clinical syndrome of cough, dyspnea, chest discomfort, and fever.

Byssinosis   An asthma-like pulmonary syndrome resulting from inhalation of textile dust (e.g., cotton dust).

Capitation basis for payment   Payment of primary care physicians on a "per head" basis. Although patients vary in their need for and use of medical services, the physician receives the same amount of money per patient per year.

Case definition   Characterizes the clinical manifestations of the condition under investigation. The case definition provides the inclusion and exclusion criteria that are used to determine which subjects are cases and which are not cases in an outbreak investigation.

Case fatality ratio   The proportion of clinically ill persons who die of the condition under study. This is a marker of virulence.

Case finding   The process of searching for asymptomatic diseases or risk factors among people while they are in a clinical setting (i.e., among people who are under medical care). The distinction between screening and case finding is frequently ignored in the literature and in practice; the distinction is important because many of the criteria for community screening do not need to be met during the process of case finding.

Case-control study   Study groups are defined on the basis of disease (or outcome) status. The frequency of the risk factor (exposure) in the cases (diseased) is compared with the frequency of the risk factor (exposure) in the controls (nondiseased).

Causality   A factor produces or contributes to the production of a specified outcome. *See also* Direct causality and Indirect causality.

Cause-specific rates   Rates that provide numerators that are comparable with regard to diagnosis.

Cell-mediated immunity A tissue-based cellular response to foreign antigens. The response involves mobilization of killer T cells.

Central limit theorem For reasonably large samples, the distribution of the means of many samples is normal (gaussian), even though the data in individual samples may have skewness, kurtosis, or unevenness.

Chemical substance abuse Both physical dependence (including tolerance) and psychologic dependence on the use of chemicals such as alcohol or illegal drugs to modify mood and performance and to escape from anxiety. Cigarette smoking is also a form of chemical dependence or substance abuse.

Chickenpox An illness that occurs most frequently during childhood, is caused by varicella-zoster virus (VZV) infection, and is characterized by fever and a papulovesicular rash. Chickenpox is also called varicella.

Chi-square test of independence A statistical significance test used to analyze nominal or dichotomous data in a contingency table. The first step is to determine the chi-square value for each cell in the table. This is done by calculating the square of the observed count (O) minus the expected count (E) in a cell and dividing the result by the expected count for that cell. The next step is to add the values for all cells in the table. The standard chi-square formula is $\Sigma[(O - E)^2/E]$.

Cholera An acute and sometimes fulminant diarrheal illness that is due to an enterotoxin produced by the bacterium *Vibrio cholerae*.

Chronic renal disease A nonspecific term referring to a gradual decline in the functional capacity of the kidney, as measured by the creatinine clearance and glomerular filtration rate. The term is conventionally applied to renal insufficiency that is irreversible.

Coal worker's pneumoconiosis A disease that is caused by chronic inhalation of coal dust, is characterized by pulmonary inflammation or fibrosis, and is also known as black lung disease.

Coefficient A weighting factor used in an equation, with the weight based on the relative importance of the factor in predicting the outcome.

Cohort A clearly defined group of persons studied over time.

Cohort study A study in which a clearly identified group is characterized by exposure and is followed for the outcome.

Completeness of medical care Adequate attention to all aspects of a medical problem, including prevention, early detection, diagnosis, treatment, follow-up measures, and rehabilitation.

Comprehensiveness of medical care The extent to which care is provided for all types of health problems, including dental and mental health problems.

Confounding Confusion of two supposedly causal variables, so that part or all of the purported effect of one variable is actually due to the other.

Contingency table Used to determine whether the distribution of one variable is conditionally dependent (contingent) upon the other variable.

Continuity of medical care Management of a patient's care over time is coordinated among providers.

Continuous variables Variables in which data are measured over the range of an uninterrupted numerical scale. Examples are height, weight, and age.

Convalescent sera *See* Acute and convalescent sera.

Coronary artery disease The accumulation of atherosclerotic plaque in the coronary arteries, which reduces perfusion of the myocardium and sometimes causes ischemia, infarction, or both.

Cost-benefit analysis Measures and compares the costs and benefits of a proposed course of action in terms of the same units, usually monetary units such as dollars.

Cost-effectiveness analysis Provides a way of comparing the cost of different proposed means to a particular end in terms of the most appropriate measurement units. Assesses the least costly means of achieving a fixed goal.

Covariance The product of the deviation of an observation from the mean of the x variable, multiplied by the same observation's deviation from the mean of the y variable.

Cox method *Same as* Proportional hazards method.

Cox model *Same as* Proportional hazards model.

Crack cocaine Freebase cocaine, which is usually smoked and is the most potent and addictive form of cocaine.

Critical ratios A class of tests of statistical significance that depend on dividing some parameter (such as a difference between means) by the standard error of that parameter.

Cross-sectional ecologic study A study of the frequency with which some characteristic (e.g., smoking) and some outcome of interest (e.g., lung cancer) occur in the same geographically defined population at one particular time.

Cross-sectional survey A survey of a population at a single point in time.

Crude rates Rates that apply to an entire population, without reference to any characteristics of the individuals in it.

Cumulative incidence The total number of incident cases over a specified period of time. Incident cases resulting in death would be included in the cumulative incidence measure but not in the prevalence.

Data dredging The analysis of large data sets with modern computer techniques, permitting the assessment of hundreds of possible associations among the study variables. Unless alpha is adjusted, the testing of multiple hypotheses raises the risk of false-positive error.

Decision analysis A type of analysis intended to improve clinical decision making under conditions of uncertainty.

Deductive reasoning Reasoning that proceeds from the general (i.e., from assumptions, from propositions, and from formulas considered true) to the specific (i.e., to specific members belonging to the general category).

Degrees of freedom The number of observations in a data set that are free to vary once the parameters of the data set (e.g., the mean) have been established.

Denominator data Data that define the population at risk.

Diabetes mellitus An impairment in glucose metabolism that results from lack of insulin production (type I disease) or from insulin resistance (type II disease). Hyperglycemia is the principal expression but not the only expression of the metabolic derangements associated with diabetes mellitus.

Dichotomous variables Variables with only two levels.

Differential error Nonrandom, systematic, or consistent error in which the values tend to be inaccurate in a particular direction. *Same as* Bias.

Dimensional variables *Same as* Continuous variables.

Diphtheria Acute infectious disease caused by *Corynebacterium diphtheriae* and acquired from a person who has the disease or is a disease carrier. Diphtheria usually involves the upper respiratory tract and is characterized by the formation of a pseudomembrane attached to the underlying tissue.

Direct causality The factor under consideration exerts its effect without intermediary factors.

Direct standardization Two populations to be compared are given the same age distribution. Then this distribution is applied to the observed age-specific death rates to determine the number of deaths that would have occurred in each of the two populations if they had been identical in age distribution.

Disability A social definition of limitation, based on the degree of impairment. The formal categories of disability used in most states for reimbursement of workers who have job-related injuries or illnesses covered under a workers' compensation program are permanent total disability, permanent partial disability, temporary total disability, temporary partial disability, and death.

Disability limitation Medical and surgical measures aimed at controlling or correcting the anatomic and physiologic components of disease in symptomatic patients and preventing resultant limitations in functional ability.

Discounting A reduction in the present value of delayed benefits (or an increase in the present costs of benefits) to account for the time value of money (i.e., inflation).

Discrete variables Dichotomous variables and nominal variables are sometimes called discrete variables because the different categories are completely separate from each other.

Disease A medically definable process characterized by pathophysiology and pathology. *Compare* Illness.

Dose-response relationship Exists when an increase in the intensity or duration of exposure increases the risk of an adverse outcome. The relationship is often demonstrated in studies of chronic exposure, such as studies of the relationship between the quantity of cigarette smoking and the risk of lung cancer. In research involving a potential carcinogen, the dose-response relationship is measured beyond the usual latent period for the carcinogen, which is the period between the onset of exposure and the development of cancer.

Double-blind study A study in which neither the subjects nor the investigators are aware of the treatment assignment (active agent or placebo) until the trial is terminated.

Drug abuse *See* Chemical substance abuse.

Dystress A harmful form of stress, the level of which must be low in order for an individual to have good health.

Early fetal death Delivery of a dead fetus during the first 20 weeks of gestation.

Ebola virus infection A virulent hemorrhagic disease with a high case fatality ratio.

Ecologic fallacy The use of ecologic data to draw inferences about causal relationships in individuals. If the frequency of an exposure and the frequency of an outcome are determined in the same population but no information regarding the occurrence of exposure and outcome in the same individual is provided, the data cannot be construed to establish causality.

Effect modification Occurs when the strength (or even the direction) of the influence of a causal factor on outcome is altered by a third variable, the effect modifier.

Endemic disease Disease that is occurring regularly in a defined population.

Enzootic disease Disease that is occurring regularly in animal populations.

Eosinophilia-myalgia syndrome A syndrome of muscle pain and hypereosinophilia caused by a contaminant in one commercially prepared brand of the amino acid L-tryptophan.

Epidemic The occurrence of any disease at a frequency that is unusual (compared with baseline data) or unexpected.

Epidemic threshold The necessary degree of variation from usual patterns required for a disease to qualify as an outbreak.

Epidemiologic year Runs from the month of lowest incidence of a particular condition in one year to the same month in the next year.

Epidemiology The study of factors that influence the occurrence and distribution of disease in human populations.

Epizootic disease Disease outbreak in animals.

Error term A term that is needed to make an equation true if the prediction is not perfect. The error term is the portion of variation in the dependent variable that is not explained by the statistical model.

Eustress A helpful form of stress that must be present in order for an individual to have good health.

External validity Is present when the results of a study are true and meaningful for a larger population and not just for the study participants.

False-negative error *Same as* Type II error.

False-positive error *Same as* Type I error.

Fee-for-service method of payment Physicians are paid for each major item of service provided.

Fetal death Delivery of a dead fetus at any time during gestation.

Fisher exact probability test A statistical significance test that is used to analyze data in 2×2 contingency tables in which one or more of the expected counts are too small to satisfy conditions for the use of chi-square analysis.

Frequency distribution A plot of data displaying the value of each data point on one axis and the frequency with which that value occurs on the other axis.

***F*-Test** The test of statistical significance used with ANOVA. The F ratio is the test statistic or critical ratio. It is the ratio of between-groups variance to within-groups variance.

General linear model The general model depicting the linear (first-order) relationship between multiple independent variables and one dependent (outcome) variable. ANOVA, ANCOVA, multiple linear regression, and other multivariable techniques are variations of this basic model.

German measles *Same as* Rubella.

Ghon complex A characteristic abnormality seen on chest x-ray following resolution of initial infection with *Mycobacterium tuberculosis*.

Gonorrhea Various clinical manifestations of infection with the sexually transmitted pathogen *Neisseria gonorrhoeae*.

Goodness-of-fit test A general term used to describe the comparison of actual data with the results predicted by a particular statistical model, such as the expected counts generated by the use of chi-square analysis.

Granuloma A collection of inflammatory cells in a nodular formation that isolates the inflammatory agent (e.g., pathogen) within the complex.

Ground water Water that is found in underground spaces called aquifers. When adequately protected from surface pollutants, aquifers represent an important source of potable water.

Hantavirus pulmonary syndrome A newly emergent, life-threatening syndrome that is characterized by respiratory distress and is caused by infection with particular serotypes of hantavirus.

Health A difficult term to define. The World Health Organization defines it as "a state of complete physical, mental, and social well-being and not merely the absence of disease or infirmity."

Health belief model Before seeking preventive measures, people generally must believe that the disease at issue is serious, if acquired; that they or their children are personally at risk for the disease; that the preventive measure is effective in warding off the disease; and that there are no serious risks or barriers involved in obtaining the preventive measure. In addition, there need to be cues to action, consisting of information regarding how and when to obtain the preventive measure, as well as the encouragement from or support of other people.

Health maintenance organizations (HMOs) Prepaid group practices consisting of a legal and fiscal entity that does the contracting and financial transactions and seeks to control the costs of medical care; a group of physicians that provides the outpatient and inpatient medical care; and an associated hospital or hospitals.

Health risk assessments (HRAs) Use of questionnaires or computer programs to elicit and evaluate information concerning individuals in a clinical or industrial medical practice. Each assessed person receives information concerning estimates of his or her life expectancy and the types of interventions that are likely to have a positive impact on health or longevity.

Healthplan Employer Data and Information Set (HEDIS) A national data set of information about the performance of selected services by each managed care organization. HEDIS emphasizes data on preventive services.

Healthy worker effect Because people with jobs must be in reasonably good health to remain employed, their risk of death and illness is lower than that of the population as a whole. A carrier that insures a group of workers will benefit from this effect.

Hepatitis A nonspecific term referring to inflammation of the liver. Common causes include viruses and toxins, especially excess alcohol consumption.

Herd immunity Immunity that results when a vaccine not only prevents the vaccinated person from contracting the disease but also prevents him or her from spreading the disease and thereby protects even the unimmunized persons in the population.

Heritability The degree to which acquisition of a disease is influenced by genetic predisposition.

Herpes zoster A painful dermatomal rash that results from the reactivation of latent varicella-zoster virus, often many years after a case of chickenpox. Herpes zoster is also called shingles.

Hospice A nursing home that specializes in providing terminal care, especially for patients with cancer or AIDS.

Human immunodeficiency virus (HIV) A retrovirus that has a particular trophism for CD4 helper cells and is the infectious agent responsible for AIDS.

Hyperlipidemia A level of circulating lipoprotein particles or total cholesterol that exceeds the established reference range for a given population.

Hypersensitivity pneumonitis Pulmonary inflammation resulting from an allergic response to an inspired antigen.

Hypertension An average systolic blood pressure of 140 mm Hg or higher or an average diastolic blood pressure of 90 mm Hg or higher in an otherwise healthy person.

Iatrogenic diseases and injuries Diseases and injuries generated during the process of treatment.

Iceberg phenomenon The earliest identified cases of a new disease are often fatal or severe (representing the tip of the iceberg); however, as more becomes known about the disease, less severe cases and asymptomatic cases are usually discovered.

Illness What the patient experiences when he or she is sick. *Compare* Disease.

Immunodeficiency A deficiency of the immune system, which may be long-term (as in AIDS) or may be transient (lasting for a short period following some types of infections or the administration of chemotherapy for certain types of cancer).

Impairment A limitation of capacity or functional ability, usually as determined by a licensed physician.

Incidence The frequency (number) of new occurrences of disease, injury, or death in the study population during the time period being examined.

Incidence density The frequency (density) of new events per person-time. Incidence density is especially useful in studying the frequency rates of diseases or events that occur more than once for an individual, such as otitis media, colds, or hospital admissions.

Incidence density measures Measures of the frequency of adverse health events that are used, for example, to determine the optimal timing for administration of a new vaccine and the duration of the immunity produced.

Incidence rate The number of incident cases over a defined study period, divided by the population at risk at the midpoint of that study period.

Independent practice association (IPA) A form of health maintenance organization (HMO). Patients enrolled in an IPA can choose a primary care physician from a list of physicians who have contracted to provide services for the IPA. The IPA pays an individual physician on a fee-for-service basis whenever a member uses that physician's services. The IPA physicians limit their fees to the rates specified in the contract, and they agree to certain kinds of quality review and practice controls that are often similar to those of managed care.

Index case The case in which the condition under investigation was first identified.

Indirect causality One factor influences one or more other factors that are, in turn, directly causal.

Indirect standardization Used if age-specific death rates are not available in the study population or if the study population is small and would therefore yield age-specific death rates that would be statistically unstable. Death rates from the standard population are applied to the known age distribution of the study group.

Individual practice association *See* Independent practice association.

Inductive reasoning Reasoning that proceeds from the specific (i.e., from data) to the general (i.e., to formulas or conclusions).

Infant death The death of a live-born child before that child's first birthday.

Infectiousness of an organism A measure that is calculated as the proportion of exposed persons who become infected, although it is also influenced by the conditions of exposure and the immune status of the exposed person.

Influenza Infection of the upper respiratory tract by an influenza virus, resulting in an illness generally characterized by fever, sore throat, dry cough, and severe myalgia.

Interaction *See* Effect modification.

Intermediate care facility (ICF) A facility that is suitable if the patient's primary need is for help with the activities of daily living. An ICF is not required to have a registered (skilled) nurse on duty at all times.

Intermediate fetal death Delivery of a dead fetus between 20 and 28 weeks of gestation.

Intermediate hospital A medium to large community hospital that has a considerable amount of the latest technology but less research and investigational activity than a tertiary medical center.

Internal validity Is present when the results of a study are true and meaningful for the participants.

Interobserver variability A measure of disagreement between or among different observers.

Intervening variables Intermediary factors involved in indirect causality.

Interview survey A type of cross-sectional survey.

Intraobserver variability A measure of inconsistency in repeated assessments by a single observer.

Joint distribution graph A plot of two continuous variables that can be used to visualize the relationship between the two variables (if one exists) and to determine the direction (positive or negative) and linearity of such a relationship.

Kaplan-Meier method of life table analysis The most commonly used approach to survival analysis in medicine. The Kaplan-Meier method is different from the actuarial method in that the occurrence of each death defines the end of one observation period and the beginning of the next. Therefore, with this method, the duration of observation periods for which survival is determined varies throughout. *See also* Life table analysis.

Kappa test A measure of the extent to which agreement between two observers improves on chance agreement.

Kendall rank correlation test A nonparametric significance test of correlation used for ordinal data.

Kruskal-Wallis one-way ANOVA A nonparametric significance test used to compare three or more groups of ordinal data. It is analogous to the one-way ANOVA used for three or more groups of continuous data.

Kurtosis Vertical distortion of a frequency distribution.

Kwashiorkor A disease that tends to occur in children at the time of weaning, when starchy foods replace breast milk and there is protein deficiency despite nearly adequate calorie intake. The development of ascites (fluid in the abdominal cavity) produces a distended abdomen, which suggests obesity but is actually due to severe undernutrition. Kwashiorkor is also called visceral protein malnutrition.

Late fetal death The death of a product of conception after 28 weeks of gestation but before birth.

Late look bias Bias that occurs when mild, slowly progressive cases of a disease are preferentially detected in a survey because patients with this form of the disease live longer and can be interviewed, whereas more severe cases result in death and go undetected by the survey.

Lead-time bias Bias that occurs when screening detects disease earlier in its natural history than would otherwise have happened, so that the time from diagnosis to death is lengthened. Having additional lead time does not necessarily alter the natural history of the disease and therefore may not indicate longer life.

Leavell's levels Three levels of preventive health care (primary, secondary, and tertiary levels) based on the premise that all of the activities of physicians and other health professionals have the goal of prevention. What is to be prevented depends on the stage of health or disease in the individual receiving preventive care.

Length bias Bias that occurs when milder, more indolent cases of disease are detected disproportionately in population screening programs. More aggressive cases have already resulted in death or in symptoms requiring medical intervention.

Life expectancy Traditionally defined as the average number of years of life remaining at a given age.

Life table analysis A statistical analysis of survival (or another dichotomous outcome) in which proportionate survival is assessed repeatedly over the intervals of observation. This shows the pattern of mortality, as well as the overall rates of death and survival. *See also* Actuarial method of life table analysis and Kaplan-Meier method of life table analysis (the two methods in common use).

Likelihood ratio negative The ratio of the false-negative error rate of a test to the specificity of the test.

Likelihood ratio positive The ratio of the sensitivity of a test to the false-positive error rate of the test.

Linear regression analysis A statistical test of the strength of the linear relationship between one independent and one dependent variable, both of which must be continuous.

Live attenuated vaccines Created by altering infectious organisms so that they are no longer pathogenic but are still viable and antigenic.

Live birth Delivery of a product of conception that shows any sign of life after complete removal from the mother.

Local community hospital Hospital that provides services such as routine diagnosis, treatment, and surgery but lacks the personnel and facilities for complex procedures.

Lockjaw *Same as* Tetanus.

Logrank test A significance test used to compare the rates of survival as determined by Kaplan-Meier life table analysis.

Longitudinal ecologic studies Use of ongoing surveillance or frequent cross-sectional studies to measure trends in disease rates over years in a defined population.

Lyme disease A complex disease that affects multiple systems of the body and results from exposure to the tick-borne pathogen *Borrelia burgdorferi*.

Malaria A febrile illness caused by infection with a mosquito-borne protozoan of the genus *Plasmodium*. Plasmodia are obligate intracellular parasites.

Managed care A system of administrative controls, the primary goal of which is to reduce the costs of medical care.

Mann-Whitney *U* test A nonparametric significance test used to compare two groups of ordinal data. It is analogous to the Student's *t*-test for continuous data.

Marasmus A severe wasting syndrome that affects infants and results from malnutrition. It occurs when all nutrients in the diet are deficient, causing almost total growth retardation.

McNemar chi-square test A modification of the chi-square test for use with paired data. The formula is $(|b - c| - 1)^2 / (b + c)$.

Mean The average value, calculated as the sum of all of the observed values divided by the total number of observations.

Mean deviation The average of the absolute value of the deviations of all observations from the mean.

Mean square Another name for variance, which is defined as a sum of squares divided by the appropriate number of degrees of freedom.

Measles A highly contagious infection caused by a paramyxovirus and recognized particularly by a characteristic maculopapular rash. Measles is effectively prevented by vaccination.

Measurement bias Bias resulting in distorted quantification of exposures or outcome because of improper technique or subjectivity of the measurement scale.

Median The middle observation when data have been arranged in order from the lowest to the highest value.

Medicaid A program funded by general tax revenues of the federal and state governments. The benefits are considered to be social welfare, instead of social insurance.

Medical commons Shared medical resources. An attempt by one individual or group to maximize its own welfare by using more than its fair share of the medical commons would necessarily diminish the good that others can derive from it.

Medically indigent persons People whose incomes are too high to be eligible for Medicaid, who do not receive medical insurance in their jobs, and who are not able to pay for individual medical care insurance policies.

Medicare A program that is administered by the federal government. It pays for the health benefits of most individuals who are 65 years of age or older and of individuals who receive Social Security benefits due to disability.

Meningitis Inflammation of the meninges, which are the sheaths of connective tissue surrounding the brain and spinal cord.

Meta-analysis Used increasingly in medicine to try to obtain a pooled quantitative or qualitative (methodologic) analysis of the research literature on a particular subject.

Metal fume Gaseous metal oxide that comes primarily from activities in occupational settings, such as welding without adequate ventilation.

Metal fume fever An acute syndrome that is usually characterized by flu-like symptoms occurring a few hours after exposure to metal fumes.

Miscarriage *Same as* Early fetal death.

Mode The most commonly observed value in a distribution (i.e., the value with the highest number of observations).

Multiple drug–resistant tuberculosis (MDRTB) An increasingly common type of tuberculosis that is resistant to more than one antimicrobial agent as a result of the failure of patients to complete the prescribed course of treatment with antituberculous drugs.

Multiple linear regression Method used in multivariable analysis if the dependent variable and all of the independent variables are continuous.

Multivariable analysis Analysis of the relationship of more than one independent variable to a single dependent variable.

Multivariable models Statistical models that have one dependent (outcome) variable but include more than one independent variable.

Multivariate analysis A term that is frequently used incorrectly. It refers to methods for analyzing more than one dependent variable as well as more than one independent variable.

Mumps An infectious disease that is caused by a paramyxovirus, occurs most frequently during childhood, and is characterized in particular by parotitis (painful swelling of the parotid glands). The disease is effectively prevented by vaccination.

Myocardial infarction Necrosis of the heart muscle as a result of protracted ischemia.

Natural booster phenomenon An augmentation of immunity that occurs with periodic exposure to an infectious agent. This effect may be lost when immunization prevents exposure.

Necessary cause Precedes a disease and has the following relationship with it: If the cause is absent, the disease cannot occur. If the cause is present, the disease may or may not occur.

Negative predictive value Indicates what proportion of subjects with negative test results are truly free of the disease.

Neyman bias *Same as* Late look bias.

Nominal variables "Naming" or categorical variables that have no measurement scale.

Noncausal association The relationship between two variables is statistically significant, but no causal relationship exists, either because the temporal relationship is incorrect (the presumed cause comes after, rather than before, the presumed effect) or because another factor is responsible for both the presumed cause and the presumed effect.

Nondifferential error Produces findings that are too high and too low in approximately equal amounts, owing to random factors.

Nonparametric data Data for which descriptive parameters such as the mean and standard deviation cannot be obtained, because there is no measurement scale. No assumption is made about the underlying frequency distribution.

Nosocomial infections Hospital-acquired infections, which are more common than is often supposed.

Null hypothesis The hypothesis that there is no real (true) difference between means or proportions of the groups being compared or that there is no real association between two continuous variables. *Compare* Alternative hypothesis.

Number needed to harm (NNH) The number of patients who would need to be treated, on average, for one of them to experience the adverse effects of a particular type of treatment. The NNH is based on the absolute risk increase (ARI). If, for example, the risk of harm is 0.02 without the treatment and 0.05 with the treatment, the ARI = 0.03. The NNH is calculated as 1/ARI. In this example, it would be 1/0.03 = 33.3. *Compare* Number needed to treat.

Number needed to treat (NNT) The number of patients who would need to be treated, on average, for one of them to experience the beneficial effects of a particular type of treatment. The NNT is based on the absolute risk reduction (ARR). If, for example, the risk of benefit is 0.10 with the treatment and 0.04 without the treatment, the ARR = 0.06. The NNT is calculated as 1/ARR. In this example, it would be 1/0.06 = 16.7. *Compare* Number needed to harm.

Numerator data Data that define the events or conditions of concern.

Nursing home *Same as* Skilled nursing facility.

***N*-Way ANOVA** *See* Analysis of variance (ANOVA).

Occupational asthma A bronchospastic disease whose symptoms occur during periods of exposure to respiratory tract irritants in the workplace. The symptoms are usually less pronounced during periods away from work, such as weekends.

Odds ratio (OR) The odds of exposure in the diseased group divided by the odds of exposure in the nondiseased group.

One-way ANOVA *See* Analysis of variance (ANOVA).

Ordinal variables Medical data that can be characterized in terms of more than two values and have a clearly implied direction from better to worse but are not measured on a continuous measurement scale.

Outbreak Often used to denote a local epidemic (may be considered interchangeable with the term *epidemic*).

Outliers Extreme values that are widely deviant from the mean.

Overall percent agreement The percentage of the total observations found in cells *a* and *d* of a 2×2 table.

p **Value** The probability that the observed difference could have been obtained by chance alone, given random variation and a single test of the null hypothesis.

Parametric data Data for which descriptive parameters (typically the mean and standard deviation) are known and define the underlying frequency distribution of the data. The underlying distribution is often assumed to be normal, as provided in the central limit theorem.

Particulate matter Small solid particles dispersed in air. An example is the matter that results from cigarette smoking or from fuel combustion, which often contains carcinogenic substances.

Passive immunity Protection against an infectious disease provided by circulating antibodies made in another organism.

Passive surveillance Reporting of disease by physicians, laboratories, and hospitals on a voluntary basis.

Pathogenicity of an organism Calculated as the proportion of infected individuals who are clinically ill.

Pathognomonic test A test whose results, if positive, are synonymous with having the disease.

Pearson correlation coefficient A measure of strength of the linear relationship between two continuous variables.

Peptic ulcer disease A disease that is associated with hypersecretion of gastric acid and is characterized by erosions of the stomach or duodenum. The disease is often caused by the bacterium *Helicobacter pylori*.

Period prevalence The number of persons who had the disease of interest at any time during the specified time interval. It is the sum of the point prevalence at the beginning of the interval plus the incidence during the interval.

Person-time A unit of time used in studies in which persons are observed for unequal periods. For example, when one person is observed for 3 months, another for 14 months, and another for 7 months, the amount of time can be expressed as 24 person-months or 2 person-years.

Person-time methods of analysis Methods that control for the fact that the length of observation of persons in a study will vary. These methods are used in calculating incidence density.

Pertussis An acute, highly contagious respiratory tract infection that is characterized by paroxysmal coughing, is commonly called whooping cough, and is caused by the bacterium *Bordetella pertussis*.

Pneumococcal infection An infection caused by *Streptococcus pneumoniae*. This bacterium is a common cause of community-acquired pneumonia.

Pneumoconiosis A pulmonary injury caused by deposition of respirable particulate matter in the lungs and by the resulting inflammatory response.

Point prevalence The number of cases in the study population at one point in time.

Poliomyelitis A febrile viral disease that results in paralysis in severe cases. The disease is preventable by vaccination and is targeted for eradication by the World Health Organization.

Population attributable risk The risk in the total population minus the risk in the unexposed group. The population attributable risk answers this question: Among the general population, how much of the total risk for the disease of interest is due to the risk factor (exposure) of interest?

Population attributable risk percent (PAR%) The PAR% answers this question: Among the general population, what percentage of the total risk for the disease of interest is due to the risk factor (exposure) of interest?

Positive predictive value The proportion of subjects with positive test results who actually have the disease of interest.

Posterior probability Revised estimate of the probability of disease in a given patient following a diagnostic test or intervention.

Precision The ability of an instrument to provide the same or a very similar result with repeated measurements.

Prediction model A model, complete with coefficients, for use in predicting a particular outcome given the presence of a variety of independent variables.

Preferred provider organization (PPO) Formed when a third-party payer (e.g., an insurance plan or a company) establishes a network of contracts with independent practitioners. The patients in a PPO can see practitioners who are not members of the network, although they will have to pay a surcharge for their services.

Prevalence The number of persons in a defined population who have a specified disease or condition at a point in time, usually the time a survey is done.

Prevalence rate The proportion of persons with a defined disease or condition at the time they are studied. This is not truly a rate, although it is conventionally referred to as one.

Preventive medicine A medical specialty emphasizing practices that help individuals and populations promote and preserve health and avoid injury and illness.

Prior probability The probability of disease in a given patient that is estimated prior to the performance of laboratory or other tests and is based on the estimated prevalence of a particular disease among patients with similar signs and symptoms.

Product-limit method of life table analysis *Same as* Kaplan-Meier method of life table analysis.

Prognostic stratification *Same as* Stratified allocation.

Proportional hazards method A method used to test for differences between Kaplan-Meier survival curves while controlling for other variables. The method is also used to determine which variables are associated with better survival.

Proportional hazards model A modification of multiple logistic regression to permit multivariable modeling of the data in a life table analysis.

Prospective cohort study The investigator assembles the study groups in the present time on the basis of exposure, collects baseline data on them, and follows subjects over time for the outcomes of interest.

Prospective payment system (PPS) based on diagnosis-related groups (DRGs) Each hospital admission is classified into one of 23 major diagnostic categories based on organ systems, and these diagnostic categories are further subdivided into DRGs. A DRG may consist of a single diagnosis or procedure, or it may consist of several diagnoses or procedures that, on average, have similar hospital costs per admission.

Public health (1) The health status of the public (i.e., of a defined population). (2) The organized social efforts made to preserve and improve the health of a defined population.

Qualitative characteristic A characteristic that must be described in detail but is not truly measurable.

Quantitative characteristic A characteristic that can be described by a rigid, dimensional measurement scale.

Quality-adjusted life years (QALY) A health status index that incorporates both life expectancy and the perceived impact of illness and disability on the quality of life.

Rabies A highly virulent viral infection of the central nervous system, which is spread to humans from infected animals and is usually preventable by postexposure prophylaxis.

Random error Produces findings that are too high and too low in approximately equal amounts, owing to random factors.

Random sampling Entails selecting a small group for study from a much larger group of potential study subjects.

Randomization Entails allocating the available subjects to one or another study group and is generally used in clinical studies.

Randomized controlled clinical trials (RCCTs) Studies designed to test a therapeutic measure. Subjects are randomly assigned to one of the following groups: (1) the intervention group, which will receive the experimental treatment, or (2) the control group, which will receive the nonexperimental treatment, consisting of either a placebo (inert substance) or a standard method of treatment.

Randomized controlled field trials (RCFTs) Studies that are similar to RCCTs (described above) but are designed to test a preventive measure, such as a vaccine. Susceptible persons are randomized into two groups and are then given the vaccine or a placebo, usually at the beginning of the high-risk season of the year. Testing the efficacy of vaccines by RCFTs is costly, but it may be required the first time a new vaccine is introduced.

Ranked variables *Same as* Ordinal variables.

Rapid sand filtration A technique for purifying water by adding a flocculent (usually aluminum sulfate, called alum) to the water before filtration. The flocculent coagulates and traps suspended materials, thereby preventing them from passing through the sand with the filtered water. The flocculent is removed periodically by back flushing, and new flocculent is added to the next batch of water.

Rate The frequency (number) of events that occur in a defined time period, divided by the average population at risk.

Rate difference Similar to risk difference but applied to rates.

Ratio variables The variables derived from a continuous scale that has a true 0 point.

Recall bias Bias resulting from differential recall of exposure to causal factors among those who have a disease as compared with those who do not have it.

Regression toward the mean Patients chosen to participate in a study precisely because they had an extreme measurement on some variable are likely to have a measurement that is closer to average at a later time for reasons unrelated to the type or efficacy of the treatment they are given. Regression toward the mean is also known as the statistical regression effect.

Rehabilitation An attempt to mitigate the effects of disease and thereby prevent or limit social and functional disability.

Relative risk (RR) The ratio of the risk in the exposed group to the risk in the unexposed group, which is expressed as $RR = Risk_{(exposed)} / Risk_{(unexposed)} = [a/(a+b)]/[c/(c+d)]$.

Renal disease *See* Acute tubular necrosis and Chronic renal disease.

Resource-based relative value scale (RBRVS) A method of rating the relative value of outpatient diagnosis and treatment, based on the average time that the care giver (physician or other practitioner) spends with the patient, the years of training and skill required by the care giver, and the cost of the equipment needed. The RBRVS was created to reimburse primary care practitioners more fairly in a reimbursement system that tended to pay more for procedures than for clinical time and judgment.

Retrospective cohort study Cohorts are identified on the basis of *past* exposure and followed forward to the present for the occurrence of the outcome of interest.

Rheumatic fever An immune-mediated inflammatory condition that occurs following streptococcal infection and can result in permanent damage to the kidneys and heart valves.

Risk Calculated as the proportion of persons who are unaffected at the beginning of a study period but who undergo the risk event during the study period.

Risk difference The risk in the exposed group minus the risk in the unexposed group.

Risk event Death, disease, or injury.

Risk factor A characteristic that, if present and active, clearly increases the probability of a particular disease in a group of persons who have the factor compared with an otherwise similar group of persons who do not. A risk factor is neither a necessary cause nor a sufficient cause of the disease.

Risk ratio *Same as* Relative risk.

Rubella An acute respiratory tract infection caused by a togavirus. Although the infection is usually benign and self-limited, it can cause death or severe injury to an embryo if maternal infection occurs during the first trimester. Rubella is also known as German measles and is prevented by vaccination.

Sabin oral polio vaccine (OPV) A vaccine that provides herd immunity to poliomyelitis and has resulted in the apparent eradication of wild virus from the western hemisphere. The oral vaccine is made from live virus and has produced clinical illness under certain circumstances.

Salk polio vaccine An injectable vaccine that provides individual immunity to poliomyelitis but is less effective at interrupting transmission than is the live attenuated vaccine.

Schmutzdecke *See* Slow sand filtration.

Screening The process of identifying a subgroup of people who are at high probability of having asymptomatic disease or who have a risk factor that puts them at high risk for developing a disease or becoming injured. Screening takes place in a community setting and is applied to a community population, such as students in a school or workers in an industry. *Compare* Case finding.

Selection bias Bias resulting when the allocation of individuals to a study or to a particular study group is influenced by individual characteristics that also influence the probability of the outcome.

Sensitivity The ability of a test to detect a disease when it is present.

Sentinel health event An adverse health event (death, disease, or impairment) that serves to identify a potential threat to the public health.

Shingles *Same as* Herpes zoster.

Sick building syndrome A group of workers may suffer from a constellation of symptoms (such as headache, watery eyes, and wheezing) and ascribe these symptoms to the building in which they work. The syndrome often, but not always, occurs in buildings that are tightly sealed for energy conservation or are not well ventilated. The cause of the symptoms seems to vary from one building to the next but is, in essence, unknown.

Sign of life A breath, a cry, a pulsation of the umbilical cord, or any spontaneous movement at the time of birth.

Sign test A nonparametric significance test for use with continuous, ordinal, or dichotomous data. The sign test is used to determine whether or not, on average, one group experienced a better outcome on significantly more variables than another group.

Silicosis A type of pneumoconiosis that results from inhalation of the dust of stones or sand containing silicon dioxide. *See* Pneumoconiosis.

Skewness Horizontal distortion of a frequency distribution, so that one tail of the plot is longer and contains more observations than the other.

Skilled nursing facility (SNF) Usually provides specialized care, such as intravenous fluids and medicines. A registered (skilled) nurse must be on duty at all times.

Sleeping sickness A form of trypanosomiasis endemic in parts of Africa. It is spread by the bite of the tsetse fly.

Slow sand filtration A technique for purifying water by filtering it through a large bed of packed sand, on which an organic layer (the *Schmutzdecke,* German for "dirt layer") forms and assists in the filtration process.

Smallpox An acute infectious disease characterized by distinctive skin eruptions. Smallpox has now been eradicated worldwide as a result of successful vaccination.

Spearman rank correlation test A test that is analogous to the Pearson correlation coefficient but is used for ranked data.

Specific rates Rates that pertain to some homogeneous subgroup of the population, such as an age group, gender group, or ethnic group.

Specificity The ability of a test to indicate nondisease when no disease is present.

Staff model health maintenance organization (staff model HMO) Most of the physicians in this type of HMO are salaried, full-time employees who work exclusively for the HMO or belong to a physician group that contracts to provide all of the medical services to the HMO. Some specialists may be retained on part-time contracts. The HMO may have its own hospitals or may hospitalize its patients in one or more local hospitals, in which case the local hospitals are not usually a formal part of the HMO.

Standard deviation (SD) The square root of the variance.

Standard error (SE) The standard deviation (SD) of a population of sample means, rather than of individual observations. The SE is calculated as the observed SD divided by the square root of N.

Standard error of the difference between the means (SED) The square root of the sum of the respective population variances, each divided by its own sample size.

Standardized mortality ratio (SMR)   The observed total events in the study group, divided by the expected number of events based on the standard population rates applied to the study group. The constant multiplier for this measure is 100.

Standardized rates   Crude rates that have been modified so as to allow for valid comparisons of rates. Standardization is usually necessary to correct for differing age distributions in different populations. *See* Direct standardization and Indirect standardization.

Statistical regression effect   *Same as* Regression toward the mean.

Statistical significance   A result is statistically significant whenever a significance test produces a *p* value less than the preset value of alpha, which is conventionally 0.05. The implication of statistical significance at an alpha of 0.05 is that chance would produce such a difference between comparison groups no more often than 5 times out of 100. This is taken to mean that chance is not responsible for the outcome.

Stillbirth   *Same as* Late fetal death.

Stratified allocation   Assignment of patients to different risk groups on the basis of variables such as the severity of disease (e.g., stage of cancer) and age.

Strength of association   The degree to which variation in one variable explains variation in another. The greater the strength of association between variables, the more completely variation in one predicts variation in the other.

Strep throat   Infection of the oropharynx by group A beta-hemolytic streptococci (*Streptococcus pyogenes*).

Sufficient cause   Precedes a disease and has the following relationship with it: If the cause is present, the disease will always occur.

Surface water   Surface sources of potable water, including protected surface reservoirs, lakes, and rivers.

Surveillance   *See* Active surveillance and Passive surveillance.

Synergy   Is present when the impact that two or more factors have on an individual or population is greater than the sum of the separate effects of each factor.

Syphilis   A sexually transmitted infectious disease caused by the spirochete *Treponema pallidum*. The disease is most communicable in its early stages. Early treatment with penicillin prevents disease progression to late stages but consequently permits reinfection. Reinfection may lead to greater rates of transmission if the highly infectious early stages of the disease occur repeatedly in the same individual.

Tertiary medical center   Hospital that has most or all of the latest technology and usually participates actively in medical education and even in clinical research.

Tetanus   Acute infection with the bacterium *Clostridium tetani*. The bacterium produces a neurotoxin that can cause severe muscle spasm and paralysis. Tetanus is also known as lockjaw.

Threshold level   The level below which the body can adapt to an adverse exposure successfully and with little or no harm resulting. There is such a threshold level for most chemical and physical agents and even for most microbes. Usually, nonthreshold exposures are limited to those that alter genetic material, thereby producing genetic mutations and potentially causing cancer. Ionizing radiation is currently considered a nonthreshold exposure.

Total variation   Equal to the sum of the squared deviations from the mean. It is usually called the total sum of squares (TSS) but is sometimes referred to simply as the sum of squares (SS).

Toxoids   Inactivated or altered bacterial exotoxins, such as diphtheria vaccine and tetanus vaccine.

Trypanosomiasis   Infection with protozoa of the genus *Trypanosoma*.

t-Tests   Tests that compare differences between two means.

Tuberculosis   Diverse clinical manifestations resulting from infection with *Mycobacterium tuberculosis*.

Type I error   Error that occurs when data lead one to conclude that something is true when in reality it is not true. Type I error is also called alpha error and false-positive error.

Type II error   Error that occurs when data lead one to conclude that something is false when in reality it is true. Type II error is also called beta error and false-negative error.

Typhoid   An acute febrile illness caused by ingestion of food contaminated with *Salmonella typhi*. Typhoid is also known as typhoid fever.

Unit of observation   The source of data in a medical study. The unit is usually a study participant.

Utilization management   *Same as* Managed care.

Validity   *See* External validity and Internal validity.

Variable   A measure of a single characteristic.

Variance   The sum of the squared deviations from the mean, divided by the number of observations minus 1.

Varicella   *Same as* Chickenpox.

Vector   A factor in disease transmission, often an insect, that carries the agent to the host.

Visceral protein malnutrition   *Same as* Kwashiorkor.

Whooping cough   *Same as* Pertussis.

Wilcoxon matched-pairs signed-ranks test   A nonparametric significance test used to compare paired, ordinal data. It is analogous to the paired *t*-test for continuous data.

Within-groups mean square   *Same as* Within-groups variance.

Within-groups variance   Measurement based on the variation within each group (i.e., variation around a single group mean).

Workers' compensation laws   Laws stipulating that

people with a job-related injury or illness have their medical and rehabilitation expenses paid and also receive a certain amount of cash payments in lieu of wages while they are recuperating.

Yates correction for continuity An adjustment to the chi-square value recommended when counts in the contingency table are small, because the binomial distribution is discontinuous.

Yellow fever An acute, mosquito-borne infectious disease caused by a flavivirus. The clinical manifestations are variable.

z-**Tests** Significance tests used to compare differences between proportions.

Appendix

TABLE A   **Random Numbers***

53872	34774	19087	81775	71440	12082	75092	34608	75448	13148
04226	62404	71577	00984	56056	32404	87641	53392	92561	33388
28666	44190	75524	62038	21423	46281	92238	96306	72606	80601
63817	30279	14088	86434	16183	06401	90586	80292	54555	47371
22359	16442	83879	47486	19838	32252	39560	95851	36758	36141
50968	28728	83525	16031	77583	65578	84794	51367	32535	83834
39652	24248	96617	91200	10769	52386	39559	75921	49375	22847
35493	00529	69632	29684	80284	87828	72418	80950	86311	34016
75687	53919	80439	20534	96185	72345	96391	52625	50866	45132
31509	93521	10681	44124	88345	84969	88768	48819	22311	41235
40389	76282	37506	60661	23295	67357	95419	10864	87833	09152
59244	54664	63424	97899	44153	69251	08781	18604	02312	21658
99876	17075	40934	08912	96196	58503	63613	24486	98092	45672
06457	50072	18060	71023	84349	40984	59487	77782	32107	53770
14297	07687	05517	10362	35783	62236	63764	45542	68889	03862
51661	57130	97442	29590	21634	79772	73801	70122	46467	47152
53455	41788	16117	09698	24409	05079	76603	57563	33461	46791
48086	31512	62819	27689	63744	11023	11184	87679	22218	70139
19108	01602	96950	41536	39974	88287	83546	69187	45539	78263
39001	77727	33095	58785	29179	45421	71416	20418	38558	78700
72346	55617	14714	21930	14851	38209	52202	03979	05970	74483
19094	64359	89829	10942	53101	37758	29583	26792	42840	45872
82247	77127	01652	50774	04970	83300	33760	22172	67516	62135
75968	18386	31874	52249	21015	20365	57475	32756	58268	75739
01963	38095	99960	91307	99654	74279	80145	53303	11870	50485
64828	15817	80923	55226	51893	93362	15757	47430	84855	95822
64347	61578	44160	06266	35118	52558	56436	96155	10293	67506
54746	52337	84826	39012	59118	19851	10156	78167	41473	99025
22241	41501	02993	99340	91044	67268	51088	12751	74008	33773
11906	20043	10415	44425	31712	54831	85591	62237	88797	14382
76637	07609	95378	95580	86909	50609	99008	99042	50364	36664
93896	47120	98926	30636	28136	49458	84145	79205	79517	93446
75292	88232	14360	12455	13656	65736	70428	66917	64412	38502
98792	29828	10577	48184	29433	98278	22543	76155	82107	22066
65751	91049	94127	47558	99880	79667	86254	72797	67117	44699
72064	62102	39155	79462	82975	02638	00302	79476	72656	84003
01227	35821	80607	61734	02600	45564	72344	71034	48370	96826
44768	56504	13993	59701	88238	92483	09497	66058	36651	37927
69838	91226	85736	72247	64099	86305	49877	76215	66980	30228
01800	39313	57730	84410	47637	01369	51830	43536	58937	91901
11756	45441	59948	57975	92422	70057	50210	30345	55912	31638
39056	86614	53643	62909	27198	04454	33789	86463	66603	48083
88086	93172	68311	39164	42012	10447	45933	28844	36844	57684
12648	27948	76750	19915	66815	34015	43011	27150	94264	89516
16254	87661	66181	68609	58626	58428	75051	27558	49463	66646
69682	19109	94189	94626	09299	10649	55405	54571	57855	54921
61336	86663	13010	40412	50139	30769	13048	61407	41056	60510
65727	66488	12304	70011	93324	58764	87274	43103	96002	06984
55705	34418	99410	32635	42984	40981	91750	27431	05142	77950
95402	51746	98184	38830	97590	00066	82770	42325	28778	83571
79228	94510	57711	64366	89040	43278	69072	22003	89465	61483
48103	56760	82564	33649	35176	32278	51357	05489	47462	55931
70969	27677	99621	63065	73194	70462	19316	77945	45004	39895
69931	20237	75246	59124	12484	22012	79731	82435	56301	99752
37208	22741	41946	74109	03760	24094	40210	76617	52317	50643
60151	92327	85150	27728	64813	47667	66078	03628	95240	03808
46210	47674	53747	95354	67757	75477	26396	09592	96239	50854
55399	48142	12284	95298	56399	61358	87541	12998	79639	63633
23677	64950	97041	43088	80143	34294	91468	01066	90350	78891
41947	70066	90311	17133	11674	00826	75760	37586	33621	14199

Source of data: RAND Corporation. A Million Random Digits with 100,000 Normal Deviates. New York, Free Press, 1955. Copyright 1955 and 1983 by the RAND Corporation. Used by permission.

***Instructions for use of the table:** Decide in advance how many table columns will be used and in what direction the numbers will be assigned after the starting point is identified. Then blindly put a pencil on the table, and start with the numbers nearest the pencil point, moving in the predetermined direction (e.g., moving up the columns).

TABLE B   Standard Normal-Tail Probabilities (Table of z Values)*

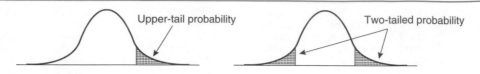

z	Upper-Tail Probability	Two-Tailed Probability	z	Upper-Tail Probability	Two-Tailed Probability
0.00	0.5000	1.0000	0.36	0.3594	0.7188
0.01	0.4960	0.9920	0.37	0.3557	0.7114
0.02	0.4920	0.9840	0.38	0.3520	0.7039
0.0251	0.49	0.98	0.3853	0.35	0.70
0.03	0.4880	0.9761	0.39	0.3483	0.6965
0.04	0.4840	0.9681	0.40	0.3446	0.6892
0.05	0.4801	0.9601	0.41	0.3409	0.6818
0.0502	0.48	0.96	0.4125	0.34	0.68
0.06	0.4761	0.9522	0.42	0.3372	0.6745
0.07	0.4721	0.9442	0.43	0.3336	0.6672
0.0753	0.47	0.94	0.4399	0.33	0.66
0.08	0.4681	0.9362	0.44	0.3300	0.6599
0.09	0.4641	0.9283	0.45	0.3264	0.6527
0.10	0.4602	0.9203	0.46	0.3228	0.6455
0.1004	0.46	0.92	0.4677	0.32	0.64
0.11	0.4562	0.9124	0.47	0.3192	0.6384
0.12	0.4522	0.9045	0.48	0.3156	0.6312
0.1257	0.45	0.9	0.49	0.3121	0.6241
0.13	0.4483	0.8966	0.4959	0.31	0.62
0.14	0.4443	0.8887	0.50	0.3085	0.6171
0.15	0.4404	0.8808	0.51	0.3050	0.6101
0.1510	0.44	0.88	0.52	0.3015	0.6031
0.16	0.4364	0.8729	0.5244	0.3	0.6
0.17	0.4325	0.8650	0.53	0.2981	0.5961
0.1764	0.43	0.86	0.54	0.2946	0.5892
0.18	0.4286	0.8571	0.55	0.2912	0.5823
0.19	0.4247	0.8493	0.5534	0.29	0.58
0.20	0.4207	0.8415	0.56	0.2877	0.5755
0.2019	0.42	0.84	0.57	0.2843	0.5687
0.21	0.4168	0.8337	0.58	0.2810	0.5619
0.22	0.4129	0.8259	0.5828	0.28	0.56
0.2275	0.41	0.82	0.59	0.2776	0.5552
0.23	0.4090	0.8181	0.60	0.2743	0.5485
0.24	0.4052	0.8103	0.61	0.2709	0.5419
0.25	0.4013	0.8026	0.6128	0.27	0.54
0.2533	0.40	0.80	0.62	0.2676	0.5353
0.26	0.3974	0.7949	0.63	0.2643	0.5287
0.27	0.3936	0.7872	0.64	0.2611	0.5222
0.2793	0.39	0.78	0.6433	0.26	0.52
0.28	0.3897	0.7795	0.65	0.2578	0.5157
0.29	0.3859	0.7718	0.66	0.2546	0.5093
0.30	0.3821	0.7642	0.67	0.2514	0.5029
0.3055	0.38	0.76	0.6745	0.25	0.50
0.31	0.3783	0.7566	0.68	0.2483	0.4956
0.32	0.3745	0.7490	0.69	0.2451	0.4902
0.33	0.3707	0.7414	0.70	0.2420	0.4839
0.3319	0.37	0.74	0.7063	0.24	0.48
0.34	0.3669	0.7339	0.71	0.2389	0.4777
0.35	0.3632	0.7263	0.72	0.2358	0.4715
0.3585	0.36	0.72	0.73	0.2327	0.4654

TABLE B Standard Normal-Tail Probabilities (Table of z Values)* *Continued*

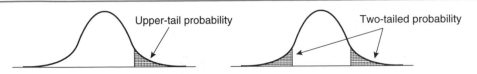

Upper-tail probability   Two-tailed probability

z	Upper-Tail Probability	Two-Tailed Probability	z	Upper-Tail Probability	Two-Tailed Probability
0.7388	0.23	0.46	1.13	0.1292	0.2585
0.74	0.2296	0.4593	1.14	0.1271	0.2543
0.75	0.2266	0.4533	1.15	0.1251	0.2501
0.76	0.2236	0.4473	1.16	0.1230	0.2460
0.77	0.2206	0.4413	1.17	0.1210	0.2420
0.7722	0.22	0.44	1.175	0.12	0.24
0.78	0.2177	0.4354	1.18	0.1190	0.2380
0.79	0.2148	0.4295	1.19	0.1170	0.2340
0.80	0.2119	0.4237	1.20	0.1151	0.2301
0.8064	0.21	0.42	1.21	0.1131	0.2263
0.81	0.2090	0.4179	1.22	0.1112	0.2225
0.82	0.2061	0.4122	1.227	0.11	0.22
0.83	0.2033	0.4065	1.23	0.1093	0.2187
0.84	0.2005	0.4009	1.24	0.1075	0.2150
0.8416	0.20	0.40	1.25	0.1056	0.2113
0.85	0.1977	0.3953	1.26	0.1038	0.2077
0.86	0.1949	0.3898	1.27	0.1020	0.2041
0.87	0.1922	0.3843	1.28	0.1003	0.2005
0.8779	0.19	0.38	1.282	0.10	0.20
0.88	0.1894	0.3789	1.29	0.0985	0.1971
0.89	0.1867	0.3735	1.30	0.0968	0.1936
0.90	0.1841	0.3681	1.31	0.0951	0.1902
0.91	0.1814	0.3628	1.32	0.0934	0.1868
0.9154	0.18	0.36	1.33	0.0918	0.1835
0.92	0.1788	0.3576	1.34	0.0901	0.1802
0.93	0.1762	0.3524	1.341	0.09	0.18
0.94	0.1736	0.3472	1.35	0.0885	0.1770
0.95	0.1711	0.3421	1.36	0.0869	0.1738
0.9542	0.17	0.34	1.37	0.0853	0.1707
0.96	0.1685	0.3371	1.38	0.0838	0.1676
0.97	0.1660	0.3320	1.39	0.0823	0.1645
0.98	0.1635	0.3271	1.40	0.0808	0.1615
0.99	0.1611	0.3222	1.405	0.08	0.16
0.9945	0.16	0.32	1.41	0.0793	0.1585
1.00	0.1587	0.3173	1.42	0.0778	0.1556
1.01	0.1562	0.3125	1.43	0.0764	0.1527
1.02	0.1539	0.3077	1.44	0.0749	0.1499
1.03	0.1515	0.3030	1.45	0.0735	0.1471
1.036	0.15	0.3	1.46	0.0721	0.1443
1.04	0.1492	0.2983	1.47	0.0708	0.1416
1.05	0.1469	0.2937	1.476	0.07	0.14
1.06	0.1446	0.2891	1.48	0.0694	0.1389
1.07	0.1423	0.2846	1.49	0.0681	0.1362
1.08	0.1401	0.2801	1.50	0.0668	0.1336
1.080	0.14	0.28	1.51	0.0655	0.1310
1.09	0.1379	0.2757	1.52	0.0643	0.1285
1.10	0.1357	0.2713	1.53	0.0630	0.1260
1.11	0.1335	0.2670	1.54	0.0618	0.1236
1.12	0.1314	0.2627	1.55	0.0606	0.1211
1.1264	0.13	0.26	1.555	0.06	0.12

Table continued on following page

TABLE B   Standard Normal-Tail Probabilities (Table of z Values)* Continued

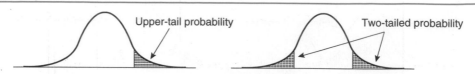

z	Upper-Tail Probability	Two-Tailed Probability	z	Upper-Tail Probability	Two-Tailed Probability
1.56	0.0594	0.1188	2.03	0.0212	0.0424
1.57	0.0582	0.1164	2.04	0.0207	0.0414
1.58	0.0571	0.1141	2.05	0.0202	0.0404
1.59	0.0559	0.1118	2.054	0.02	0.04
1.60	0.0548	0.1096	2.06	0.0197	0.0394
1.61	0.0537	0.1074	2.07	0.0192	0.0385
1.62	0.0526	0.1052	2.08	0.0188	0.0375
1.63	0.0516	0.1031	2.09	0.0183	0.0366
1.64	0.0505	0.1010	2.10	0.0179	0.0357
1.645	0.05	0.10	2.11	0.0174	0.0349
1.65	0.0495	0.0989	2.12	0.0170	0.0340
1.66	0.0485	0.0969	2.13	0.0166	0.0332
1.67	0.0475	0.0949	2.14	0.0162	0.0324
1.68	0.0465	0.0930	2.15	0.0158	0.0316
1.69	0.0455	0.0910	2.16	0.0154	0.0308
1.70	0.0446	0.0891	2.17	0.0150	0.0300
1.71	0.0436	0.0873	2.18	0.0146	0.0293
1.72	0.0427	0.0854	2.19	0.0143	0.0285
1.73	0.0418	0.0836	2.20	0.0139	0.0278
1.74	0.0409	0.0819	2.21	0.0136	0.0271
1.75	0.0401	0.0801	2.22	0.0132	0.0264
1.751	0.04	0.08	2.23	0.0129	0.0257
1.76	0.0392	0.0784	2.24	0.0125	0.0251
1.77	0.0384	0.0767	2.25	0.0122	0.0244
1.78	0.0375	0.0751	2.26	0.0119	0.0238
1.79	0.0367	0.0734	2.27	0.0116	0.0232
1.80	0.0359	0.0719	2.28	0.0113	0.0226
1.81	0.0352	0.0703	2.29	0.0110	0.0220
1.82	0.0344	0.0688	2.30	0.0107	0.0214
1.83	0.0336	0.0672	2.31	0.0104	0.0209
1.84	0.0329	0.0658	2.32	0.0102	0.0203
1.85	0.0322	0.0643	2.326	0.01	0.02
1.86	0.0314	0.0629	2.33	0.0099	0.0198
1.87	0.0307	0.0615	2.34	0.0096	0.0193
1.88	0.0301	0.0601	2.35	0.0094	0.0188
1.881	0.03	0.06	2.36	0.0091	0.0183
1.89	0.0294	0.0588	2.37	0.0089	0.0178
1.90	0.0287	0.0574	2.38	0.0087	0.0173
1.91	0.0281	0.0561	2.39	0.0084	0.0168
1.92	0.0274	0.0549	2.40	0.0082	0.0164
1.93	0.0268	0.0536	2.41	0.0080	0.0160
1.94	0.0262	0.0524	2.42	0.0078	0.0155
1.95	0.0256	0.0512	2.43	0.0075	0.0151
1.960	0.025	0.05	2.44	0.0073	0.0147
1.97	0.0244	0.0488	2.45	0.0071	0.0143
1.98	0.0239	0.0477	2.46	0.0069	0.0139
1.99	0.0233	0.0466	2.47	0.0068	0.0135
2.00	0.0228	0.0455	2.48	0.0066	0.0131
2.01	0.0222	0.0444	2.49	0.0064	0.0128
2.02	0.0217	0.0434	2.50	0.0062	0.0124

TABLE B   Standard Normal-Tail Probabilities (Table of z Values)* *Continued*

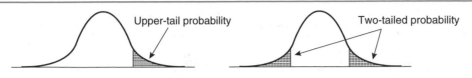

z	Upper-Tail Probability	Two-Tailed Probability	z	Upper-Tail Probability	Two-Tailed Probability
2.51	0.0060	0.0121	2.90	0.0019	0.0037
2.52	0.0059	0.0117	2.95	0.0016	0.0032
2.53	0.0057	0.0114	3.00	0.0013	0.0027
2.54	0.0055	0.0111	3.05	0.0011	0.0023
2.55	0.0054	0.0108	3.090	0.001	0.002
2.56	0.0052	0.0105	3.10	0.0010	0.0019
2.57	0.0051	0.0102	3.15	0.0008	0.0016
2.576	0.005	0.01	3.20	0.0007	0.0014
2.58	0.0049	0.0099	3.25	0.0006	0.0012
2.59	0.0048	0.0096	3.291	0.0005	0.001
2.60	0.0047	0.0093	3.30	0.0005	0.0010
2.61	0.0045	0.0091	3.35	0.0004	0.0008
2.62	0.0044	0.0088	3.40	0.0003	0.0007
2.63	0.0043	0.0085	3.45	0.0003	0.0006
2.64	0.0041	0.0083	3.50	0.0002	0.0005
2.65	0.0040	0.0080	3.55	0.0002	0.0004
2.70	0.0035	0.0069	3.60	0.0002	0.0003
2.75	0.0030	0.0060	3.65	0.0001	0.0003
2.80	0.0026	0.0051	3.70	0.0001	0.0002
2.85	0.0022	0.0044	3.75	0.0001	0.0002
			3.80	0.0001	0.0001

Source of data: National Bureau of Standards. Applied Mathematics Series—23. US Government Printing Office, Washington, D. C., 1953. Abstracted by Shott, S. Statistics for Health Professionals. Philadelphia, W. B. Saunders Company, 1990. Used by permission.
*Instructions for use of the table to determine the *p* value that corresponds to a calculated *z* value: In the left-hand column (headed *z*), look up the value of *z* found from calculations. Look at the first column to the right (for a one-tailed *p* value) or the second column to the right (for a two-tailed *p* value) that corresponds to the value of *z* obtained. For example, a *z* value of 1.74 corresponds to a two-tailed *p* value of 0.0819. **Instructions for use of the table to determine the *z* value that corresponds to a chosen *p* value:** To find the appropriate *z* value for use in confidence limits or sample size determinations, define the one-tailed or two-tailed *p* value desired, look that up in the second or third column, respectively, and determine the *z* value on the left that corresponds. For example, for a two-tailed alpha at 0.05, the corresponding *z* is 1.960; and for a one-tailed beta of 0.20, the corresponding *z* is 0.8416.

TABLE C   **Upper Percentage Points for t Distributions***

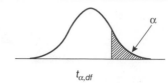

	Upper-Tail Probability						
df	0.40	0.30	0.20	0.15	0.10	0.05	0.025
1	0.325	0.727	1.376	1.963	3.078	6.314	12.706
2	0.289	0.617	1.061	1.386	1.886	2.920	4.303
3	0.277	0.584	0.978	1.250	1.638	2.353	3.182
4	0.271	0.569	0.941	1.190	1.533	2.132	2.776
5	0.267	0.559	0.920	1.156	1.476	2.015	2.571
6	0.265	0.553	0.906	1.134	1.440	1.943	2.447
7	0.263	0.549	0.896	1.119	1.415	1.895	2.365
8	0.262	0.546	0.889	1.108	1.397	1.860	2.306
9	0.261	0.543	0.883	1.100	1.383	1.833	2.262
10	0.260	0.542	0.879	1.093	1.372	1.812	2.228
11	0.260	0.540	0.876	1.088	1.363	1.796	2.201
12	0.259	0.539	0.873	1.083	1.356	1.782	2.179
13	0.259	0.537	0.870	1.079	1.350	1.771	2.160
14	0.258	0.537	0.868	1.076	1.345	1.761	2.145
15	0.258	0.536	0.866	1.074	1.341	1.753	2.131
16	0.258	0.535	0.865	1.071	1.337	1.746	2.120
17	0.257	0.534	0.863	1.069	1.333	1.740	2.110
18	0.257	0.534	0.862	1.067	1.330	1.734	2.101
19	0.257	0.533	0.861	1.066	1.328	1.729	2.093
20	0.257	0.533	0.860	1.064	1.325	1.725	2.086
21	0.257	0.532	0.859	1.063	1.323	1.721	2.080
22	0.256	0.532	0.858	1.061	1.321	1.717	2.074
23	0.256	0.532	0.858	1.060	1.319	1.714	2.069
24	0.256	0.531	0.857	1.059	1.318	1.711	2.064
25	0.256	0.531	0.856	1.058	1.316	1.708	2.060
26	0.256	0.531	0.856	1.058	1.315	1.706	2.056
27	0.256	0.531	0.855	1.057	1.314	1.703	2.052
28	0.256	0.530	0.855	1.056	1.313	1.701	2.048
29	0.256	0.530	0.854	1.055	1.311	1.699	2.045
30	0.256	0.530	0.854	1.055	1.310	1.697	2.042
40	0.255	0.529	0.851	1.050	1.303	1.684	2.021
60	0.254	0.527	0.848	1.045	1.296	1.671	2.000
120	0.254	0.526	0.845	1.041	1.289	1.658	1.980
∞	0.253	0.524	0.842	1.036	1.282	1.645	1.960

TABLE C   **Upper Percentage Points for *t* Distributions*** *Continued*

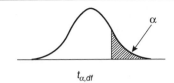

$t_{\alpha, df}$

df	Upper-Tail Probability						
	0.02	0.015	0.01	0.0075	0.005	0.0025	0.0005
1	15.895	21.205	31.821	42.434	63.657	127.322	636.590
2	4.849	5.643	6.965	8.073	9.925	14.089	31.598
3	3.482	3.896	4.541	5.047	5.841	7.453	12.924
4	2.999	3.298	3.747	4.088	4.604	5.598	8.610
5	2.757	3.003	3.365	3.634	4.032	4.773	6.869
6	2.612	2.829	3.143	3.372	3.707	4.317	5.959
7	2.517	2.715	2.998	3.203	3.499	4.029	5.408
8	2.449	2.634	2.896	3.085	3.355	3.833	5.041
9	2.398	2.574	2.821	2.998	3.250	3.690	4.781
10	2.359	2.527	2.764	2.932	3.169	3.581	4.587
11	2.328	2.491	2.718	2.879	3.106	3.497	4.437
12	2.303	2.461	2.681	2.836	3.055	3.428	4.318
13	2.282	2.436	2.650	2.801	3.012	3.372	4.221
14	2.264	2.415	2.624	2.771	2.977	3.326	4.140
15	2.249	2.397	2.602	2.746	2.947	3.286	4.073
16	2.235	2.382	2.583	2.724	2.921	3.252	4.015
17	2.224	2.368	2.567	2.706	2.898	3.222	3.965
18	2.214	2.356	2.552	2.689	2.878	3.197	3.922
19	2.205	2.346	2.539	2.674	2.861	3.174	3.883
20	2.197	2.336	2.528	2.661	2.845	3.153	3.849
21	2.189	2.328	2.518	2.649	2.831	3.135	3.819
22	2.183	2.320	2.508	2.639	2.819	3.119	3.792
23	2.177	2.313	2.500	2.629	2.807	3.104	3.768
24	2.172	2.307	2.492	2.620	2.797	3.091	3.745
25	2.167	2.301	2.485	2.612	2.787	3.078	3.725
26	2.162	2.296	2.479	2.605	2.779	3.067	3.707
27	2.158	2.291	2.473	2.598	2.771	3.057	3.690
28	2.154	2.286	2.467	2.592	2.763	3.047	3.674
29	2.150	2.282	2.462	2.586	2.756	3.038	3.659
30	2.147	2.278	2.457	2.581	2.750	3.030	3.646
40	2.123	2.250	2.423	2.542	2.704	2.971	3.551
60	2.099	2.223	2.390	2.504	2.660	2.915	3.460
120	2.076	2.196	2.358	2.460	2.617	2.860	3.373
∞	2.054	2.170	2.326	2.432	2.576	2.807	3.291

Source of data: Shott, S. *Statistics for Health Professionals*. Philadelphia, W. B. Saunders Company, 1990. Used by permission.

*Instructions for use of the table:** To determine the *p* value that corresponds to a calculated *t* value, first find the line that corresponds to the column of degrees of freedom *(df)* on the left. Then in the center of the table find the value that most closely corresponds to the value of *t* found from calculations. (1) **For a one-tailed *t*-test:** Look at the top row to find the corresponding probability. For example, a *t* value of 2.147 on 30 *df* corresponds to a *p* value of 0.02. If the observed value of *t* falls between values given, state the two *p* values between which the results of the *t*-test fall. For example, if a *t* of 2.160 is found on 30 *df*, the probability is expressed as follows: 0.015 < *p* < 0.02. (2) **For a two-tailed *t*-test:** The procedure is the same as for a one-tailed test, except that the *p* value obtained must then be *doubled* to include the other tail probability. For example, if a two-tailed *t*-test gives a *t* value of 2.147 on 30 *df*, the *p* value of that column (0.02) must be doubled to give the correct *p* value of 0.04.

TABLE D   Upper Percentage Points for Chi-Square Distributions*

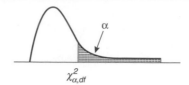

				Probability					
df	0.9995	0.995	0.99	0.975	0.95	0.90	0.80	0.70	0.60
1	0.000000393	0.0000393	0.000157	0.000982	0.00393	0.0158	0.0642	0.148	0.275
2	0.00100	0.0100	0.0201	0.0506	0.103	0.211	0.446	0.713	1.022
3	0.0153	0.0717	0.115	0.216	0.352	0.584	1.005	1.424	1.869
4	0.0639	0.207	0.297	0.484	0.711	1.064	1.649	2.195	2.753
5	0.158	0.412	0.554	0.831	1.145	1.610	2.343	3.000	3.655
6	0.299	0.676	0.872	1.237	1.635	2.204	3.070	3.828	4.570
7	0.485	0.989	1.239	1.690	2.167	2.833	3.822	4.671	5.493
8	0.710	1.344	1.646	2.180	2.733	3.490	4.594	5.527	6.423
9	0.972	1.735	2.088	2.700	3.325	4.168	5.380	6.393	7.357
10	1.265	2.156	2.558	3.247	3.940	4.865	6.179	7.267	8.295
11	1.587	2.603	3.053	3.816	4.575	5.578	6.989	8.148	9.237
12	1.934	3.074	3.571	4.404	5.226	6.304	7.807	9.034	10.182
13	2.305	3.565	4.107	5.009	5.892	7.042	8.634	9.926	11.129
14	2.697	4.075	4.660	5.629	6.571	7.790	9.467	10.821	12.078
15	3.108	4.601	5.229	6.262	7.261	8.547	10.307	11.721	13.030
16	3.536	5.142	5.812	6.908	7.962	9.312	11.152	12.624	13.983
17	3.980	5.697	6.408	7.564	8.672	10.085	12.002	13.531	14.937
18	4.439	6.265	7.015	8.231	9.390	10.865	12.857	14.440	15.893
19	4.912	6.844	7.633	8.907	10.117	11.651	13.716	15.352	16.850
20	5.398	7.434	8.260	9.591	10.851	12.443	14.578	16.266	17.809
21	5.896	8.034	8.897	10.283	11.591	13.240	15.445	17.182	18.768
22	6.404	8.643	9.542	10.982	12.338	14.041	16.314	18.101	19.729
23	6.924	9.260	10.196	11.689	13.091	14.848	17.187	19.021	20.690
24	7.453	9.886	10.856	12.401	13.848	15.659	18.062	19.943	21.652
25	7.991	10.520	11.524	13.120	14.611	16.473	18.940	20.867	22.616
26	8.538	11.160	12.198	13.844	15.379	17.292	19.820	21.792	23.579
27	9.093	11.808	12.879	14.573	16.151	18.114	20.703	22.719	24.544
28	9.656	12.461	13.565	15.308	16.928	18.939	21.588	23.647	25.509
29	10.227	13.121	14.256	16.047	17.708	19.768	22.475	24.577	26.475
30	10.804	13.787	14.953	16.791	18.493	20.599	23.364	25.508	27.442
35	13.787	17.192	18.509	20.569	22.465	24.797	27.836	30.178	32.282
40	16.906	20.707	22.164	24.433	26.509	29.051	32.345	34.872	37.134
45	20.137	24.311	25.901	28.366	30.612	33.350	36.884	39.585	41.995
50	23.461	27.991	29.707	32.357	34.764	37.689	41.449	44.313	46.864
60	30.340	35.534	37.485	40.482	43.188	46.459	50.641	53.809	56.620
70	37.467	43.275	45.442	48.758	51.739	55.329	59.898	63.346	66.396
80	44.791	51.172	53.540	57.153	60.391	64.278	69.207	72.915	76.188
90	52.276	59.196	61.754	65.647	69.126	73.291	78.558	82.511	85.993
100	59.896	67.328	70.065	74.222	77.929	82.358	87.945	92.129	95.808
120	75.467	83.852	86.923	91.573	95.705	100.624	106.806	111.419	115.465
140	91.391	100.655	104.034	109.137	113.659	119.029	125.758	130.766	135.149
160	107.597	117.679	121.346	126.870	131.756	137.546	144.783	150.158	154.856
180	124.033	134.884	138.820	144.741	149.969	156.153	163.868	169.588	174.580
200	140.660	152.241	156.432	162.728	168.279	174.835	183.003	189.049	194.319

TABLE D   Upper Percentage Points for Chi-Square Distributions* *Continued*

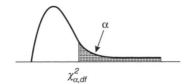

$\chi^2_{\alpha,df}$

df					Probability					
	0.50	0.40	0.30	0.20	0.10	0.05	0.025	0.01	0.005	0.0005
1	0.455	0.708	1.074	1.642	2.706	3.841	5.024	6.635	7.879	12.116
2	1.386	1.833	2.408	3.219	4.605	5.991	7.378	9.210	10.597	15.202
3	2.366	2.946	3.665	4.642	6.251	7.815	9.348	11.345	12.838	17.730
4	3.357	4.045	4.878	5.989	7.779	9.488	11.143	13.277	14.860	19.997
5	4.351	5.132	6.064	7.289	9.236	11.070	12.833	15.086	16.750	22.105
6	5.348	6.211	7.231	8.558	10.645	12.592	14.449	16.812	18.548	24.103
7	6.346	7.283	8.383	9.803	12.017	14.067	16.013	18.475	20.278	26.018
8	7.344	8.351	9.524	11.030	13.362	15.507	17.535	20.090	21.955	27.868
9	8.343	9.414	10.656	12.242	14.684	16.919	19.023	21.666	23.589	29.666
10	9.342	10.473	11.781	13.442	15.987	18.307	20.483	23.209	25.188	31.420
11	10.341	11.530	12.899	14.631	17.275	19.675	21.920	24.725	26.757	33.137
12	11.340	12.584	14.011	15.812	18.549	21.026	23.337	26.217	28.300	34.821
13	12.340	13.636	15.119	16.985	19.812	22.362	24.736	27.688	29.819	36.478
14	13.339	14.685	16.222	18.151	21.064	23.685	26.119	29.141	31.319	38.109
15	14.339	15.733	17.322	19.311	22.307	24.996	27.488	30.578	32.801	39.719
16	15.338	16.780	18.418	20.465	23.542	26.296	28.845	32.000	34.267	41.308
17	16.338	17.824	19.511	21.615	24.769	27.587	30.191	33.409	35.718	42.879
18	17.338	18.868	20.601	22.760	25.989	28.869	31.526	34.805	37.156	44.434
19	18.338	19.910	21.689	23.900	27.204	30.144	32.852	36.191	38.582	45.973
20	19.337	20.951	22.775	25.038	28.412	31.410	34.170	37.566	39.997	47.498
21	20.337	21.991	23.858	26.171	29.615	32.671	35.479	38.932	41.401	49.011
22	21.337	23.031	24.939	27.301	30.813	33.924	36.781	40.289	42.796	50.511
23	22.337	24.069	26.018	28.429	32.007	35.172	38.076	41.638	44.181	52.000
24	23.337	25.106	27.096	29.553	33.196	36.415	39.364	42.980	45.559	53.479
25	24.337	26.143	28.172	30.675	34.382	37.652	40.646	44.314	46.928	54.947
26	25.336	27.179	29.246	31.795	35.563	38.885	41.923	45.642	48.290	56.407
27	26.336	28.214	30.319	32.912	36.741	40.113	43.195	46.963	49.645	57.858
28	27.336	29.249	31.391	34.027	37.916	41.337	44.461	48.278	50.993	59.300
29	28.336	30.283	32.461	35.139	39.087	42.557	45.722	49.588	52.336	60.735
30	29.336	31.316	33.530	36.250	40.256	43.773	46.979	50.892	53.672	62.162
35	34.336	36.475	38.859	41.778	46.059	49.802	53.203	57.342	60.275	69.199
40	39.335	41.622	44.165	47.269	51.805	55.758	59.342	63.691	66.766	76.095
45	44.335	46.761	49.452	52.729	57.505	61.656	65.410	69.957	73.166	82.876
50	49.335	51.892	54.723	58.164	63.167	67.505	71.420	76.154	79.490	89.561
60	59.335	62.135	65.227	68.972	74.397	79.082	83.298	88.379	91.952	102.695
70	69.334	72.358	75.689	79.715	85.527	90.531	95.023	100.425	104.215	115.578
80	79.334	82.566	86.120	90.405	96.578	101.879	106.629	112.329	116.321	128.261
90	89.334	92.761	96.524	101.054	107.565	113.145	118.136	124.116	128.299	140.782
100	99.334	102.946	106.906	111.667	118.498	124.342	129.561	135.807	140.169	153.167
120	119.334	123.289	127.616	132.806	140.233	146.567	152.211	158.950	163.648	177.603
140	139.334	143.604	148.269	153.854	161.827	168.613	174.648	181.840	186.847	201.683
160	159.334	163.898	168.876	174.828	183.311	190.516	196.915	204.530	209.824	225.481
180	179.334	184.173	189.446	195.743	204.704	212.304	219.044	227.056	232.620	249.048
200	199.334	204.434	209.985	216.609	226.021	233.994	241.058	249.445	255.264	272.423

Source of data: Copyright 1982, Novartis. Reprinted with permission from the Geigy Scientific Tables, 8th ed., edited by Lentner, C. All rights reserved. Abstracted by Shott, S. Statistics for Health Professionals, Philadelphia, W. B. Saunders Company, 1990.
*Instructions for use of the table: Determine the degrees of freedom *(df)* appropriate to the chi-square test just calculated, and go to the line that most closely corresponds, using the left-hand column (headed *df*). On that line, move to the right in the body of the table and find the chi-square value that corresponds to what was calculated. The corresponding *p* value is found at the top of that column. For example, on 6 *df*, a calculated chi-square of 12.592 corresponds to a *p* value of 0.05. If the calculated chi-square value falls between two columns in the table, state the two *p* values between which the results of the chi-square test fall. For example, on 6 *df*, the probability of a chi-square of 13.500 is expressed as follows: $0.025 < p < 0.05$.

Index

COLLEGE OF OSTEOPATHIC MEDICINE
LEARNING CENTER